W9-APZ-606

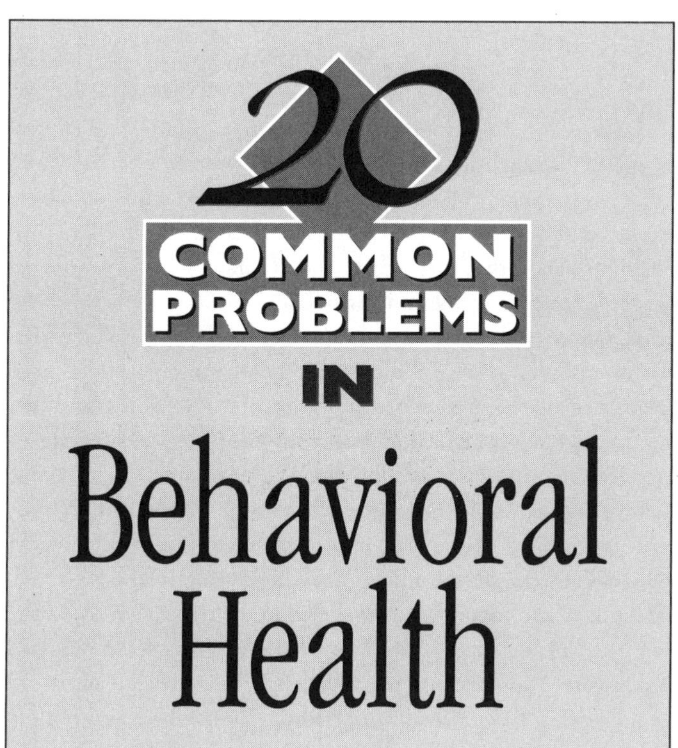
20
COMMON
PROBLEMS
IN
Behavioral
Health

Notice

Medicine is an ever-changing science. As new research and clinical experience broaden our knowledge, changes in treatment and drug therapy are required. The editors and the publisher of this work have checked with sources believed to be reliable in their efforts to provide information that is complete and generally in accord with the standards accepted at the time of publication. However, in view of the possibility of human error or changes in medical sciences, neither the editors nor the publisher nor any other party who has been involved in the preparation or publication of this work warrants that the information contained herein is in every respect accurate or complete, and they disclaim all responsibility for any errors or omissions or for the results obtained in this work. Readers are encouraged to confirm the information contained herein with other sources. For example and in particular, readers are advised to check the product information sheet included in the package of each drug they plan to administer to be certain that the information contained in this work is accurate and that changes have not been made in the recommended dose or in the contraindications for administration. This recommendation is of particular importance in connection with new or infrequently used drugs.

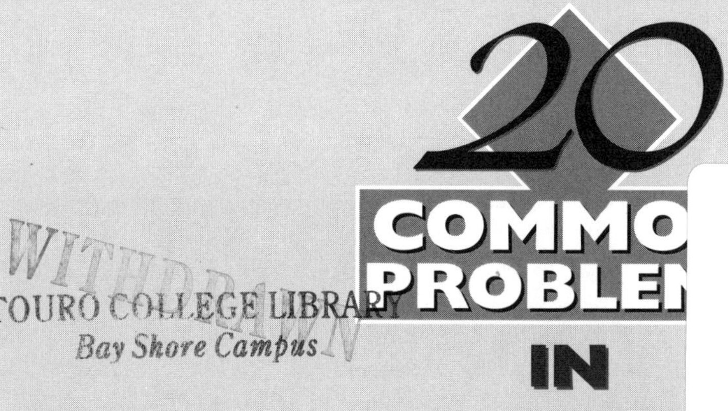

20 COMMO
PROBLE
IN
Behavioral Health

EDITORS

FRANK VERLOIN DEGRUY III, M.D., M.S.F.M.
Professor and Chair, Department of Family Medicine
University of Colorado Health Sciences Center, Denver, Colorado

W. PERRY DICKINSON, M.D.
Professor of Family Medicine and Director of Research, Department of Family Medicine
University of Colorado Health Sciences Center, Denver, Colorado

ELIZABETH W. STATON, B.A.S.
Professional Research Assistant, Department of Family Medicine
University of Colorado Health Sciences Center, Denver, Colorado

SERIES EDITOR

BARRY D. WEISS, M.D.
Professor of Clinical Family and Community Medicine
University of Arizona College of Medicine, Tucson, Arizona

McGraw-Hill
Medical Publishing Division

New York Chicago San Francisco Lisbon London Madrid Mexico City
Milan New Delhi San Juan Seoul Singapore Sydney Toronto

BS

McGraw-Hill

A Division of The ***McGraw-Hill*** *Companies*

20 COMMON PROBLEMS IN BEHAVIORAL HEALTH

1 2 3 4 5 6 7 8 9 0 DOCDOC 0 9 8 7 6 5 4 3 2

ISBN 0-07-016438-X

This book was set in Garamond by V&M Graphics, Inc.
The editors were Andrea Seils, Susan Noujaim, and Nicky Panton.
The production supervisor was Richard Ruzycka.
The cover designer was Marsha Cohen/Parallelogram.
The index was prepared by Geraldine Beckford.

R. R. Donnelley & Sons Company was printer and binder.

This book is printed on acid-free paper.

Cataloging-in-Publication Data is on file for this book at the Library of Congress.

10/29/23

We dedicate this book to three great physicians
whose traces run through everything we write:
Jack Medalie, Moon Mullins, and Gayle Stephens.

And with love and affection we also dedicate this
to our three families, near and far.

Contents

Contributors

BEHAVIORAL PROBLEMS IN CHILDHOOD AND ADOLESCENCE (CHAPTER 3)

Sara C. Hamel, M.D.
Assistant Professor of Pediatrics
Department of Pediatrics
University of Pittsburgh School of Medicine
Pittsburgh, Pennsylvania

Kelly J. Kelleher, M.D., M.P.H.
Staunton Professor of Pediatrics and Psychiatry
Departments of Pediatrics and Psychiatry
University of Pittsburgh School of Medicine
Pittsburgh, Pennsylvania

CARING FOR PATIENTS EXPERIENCED AS DIFFICULT (CHAPTER 12)

Steven R. Hahn, M.D.
Professor of Clinical Medicine and Instructor in Psychiatry
Departments of Clinical Medicine and Psychiatry
Albert Einstein College of Medicine
Bronx, New York

DEVELOPMENTAL AND PARENTING ISSUES IN CHILDHOOD (CHAPTER 2)

W. Perry Dickinson, M.D.
Professor of Family Medicine and Director of Research
Department of Family Medicine
University of Colorado Health Sciences Center
Denver, Colorado

EATING AND WEIGHT DISORDERS IN ADULTS (CHAPTER 14)

Carlos M. Grilo, Ph.D.
Associate Professor of Psychiatry
Department of Psychiatry
Yale University School of Medicine
New Haven, Connecticut

END OF LIFE (CHAPTER 11)

Tillman Farley, M.D.
Assistant Professor of Family Medicine
Department of Family Medicine
University of Colorado Health Sciences Center
Denver, Colorado

FAMILY PROBLEMS (CHAPTER 1)

Susan H. McDaniel, Ph.D.
Professor of Psychiatry and Family Medicine
Director of the Wynn Center for Family Research
Departments of Family Medicine and Psychiatry
University of Rochester School of Medicine and Dentistry
Rochester, New York

David B. Seaburn, M.S.
Assistant Professor of Psychiatry and Family Medicine
Departments of Family Medicine and Psychiatry
University of Rochester School of Medicine and Dentistry
Rochester, New York

Thomas L. Campbell, M.D.
Professor of Psychiatry and Family Medicine
Associate Chair, Family Medicine
Departments of Family Medicine and Psychiatry
University of Rochester School of Medicine and Dentistry
Rochester, New York

GRIEF AND LOSS (CHAPTER 10)
Tillman Farley, M.D.
Assistant Professor of Family Medicine
Department of Family Medicine
University of Colorado Health Sciences Center
Denver, Colorado

IDENTIFYING AND CHANGING HEALTH-RISK BEHAVIORS (CHAPTER 8)
Deborah S. Main, Ph.D.
Associate Professor of Family Medicine
Department of Family Medicine
University of Colorado Health Sciences Center
Denver, Colorado

Jo Ann Rosenfeld, M.D.
Associate Professor
Johns Hopkins School of Medicine
Franklin Square Family Practice
Baltimore, Maryland

Elizabeth W. Staton, B.A.S.
Professional Research Assistant
Department of Family Medicine
University of Colorado Health Sciences Center
Denver, Colorado

MENTAL SYMPTOMS (CHAPTER 20)
Frank Verloin deGruy, III, M.D., M.S.F.M.
Professor and Chair of Family Medicine
Department of Family Medicine
University of Colorado Health Sciences Center
Denver, Colorado

NONCOOPERATION (CHAPTER 13)
Kelly Derbin, M.D.
Assistant Director
Residency Program
Hinsdale Family Medicine Residency
Hinsdale, Illinois

Allen Perkins, M.D., M.P.H.
Associate Professor and Vice Chair of Family Medicine
Department of Family Practice and Community Medicine
University of South Alabama College of Medicine
Mobile, Alabama

PANIC DISORDER (CHAPTER 18)
David A. Katerndahl, M.D., M.A.
Professor of Family Medicine
Department of Family Practice
University of Texas Health Science Center at San Antonio
San Antonio, Texas

POST-TRAUMATIC STRESS SYNDROMES IN PRIMARY CARE PATIENTS (CHAPTER 19)
L. Miriam Dickinson, Ph.D.
Assistant Professor of Family Medicine
Department of Family Medicine
University of Colorado Health Sciences Center
Denver, Colorado

W. Perry Dickinson, M.D.
Professor of Family Medicine and Director of Research
Department of Family Medicine
University of Colorado Health Sciences Center
Denver, Colorado

PROBLEM DRINKING AND TOBACCO USE (CHAPTER 9)
Carlos Roberto Jaén, M.D., Ph.D.
Professor and Chair of Family Medicine
Department of Family Practice
University of Texas Health Science Center at San Antonio
San Antonio, Texas

Daniel C. Vinson, M.D., M.S.P.H.
Professor of Family Medicine
Department of Family Medicine
University of Missouri-Columbia
Columbia, Missouri

REACTIONS TO ILLNESS (CHAPTER 5)
Clydette Stulp deGroot, Ed.D.
Assistant Professor of Family Medicine
Department of Family Medicine
University of Colorado Health Sciences Center
Denver, Colorado

Elizabeth W. Staton, B.A.S.
Professional Research Assistant
Department of Family Medicine
University of Colorado Health Sciences Center
Denver, Colorado

SEXUAL PROBLEMS (CHAPTER 7)

Sharon J. Parish, M.D.
Assistant Professor of Medicine
Department of Medicine
Albert Einstein College of Medicine;
Department of Medicine
Montefiore Medical Center
Bronx, New York

William H. Salazar, M.D.
Associate Professor
Departments of Medicine and Psychiatry and Health Behavior
Medical College of Georgia
Augusta, Georgia

STRESS IN PRIMARY CARE PATIENTS (CHAPTER 4)

Deborah J. Seymour, Psy.D.
Assistant Professor and Director of Behavioral Science
Department of Family Medicine
University of Colorado Health Sciences Center
Denver, Colorado

Kirsten Black, M.P.H., R.D.
Instructor in Family Medicine
Department of Family Medicine
University of Colorado Health Sciences Center
Denver, Colorado

THE MANAGEMENT OF DEPRESSION AS A CHRONIC DISEASE (CHAPTER 16)

W. Perry Dickinson, M.D.
Professor of Family Medicine and Director of Research
Department of Family Medicine
University of Colorado Health Sciences Center
Denver, Colorado

UNEXPLAINED PHYSICAL SYMPTOMS AND SOMATOFORM DISORDERS (CHAPTER 15)

Kurt Kroenke, M.D.
Professor of Medicine
Regenstrief Institute for Health Care and the Department of Medicine
Indiana University
Indianapolis, Indiana

VIOLENCE AND ABUSE AS PRIMARY CARE PROBLEMS (CHAPTER 6)

W. Perry Dickinson, M.D.
Professor of Family Medicine and Director of Research
Department of Family Medicine
University of Colorado Health Sciences Center
Denver, Colorado

L. Miriam Dickinson, M.D.
Assistant Professor of Family Medicine
Department of Family Medicine
University of Colorado Health Sciences Center
Denver, Colorado

WORRIES AND ANXIETY (CHAPTER 17)

Larry Culpepper, M.D., M.P.H.
Professor and Chair of Family Medicine
Department of Family Medicine
Boston University
Boston, Massachusetts

Preface

This book is part of McGraw-Hill's *20 Common Problems* series, and takes its place in a series that is divided by topic to collectively cover the full range of problems commonly seen by primary care clinicians. In some cases the *20 Common Problems* books stand side-by-side in relation to one another, such that a problem found in one volume will not appear in another. This book does not work like that. Just as primary care itself cuts across the content areas of many medical and surgical specialties, so the material presented here cuts across the medical content areas of all of primary care. The coverage and organization of this book reflect our belief that clinical medicine is a fundamentally behavioral proposition. Accordingly, we have provided content that bears on every clinical encounter. It makes no more sense to speak of a clinical problem or encounter apart from the behavior that gives it shape and substance than to speak of the life of a fish apart from water. Behavior is the matrix out of which clinical medicine issues and upon which it operates. Thus, the material here is rendered in terms that emphasize the behavioral issue under consideration, but always within the context of ordinary primary care practice.

We have felt the need to take certain liberties with the concept of "problem." Because of the behavioral basis of clinical medicine, we have defined a behavioral problem more broadly than one might define a renal problem, for example. On some points we have discussed behavior itself as problematic, such as with some of the mental disorders described at the end of the book. On other points we have assumed that the behavior is a normal response to events or circumstances, but that attending to this normal response can reduce limitations or suffering for the patient. This assumption is perhaps most apparent in the chapter on *Violence and Abuse* and the chapter on *Post-Traumatic Stress Syndromes*, both of which guide clinicians in addressing and intervening with patients whose life circumstances cause them suffering.

As with the other volumes in this series, *20 Common Problems in Behavioral Health* is a book for clinicians. After reading this material, the reader should be able to recognize the most common behavioral problems and the circumstances that evoke important behavioral responses, and know how to manage these problems. Insofar as possible, the recommendations in this volume are based on sound evidence; however, the research literature that supports these topics is somewhat unevenly developed. In many instances the authors have noted that they had to rely on logic, experience, consensus, and judgment to tender the recommendations offered. We are proud to have a panel of extraordinarily expert authors for this effort, which has enabled us to produce a volume more useful than the state of evidence led us to even hope for. While many details of management will change over the years, we are confident that the principles upon which the authors of this volume have built their chapters will endure.

The book is organized according to the following logic. The first chapter, by McDaniel, Seaburn, and Campbell, addresses family problems. This chapter serves notice to the reader that the biopsychosocial model forms the basis on which behavioral problems are best understood in primary care. This model firmly establishes the context for all of clinical medicine. All subsequent chapters should be read through this filter, and many of the connections drawn out in the first chapter apply to the subsequent material.

This first chapter is followed by a group of chapters, two through eleven, presenting problems that may arise during the course of a normal life. We have put these in a rough developmental perspective, such that this section begins with problems arising in childhood and ends with problems arising at the end of life. Between birth and death people have to contend with many complex experiences, including stress, illnesses, violence, and sexual problems. Throughout these chapters, much of what we are calling behavioral problems are reactions to the vicissitudes of life that could be construed as normal reactions, but which nevertheless prolong, perpetuate, or exacerbate the patient's distress, impairment and suffering. We take the position that the primary care clinician has something important to offer patients in these circumstances and has the obligation to offer it—that this is part of the fundamental business of primary care.

Main, Rosenfeld, and Staton make it clear in Chap. 8 that a certain measure of harm befalls us as a result of risky or harmful behaviors. Addressing and changing these behaviors is incredibly important and is generally manageable within the primary care setting. Smoking and drinking are two significant instances of harmful behaviors—so important that they have been given their own chapter, Chap. 9 by Jaén and Vinson.

The partnership between patients and clinicians is not always comfortable and easy. This is true irrespective of patients' stage of life or the nature of their problems. Two chapters are devoted explicitly to problems within the clinician-patient relationship. Chap. 12, by Steve Hahn, provides a framework for understanding and learning to care for patients we experience as difficult. Chap. 13, by Derbin and Perkins, discusses patients who do not agree to or do not follow a therapeutic plan. This chapter will help the clinician understand some of the reasons that patients appear noncooperative and discusses how to care for them.

The last seven chapters of this book contain what many think of as the actual behavioral problems: mental disorders and their constituent symptoms. It is no accident that this DSM-oriented material takes up only one-third of this volume and that it comes last. We believe that most of the behavioral work inherent in the practice of primary care occurs in the context of care for ordinary, common primary care medical problems, and that when one has learned to do this well, one has the basis for attending competently to explicitly psychological symptoms and syndromes. Thus, these final chapters represent a sort of climax, consisting of the purest, most florid behavioral problems a primary care clinician will ordinarily be called on to deal with. These chapters offer practical advice on how to manage these most psychological of problems in the course of ordinary primary care.

The last chapter is an exception to this pattern, coming round as it does to subthreshold psychological syndromes and individual psychological symptoms. In a sense, it ends where we began—with the assertion that behavioral problems are part of every encounter, and that ordinary primary care is colored by this behavioral dimension. The clinician who looks for and deals with this dimension in every clinical problem is more likely to practice effective and rewarding primary care.

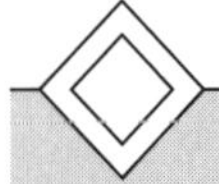

Acknowledgments

This book would not be a book were it not for the extraordinary efforts of the contributing authors. We gratefully acknowledge their contributions, which often went beyond their individual chapters as we struggled to make this into a coherent whole. Susan Noujaim at McGraw-Hill did the impossible: she retained her composure in the face of delays, complications, and changes of address, and simply stayed on task; her relentlessness was of the kindest and most encouraging order. We also express our thanks to a large group of primary care clinicians, mental health professionals, and, especially, patients who have contributed so much over the years to our understanding of behavioral problems in primary care. Without them, none of our work in this area would have much meaning or relevance.

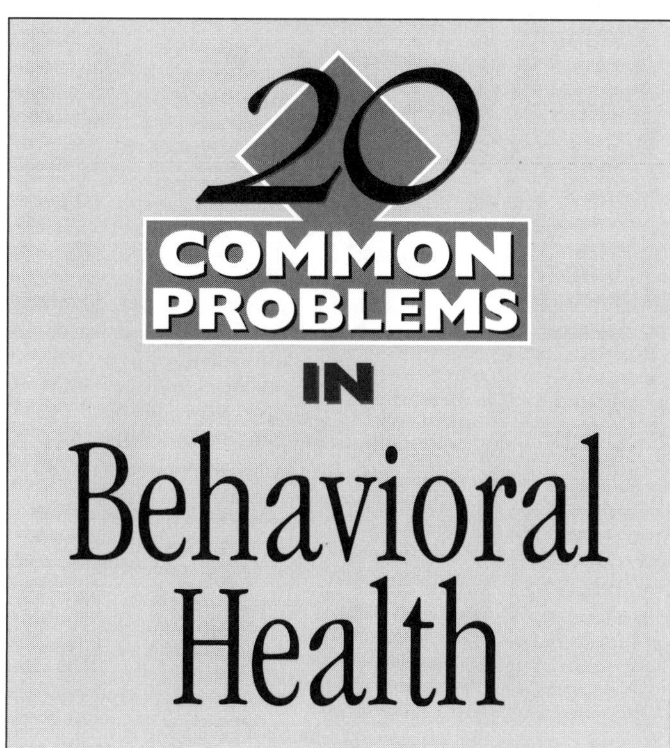
20
COMMON
PROBLEMS
IN
Behavioral
Health

Part 1

Normal Life Problems

Susan H. McDaniel
David B. Seaburn
Thomas L. Campbell

Family Problems

Introduction

Primary care clinicians are in an excellent position to address many family problems because of the continuity of their relationships with patients and families. Primary care clinicians are part of a family's life through myriad developmental transitions, such as marriage, childbirth, child rearing, adolescence, leaving home, separation and divorce, remarriage, midlife, old age, dying, and death. Any of these family transitions can create stress that may contribute to symptoms ranging from headaches to chronic pain and depression. Most patients with these symptoms, as well as other symptoms of mental health disorders, are seen in the privacy of primary care clinicians.

Although many patient problems have roots in family distress, the family most often is a valuable resource to the clinician in addressing a patient's difficulties. Research by Fiscella and Campbell has documented that enlisting family members' involvement can be pivotal in understanding patient problems and improving treatment outcomes. The family has influence on how an individual thinks, feels, and behaves about health. The family also has primary responsibility for individuals when they are ill.

This chapter presents common family problems that can be addressed in primary care practice. We will discuss how to involve family members when necessary, how to include the family when a patient is chronically ill, and other specific family difficulties that can arise during the life cycle, such as sexual or marital issues, child or adolescent concerns, problems of aging, and end-of-life decisions. The chapter also describes practical considerations in making mental health referrals, as well as how to collaborate with mental health professionals.

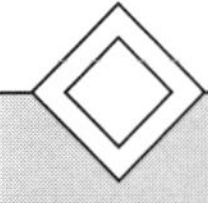

Enlisting Family Members' Involvement

When family factors are part of a patient's problem, whether it be a change in diet after an myocardial infarction, a marital conflict, or a concern about nursing home placement, it is often difficult to assess or treat the problem without the direct involvement of the patient's family. Medalie and colleagues found that family members attend a patient visit about one third of the time, and another 39 percent of patients come to the family physician's office with a family member or friend. Two thirds of the time, these people accompany the patient into the examination room. The majority of all patients surveyed by Botelho and associates indicated they prefer to have the family member or friend with them during the visit.

However, sometimes the patient is hesitant to involve family members for many reasons, and the patient must agree to involve family members before they are invited into the exam room. A planned approach involving family members, whereby this involvement is discussed with the patient, is best. It enables the clinician to address concerns that the patient or family member may have, such as whether the family members or the patient will be blamed for the problem or whether the family members will be told they too have a problem. The following are some basic guidelines for preparing patients and family members for an office visit that involves the family.

- *Communicate a clear rationale for involving the family.* This rationale should specify how family involvement might aid in addressing a health issue, and how it will enable you as the clinician to provide better care for the patient.
- *Be supportive, empathic, and impartial.* Do not take sides with the patient against other family members. Even if the family member has been critical, the patient may have a negative reaction to criticism of family and be protective of them.

The patient may be reluctant to invite family members because it results in a loss of confidentiality, or the patient may be eager to invite family members, hoping the clinician will side with him or her and "defeat" other family members. In these cases, family members may be unlikely to come, perhaps sensing patients' reluctance to their involvement. Although the physician should generally be neutral about such issues, neutrality in family issues should be abandoned in cases of high risk to patients—typically, situations of physical or sexual abuse, suicidality, or homicidality. In such situations, it is important to advocate for the patient at risk and to act in ways that ensure the patient's safety. This may include convening a family "safety watch" for the patient who is suicidal. It may also include not inviting the abusive family member to come to a visit if the clinician is unsure whether such a visit could escalate conflict within the family.

- *Emphasize concern for the patient and for the family as a whole.* This involves communicating understanding of the patient's dilemma as well as sensitivity to the possible stresses of other family members.
- *Involve family or significant others* to better understand what the patient and family are facing. This communicates both sensitivity to the family's distress and respect for each family member's view of the situation.
- *Stress the benefits of including others.* There may be greater likelihood that change can occur if the family works together.
- *Clarify what the patient can expect* in a meeting with other family members. The meeting is not a time for reporting to the family everything the patient has said. Confidentiality must be maintained. Rather, the meeting will be an opportunity for everyone to share views and make plans for how to address any problems.
- *Offer to invite family members* by phone or letter. This technique is effective when the clinician is unsure whether the patient will be able or willing to invite the family. A phone call to a partner or other significant family member during the patient's visit has the benefit of ensuring that the patient and the family hear the same message at the same time. With difficult patients or serious family problems, the invitation process can take several office visits with the patient to answer any questions before a family visit can be arranged.

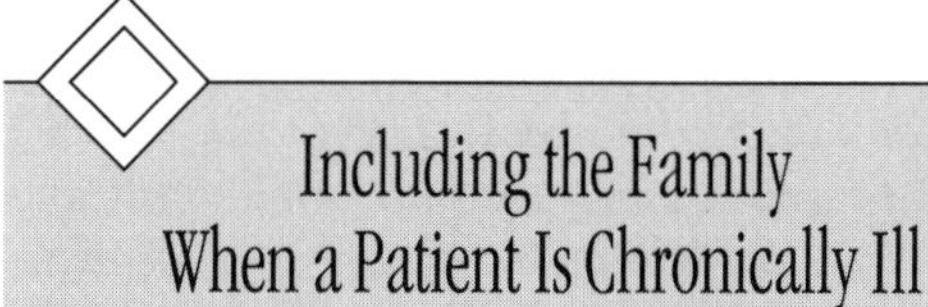

Including the Family When a Patient Is Chronically Ill

Family difficulties can arise when a member of the family is chronically ill, and difficulties often have to do with the degree and nature of other family members' involvement in treatment. This involvement can influence whether or not patients are motivated for treatment or capable of carrying out a treatment plan. Some common patterns of family involvement recognized by McDaniel and colleagues follow.

The Family Member as Customer

When a patient is unclear about the reasons for a visit, it may be because the patient has been sent to the doctor by a family member. The family member may have greater concern about the patient's health than the patient does, and may be more motivated for treatment to occur. In such situations, the concerned family member can be thought of as the "customer." For example, middle-aged men who come for physical examinations are often sent by spouses who are worried their husbands are overworking or are not taking care of themselves. It is tempting to dismiss the spouse's (i.e., the customer's) concerns because the patient seems unconcerned. It is best, though, to get permission from the patient to invite the spouse in to better assess the situation and ensure that the customer's concerns are met.

The customer can often be a valuable reporter on the patient's health, unless the couple is in a struggle that makes the patient feel attacked or intruded upon. Should this be the case, significant family problems are likely, and the family may benefit from referral to a marriage and family therapist.

HARVEY AND ELEANOR KASPAR *Harvey Kaspar, a patient with early, undiagnosed Alzheimer's disease, comes in for a physical. When you ask why he decided to have a check-up, he said, "I don't know. My wife seemed to think something was wrong." You learn that Mrs. Kaspar is in the waiting room. You invite Mrs. Kaspar to join you in the examination room, whereupon Mrs. Kaspar reports that Harvey has become more forgetful and irritable over the past few months.*

Overinvolved Family Members

The family may be overly involved with the patient's problem for many reasons. Overinvolvement of family members can manifest itself as contentious disagreeing with the clinician over how the patient should be treated, or as a constant prodding of the patient to "do what the doctor says." The patient may respond by passively resisting one side or the other, usually the clinician. Family member overinvolvement is often, but not necessarily, pathological. Woods reports evidence that parental overinvolvement in some childhood chronic illnesses may have a positive influence on the course of the illness.

Whether the effect is positive or negative, intense involvement of family members can influence the course of a patient's illness and the patient's decisions about treatment. Signs of dysfunctional family overinvolvement include patient passivity toward treatment, greater knowledge about the illness by family members than by the patient, reluctance on the part of the patient and/or family members for the patient to be seen alone, and reports of family member "overfunctioning" on behalf of a patient who is not incapacitated.

VALERIE AND LOIS SINGER *Valerie Singer is a single mother in her mid-20s who has insulin-dependent diabetes mellitus. Valerie lives with her mother, Lois, who has primary responsibility for Valerie's son while Valerie goes to business school. Valerie's sugar levels are often uncontrolled, and Lois calls you to say she is frustrated with her daughter and worried about her diabetes. Lois' brother died of complications from untreated diabetes, and she hopes you can make Valerie take care of herself.*

With Valerie's consent, you invite Lois to her next appointment. You learn that Lois monitors Valerie's diet constantly, keeping a chart on the refrigerator and leaving notes everyday about her insulin. Valerie appreciates her mother's concern and efforts to help, especially with her son, but she resents her mother's effort to "control everything." Reassuring Lois that the best way to ensure Valerie's health might be to leave the diet and insulin decisions in her daughter's hands relieves Lois of her sense of responsibility and creates space for Valerie to take charge of her health. You acknowledge that Lois is likely to feel anxious about her Valerie's health until Valerie can prove her ability to take good care of it on her own. Another conjoint session is scheduled for 6 months later, to check on Valerie's progress with Lois present. Several individual visits were scheduled in the interim for Valerie alone.

It is best to talk directly to overinvolved family members to understand their concerns and to enlist their help in a more constructive way. In the case of Valerie, you spoke with her mother and learned there was a family history of diabetes that increased her worry and protectiveness. Lois was willing to negotiate with her daughter about the management of her diabetes. Valerie's mother was relieved to interact directly with you and be advised about how best to approach her daughter's illness.

Underinvolved Family Members

Lack of comment by patients about their families can be mistaken as evidence that everything is fine. In some instances, lack of comment reflects a lack of involvement that may negatively affect the course of the illness.

However, lack of involvement should not always be considered lack of interest or concern. Rather, family members may feel helpless and expect clinicians to take full responsibility for their family member's illness. They may not understand the illness and the beneficial role they might play in its treatment.

MARTIN BLANCHARD *Martin Blanchard is in his late 50s. He is obese and has hypertension. You have tried unsuccessfully for 6 months to encourage him to lose weight. Martin appears motivated and has met with a dietitian several times, but has not lost weight. You are also treating Martin with an antihypertensive, and are concerned that he could have a stroke. Given these risks, with permission, you invite Martin's wife, Tina, to the next visit. At that time you learn that Tina cooks all the family meals. She uses salt in her cooking, and Martin's favorite meals are high in fat content. She did not worry about her husband's hypertension because Martin always said he was doing fine after each doctor visit. You describe hypertension in detail and also discuss diet with Tina. Once she understands the role she can play in her husband's health, she is willing to make changes in her cooking.*

The best approach with chronic illness is to involve family members early and repeatedly. This enables the clinician to assess the degree and nature of family member involvement, its impact on the illness course, and how to enlist family members as allies in treatment. Family involvement must be balanced by maintaining or enhancing the patient's autonomy.

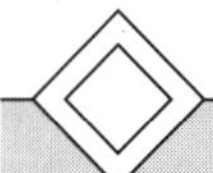

Parent Child Conflict

One of the most challenging roles in life is that of being a parent, and parent–child conflict is a routine part of raising a child. Parents bring questions to the clinician about their children's development and their functioning as a parent. It is important for the primary care clinician to know when to provide support for normal conflict been parent and child, when to provide advice or intervene, and when to refer to a child-oriented family therapist. It is also important to gather information about the child and family's strengths and resources.

Parenting, and especially discipline, takes a lot of time and energy for the adults involved. Work and other obligations of modern life provide competition for this time and energy. Frequently, problems with a child's misbehavior require some sort of intervention that involves increased attention to the child by the adult.

BETTY AND DANIEL SAMUELS *Betty Samuels is at her wits' end. She has brought her son, Daniel, in for a visit with you after his grades for this quarter dropped and his teacher complained of his disruptive behavior in school. Mrs. Samuels wonders if Daniel is "hyperactive" and needs to be put on Ritalin. When asked about what she had tried to solve the problem, she said that her son did not respond to "time-outs" and that she does not know what to do.*

Daniel sits quietly and attentively while his mother describes the problem; there are no signs of hyperactivity. When asked if he is aware that his mother and teacher are concerned about his grades and behavior, he says "yes," but is unable to offer an explanation other than "My friends are worse in school that I am. I don't know why you're picking on me." Betty then says that she returned to full-time employment this year and worries that this change is bothering Daniel. When questioned further, it sounds as if Mrs. Samuels retained all the household responsibilities she carried while working part time and is both busy and exhausted by the end of the day. The time she previously spent attending to Daniel and structuring his homework is now spent on household chores. It seems likely that Daniel's behavior is signaling his own difficulty doing without this kind of attention from a parent, as well as the difficulty the family was having reorganizing to meet the challenges of this transition.

Given all this, you ask Betty and Daniel to return in a week to continue the assessment. You asked that Mr. Samuels accompany them so you can hear his views about the problems with Daniel and the changes since his wife increased her work hours. You say that you will call the school and speak with Daniel's teacher to get a better understanding of the school problems. You indicate that it does not sound as if Daniel has an attention deficit problem, but want to gather more data from the family and the school before ruling it out entirely. In the meantime, you ask Mrs. Samuels to set a regular homework time for Daniel each night, with homework supervised alternately by her and Daniel's father. After the next assessment session, depending on how flexible the parents are in reorganizing the parenting and household tasks and how Daniel responds to the increased structuring and attention from his parents, you will make a decision about whether or not to make a referral for child and family therapy.

Children like Daniel often let parents know when they need to change their parenting style, either because the child has outgrown what worked in earlier stages, or because the demands on the rest of the family mean that the child is not getting his or her needs met. Of course, some children are temperamentally difficult, or the match between the child and parents' temperaments is poor, and the family may benefit from advice from the clinician. Often, however, the family has the strengths and resources to come up with their own solutions to a child's behavior problems. The clinician's role is to provide support and a safe place to discuss the parent's concerns.

Divorce and serial adult relationships are a normative part of life for many children today. On the one hand, multiple relationships mean multiple opportunities for adult love, attention, and guidance for children. On the other hand, it may also mean multiple opportunities for children to experience difficulty in establishing loyalty to adults, and to get caught in the crossfire of adult conflict. Especially when parents do not live together, a child's behavior problems can signal interpersonal problems among the adults that care for them.

SHAWNA, MARTIN, AND STEPHANIE BROWN *Shawna's parents divorced when she was 5. Her father remarried about 6 months ago, and Shawna is now 8 years old. Mrs. Brown complains to you that Shawna is "impossible to live with" for a full 2 days after each weekend she spends with her Dad. Shawna is also awakening several times at night and having nightmares. Mrs. Brown thinks Shawna should not spend any more time with her father; she says that her ex-husband refuses to acknowledge any behavior problems at his house and the problem must be that the new Mrs. Brown does not know how to be a good mother. When asked how long this had been a problem, Mrs. Brown said, "About 6 months. It wasn't so bad before that."*

You say that it sounds like there had been some new stress for Shawna and Mrs. Brown in the last 6 months and ask if Mrs. Brown would feel comfortable discussing the problems with her ex-husband during an office visit. She agrees to ask him, but says she does not feel comfortable asking his new wife. You note this response and say that the next step is to conduct a more complete assessment with Shawna and her parents. Perhaps together they will arrive at a plan that can help both Shawna and Mrs. Brown feel more comfortable, and allow Shawna to have continued access to both her parents. If not, then they can consider other possibilities, such as involving Mr. Brown's new wife or possibly making a referral for Shawna and her parents to a child-oriented family therapist. Mrs. Brown seems nervous about discussing these issues with her ex-husband, but is also relieved that they might get some help with Shawna's recent behavior problems.

Not infrequently, convening one family meeting to discuss a recent childhood behavior problem with the child and the adults who care for the child will result in a plan that helps the child through a difficult time. Long-standing or serious parent–child conflict, however, requires referral to an appropriate mental health professional, because such problems do not usually remit with a family meeting or primary care family counseling. Serious parent–child conflict, such as abuse, may present in the child as somatizing behavior (such as abdominal pain), injury reported as an accident, running away, deteriorating school performance, eating disorders, or other behavior problems. Any suspicion of child physical or sexual abuse must be reported to state authorities; the child and involved adult should be referred for psychotherapy.

A specific approach to dealing with parent–child conflict includes the following.

1. *Take a detailed history of the problem,* noting any repetitive patterns of behavior. Ask what happens in the family before and after the child misbehaves.
2. *Ask in detail about attempted solutions to the conflict.* It is common for parents to say, for example, that their child does not respond to "time-out." It is also common to find out that the parent is not supervising the time-out, but rather, is expecting the child to stay put without requiring further attention. Emphasizing that any discipline will take more energy from the parent than from the child is an important part of setting appropriate expectations for what it takes to teach children to manage their impulses.
3. *With conflict that does not resolve quickly, involve all relevant caretaking adults in constructing a plan to help the child.* This includes the mother, father, and any other relatives or other people who care regularly for the child. Contact with the school is also an important part of the assessment.
4. *Work closely with a family therapy colleague or colleagues in cases of serious or long-standing parent–child conflict.* With serious symptoms or conflict, it is important to rule out substance abuse, suicidality, physical or sexual abuse, and psychosis or other serious mental illness.

Adolescent Health Care Problems: Secrets and Confidentiality

Parental care of children requires balancing nurturance with appropriate limit setting. For adolescents, the same holds true, but it must occur with increasing respect for the adolescent's sense of identity and growing need for autonomy and independence. Some believe that the absence of the parent from the examination room is essential to developing a relationship with the clinician and that according to Cogswell, the clinician can play a role in "accelerating the process of children becoming independent patients." However, it is also important for the clinician to balance this autonomy with respect for the parents' ongoing role in the overall health and development of the adolescent.

Despite the common view of adolescence as a period of rebellion against parental values, most adolescents derive much of their self-esteem from parental support and approval. It is recommended that the clinician remain adolescent focused, but with a family orientation. In the end, it is important to work with adolescents and their parents in a balanced way. Three general guidelines for caring for adolescents are:

1. *Maintain a relationship with both the adolescent and the parents, provided the adolescent tolerates this.* Avoid taking sides where possible. Siding with either the adolescent or the parent may result in the clinician losing the trust of either or both.
2. *Be sensitive to emotional issues that can arise when working with adolescents.* The natural pull to side with the adolescent or the parents can reflect the clinician's own views on adolescence. Such responses are normal, but it is important to recognize how they may influence the clinician's work with adolescent patients.
3. *Be aware of how adolescents' efforts to become independent individuals play a part in adolescent health care.* "Individuation" can play a part in everything from discussions about who will enter the examination room, to physical examinations, to requests for contraceptives, to pregnancy tests. The clinician is in an excellent position to help adolescents and parents address these issues together, if appropriate and helpful. A balanced approach to adolescent health problems is challenged most when issues of confidentiality arise. The following

illustrates a common dilemma that may arise and upset the balance.

ALEX AND PATRICIA DUMAS *Mrs. Dumas asks to speak with you privately before you see Alex, age 17. She explains that she and her husband are worried that Alex might be using drugs. A family friend reported seeing Alex smoking marijuana at a party. Mrs. Dumas hopes you can explore this issue with Alex during his work physical to find out if he has been smoking marijuana, drinking heavily on weekends, or both. Alex is very open about his behaviors, but adds, "You aren't going to tell my mother, are you?"*

Clinicians are often given information about patients and family members and then asked to keep the information secret. Some clinicians feel that all information shared by patients must be kept as confidential, without question. Others see secrets between physicians and adolescent patients as posing both ethical and clinical dilemmas. As Newman indicates, blanket acceptance of secrets may draw the clinician into dysfunctional family patterns of relating. Furthermore, colluding in a secret may "limit our freedom to provide appropriate health care and force us to compromise our own integrity."[1] However, legitimate requests for confidentiality may be essential for some patients to pursue treatment for such conditions as sexually transmitted diseases, drug use, HIV, and pregnancy.

The issue again is one of balance and sensitivity to the adolescent's needs for care and confidentiality. The clinician's task is to maintain confidentiality where appropriate without entering into bonds of secrecy that may influence the provision of health care or contribute to unhealthy family relations. This task is perhaps most daunting when working with adolescents. The adolescent's process of forming an identity may include experimentation with drugs, sex, or other activities that can pose health risks. Adolescent individuation often includes an effort to limit the information that parents have about such behavior. On the other hand, parents are often struggling with issues of control while trying to maintain a relationship with their adolescent. An encounter with a clinician offers an opportunity to facilitate communication.

In the case of Alex and Mrs. Dumas, the clinician is asked to keep two secrets. Mrs. Dumas does not want you to divulge their conversation, but she does want you to investigate Alex's "drug problem." Alex wants you to keep his drug use a secret, because he does not want his parents to know about his drug and alcohol use. This poses a dilemma for you. Both secrets influence how you provide care for Alex. Both secrets also reflect family issues concerning communication between Alex and his parents. With regard to Mrs. Dumas' request, you encouraged Mrs. Dumas to share her concerns with Alex present. Mrs. Dumas did so, but had she refused, you could have pushed for permission to share their conversation with Alex. In this way, you could avoid keeping a binding secret and simultaneously facilitate communication between Mrs. Dumas and her son. When dealing with adolescent health care problems that raise issues of confidentiality, the following guidelines may be helpful in promoting healthy communication between the adolescent, the parents, and the provider.

Structure adolescent health care visits in a way that maximizes open communication, minimizes secrecy, and respects both the adolescent's autonomy and need or demand for privacy and the parent's role. Many adolescents simply reject the doctor as their doctor if the physician is also is dealing with the parents. As with the Dumas example, one successful format when parents accompany the adolescent is to see the parents with the adolescent at the beginning of the visit. Explain that the visit includes time together, time alone with the adolescent, and time at the end with everyone to discuss some treatment directions (others may be confidential) and answer questions. See the adolescent alone for the majority of the visit. Negotiate with the adolescent what to share with the parents at the end of the visit. End by discussing some findings and treatment directions with the adolescent and the parents together.

[1]Newman NK: Family secrets: A challenge for family physicians. *J Fam Pract* 36:494, 1993.

Discuss confidentiality with the parents and the adolescent together. In a series of decisions between 1976 and 1983, the Supreme Court established the adolescent's right to confidential treatment in many areas, including the purchase and use of contraception and requests for abortions. With suicidal or homicidal behavior, or threat of felony, however, confidentiality must be broken and the problem reported in most states.

Finally, despite the adolescent's legal rights to consent to his or her own treatment, the responsibility for judging the adolescent's capacity to make clear decisions often falls to the clinician. Confidentiality remains a complex issue that is best dealt with honestly and directly. Confidentiality should be presented as a multifaceted issue that deserves discussion and often requires negotiation. In the Dumas case, you can take the opportunity to address confidentiality with Mrs. Dumas and Alex together.

ALEX AND PATRICIA DUMAS (CONTINUED) *"When I see adolescents with their parent(s), I like to take the opportunity to discuss confidentiality. Patients often share information with me that they would like to keep confidential. In most cases I honor that request. In several areas I cannot extend confidentiality. For example, if either of you were at risk of hurting yourself or someone else, I would have to inform others for the sake of your safety or the safety of others. In all requests for confidentiality, I may feel as a clinician that it would be better, for health reasons, if the information was shared with others, particularly family. In those instances, I encourage the adolescent or family member to talk with other family members, and I offer to assist in whatever way I can. But I do not communicate confidential information to other family members without the patient's consent. And I never refuse treatment, even if a patient does not want to talk with others about their problems. My main concern is to provide necessary and adequate health care for any patient."*

This approach has the benefit of modeling openness, honesty, and directness. It allies the clinician, not only with the parents and the adolescent, but also with the goal of quality health care for the adolescent. Furthermore, if raised early in patient care, it avoids the problem of raising the issue of confidentiality after confidential information has already been shared with the clinician.

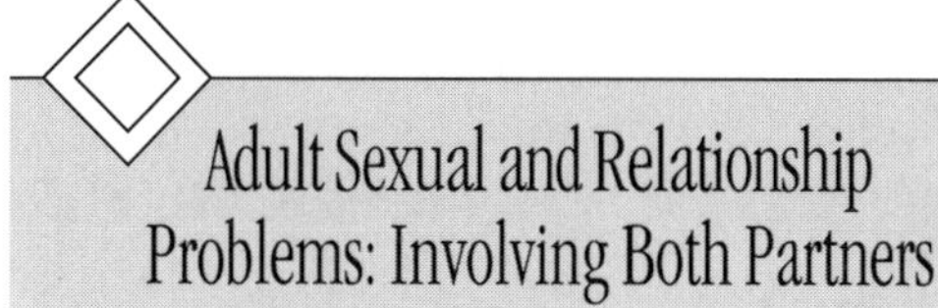

Adult Sexual and Relationship Problems: Involving Both Partners

Like adolescent problems, adult sexual problems often require special interviewing skills. Patients who present with low back pain, abdominal pain, urinary difficulties, and other somatic complaints may have underlying sexual complaints that they are hesitant to voice. Assessment of sexual problems in primary care, whether heterosexual or homosexual, depends largely on the clinician's initiative in discussing the matter. Masters and Johnson estimated that 50 percent of all marriages experience sexual problems at some time. Laumann and Rosen found that sexual dysfunction is more prevalent for women (43 percent) than men (31 percent), and is highly associated with negative experiences in sexual relationships and overall well-being. Pauly found that clinicians who do not inquire about these problems will learn about them only 10 percent of the time, while clinicians who routinely inquire identify sexual problems 50 to 100 percent of the time.

Problems with sexual function may arise because of organic factors that, in turn, affect the couple's overall relationship. Such problems may also arise because of general relationship problems that then affect sexual functioning. For this reason, a biopsychosocial approach should always be used when assessing sexual intimacy. Some evaluation questions that address the nature of the problem include the following:

- Are you satisfied with the degree of intimacy in your relationship?
- Are you satisfied with your sex life?

- If not, what difficulties are you having?
- Do these problems occur all the time or just under certain circumstances?
- *For men:* Do you have problems obtaining or maintaining an erection?
- *For women:* Do you have difficulty becoming sexually aroused?
- Do you ever have pain during intercourse or difficulty achieving an orgasm?
- What do you feel is the reason for these problems?
- Have either of you been ill recently?
- Are you on medication?
- Do you drink alcohol or use drugs?
- How would you like your sexual relationship to be?

The following case illustrates how sexual and relationship problems are frequently intertwined.

JEANETTE AND STEVE GUADINO *Mrs. Gaudino comes in complaining that her marriage is stale and lifeless. You say you would be happy to explore this problem further, but that it would be best if her husband could join her. Mrs. Gaudino appears apprehensive, but agrees to a session with her husband to identify what would be most likely to lead to improvements in the relationship. Mr. Gaudino surprises his wife with his willingness to come in. He hopes the clinician will ask about their sexual relationship, his primary concern; he is not sure he can bring it up himself.*

When Mr. and Mrs. Gaudino come in for their appointed visit, after discussing some work issues, you ask if their relationship stress had affected their sexual relationship. At first both are nervous and say "No." When you ask if they are satisfied with their sexual relationship, Mrs. Gaudino says, "Not really." She says they are not "close" often enough. When asked what she means by close, Mrs. Gaudino says, "You know, we don't have sex enough." The Gaudinos say they have been having sex approximately once a month during the past 6 months. They agree it was more frequent before, but cannot be specific. Mr. Gaudino says he is often too tired from his new job, and when he is not tired his wife sometimes "turns a cold shoulder." The last two times they tried to have intercourse, Mr. Gaudino could not maintain an erection. They have not tried again in the past 6 weeks. Mr. Gaudino has not been ill, he drinks alcohol in moderation ("3 to 4 beers a week"), and he was able to have erections at other times. The couple speculates that relationship problems are the cause of their sexual difficulties. You refer the couple for sexual counseling with an appropriately trained couple's therapist.

While a patient may not raise sexual problems directly, it is not uncommon for patients to complain about other aspects of the primary relationship to their clinician. As early as possible, it is important to *involve the partner in discussions.* Offering to do so will test the patient's interest in making changes. Listening to one patient complain about another family member, especially a spouse, over a long period of time, can signal to the patient that the clinician sides with the patient against the spouse and can prevent an accurate and comprehensive assessment of the relational problem. Taking sides can actually escalate the problem, as when the patient goes home and reports to her husband, "The doctor agrees with me that I ought to cut back my work hours and stay home with the children. He thinks my headaches are related to work stress, and that you are being too rigid about this." Although there may be a reason for this patient to push her point, doing so likely represents a long-standing marital conflict. It is much safer to see this couple together, hear the husband's concerns as well, and facilitate a discussion oriented toward problem solving that may lead to a healthier outcome for the family overall.

One area of particular concern in primary care practice is domestic violence. When patients present with unexplained bruising or other injuries, or repeatedly complain about relationship problems, it is important to ask if their partner has ever punched, kicked, bruised, or scratched them before. If domestic violence has occurred recently, it is important to evaluate the woman's safety, counsel her to use a women's shelter if appropriate, and refer her to a psychotherapist who will be able to decide upon the needed individual, group, and/or couples treatment for both parties involved in the conflict. Anger management groups for batterers may also be useful.

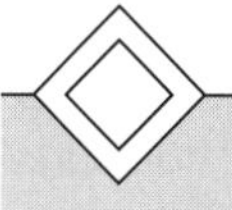

Families and the Elderly: Caring for the Caregiver

The fastest growing segment of the population is the elderly. Contrary to popular belief, most elders are close to their families. The majority live near one of their children and visit them often; only 5 percent live in nursing homes or other institutional settings.

The importance of family connections increases with age. Physical deterioration and social and financial changes often push people back to their families, despite a desire to remain independent. The majority of caregivers for the elderly are family members, typically women. There are important gender differences between male and female caregivers. Because women are socialized to assume caregiving responsibilities, they are more likely to feel responsible for all the caregiving and have difficulty asking for or receiving help. Men often have more difficulty accepting caregiving responsibilities and are more likely to ask or pay for help. For example, women who are recovering from a myocardial infarction (MI) often continue household responsibilities, such as cooking and cleaning, whereas men are usually cared for by their wives during the post-MI period.

Caregiving to elder family members is very demanding and often highly emotional, as the specter of death and grief highlights long-standing family processes, loyalties, obligations, and responsibilities. When there is intense involvement of family caregivers, medical care of the elderly needs to be consciously family oriented.

The clinician's role at this stage of life may be powerful. The clinician is seen as a supporter, advisor, healer, social contact, lifeline, and guide to the patient and family. With regard to the family, one of the clinician's most important roles is to involve, assess, and support any primary family caregiver(s). To overlook this can lead to a downward spiral that can greatly affect the elder family member. The caregiver becomes more distressed and is less able to meet the elder family member's needs. The elder family member may then deteriorate physically and emotionally, thus putting greater demands on the caregiver who may then "burn out."

DONALD BENJAMIN AND SARAH YOLOM *Mr. Benjamin gradually developed serious Parkinson's disease with accompanying dementia. He came to live with his daughter and son-in-law 6 months ago. They were committed to caring for him. Mrs. Yolom, Mr. Benjamin's daughter, accompanies him to every office visit. At one visit, Mrs. Yolom appears lethargic. She has little to say and often yawns during the interview. When asked how she is doing, Mrs. Yolom says she is losing sleep because her father was up each night for the past week. Her husband offered to help, but she felt guilty allowing his involvement. Mr. Benjamin is her father, she says, and she should take care of him.*

Depression can accompany the demands of caregiving. The risk of depressive symptoms increases when the caregiver has little support or refuses to accept available help. The clinician should assess several aspects of the caregiver's experience.

The Caregiver's Relationship to the Patient

Can the caregiver express affection with the patient or is it withheld? Does the caregiver feel solely responsible for the patient? Was the previous relationship with the patient positive or negative?

The Patient's Condition

How impaired is the patient, physically and emotionally? Is the patient's behavior disruptive? How independent is the patient? How knowledgeable is the caregiver about the patient's condition?

The Caregiver's Condition

How is the caregiver's physical health? Is the caregiver depressed? Does the caregiver have support? Does the caregiver take time for himself or herself? Can the caregiver delegate responsibilities to other family members? Does the caregiver have a realistic sense of his or her responsibility for the patient's health?

Family Resources

Can the family afford assistance with caregiving? How is the family coping with the patient's needs? Do family members maintain some degree of social activity? Can family members talk with and support each other?

Community Resources

Is a day care program available for the patient? Are there support groups available for the caregiver and family? Is respite care available? Is psychological and family therapy available for the patient, caregiver, and family?

By addressing how the caregiver is doing, the clinician is making a powerful statement to the patient and family—that the caregiver has legitimate needs. This often results in other family members providing more support and assistance. By preventing caregiver burnout, the clinician is able to help the patient remain at home with the family.

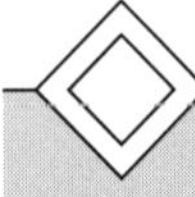

Mental Health Referral and Collaboration

Family problems that do not abate once they are identified and discussed often should be referred to a family-oriented mental health professional. Among the most common signals for a referral, in addition to a patient's request, are the following.

Serious Problems

Sometimes the severity of the problem is not clear initially. If the family's difficulties include a history of psychiatric problems, suicidal or homicidal ideation, physical or sexual abuse, substance abuse, or most sexual problems, a referral or consultation may be helpful.

Chronic Problems

If the family reports having problems for longer than 6 months, a mental health consultation or referral may be indicated.

A Multiplicity of Problems

Families that report more than one problem occurring at the same time may warrant a referral even if the individual problems are not severe or chronic. The complexity of multiple psychosocial problems may be best handled by involving a family-oriented mental health professional.

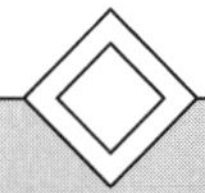

Successful Referral and Collaboration

Many primary care mental health referrals are not just made at one visit, but are accomplished over time. Except when a patient or family directly requests a referral, successful referrals are usually part of a process rather than being a single event. The effectiveness of a mental health referral also depends on the relationship between the clinician and mental health professionals. A collaborative relationship enhances both the referral and the course of treatment. A successful referral and collaboration includes the following:

- *Introduce the idea of referral gradually over time.* First, help the patient identify and discuss the problem. Second, involve relevant family members. Third, introduce the idea of referral as a resource that may benefit everyone in the family.
- *Refer to a specific individual, if possible.* Patients are more likely to transfer the trust they have in you to a specific person that you recommend rather than an impersonal clinic or agency.
- *When possible, consult early with the therapist to whom you are referring.* The therapist may have ideas about how to make the referral, and the contact sets the stage for ongoing collaboration during treatment. With patients very resistant to referral, a conjoint session with you and the mental health professional may provide the necessary bridge for a successful referral.
- *Maximize the patient's and family's motivation* by using language that is meaningful to them and that reflects their concerns when presenting the idea of referral. "You both have demonstrated your commitment to making things better, and are working very hard. Your efforts deserve the support of someone who specializes in the issues you are addressing." It is helpful not to "pathologize" the patient or family when discussing referral.
- *Give the patient and family time to consider the referral.* Give the process time. Schedule a follow-up visit to discuss the decision. When a patient and family are ambivalent about referral, such discussions allow families time to make their own decisions while maintaining a connection with you no matter what the decision.
- *When the patient and family accept the referral, call the therapist for an appointment before they leave the office.*
- *Make explicit what kind of communication you want from the therapist.* The number one complaint clinicians have about therapists is that clinicians never hear from them once the referral is made. It is best to be direct about the communication you desire.
- *Clarify your own availability regarding the case.* Will you be available? How can you be contacted? When is it best to call you?
- *Negotiate and clarify areas of responsibility.* What issues are best discussed with the therapist (e.g., relationship issues)? What issues should the therapist refer back to the clinician (e.g., possible physiologic factors in sexual dysfunction)? What issues should the clinician and therapist discuss together (e.g., when the patient and family are somatically fixated)? In difficult cases the process can be aided by a face-to-face meeting between the clinician, therapist, and family.

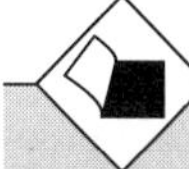

Summary

Family problems may be a factor in a patient's decision to see a primary care clinician. Early recognition of relationship problems by the primary care clinician may decrease the frequency of medical visits by patients whose symptoms are grounded in family stress. Engaging family members in addressing such problems can be an effective intervention. Involving family members also protects the clinician from entering into exclusive individual relationships with patients that do not address the familial roots of problems.

When family-based problems require more than primary care counseling, the primary clinician is in a central position to prepare patients and families for referrals to family-oriented mental health providers. Collaboration with a family-oriented mental health professional may help facilitate effective treatment and can be professionally rewarding for both the therapist and the clinician.

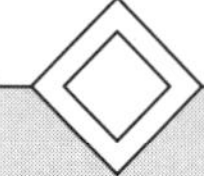

Acknowledgment

This chapter is an updated adaptation of a chapter previously published by Seaburn DB, McDaniel SH, and Campbell TL: Common family problems.

In: Noble J (ed): *Primacy Care Medicine*, 2nd ed. New York: Little, Brown; 1966, with permission.

Suggested Reading

Campbell TL: Family's impact on health: A critical review and annotated bibliography. NIMH Series DN, No. 6 DHHS Publ. No. (ADM) 86-1461, 1986. Also published in *Fam Sys Med* 4(2,3):135, 1986.

This monogragh and special issue of Family Systems Medicine *reviews the research literature on how family factors, especially family relationships, influence health. It also includes an annotated bibliography of the reviewed studies.*

Doherty WJ, Baird MA: Family therapy and family medicine. New York: Guildford Press; 1983.

This landmark book outlines the theory and practice of a family systems approach to health care. It has excellent chapters on how to assess, refer, and counsel families in primary care.

Doherty WJ, Campbell TL: Families and health. Beverly Hills, CA: Sage Publications; 1988.

This book is part of the Sage Family Studies literature and is written for family professionals as well as medical providers. It reviews the literature on families and health and its implications for health professionals. It is organized around the Family Health and Illness Cycle.

McDaniel SH, Campbell TL, Seaburn DB: Family-oriented primary care: A manual for medical providers. Berlin: Springer-Verlag; 1990.

This practical guide to implementing a family-oriented approach in primary care has chapters on how to convene a family conference and conduct a family interview and contains specific practical guidelines for dealing with numerous life-cycle and health-related issues.

McDaniel SH, Hepworth J, Doherty WJ. Medical family therapy: A biopsychosocial approach to families with health problems. New York: Basic Books; 1992.

This book defined the field of family-oriented psychotherapy for patients with health problems. There are chapters on childhood health problems, infertility, somatization, lifestyle behaviors, terminal illness, and others.

Families, Systems & Health: *The Journal of Collaborative Family Healthcare*. www.fsh.org

This journal publishes articles that describe and evaluate an integrated, systemic view of health, illness, and the health care system with particular interest in new models of collaboration between families, health professionals, and mental health teams in different community and healthcare settings.

The Collaborative Family Healthcare Coalition Web Site. www.cfhcc.org

The Collaborative Family Healthcare Coalition, founded in 1993, is a diverse group of physicians, nurses, psychologists, social workers, family therapists, and other health care workers, working in both primary and tertiary care settings, who study, implement, and advocate for the collaborative family health care paradigm. It also includes researchers, educators, health care policy workers, and consumer group representatives. The Coalition functions as a communication network and information clearinghouse by holding a biennial conference, maintaining web site database listings and a list server, including a subscription to Families, Systems & Health *with membership.*

Integrated Primary Care. www.integratedprimarycare.com

This site describes what Integrated Primary Care is like in practice. It puts visitors in contact with books, journals, organizations, and web resources for getting started. The site describes existing programs of Integrated Primary Care (IPC) and offers evidence on the clinical effectiveness and cost effectiveness of IPC. There is special attention paid to integrating care for low income and underserved populations, and discussions of training programs for professionals. A summary of research of progress and a bibliography are provided.

Bibliography

Botelho RJ, Lue BH, Fiscella K: Family involvement in routine health care: A survey of patients' behaviors and preferences. *J Fam Pract* 42:572, 1996.

Cogswell BE: Cultivating the trust of adolescent patients. *Fam Med* 17:254, 1985

Doherty WJ, Baird WA: *Family Therapy and Family Medicine*. New York: Guilford Press; 1985.

Fiscella K, Campbell TL: Association of perceived family criticism with health behaviors. *J Fam Pract* 48:128, 1999.

Holder AR: Minors' rights to consent to medical care. *JAMA* 257:3400, 1987.

Kaplan HS: *The New Sex Therapy*. New York: Brunner/Mazel; 1974.

Kolodny RC, Masters WH, Johnson VE: *Textbook of Sexual Medicine*. Boston: Little, Brown; 1979.

Landau-Stanton J, Stanton MD: Treating suicidal adolescents and their families. In: Mirkin M, Koman S (eds): *Handbook of Adolescents and Family Therapy*. New York: Gardner Press; 1985.

Laumann EO, Paik A, Rosen RC: Sexual dysfunction in the United States: Prevalence and predictors. *JAMA* 281:537, 1999.

Masters WH, Johnson VE: *Human Sexual Inadequacy*. Boston: Little, Brown; 1970.

McDaniel SH, Campbell TL, Seaburn DS: *Family-Oriented Primary Care: A Manual for Medical Providers*. New York: Springer-Verlag; 1990.

Medalie JH, Zyzanski SJ, Langa D, et al: The family in family practice: Is it a reality? *J Fam Pract* 46:390, 1998.

Newman NK: Family secrets: A challenge for family physicians. *J Fam Pract* 36:494, 1993.

Pauly IB: Human sexuality in medical education and practice. *Aust N Z J Psychiatry* 5:206, 1971.

Schurman RA, Kramer PD, Mitchell JB: The hidden mental health network. Treatment of mental illness by nonpsychiatrist physicians. *Arch Gen Psychiatry* 42:89, 1985.

Woods B: Beyond the "psychosomatic family": A biobehavioral family model of pediatric illness. *Fam Process* 32:261, 1993.

Chapter 2

W. Perry Dickinson

Developmental and Parenting Issues in Childhood

Introduction

Primary care clinicians deal with many mental health issues that do not involve major psychopathology and often do not result in the clinician making and coding a specific psychiatric diagnosis. The majority of these generally mild but significant mental health problems derive directly or indirectly from normal developmental issues all people face as they proceed through life. A working knowledge of normal human psychosocial development, therefore, is a vital tool that primary care clinicians need to have to deal with mental health issues. When combined with an understanding of family systems dynamics and knowledge of individual patients' life contexts, a developmental approach allows clinicians to make clear sense out of mental health issues that otherwise can be very confusing, and also allows for a level of preventive mental health care that otherwise is not possible.

In this chapter, we will focus on a developmental approach to childhood mental health issues. Childhood is the stage of life in which the utility of a developmental approach is most clear, although this by no means should imply to the reader that psychosocial developmental issues are not important in adults. Because child discipline issues commonly arise and are intimately intertwined with psychosocial development, we also will include an approach to counseling parents about parenting skills. After a general discussion of the basic principles and framework of a developmental approach, the influence of family dynamics on development, and basic parenting skills, we will take a tour of childhood from birth through adolescence, covering the development issues that are specific to each stage.

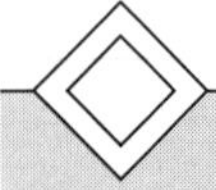

Basic Concepts of a Developmental Approach

There are a few basic developmental concepts that must be understood before specific issue can be addressed. First, people (and families) go through predictable stages of life with specific issues that must be resolved and patterns of behavior that occur at each stage. Second, if an issue is not resolved during a particular stage, it may have both immediate and long-term consequences. Development may be arrested at that stage, at least for that particular area of development, or it will proceed with the unresolved issue returning to negatively affect subsequent developmental stages. The third concept is that how these issues are dealt with strongly influences a person's future personality and psychological well-being. Note that this says influences, not determines; future environment, events, or stages of development may temper the effects. Finally, issues tend to repeat at different stages. This builds a certain amount of plasticity into the system; issues that are unresolved at one stage of life can be dealt with again at a subsequent stage, when the circumstances may be more favorable to successful resolution of the issues.

There are several ways to view the passage of an individual through the various periods of life and developmental stages. One would be to view the developmental stages and issues in a strictly linear, stepwise fashion, with some form of resolution of the developmental tasks at one stage required for passage to the next stage. However, this view does not appear to be strictly the case. Over recent years, many developmental experts have started to view each developmental stage as a sensitive period, when particular issues can be most optimally resolved, rather than a critical period, when the issues must be resolved before going on to the next stage. There also has been increased recognition of the individual nature of each person's passage through the stages.

Tyson describes a "play dough" view of development, in which new abilities add to the overall developmental structure to gradually transform the child's abilities and maturation. In this view, new pieces of clay can "patch" defects that persist from issues that were not resolved at earlier stages, in contrast to the "Lego" view, in which unresolved issues cause ongoing problems. The developmental stages and issues that are presented in this chapter should thus be considered to be a general model that applies to most children, but with individual variability.

There have been a number of theorists who have made major contributions to our knowledge of human development, but three particularly stand out. Erik Erikson's framework of psychosocial development is very practical and useful in primary care and is the primary model used in this chapter. Sigmund Freud's theories of psychosexual development provided much of the basic framework for a developmental approach to mental health and in many ways gave rise to modern psychiatry. Although some aspects of his theories have been discredited in recent years, they still describe aspects of child behavior that can be important for parents and clinicians. Piaget focused on cognitive development through detailed observation and description of child behavior. His theories have been extremely influential in modern education, but also describe behaviors that are important in primary care. All three of these conceptual models of development—psychosocial, psychosexual, and cognitive—are incorporated into the descriptions of the developmental issues for each stage of childhood that follow later in this chapter.

Preventive Counseling

Using a developmental framework, primary care clinicians can anticipate that certain behavioral issues will arise at particular stages of life. The struggle of the individual and family to resolve these issues may result in certain predictable problems that may be preventable or diminished with effective counseling. Preventive counseling implies that a clinician identifies the mental health issues that are likely to arise in the near future for a patient or family and attempts to facilitate successful resolution of these issues so that major problems do not develop. Simply warning patients in advance as to what they may expect at particular stages, and giving assurance of the normalcy of what they are or will be going through, is often very therapeutic. If, on the other hand, the clinician waits until problems actually develop, intervention may be more difficult.

Family Influences

The past and present family environments affect individual development. This is especially true in early childhood, when the family represents almost the whole of the child's social environment. The family approach described here is especially influenced by the work and theories of Murray Bowen. It is beyond the scope of this chapter to discuss the complete range of family circumstances that can affect the development of individual family members. However, we have found several areas of family issues or functioning that seem to have particular importance in childhood development.

1. *Intimacy* is one of the basic components of family relationships, referring to the amount of closeness, caring, sharing, and trust among family members. It also includes the quality and quantity of their interactions.
2. *Individuation* is the process through which a person develops and maintains a sense of self-identity in a relationship. Families are variable in how well they promote a high level of individuation among family members. In families that have a low level of individuation, family members have great difficulty in identifying and maintaining their own ideas, feelings, and values, separate from other family members.
3. *Family criticism* is used in many families to deal with virtually any situation where a child

"gets out of line" by doing something that is contrary to the family's concept of what a member should do or how a member should behave. Such criticism can be extremely destructive and damaging to a child's self-image, trust in relationships, self-esteem, confidence level, and ability to successfully complete developmental tasks.

4. *Triangulation* is the process by which two people in a relationship who are in conflict involve another person in such a way that the conflict is diminished in the relationship and displaced onto the third person. Children are often triangulated into parental conflicts or problems, and one child may be the focus of most of the triangulation. Multiple interlocking triangles often exist in extended families as a way of dispersing stress and avoiding conflict.
5. *Family structure* may influence childhood development. This includes single parent families, teenage parents, families with both parents working, adoption, children being raised by grandparents or other relatives, and other variations on family structure.
6. *Multigenerational family patterns or traditions* may be important in setting the stage for problems with a particular developmental issue. Often, a primary care clinician who has a long-term relationship with a family can predict difficulties with a specific issue through knowledge of prior family problems, the family's expectations, or patterns of behavior in the family over generations.
7. A *"special child"* may be the focus for increased attention or expectations and is particularly vulnerable to dysfunctional family processes. This special status can result from illness, prematurity, congenital problems in the child, or an unwanted or unplanned pregnancy. Previous spontaneous or induced abortions, stillbirths, or infertility problems can greatly increase the family's anxiety about a pregnancy, thus putting the child at risk. A death in the family can be significant in this regard, especially the death of a child or the recent death of a close family member. In these situations, the child may be viewed, consciously or unconsciously, as a "replacement" for the deceased person, with the consequent burden of unusual family expectations. If separation and individuation of the parents from their family of origins has been difficult or traumatic, the birth of their first child may have special significance in completing the separation process, producing a great deal of stress in the extended family. Even when there have been previous children or grandchildren, the first child of a particular gender may have added meaning in some family situations.

Parenting and Discipline Issues

Parenting and discipline issues can be seen as a subsection of family influences, but the subject is important enough to be dealt with separately. Many child discipline problems arise around child development issues. Parents often have unrealistic expectations of what their child's behavior should be and, therefore, get into battles with the child that can be counterproductive. Parents may not have had good role models for dealing with child discipline issues and either repeat the patterns of discipline from their own families or react to those patterns negatively and do the opposite. Neither strategy is truly effective.

Primary care clinicians are in a position to provide brief interventions around child discipline issues that can assist parents and children in more effectively dealing with these problems, thereby heading off secondary behavioral problems. In this section, we discuss an overall approach to child discipline that is practical and easy to present to parents, with more specific examples presented around issues arising at various developmental stages in the subsequent sections.

One of the most important roles that those of us with children have is child rearing, but few people have any formal training in this role. And, unfortunately, the instructions do not come printed on the back of the child. Furthermore, every child and every parent are different from every other child and parent. For example, some children are more sensitive, energetic, or impulsive than others, and parents are highly variable in their expectations of their children. This is an area where primary care clinicians can really be of assistance to the families. That does not mean that the clinician should prescribe a specific solution for a family's discipline issues. However, it helps for parents to understand some principles of child behavior and discipline.

1. A primary guiding principle should be that children deserve to be wanted and loved. The ideal is for children to be loved and wanted as they are.
2. No child wants to fail or misbehave, but every child will do so at times.
3. All children need limits. However, children also need to be comfortable with exploring the limits. Limits that are set too tightly can cause major problems.
4. A key purpose of discipline is to assist children in reaching their maximum potential.
5. Parents need to carefully think about their expectations for their child's behavior. The parents need to agree on their expectations so that they can be consistent. The expectations and rules should then be clearly communicated to the child. Those expectations will need to evolve constantly, as the child grows and develops.
6. Every child is different, and it is not productive to compare one child's behavior to another's. Expectations need to be appropriate for the child.
7. Rewards are almost always more effective than punishment in changing behavior. As a matter of fact, in situations in which the child is misbehaving as a way of getting attention, punishment can often serve to reinforce the negative behavior. The best management of a negative attention-seeking behavior is to ignore it and then reward the parallel positive behavior. If any discipline is needed to control totally unacceptable or dangerous behavior, it should be done with minimal interaction with the child. This is one of the places where isolation or "time out," with the child sitting in a quiet place for a defined period of time, works well. But remember that love, praise, and positive attention are the best ways to change behavior.
8. A reward system is often effective in changing behavior and getting tasks done, especially for older children who can understand the system. A contract should be drawn up and agreed upon, specifying the expected behavior, time frame, specific responsibility, rewards for accomplishing the task or behavior, and consequences for failing to accomplish to task. Realize that children are infinitely creative in their ability to circumvent the system and then plead ignorance; the more specific the contract, the less room for this type of creativity.
9. Punishment should be used as a last resort. The punishment should always fit the misbehavior and should be immediate. It also should be directly tied to a specific behavior. It is not fair to let small problems accumulate until a behavior or action becomes "the straw that broke the camel's back," resulting in an overreaction that is too general and is often ineffective.
10. Punishment should be private and rewards public.
11. Spanking is the lowest form of discipline and is not very effective in the long run. However, there may be times when it is useful, within limits. It can be particularly useful with young children as a way of getting their attention with very bad or dangerous behavior. When used, one spank with an open hand on the buttocks is enough. Overuse of spanking or other physical punishment usually results in angry, aggressive behavior in the child. It is hard to stress to a child that violent behavior is unacceptable when the parent is using violent behavior to punish the child.

When the clinician identifies that there are issues around child discipline, the best initial strategy may be to discuss some of the basic principles listed above with the parents. Discipline issues should be discussed in the context of the child's developmental stage and individual characteristics. This strategy will suffice much of the time. If further counseling is needed, the clinician could choose to refer the family for counseling or to try a brief intervention over three to four office visits. The first step in such a primary care intervention would be to have the parents jointly derive a list of the two or three primary behaviors or issues that need work and then develop a strategy for addressing those areas, proceeding to a set of rules and a reward system. If the child is old enough to have input into this process, the clinician should then request that the parents and child negotiate a contract, including a system for monitoring success, and then check the progress in a follow-up session. If the family is unable to progress through this process, referral for family counseling may be indicated.

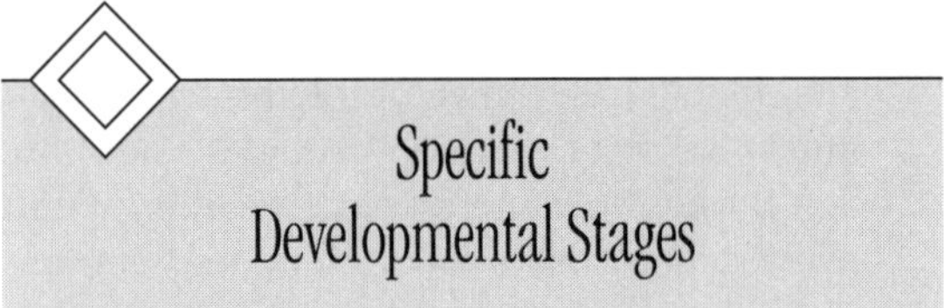

Specific Developmental Stages

In this section, we review the major psychosocial developmental issues for infants, toddlers, preschool children, school-age children, and adolescents. We will focus on the developmental tasks that result in behaviors that are likely to come up in primary care clinical encounters. There are numerous issues related to a psychodynamic viewpoint, such as the development of defense mechanisms and the root causes of certain mental health issues, that are more complex and beyond the scope of this chapter. The effects of specific family influences on some of the most important developmental tasks at each stage will also be discussed. It should be noted that the ages for the beginning and end of each stage are generally quite variable, with each individual child progressing through the stages at his or her own rate. The age range given should be taken as a general average rather than an absolute.

Infants (Birth to 15 Months)

Infancy is a time of rapid physical, psychomotor, cognitive, and psychosocial growth and development. There is a tendency to lose sight of psychosocial issues at this stage because of the more obvious changes in other areas. However, this stage establishes many of the patterns for subsequent psychosocial and personality development.

Developmental Tasks

The primary psychosocial developmental tasks for infancy have to do with the bonding and attachment of the infant to the parents or primary parental figures, and the meeting of the child's basic needs. In Eriksonian terms, this is the stage at which a sense of "basic trust versus mistrust" is formed depending on the manner in which the child's basic needs for food, shelter, protection, and nurturing are met. The bonding process begins at or before birth, and the degree of bonding and the level of trust in the parent–child relationship strongly influence the child's later ability to form close, nonanxious, trusting relationships with other people.

Klaus and Kennel's study in the mid-1970s pointed out the importance of the initial bonding that occurs between mother and child immediately after birth. There are a number of things that can interfere with the early bonding process and cause later problems, including illness or prematurity of the newborn infant. When the baby has to be swept away to the nursery because of problems that may result in IV lines, respirators, feeding tubes, or other medical interventions, the initial bonding process is disrupted, and the parents may not be able to take on much responsibility for taking care of the baby's basic needs for a fairly prolonged period of time. In such a situation, the parents should be encouraged to participate in caring for the infant to the fullest extent possible, and the clinician may have to work actively to remove barriers to such participation.

Temperament

A child's temperament is the style in which the child acts, reacts to the environment, expresses emotions, and interacts socially with others. There is clear evidence that infants' basic temperamental characteristics are present at birth and tend to persist over time, although they modify and mature with development. Of particular importance is the fit of the parents' personalities and parenting styles with the infant's basic temperament. For example, when very anxious parents are coupled with an infant who is very irritable and reactive, there tend to be problems, often presenting to the primary care clinician as colic or feeding difficulties. During this stage, the basic building blocks are being laid for future social and intimate relationships.

Cognitive Development

Cognitive development is very interesting during infancy and can be tracked through stages that can be observed in the child's behavior. During this early, preverbal stage, the infant obtains new knowledge by direct sensorimotor contact. One area in which you can see the child's cognitive development clearly is the developing sense of self and others. At birth, an infant has little or no ability to discriminate where its body and self begin and end. This is seen in the infant's primitive suck reflex; an infant will attach onto and suck any object placed in the mouth or against the cheek, whether the mother's breast, bottle nipple, or the baby's fist. Over time, however, the child progressively begins to differentiate "self" from its surroundings, as seen in a baby's sense of fascination and discovery in exploring his or her own hands, feet, and other appendages.

As the infant becomes more comfortable with what is self, the infant also begins to recognize and respond to specific portions of the surroundings, usually starting with the parents. An important early milestone of this process is the social smile, which should be present by 2 or 3 months of age. If the smile is delayed or does not appear, it may be a sign of neurologic or visual dysfunction, retardation, or problems in interactions with the parents or other caregivers.

The next major cognitive issue is the development of a sense of object permanence, the understanding that just because an object is out of one's field of vision, it does not cease to exist. This begins to emerge at 5 to 6 months of age. The child's budding sense of object permanence can be seen in the hilarious response to peek-a-boo games, and in the game of "throw down the toy 50 times and laugh uncontrollably each time Dad gives it back to me."

The developing ability to discriminate among people in the environment and to become concerned when key people are not there is expressed as stranger anxiety, which becomes an issue at around 5 to 6 months, and separation anxiety, beginning around 7 to 8 months. Parents can help to reduce their infant's separation anxiety by alleviating and soothing the child's anxiety and by shaping the separation anxiety by not overreacting to it. Parents who themselves are not comfortable with separation do not do this very well and may have to be coached.

BEN CARROLL *Ben Carroll, a 9-month-old infant, is brought in for a check-up by his 22-year-old mother. Physically, everything is going well. Because you know that separation and stranger anxiety can commonly cause parental concern, you ask Mrs. Carroll about this. She indicates that she has been having a lot of difficulty dealing with this, because Ben wants to be close to her all the time, clinging to her constantly and screaming whenever anyone else tries to pick him up. You know from previous conversations that Mrs. Carroll is staying home from work for a year to take care of Ben and that she has not left him in day care because of concerns about him getting sick. You ask her whether she ever leaves Ben with anyone else, and she indicates that she does not. You explain that separation anxiety is a normal developmental stage, but that this anxiety appears to be excessive for Ben. You suggest that he needs to experience contact with other people for periods of time, and that she very much needs a break from taking care of Ben all of the time. You discuss options for this with her, and she decides that a small mother's "day out" program at her church would work well for her. You counsel her to not* *overreact when Ben cries when he is left, but to do things to soothe him as soon as she picks him up. You tell her that it is important for Ben to develop experiences that will help him get through this stage, and that she should not feel guilty for leaving him. You also schedule a follow-up visit in a month to monitor their progress.*

Hopefully, by the end of the infancy stage the child will have developed an initial sense of self, separate from the parents and the rest of the environment. The child also will have formed a secure and trusting relationship with the most important people in his or her life. At that point the process of separation and individuation becomes a primary concern, with entry into the toddler stage that follows.

Family Influences During Infancy

INTIMACY The amount of intimacy in family relationships strongly influences parent–child bonding and attachment processes. Parents from families in which disengaged and distant relationships are the norm will probably perpetuate that pattern in their relationships with their own child. This disrupts bonding and compromises basic trust, resulting in the child continuing the pattern with distant and distrustful future relationships. The clinician can do a number of simple things to promote bonding, including spending additional time during prenatal care to engage the expectant parent(s) in the development of the fetus, making certain that the parents are encouraged to hold and interact with the child as much and as soon after birth as possible, and encouraging breastfeeding.

FAMILY STRUCTURE Family structural issues can often affect the family's ability to provide for the child's basic physical and emotional needs. It is important that there be at least one primary caregiver who is able and willing to nurture the child and provide a focus for the child's bonding. Clinicians are often faced with situations in which it is not clear who the primary caregiver of the child may be. This is especially common in early teenage pregnancies. In situations where the teenage mother is clearly engaged with the pregnancy and is planning to be the primary caregiver, the clinician should do everything possible to empower her in that role and to promote bonding with the baby. In some situations, however, it becomes clear that the teenage mother will return to school and her "former" life after the pregnancy, and that her mother (the baby's grandmother) will actually be the primary caregiver. In that situation, the clinician should strive to promote the involvement of the grandmother in prenatal care and with bonding after birth. The teenage mother should not be shut out of the process, but it is very important that the person who will be the primary caregiver bond with the baby.

INDIVIDUATION Poorly individuated parents have a great deal of difficulty with their child's attempts at separation and individuation. In infancy, this generally presents with problems beginning in the second half of the infancy period, when the child begins to grapple with separation issues. This may produce an exaggerated separation or stranger anxiety, which may be seen in the clinician's office. It can also be seen with the extremely overanxious parent who is constantly calling the physician for a myriad of minor concerns about the infant. When this problem is identified, efforts at decreasing parental anxiety about the child, educating parents to value and nurture child autonomy, and encouraging the parents to develop other areas of their own lives can often decrease the intensity of the focus on the child and decrease future difficulties.

TRIANGULATION The triangulation process involves the child in the family's conflicts or stresses. Parents or family members who focus on the child's problems or behavior do not have to focus on or deal with their own problems. This process may have particular intensity when the child is "special" and can greatly affect the child's ability to successfully deal with his or her own developmental issues. Physicians often unintentionally support this by not looking beyond the child's presenting symptoms at the larger family context. It is important to identify this triangulation process so that inappropriate attention to the child's problems can be redirected to the real problems in the family.

OTHER ISSUES Multigenerational family patterns can help the physician to predict potential problem areas. Thus, in a family where child abuse or neglect or other forms of violence is a repeating pattern, the clinician should expend extra effort to encourage bonding and work on basic parenting skills. Programs involving home visits by various clinicians, usually nurses, have been shown to be successful at decreasing abuse and neglect and improving other outcomes.

The birth of a first child may have great significance as a milestone in the separation of the parents from their own families of origin. The birth can cause a strong reaction in the family of origin, especially when the separation of the parents has been made difficult by low levels of individuation in the family of origin. The issues of separation of the parents often expresses itself soon after birth with subtle interference from the grandparents and a great deal of stress throughout the family. The new mother is often already insecure in her role as a parent, and the interference from her mother or other family members serves to increase her anxiety. This results in phone calls to the clinician regarding feeding problems, sleeping, stooling, or other concerns about the newborn infant.

An especially common and potentially harmful problem can arise around breast-feeding, with the grandparent(s) expressing concern that the baby is not getting enough milk. Because of this, the common suggestion from the grandparent is "Why don't you go rest and let me give the baby a bottle." The mother feels like she is a failure and cannot produce enough milk for her baby. The baby gets milk out of the bottle much more easily and learns to prefer it over breast-feeding. The bottle feedings decrease the demand on the breast, and the milk supply never does really catch up, especially in an increasingly anxious mother. The grandparent gets to exert a continued presence and control. Breast-feeding is abandoned, and the new mother's self-confidence in her new role is diminished. No one really intends for this to happen, and it occurs at an unconscious level. However, it happens very commonly. The clinician should anticipate the potential for this problem in a first-time breast-feeding mother, especially one who has not successfully separated from her family of origin and particularly when the family of origin shows signs of being controlling and interfering during the prenatal course. The clinician can then counsel the expectant mother to anticipate possible problems of this type, work with her to strengthen her confidence, support and encourage her breast-feeding efforts, and monitor the situation so as to intervene early in any problems.

Toddlers (15 Months to 3 Years)

The labeling of the toddler stage as the "terrible twos" is certainly not without justification. Toddlers push the limits, explore the environment, and get into everything. They tend to do things that put them in frequent peril, like climbing on top of counters and sticking spoons into the electrical sockets. However, they also are actively working on their self-identity and autonomy, and they do not react well to their parents interfering with their explorations. Toddlers are among the great challenges of parenthood.

TIM HOLT *Tim Holt is an 18-month-old boy who is brought to your office by his mother for a well-child visit. In the course of the visit, Tim constantly is exploring the office, pulling on the paper on the exam table, tugging at electrical cords, and opening every drawer in the room. This leads to an ongoing battle with his mother, who tries valiantly to get him to stay quietly in his chair, to no avail. After watching the mother grow increasingly frustrated in her efforts, you say, "You know, kids this age can be really hard to take care of. They get* *into things constantly; that is what a toddler does for a living! It can be really frustrating trying to keep them from hurting themselves and tearing up the house while at the same time allowing them to satisfy their need to explore. How has this been going for you?"*

This leads to a conversation in which you discover that the mother has become convinced that she is a bad mother because of her inability to control Tim's behavior. He has temper tantrums in public, the house is in shambles, and the parent's friends rarely come over any more. Her husband has grown increasingly negative, saying that Tim is a bad child and she is a bad mother. You discuss discipline with the mother and discover that she does not have a very good idea of how to deal with Tim's behavior. She has resisted physical punishment, but some of her family members have been telling her that she is too lax and that she needs to spank Tim when he misbehaves.

You discuss the normal developmental issues of this stage with the mother, telling her that Tim's behavior is normal and that he is not a "bad child." You also try to bolster the mother's self-confidence in her parenting abilities, telling her that her love and nurturing of Tim are most important and that the difficulties she is having are not unusual. Because it is apparent that Tim's father is also becoming frustrated and having difficulties with the situation, you suggest a return visit in 2 weeks when he can also come, to discuss parenting and discipline issues in more detail.

With the emphasis on individuation and the development of limits, Erikson termed the primary psychosocial issue of this stage as the establishment of a sense of "autonomy versus shame and doubt." Toddlers who have achieved a sense of basic trust and established a good relationship with their parents should be well prepared for this step. A toddler's curiosity about the world and excitement in exploration should be actively supported by the parents. Children who are not allowed to pull away, establish their own identity, and develop a sense of their own limits come out of this stage lacking self-confidence and with stifled creativity.

Toilet training usually becomes an issue during this stage. This involves the initiation of a social expectation and norm that is encouraged by the parents and others. Most toddlers respond to this positively, with a need both to have mastery over their own bodily functions and to have a positive interaction with their parents. A positive and loving approach from the parents, with active reinforcement and approval of desired performance, will generally yield good results. However, toilet training can also become a battleground, with the toddler exercising his or her developing sense of autonomy or using this as a way of getting attention, even if negative, from the parents. Clinicians can help parents by counseling them to be realistic about their expectations and to be positive in their approach.

Between the ages of 18 and 24 months, toddlers also begin constructing their gender identity. Parental attitudes and beliefs about gender have a strong affect at this point. Before 18 months, children explore their genitals as part of their general body exploration. However, at around 18 months toddlers become very curious about sex-based anatomic differences. They also begin to identify with the parent of the same sex and to incorporate gender-specific behaviors into their own repertoire.

Cognitive skills develop rapidly during this stage. The toddlers' understanding of themselves and their environment expands with exploration. The maturation of the toddler's conceptual thinking gives rise to the ability to think in terms of symbols. The ability to think symbolically helps the toddler to begin to understand concepts expressed verbally.

Speech development typically makes great strides during the toddler stage. Although children vary considerably in the pace and timing of their speech development, by 18 months most children can comprehend short commands, use about five words, and point to one body part. At 24 months most toddlers can use two-word sentences, have about a 50-word vocabulary, and can point to four body parts. By the end of this stage, toddlers usually can carry out interactive conversations with their parents, although some children will lag slightly. However, their understanding of what is going on around them is certainly different from that of older children or adults. Toddlers do not understand the principle of cause and effect, and their concept of their environment is strongly colored by magical thinking and fantasy.

Discipline

Discipline becomes important during the toddler stage. Parental expectations can be very much at odds with the child's developmental capabilities. Parents commonly overestimate their toddler's ability to understand parental explanations of why the toddler should not do certain things. The toddler may display an understanding of the words, but the concepts do not really make sense. Lengthy explanations of why the child should not wander out into the street do not have long-term influence on the toddler's behavior, and some parents do not understand this. Parents also commonly interpret their child's explorations as bad behavior, and their attempts to control those explorations lead to battles of will. It is very hard to win a battle of wills with a toddler. Many parents start using spanking and other forms of punishment at this point, which only lead to more rebellious and negative behavior, and a negative cycle may result. Parents need to have their toddler's behavior normalized for them, put into the appropriate developmental perspective so that the parents see it as normal behavior rather than something that needs to be corrected. If that can occur before the negative cycle becomes established, many problems can be averted.

That is not to say that limits are not important. Toddlers push to find the limits. If there are no limits, it creates problems. Children need to know that there are limits beyond which they cannot or should not push. Parenting at this stage involves a constant balance between protecting toddlers from harm while still encouraging them to explore their surroundings; between controlling unacceptable behavior and allowing their own autonomy to develop. It is a very difficult balance to achieve, and a primary care clinician can assist the parents of a toddler through support, information regarding the appropriate behavior at this stage, counseling regarding discipline, and reassurance.

Family Influences

With the emphasis at this stage on autonomy and the development of a sense of individual identity, it is not surprising that families with low levels of individuation will have many problems. For some parents it is not acceptable for their child to pull away from them. It does not fit with their model of how parent–child relationships should work, and it threatens their own self-image. In response to the parents' high level of control, the toddler is likely to either rebel, leading to negative behavior and battles with the parents, or conform, leading to a meek and quiet child who lacks self-confidence and any sense of self-identity separate from the parents. Either reaction is undesirable. A clinician who identifies this problem in a family should attempt to make small interventions over time, instructing the family about normal toddler behavior and important developmental issues, educating the parents about appropriate parenting and discipline techniques, and considering the possibility of referral for family counseling if problems develop.

Parents commonly start considering having another child about the time their youngest child is in the toddler stage. The birth of a baby into a family with a toddler typically gives rise to sibling rivalry, with the toddler's behavior regressing and often falling into patterns of negative attention-seeking behaviors. Aggressive behavior toward the baby is also common. Parents need to be made aware that this is an almost universal reaction for a toddler with a younger sibling. They should plan special quality time with the toddler and attempt to ignore attention-seeking behavior.

Preschool (3 to 6 Years)

During the preschool years, there is a strong undercurrent of sexual issues. This is the stage in which Freudian theories have perhaps their clearest expression in observable behavior. In Freudian terms, the preschool phase is the oedipal phase, when children must come to grips with sexual urges and, in particular, the sexual attraction toward the parent of the opposite sex. Freud indicates that the suppression of these urges as being unacceptable leads to the development of the superego (conscience). Erikson terms this as the stage in which a sense of initiative versus guilt is developed, related to the development of a superego and expressed through the child's choice of good instead of unacceptable behaviors.

Psychosexual issues are expressed in the child's behavior in several ways. Aggressive behavior may surface, especially but not exclusively directed toward the parent of the same sex. The child may express a great deal of curiosity about sexual issues throughout the preschool stage. Interestingly, this sexual curiosity generally disappears completely at the end of the preschool stage, which is consistent with Freudian theory. Parents faced with sexual acting out and questions about sexual topics for the first time may present to the primary care clinician with concerns about sexual abuse. In such situations, the child should be carefully screened for any evidence of abuse. If there is no other evidence of abuse, the parents can be reassured that the child's sexual curiosity probably represents a normal developmental stage rather than a symptom of abuse in this case.

Concomitantly, this is the stage in which gender identification and roles are most strongly determined. Children usually can clearly identify their gender appropriately and describe aspects of what that means by the mid- to late-toddler stage, but the preschool phase is the period when gender roles are primarily learned. Privacy and modesty suddenly develop in children who previously had no compunction about taking off their clothes and running around naked.

In terms of cognitive development, children display a gradual shift from magical thinking to logical thinking late in the preschool phase, beginning to understand cause and effect relationships. Storytelling takes on great importance, as the child uses stories and fantasy to work out an acceptable vision of reality. These children commonly have vivid nightmares and may develop a variety of fears and phobias as they grapple with this transition. They also will commonly get into trouble with their parents over the lies and "tall tales" that they may tell. Parents should be reassured that this is normal behavior for this age that should resolve with gentle but firm correction. Certainly, harsh punishment for lying at this stage is not indicated and may actually be harmful and counterproductive.

Family Influences

Sexual abuse may be most likely and especially harmful at this stage. Children who are trying to resolve issues of appropriate expression or suppression of their own sexual urges definitely do not need to be confused by becoming involved in the sexual behavior of parents or other adults. Families with a history of abuse should be watched closely for any signs of a recurrence of abuse, especially during this stage (but, of course, also at all stages of child development).

Grade School (6 Years to Puberty)

In Freudian psychosexual developmental theory, grade school is a quiet stage of development, labeled as the latency stage. However, in other developmental frameworks it is an extremely active and important stage.

From a cognitive perspective, grade school is the period in which logical thinking develops, termed by Piaget as the concrete operational phase of cognitive development. Children at this stage develop an ability to carry out complex thinking processes around concrete events. There is a strong emphasis on learning and school achievement, which gives rise to the major psychosocial issue of the period. Grade school is generally the first time that children start measuring themselves against other children. The development of peer and social identity and relationships generally begins during the preschool stage, but is greatly accelerated during grade school. Grade school is a period when children develop a sense of their own talents and of what they may be able to accomplish. Much of the basic underpinnings of a person's self-esteem and self-image forms during this stage.

Erikson describes grade school as the stage when the child develops a sense of "industry versus inferiority." Children who struggle academically may become discouraged and lose confidence in their abilities. This can lead to behavioral problems; acting out is a common way in which children may channel the negative emotions surrounding their failures. Some children can achieve more physically than mentally, and athletic and other such pursuits can be areas of success. It is important that children be encouraged to perform to their fullest potential at this point, as it sets the stage for subsequent achievement.

AMY PERKINS *Amy Perkins, 8 years old and in the second grade, is brought in by her parents for a follow-up visit for a second episode of otitis media within a month. Her symptoms have resolved, and physical exam reveals that her ears now appear normal. You decide to use the visit to see how Amy is doing otherwise. In response to your questions, it becomes apparent that Amy has been having increasing behavioral problems, both at school and at home. While she formerly was an outgoing, happy child, she has become sullen and reactive, and she recently has gotten into trouble at school for fighting. Her school performance was acceptable overall during kindergarten and early first grade, and her parents always thought that she was at least as intelligent as her two older siblings, who have been excellent students.*

However, Amy has had increasing problems over the past year. She is especially behind in reading, despite having excellent comprehension of things that are read to her. You look for signs and symptoms of abuse, but find no indication that either physical or sexual abuse is occurring. Her father has a history of difficulty in school, finally diagnosed as dyslexia during an evaluation in early high school. You suggest to the parents that Amy should be evaluated for a possible learning disorder, and they agree to referral to an educational psychologist who specializes in this area. You schedule a follow-up visit with the family when that evaluation is completed.

It is extremely important that parents and primary care clinicians be alert for the possibility of learning problems. Children who appear to be performing at a lower level than expected or who seem to have specific areas of problems should be referred for testing early, before a pattern of failure can become established. Clinicians should not rely on overburdened schools to take responsibility for this, and parents often do not realize the extent or importance of the problem without prompting.

The other major psychosocial developmental issue during this stage involves the internalization of rules, structure, and organization. This is a period when the child's social focus turns from her family to a larger social context, with peers, teachers, and others in the environment becoming increasingly important. This stage is especially important in the area of value formation. Rules and values that have been learned from the family are tested and reshaped in this context. The child exits this stage of life with his or her values relatively fixed. Events happening later in life can change these values, but with difficulty.

FAMILY ISSUES

As related above, the most important developmental issue at this stage involves school achievement, with the development of a sense of one's capabilities as compared to others. If there is a history in the parents or siblings of learning problems, attention deficit hyperactivity disorder, or poor school performance, the parents should be counseled to watch the child's school performance closely and to come in for evaluation if problems are apparent.

Family violence also can have profound effects at this stage. Children who are being abused, or who are witnessing domestic violence in their homes, often have poor self-esteem and low self-confidence, and their school performance may suffer. They also may act out at school, relating to other children with the aggressive behavior to which they have been subjected. Thus, poor school performance, poor self-esteem, and behavioral problems at school all should be indicators for the clinician to look more closely for child abuse or other forms of family violence.

Families who have had difficulty with the individuation of family members will often have problems with the child going to school, developing a social context outside the family, or displaying different values and ideas than those that are acceptable within the family. Children can express this in two different, almost opposite, ways. They can rebel against the family's rules and over-control, often presenting with behavioral problems, with the parents complaining of not being able to control his or her behavior. Or, they may continue to be controlled by the family, causing poor socialization at school. School phobia can sometimes result, with the child's desire to avoid going to school receiving unconscious support from the family. Thus, any illnesses that the child may develop cause prolonged school absences, and the child may develop psychosomatic complaints. Occasionally, school phobia can be seen when a child is somehow traumatized at school, but a low level of family individuation is much more commonly the underlying issue.

Clinicians can often predict families and children that may have difficulty with this problem and institute preventive intervention. This might include encouraging parents to start sending their child to day care for increasing periods of time even before school begins or making the child's need to succeed in school a major, conscious issue for the families to deal with. Clinicians can also intervene early in the process by paying close attention to which children are requiring school excuses for prolonged and unreasonable absences or by asking high-risk families about school attendance.

When school phobia is identified, the intervention is to strongly encourage the parents to put the child back in school unless there are major reasons for the child not to be there. This intervention can include (1) setting clear guidelines for absences due to illness, (2) ensuring that there is no abuse or traumatization of the child at school, (3) working with the parents and the school to facilitate an easy dropping off of the child at school, and (4) supporting the parents in not responding to the child's attempts to stay home and miss school or to come home from school in the middle of the day.

Adolescence (Puberty to 18 Years)

Adolescence is a transitional stage that is full of change. It starts at puberty rather than any particular age. Through adolescence, there is a rehashing of most of the major previous developmental issues, as the previous resolutions of these issues may no longer work. Those developmental issues that were previously inadequately resolved may cause particular problems. However, rehashing of previous issues also provides a certain amount of plasticity, as issues may be resolved more successfully the second (or third!) time around.

The nature of some of the issues of adolescence are culturally influenced. In primitive cultures, rituals or rites of passage marked the transition into adulthood, sometimes resulting in a very abrupt change. In most modern cultures, the prolonged educational process causes children to be dependent on their families for longer periods of time, resulting in a prolonged adolescent period.

The primary marker used for puberty in boys is sperm production, which typically appears sometime between 12.5 and 16.5 years, with a mean age of 14. In girls, menarche is the most useful marker for puberty, occurring between 10.5 and 15.5 years, with a mean of 12. Thus, girls enter this stage at an age that is approximately 2 years younger than boys. There is a trend toward an earlier onset of puberty, especially in girls, so these ages may be changing somewhat. The average age at onset of menstruation has shifted from 15 to 16 in 1880, to 13 to 14 in 1925, to 12 in 1985.

Preadolescence

Actually, a number of early changes occur approximately 1 to 2 years before puberty, in a stage labeled as preadolescence. At this stage, there is a tremendous increase in nonspecific tension in the child, expressed in various ways. Preadolescents may display boundless energy at times, although their energy levels fluctuate wildly. They may become irritable and anxious. They enter a period of rapid growth and body changes that result in them becoming very self-conscious and preoccupied with their bodies and appearance.

Preadolescent boys tend to run in packs; peer support is very important to them. They generally do not relate well to girls and often belittle them. They may be short tempered and argumentative. They commonly have behavioral issues that are especially expressed at their mothers, whom they may reject as a means of asserting their independence.

Preadolescent girls also tend to have issues around their separation and independence from their mothers. Close relationships with one or possibly two other girls tend to be the norm, taking the place of the previously close relationships with their mothers. Clearly, preadolescent girls have more one-on-one friendships, as compared to the group friendships seen in preadolescent boys. Girls this age are attracted to males, but boys their age tend to lag behind the girls developmentally. Preadolescent girls often develop idealized "crushes" on older males, commonly older boys, teachers, or entertainers.

Adolescent Developmental Tasks

Adolescence essentially provides a transition from childhood to adulthood. There are three major themes of the issues of adolescence, as shown in Table 2-1.

INDEPENDENCE Adolescents have to gradually assume responsibility for their own needs, and there tends to be a great deal of conflict over this. There is a tendency for adolescents to rebel against limits, but they also clearly need and want limits, similarly to toddlers. In preadolescence or early adolescence, this conflict tends to be acted out around control over the adolescent's body and appearance. Haircuts, baths, and choice of clothing all can become major battlegrounds, with the adolescent insisting on the right and ability to handle these choices alone, but then often not following through with the responsibility.

Table 2-1

Main Developmental Tasks of Adolescence

1. Independence from childhood parental ties
2. Achievement of a capability for intimate sexual relationships
3. Consolidation of a firm sense of identity

Adolescents often are very ambivalent, wanting to be treated as adults and given freedom, but at the same time wanting to be taken care of like a child. For parents, this stage presents a very difficult balance between granting increasing freedom and responsibility while still imposing appropriate limits. It is important that developing adolescents complete this stage with the ability to impose limits on their own behavior and take responsibility for their own actions. Fostering this ability is a large part of the successful launching of the child into adulthood, and this should be a major goal for the family.

INTIMATE RELATIONSHIPS Adolescence is the stage in which a person develops an ability to have intimate relationships involving feelings of love as well as sexual feelings. This development occurs in stages. Early in adolescence, idealistic crushes or narcissistic choices based on how it makes adolescents look to their peers are the norm. Young adolescents tend to be very curious, but are self-conscious and embarrassed about discussing sexual topics. Early relationships may be very romanticized, stereotyped as "puppy love." Homosexual experiences are not uncommon, especially early in adolescence, and are not necessarily associated with adult homosexuality.

In boys you often see a split emerge between feelings of affection and tenderness and sexual feelings, with different individuals being the object of each. In psychosexual developmental terms, this probably represents a stage in which the boy has not yet reconciled the recapitulation of issues surrounding his sexual attraction to his mother, and having sexual feelings toward a girlfriend may not be acceptable to him at this stage. Later, as this conflict is resolved, there is a gradual integration of sexual feelings and experiences into intimate relationships. Girls tend to be able to integrate sexual feelings into intimate relationships more easily, so this form of splitting is not commonly seen in their relationships.

IDENTITY Identity consolidation is perhaps the central developmental issue for adolescents. This involves the development of a firm sense of their own identity, separate from parents and peers, including both who they are and what they wish to do with their lives. This process often involves a search outside of the family for new role models, who may become the objects of intense admiration and idealization. Previously accepted values and behavioral models are examined and challenged, and new ones are considered. Erikson terms this as the stage of "identity versus role diffusion." If this search for identity is not successfully carried out, it may result in role diffusion, with confusion and uncertainty regarding the definition of role and identity.

Cognitive Development

Piaget formulates the adolescent period as the formal cognitive phase, beginning at age 11 or 12, during which the capacity for formal, logical reasoning develops. This development includes the ability to reason hypothetically, to be increasingly creative in thinking, and to better use symbolic thinking. These abilities tie into some of the other developmental issues as well, with the adolescent able to apply these skills in examining the logic of his or her beliefs and values.

Emotional Problems in Adolescence

As in adults, depression is the most common mental health problem in adolescence, often tied to difficulty in establishing a sense of identity and autonomy. Adolescent depression is often masked by other behaviors, such as promiscuity, drug or alcohol problems, change in school performance, or behavioral problems. Delinquency and antisocial personality patterns also can be seen in adolescents. Although isolated experiences of breaking laws are not infrequent in normal adolescents, more extensive and long-lasting patterns are not common. Anorexia and bulimia often have their onset in early adolescence, possibly tied into identity conflicts related to the rapid bodily changes. They are seen more commonly when there is a pattern of sexual abuse.

TOM ROGERS *Tom Rogers, a 17-year-old high school senior, is brought in by his mother for increasing fatigue and lack of interest in doing anything. She says that he sleeps about 10 to 12 hours a day and spends most of his free time in his room playing computer games. The mother indicates that she and his father have become concerned that Tom may be taking drugs and want him to have a urine drug test. However, she says that other than the symptoms related above, they do not have any direct evidence of drug use.*

Through all of this, Tom sits quietly in his chair, looking embarrassed and not making eye contact. When you ask him what he thinks the problem may be, he says "I don't know. I don't think there is a problem." His mother shakes her head at that and says that she can never get him to talk any more, so she does not know what is going on. She relates that Tom has always been a good student and never has given them any problems at all up until now. You decide that you need to talk with Tom by himself and ask his mother to wait outside while you do the physical exam.

Before proceeding to the physical exam, you tell Tom that you wanted to talk with him privately to get his perception of what is going on. You have taken care of Tom for over 10 years and have been able to build a good relationship with him. With his mother out of the room, Tom sits up in his chair, looks more engaged in the process, and makes eye contact with you. He indicates that he has been increasingly feeling down and depressed, particularly worrying about what he is going to do with his life. He is having a great deal of difficulty deciding where to go to college and actually does not feel very interested in college at all. However, he does not know what else to do. He has done well at school, but he is not very socially active, and he does not feel that he fits in with the other kids his age. He has tried marijuana on two occasions, but did not like it, and he has not used any other drugs. He has used alcohol on a few occasions, but only once recently, when he got drunk at home by himself. He feels completely controlled by his parents, who have his life planned out for him, but he has no plans for himself.

After further questioning, your assessment is that Tom is suffering from an acute depressive episode related to extreme problems with role diffusion and difficulty in developing his own identity separate from his parents. You explain this to Tom, and he agrees with the assessment. You bring his mother back in and explain your reasoning to her, indicating that you think that Tom needs a great deal of family support for finding his own path in life at this point and that he will probably need individual counseling as well as family counseling. You start him on an antidepressant, refer him to a counselor who works well with adolescents and their families, and schedule a return visit in 2 weeks.

Family Influences

Adolescence can be a difficult stage for parents. They see their child changing before their eyes, moving toward an identity and life separate from them. They may think that their child is making unwise decisions, and some degree of generational conflict and rebellion is normal for this stage. Families that have a low level of tolerance for the individual identities of family members may have a great deal of difficulty with the adolescent's change process. The issues for this type of family are similar to those expressed earlier, in the toddler stage, for autonomy and identity issues and in the grade school stage regarding the importance of the larger social context in the testing of rules and the formation of relationships. Parents still have to maintain rules and limits, but also have to make sure that those rules are appropriate for the age of the adolescent and allow the necessary freedom for the adolescent to develop his or her own identity and rules. Excessive rigidity and rules that are too restrictive will result in poor identity consolidation for the adolescent. This may be expressed by either excessive rebellion or excessive reliance on the parents for direction, both resulting in problems in identity formation for the adolescent.

Adolescence is another stage during which sexual abuse is both common and potentially very harmful. As adolescents develop sexually, they become increasingly attractive to potential perpetrators. Incest, extrafamilial abuse, date rape, and other forms of sexual assault can all cause multiple problems, as detailed in Chap. 7. Abuse victims have difficulty consolidating a solid sense of their own identities, both in general and sexually. Clinicians should stay very alert to the possibility of victimization.

Discipline

Discipline issues often arise during adolescence. Clinicians can assist by first making sure that the parents have realistic expectations as to the level of rules that are necessary for the particular child. Parents may have difficulty relaxing the rules appropriately as their adolescent children become better able to control their own behavior, and some reality testing can help.

Next, the clinician may be able to facilitate a process whereby the parents and adolescent negotiate a set of rules that all can agree to. This should include clear written rules with performance criteria, established consequences for not following the rules, and rewards for good behavior. To achieve this, the clinician has to pay careful attention to establishing or reestablishing a trusting and therapeutic relationship with the adolescent. In situations where the parents bring the adolescent in to "be fixed" and triangulate the clinician into the conflict, the trust building process can be difficult. The clinician should also stress to the parents that the rules will need to change as the adolescent grows and develops. It is often helpful to develop a rules "contract" that includes specific plans for relaxing the rules as adolescents succeed in controlling their own behavior.

Despite the common view of adolescence as an extremely turbulent period, there are many data that indicate that most adolescents actually survive this period well! Most adolescents are successful in separating from their parents and establishing a solid, separate identity, but still value and use the wisdom of their parents. In an international study of about 20,000 middle-class adolescents, Offer and Offer found that 98 percent were actually very task oriented, most had good feelings toward their parents, most felt loved, most were not rebellious, and 90 percent felt optimistic about their future jobs.

Summary

Obviously, a person does not stop developing upon the completion of adolescence. Psychosocial developmental issues continue to be very important throughout life and are related to clinical issues that patients bring to their primary care clinicians. Families go through developmental stages as well, and the family life cycle can interact with individual family members' life cycle issues in very interesting ways. However, developmental issues have perhaps their clearest and clinically most important expressions during childhood, and it is important that primary care clinicians who take care of children thoroughly understand child development and its clinical manifestations. Hopefully, this chapter can give clinicians an introductory framework for exploring these issues.

Suggested Reading

Gemelli R: Normal Child and Adolescent Development. Washington DC: American Psychiatric Press; 1996.

This is an excellent text that explores the stages of child development in much more detail than could be done here in one chapter. It is oriented more toward psychiatry than primary care, but it still could be very useful for primary care clinicians wanting to explore this area in more depth.

Erikson E: Childhood and Society, revised edition. New York: Norton; 1963.

Erik Erikson's work especially influenced the approach presented in this chapter and is very appropriate for primary care clinicians.

American Academy of Pediatrics: *The Diagnostic and Statistical Manual-Primary Care (DSM-PC) Child and Adolescent Version*. Elk Grove Village, IL: American Academy of Pediatrics Press; 1996.

This is a useful resource for primary care clinicians, both to help in the diagnosis and management of childhood psychosocial and developmental issues and for classification for reimbursement purposes. It is available from the American Academy of Pediatrics at 1.800.433.9016.

Bibliography

Bowen M: *Family Therapy in Clinical Practice*. New York: Jason Aronson; 1978.

Chess S, Thomas A: *Temperament in Clinical Practice*. New York: Guilford; 1986.

Emde RN: The prepresentational self and its affective core. *Psychoanal Study Child* 38:165–192, 1983.

Erikson E: *Childhood and Society*, revised ed. New York: Norton; 1963.

Goldsmith H, Buss A, Plomin R: Roundtable: What is temperament? Four approaches. *Child Dev* 58:505, 1987.

Kestenbaum CJ: Current sexual attitudes, societal pressure, and the middle-class adolescent girl. In: Feinstein SC, Giovacchini PL (eds): *Adolescent Psychiatry*. Chicago: University of Chicago Press; 1979, 147.

Klaus MH, Kennell JH: *Maternal–Infant Bonding*. St. Louis: Mosby; 1976.

Mitchell SA: Aggression and the endangered self. *Psychoanal Q* 62:351, 1993.

Offer D, Offer JB: *From Teenage to Young Manhood: A Psychological Study*. New York: Basic Books; 1975.

Olds DL, Eckenrode J, Henderson CR, et al: Long-term effects of home visitation on maternal life course and child abuse and neglect. *JAMA* 278:637, 1997.

Olds DL, Henderson CR, Chamberlin R, et al: Preventing child abuse and neglect: A randomized trial of nurse visitation. *Pediatrics* 78:65, 1986.

Olds DL, Henderson CR, Kitzman H: Does prenatal and infancy nurse home visitation have enduring effects on qualities of parental caregiving and child health at 25 to 50 months of life? *Pediatrics* 93:89, 1994.

Piaget J: *The Origins of Intelligence in Children*. New York: International Universities Press; 1952.

Tyson R: The roots of psychopathology and our theories of development. *J Am Acad Child Adolesc Psychiatry* 25:12, 1986.

Sara C. Hamel
Kelly J. Kelleher

Chapter 3

Behavioral Problems in Childhood and Adolescence

Introduction

The care of children has changed dramatically in recent years due to improvements in public health and reductions in acute infectious diseases. Although today's primary care clinicians still see children with acute concerns, such as respiratory illnesses and otitis media, the focus of well-child visits has shifted to improving the quality of life for children. This focus includes not only vaccines and safety practices, but also early detection and treatment of developmental differences and behavioral problems. This new focus on behavioral and developmental issues may be difficult for primary care clinicians for several reasons. Behavioral and developmental disorders are chronic conditions that are managed more often than cured. The presentations are complex, and diagnoses must be determined from detailed and often time-consuming history taking and evaluation. No laboratory or radiologic studies are usually available to confirm a diagnosis. Adequate assessment and management involves interfacing with professionals in a number of other disciplines and systems, which takes time and is not usually seen as the role of a health care provider. Last, reimbursement to primary care clinicians for addressing issues may not be adequate.

Despite these drawbacks, families frequently look to their primary care clinician for help in assessing and managing behavioral problems, and the majority of children with behavioral problems seen by primary care clinicians are not seen by mental health specialists.

The purpose of this chapter is to provide an overview of the assessment and management of common behavioral problems of children and adolescents, with emphasis on a practical, primary care, family-centered approach to these disorders. After reading this chapter, the clinician should be able to (1) evaluate the child and family that present with a behavioral complaint, (2) establish a working diagnosis using the *Diagnostic and Statistical Manual*, 4th ed. *Primary Care DSM-*IV*-PC*, (3) devise and execute a treatment plan, and (4) provide ongoing support for the child and family as well as evaluation of the treatment. To accomplish these aims, we present an overview of the effect of behavioral problems in primary care, two vignettes, and a review of assessment and management practices for children with behavior problems seen in primary care settings.

In this chapter, the term "psychosocial" means behavioral problems or differences that affect the child's functioning within a family, with peers, or at school. We focus on the category of psychosocial problems known as "disruptive" behavior problems, because they are the most common and often most exasperating for families and clinicians. These problems may represent a developmental variation that requires reassurance and follow-up, or they may result in significant functional impairment, warranting a diagnosis such as conduct disorder, oppositional-defiant disorder, or attention deficit hyperactivity disorder (ADHD). Complete descriptions of the range of presentations of these disorders in children and adolescence are contained in the DSM-IV-PC.

This chapter will explain in detail how to use the DSM-IV-PC for assessment of children presenting with behavioral complaints. It will not, however, address two other important areas of child mental health: treatment of parent–child interaction problems and internalizing problems (e.g., depression and anxiety). These areas are covered in detail in Chap. 2 (parenting), 16 (depression), and 17 (anxiety). Finally, while reading this chapter, it should be noted that roughly half of all children with psychosocial problems in primary care practice have other "comorbid" behavioral problems. Therefore, the presence of any behavior disorder should precipitate an evaluation for others.

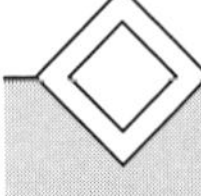

Effects of Child Behavior Problems

An understanding of the diagnosis and management of children with disruptive behavior problems is essential for primary care clinicians because these problems are common, disabling, and costly.

Epidemiology

The Surgeon General recently reported that behavior disorders occur in up to 20 percent of children in community samples, with at least half of these children demonstrating impaired functioning. Five to ten percent of school-age children have disruptive disorders as their principal diagnosis, although comorbidity with mood disorders (depression or anxiety) commonly occurs. Disruptive behaviors are more likely to occur in boys and their incidence increases with age. They are also more often diagnosed in the winter and among early school-age children, a fact likely due to the "discovery" effect of school entry.

In the practice setting, Kelleher and colleagues found psychosocial problems of all types are identified in about 18 percent of children's primary care visits. The epidemiology of disruptive disorders in primary care settings parallels that in community settings. Disruptive disorders are the most common behavioral diagnoses among children seen by primary care clinicians and account for more than half of all children with identified psychosocial problems. ADHD alone as a new or existing diagnosis is involved in 8 percent of all primary care visits for children between 4 and 15 years according to Wasserman and associates. Although severity of parent-reported symptoms and comorbidity are the best predictors of who receives this diagnosis, boys and those seen by older clinicians are more likely to be diagnosed with ADHD.

Early studies in primary care settings compared clinicians' diagnoses obtained in routine practice to psychiatric interviews. Uniformly low rates of detection of mental disorders were found. Newer studies, however, suggest a more complex picture. Primary care clinicians still do not detect one-third to one-half of children with significant impairment from specific diagnosable disorders, but if broader definitions are used (psychosocial problem rather than specific disorder), clinicians report such problems as a large proportion of their visits by children. Many children with psychosocial problems identified by primary care clinicians do not have diagnosable psychiatric disorders or high scores indicating problems on parent-reported checklists. It is not clear whether clinicians detecting problems in children are detecting early problems that do not yet meet the threshold for a diagnosis, identifying family and social situations that affect the child but do not meet criteria for a diagnosis, or actually overdiagnosing behavior disorders.

Disability

Research on the extent of disability associated with disruptive behavior disorders in primary care settings is lacking. However, psychosocial problems in children, as in adults, account for a large proportion of all disability in childhood. In fact, Newacheck found that among adolescents, emotional and behavioral symptoms account for more missed school days than any other conditions combined. In addition, children with emotional and behavioral disorders are the group most likely to drop out of school when compared to youth with other cognitive and medical disabilities. Moreover, Jellinek reports that poor family function is highly correlated with childhood and adolescent behavior problems.

These short-term disabilities are matched by long-term problems with social functioning, employment difficulties, and marital difficulties among persons with disruptive behavior disorders followed into adulthood. Although disruptive behavior disorders cannot be separated from other child psychosocial conditions, it is clear that all of these problems create chaos and associated distress for children, families, schools, and society.

Treatment and Costs

Treatment of childhood behavior problems in primary care is not well described. Only one-fourth of all children with recognized psychosocial problems in primary care are receiving specialty mental health services. Primary care clinicians report brief counseling (5 to 10 min) in 65 percent of visits with youth who have psychosocial problems. Referrals to specialists are made for slightly more than one-fifth of these patients, although children with behavior problems are less often referred than those with diagnosable psychiatric problems like anxiety and depression. Stimulants prescribed for treating ADHD are among the most common psychotropic medications administered to children in primary care settings.

Limited data exist on the costs of disruptive behavior disorders in primary care. Numerous calls for additional cost studies have gone largely unheeded. However, preliminary data by Kelleher and Childs on the effect of ADHD alone suggest that the overall costs are substantial. In examining direct or treatment costs, ADHD was found to be as expensive as asthma, the most common chronic condition of childhood. Children with ADHD have comparable direct costs, although they generally have greater use of ambulatory services and lower costs for pharmaceuticals than children with asthma do. ADHD is much more common in primary care practice and accounted for greater expenditures than depression on a practice-wide basis, even though the costs per patient for depression treatment are much higher. These studies included only an assessment of the direct costs of treating ADHD. Not considered in these numbers are the indirect costs to families and society or the excess use of educational, correctional, and other services by youth with behavior problems.

JOHNNY *Johnny is a 5-year, 3-month-old boy who is brought to your office for an acute visit because he has been suspended from his kindergarten class. School personnel advised his parents to take him to the doctor to see if he had a neurologic problem and could be put on medications. This child entered kindergarten 1 month ago and has had difficulty staying seated, pays little attention to class activities, and hits and kicks other children. He seems also to be uninterested in learning activities.*

JULIE *Julie is an 8-year-old girl who has entered your practice after switching insurance coverage. She has been previously diagnosed with ADHD, and is being prescribed methylphenidate (Ritalin) and clonidine by a psychiatrist at the local mental health agency, whom she sees once every 4 months. She has had difficulty learning in school, repeated first grade, was tested for special education, and was placed in a learning support setting in the second grade. Julie lives with her paternal grandmother, age 56, her two siblings, age 10 and 3, and two cousins, age 11 and 7 months. There are no other adults in household. She comes today with grandmother and grandmother's sister, who lives close by and provides support. Julie's grandmother wants a second opinion from you about the ADHD diagnosis and the medications that Julie is taking.*

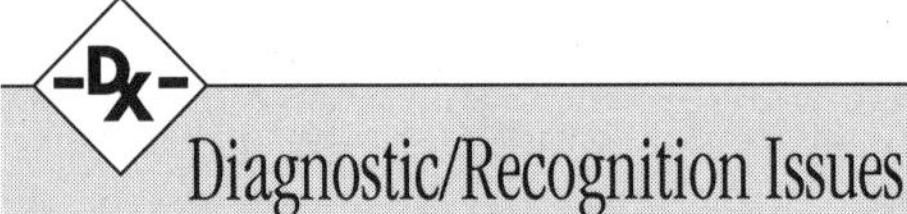

Diagnostic/Recognition Issues

When children and families arrive with a chief complaint of a behavioral problem, the clinician will benefit from using a standardized approach. Having a "routine" way of handling such issues will alleviate the clinicians' anxiety and save time. It also provides a frame of reference derived from a series of case experiences that can be used as a body of knowledge to inform the clinician. Such a standard, noncategorical (i.e., independent of the type of behavioral complaint) approach can be executed in a variety of ways and at a variety of levels.

This section of the chapter provides such a standard approach. It first presents a description of fundamental or necessary practices to address child behavior problems. It then outlines a comprehensive approach to the evaluation for those who wish to devote more time and effort to dealing with patients with behavioral problems.

Fundamental Approach

At the most fundamental level, the clinician must address the complaint with the patient and family, just as it is necessary to address a complaint of abdominal pain. The basic questions to ask include:

- What exactly are the problem behaviors?
- Where do they occur?
- When did they start?
- How long have they lasted?
- What brings them on?
- What has been done in response to them?

Asking such fundamental questions accomplishes two basic goals. First, it gives the family a sense that you take their behavioral or psychosocial concerns seriously and want to help. This is important because many families complain that their clinicians do not listen to their concerns about behavioral problems in the same way they would if they had a medical concern. Listening to families acknowledges the gravity of the situation, and your attempts to understand it validate the family's concern. If you have listened carefully and then decide to refer the patient to a mental health professional for further assessment, the family will be less likely to feel as if you are trying to avoid the issue and more likely to understand that you are referring appropriately after carefully considering their situation.

Second, you will establish whether the situation does or does not involve a safety problem for the child or family. Many children who present with the complaint "he's getting out of hand" may be committing serious aggression toward family members or angering family members, who in turn may be applying excessive physical punishment. Children with disruptive behavior problems are at higher risk for child abuse, and primary care clinicians must assess this risk with every family that presents with a behavioral complaint. Children who you suspect may be experiencing physical or sexual abuse must be immediately referred to child protective agencies. Children who are engaging in unsafe behaviors, such as setting fires, or who have expressed suicidal thinking or actions, should always be referred for immediate psychiatric evaluation.

JOHNNY (CONTINUED) *Johnny's parents tell you that at home, Johnny is difficult but manageable. The principal difficult behavior they identify is his high activity level. He has been active since "in utero" and once he learned to walk, he ran. His parents have carefully double locked doors, cabinets, and windows to keep him safe, and they make sure to provide many activities to keep him occupied. Still, they have trouble finding a babysitter who will stay with him, and at family gatherings they are embarrassed by his boisterous behavior. He has trouble playing with other children because fights break out. Other family members have told them that they are too soft on him and perhaps need to apply more physical punishment to get him under control. You ask about spanking, and they tell you they tried it but stopped because it did not change his behavior.*

The clinician should next be able to interpret the initial information obtained by grouping the symptoms into one or more "presenting complaints." The use of the DSM-IV-PC can be extremely helpful. Appendix A of the DSM-IV-PC contains a representative list of common presenting behavioral complaints in children. One should be able to match presenting complaints about the child with the categories or clusters of behaviors listed in the DSM-IV-PC. For example, the presenting complaint "difficulty staying seated" is a part of the Hyperactive/Impulsive Behaviors Cluster. One then turns to the section in the DSM-IV-PC with the description of that cluster.

A useful approach is to decide which one of three DSM-IV-PC categories the behaviors represent: (1) developmental variation, (2) problem, or (3) disorder. *Variations* are defined in DSM-IV-PC as behaviors that are "within the range of expected behaviors for the age of the child." These will usually be addressed in a brief discussion with parents and with follow-up visits to monitor the situation. *Problems* are "serious enough to disrupt the child's functioning with peers, in school, and/or in the family but do not involve a sufficient level of severity/impairment to warrant a diagnosis of a mental disorder." Problems may be treated in a primary care setting or referred to mental health professionals. *Disorders* are more serious and pervasive problems that significantly and over time affect many areas of functioning for the child. *Disorders* are defined in the *Diagnostic and Statistical Manual,* fourth edition (DSM-IV) as well as in DSM-IV-PC and may require the services of a mental health professional. A sample of how these three levels of functional impairment appear in DSM-IV-PC is given in Table 3-1, using the example of soiling as a presenting complaint.

In considering the extent of the behavior problem, evaluate how the child is functioning in school,

Table 3-1
Example of DSM-IV-PC Format

Developmental Variation	Common Developmental Presentations
Developmental Variation: V65.49 Soiling Variation The occasional passage of a small amount of feces inappropriately such that it soils the child's clothing or bedding. This situation usually will be associated with some circumstances such as not having access to toilet facilities.	Infancy Not relevant at this age. Early childhood Toilet training for bowel movements usually begins around 2 years of age but wide variation up to 4 years of age can occur. The child passes stool in places other than in the toilet. Middle childhood Occasional accidents can occur when children are preoccupied with other activities and do not have immediate access to toilet facilities. Adolescence Accidents in soiling are not likely to happen in normal situations unless there is a gastrointestinal illness such as diarrhea.
Problem: V40.3 Soiling Problem This symptom is a problem if it increases in frequency or causes disruption in parent–child or peer interactions but is not sufficiently intense to qualify for the diagnosis of encopresis.	Infancy Not relevant at this age. Early childhood The child frequently has constipation, with or without soiling, and begins to fear or is preoccupied with toileting. Middle childhood The child frequently has constipation, with or without soiling, and begins to fear or is preoccupied with toileting, has irregular stools, and has accidents; parents are concerned. Adolescence The adolescent frequently has constipation, with or without soiling, and begins to fear or be preoccupied with toileting.

Table 3-1

Example of DSM-IV-PC Format (*continued*)

DEVELOPMENTAL VARIATION	COMMON DEVELOPMENTAL PRESENTATIONS
Disorder: 307.7 Encopresis Without Constipation and Overflow Incontinence; 787.6 Encopresis With Constipation and Overflow Incontinence Repeated passage of feces into inappropriate places (e.g., clothing or floor) whether involuntary or intentional. At least one such event a month for at least 3 months. Chronological age is at least 4 years (or equivalent developmental level). Only diagnose encopresis when the behavior is not due exclusively to the direct physiologic effects of a substance (e.g., laxatives) or a general medical condition except through a mechanism involving constipation.	Infancy Not relevant at this age. Early childhood The child experiences soiling, with or without constipation. Middle childhood The child experiences constipation and soiling, avoiding potential situations that may lead to embarrassment. The child may deny having accidents. Adolescence The adolescent experiences constipation and soiling and may be more subtle in how symptoms are hidden.

at home, and with peers. The level of impairment will depend on the extent of dysfunction of these areas. Key questions developed by Wender include

1. Are the behaviors more intense, and do they occur more frequently than in other children of the same age?
2. Do the behaviors change in different settings and with different kinds of activities?
3. Are the behaviors getting worse or better?
4. Do the behaviors occur in many different settings?
5. Are there several people who notice the characteristic behaviors?

Behaviors that occur in only one setting and with only a few of the adults with whom the child interacts are more likely to represent a child's unique reaction to a specific environment or context—a developmental variation or problem, rather than an intrinsic, chronic disorder. In contrast, longer duration of symptoms more likely indicates a disorder.

JOHNNY (CONTINUED) *In discussion with the family, you find that Johnny's behaviors stand out as more intense and frequent than same-age peers at school and at home. They are consistently present; although he does well in one-on-one situations, he does very poorly in situations with many people or high stimuli, such as restaurants and malls. His parents feel the behaviors are worsening over time, rather than improving as he matures (as they had hoped). Johnny's parents tell you that many adults, including other family members, babysitters, and neighbors, have commented on his high activity level, even before he entered kindergarten. Based on this information, you decide that Johnny has a significant level of functional impairment, consistent with a disorder. The disorder you identify is Attention Deficit Hyperactivity Disorder, combined subtype.*

In summary, to perform an initial evaluation of behavioral complaints in children, primary care clinicians should listen carefully to families and refer to the DSM-IV-PC to determine the type of behavior problem and the extent of the problem (variation, problem, or disorder). Decisions about proceeding with further evaluation versus referring to mental health professionals can be guided by DSM-IV-PC definitions and will also be determined by the clinician's own level of comfort and expertise with behavioral problems. If the behaviors are categorized as variations or problems, the clinician may want to proceed with further office-based management and follow-up. For conditions that represent a disorder, the primary care clinician may be more likely to refer or consult with mental health professionals, although many children with ADHD can be managed in the primary care setting.

Comprehensive Approach

The following guidelines are for those who would strive to become more skilled in performing office-based behavioral assessments of children and families. The essential elements of an "in-depth" approach are described below (and summarized in Table 3-2). In this approach, we will continue to focus on the evaluation of children with disruptive behavioral symptoms.

Steps 1 Through 4: Information Gathering

Step 1: Office Preparation

Office preparation in anticipation of behavior problems is an important first step. A growing number of clinicians practice with on-site behavioral health trained professionals, such as social

Table 3-2

Essential Elements of "In-Depth" Primary Care Approach to Child Behavior Problems

Information gathering	**Synthesis of information and feedback**
1. Office preparation Onsite availability of behavioral health support personnel, such as clinical social workers or psychologists Use routine screening instruments Establish collaborative mechanisms in the community with schools and mental health professionals Learn about mental health benefits and management strategies by local insurers Know local parent support groups, classes, and therapists	5. Categorize type of behavior problem Refer to DSM-IV-PC Use Appendix A for initial symptoms Find behavior or cluster chapters Determine level of problem: variation, problem, or disorder
2. Interview with family Elaborate on the principal symptoms Assess resources available Understand the family perspective on the problems	6. Consider etiologic factors
3. Assess child's developmental/learning status and current behavior Review developmental milestones/past concerns Review early intervention, preschool, or school information Consider office-based screening or assessment Obtain further psychological assessment if needed	7. Determine comorbidity
4. Medical considerations Review past medical history and family history Physical examination Screening tests for head, hearing, and vision	8. Feedback with families

Table 3-3

Sample of Resource List for Referrals/Community Coordination

	Phone #	Expertise/Contact
A. Mental health providers		
1. Local community mental health agency	______	______
2. Private practice		
Psychiatrist	______	______
Psychologist	______	______
Social worker	______	______
3. Other types of mental health programs		
Catholic Charities	______	______
B. Schools		
Early intervention programs		
0 to 3	______	______
3 to 5	______	______
School-aged special education department	______	______
C. Other community resources		
WIC program	______	______
Head Start	______	______
Parent to Parent	______	______

Note: All these are listed in the telephone book.

workers, psychologists, or early childhood or developmental specialists. For visits scheduled because of behavioral complaints, joint evaluations by primary care clinicians and these other professionals may be especially effective.

Many practices routinely use instruments to screen for psychosocial problems. These instruments can be mailed to families prior to appointments or completed after registration at the office. Some take as little as 2 to 3 min to complete and may be more sensitive to parental concerns than clinicians' interviews. Ninety-seven percent of families in a national study by Jellinek, Murphy, and Burns were able to complete such instruments in the office setting with little or no assistance.

An essential element of the assessment and management of child behavior problems is close contact with educational and specialty mental health professionals. Components of coordinated services that can be arranged proactively include establishing referral patterns, determining the level of expertise and interest in children's health issues, identifying expected feedback mechanisms, and reviewing the adequacy of referral mechanisms. A sample list of types of useful resources is included in Table 3-3.

Equally important, primary care clinicians should be aware of mental health insurance benefits available to patients in their communities. Many insurance companies require either assessment or referrals to be conducted through preferred mental health networks. Office staff and primary care clinicians should know these processes ahead of time to ease the coordination of services for families dealing with child behavior problems. Last, knowledge of local parent support groups and parenting classes will be particularly useful for many families. Such information often can be posted in waiting rooms.

In addition to the above issues, it is important for office staff to use a candid but nonstigmatizing approach to discuss behavior problems and mental disorders. This approach is especially important because staff discomfort with a topic may cause parents to not disclose symptoms or adhere to treatment plans for their child's psychosocial problems. Office preparation is further described in *Bright Futures in Practice: Mental Health Promotion*.

Step 2: History Taking

History taking or an interview with the child's parents or caregivers is the next important step. The three components of the interview include (1) elaboration of the principal symptoms, (2) understanding the families' perspective on the problem, and (3) assessment of resources available to the child and family.

ELABORATION OF THE PRINCIPAL SYMPTOMS Techniques for this process have been previously discussed in the Fundamental Approach section. Disruptive behavior disorder symptoms generally fall into the broad categories of overactivity, impulsivity, aggression, defiance, and inattention. Once the key symptoms are determined, refer to DSM-IV-PC to determine diagnostic categories. Many clinicians use a simple checklist of the DSM-IV or DSM-IV-PC criteria for ADHD, oppositional-defiant disorder, or conduct disorder, and check off which ones fit. Parents can participate in completion of checklists.

Clinicians can use additional structured instruments to further elaborate many of the behavioral symptoms identified as parental, school, or community concerns, or to further evaluate symptoms identified through screening. These structured instruments are different than screening instruments in that their purpose is to help the clinician refine diagnoses, consider comorbidity, and define a management plan. The most commonly used structured instruments are behavioral checklists. They may be condition specific (e.g., Conners Parent and Teacher Rating Scales) or broad symptom lists (e.g., Child Behavior Checklist) (Table 3-4). Because such instruments involve scoring, they are usually best done with computerized scoring pro-

Table 3-4

Instruments for Use in Office Evaluation

1. Routine screening instruments
   - A. For psychosocial problems
     1. Pediatric Symptoms Checklist (Jellinek et al, 1988)
     2. Eyberg Child Behavior Inventory (Eyberg, 1980)
   - B. For developmental problems
     1. Child Development Inventories (Ireton, 1992)
     2. Parents' Evaluation of Developmental Status (Glascoe, 1997)
2. In-depth assessment questionnaires/checklists
   - A. General psychological (behavioral) symptoms
     1. Child Behavior Checklist (CBCL) (Achenbach, 1988)
     2. Teacher Report Form (TRF) (Achenbach, 1980)
     3. Youth Self-Report (Achenbach, 1988)
   - B. Specific for disruptive behaviors
     1. Conner's Parent Rating Scale—Revised (Multi-Health Systems)
        Conner's Teacher Rating Scale—Revised
        Conner's Abbreviated Parent–Teacher Questionnaire
     2. ADHD Rating Scale for Parents and Teachers (DuPaul)
     3. Disruptive Behavior Rating Scale (Barkley and Murphy, 1998)
   - C. Specific for comorbidity
     1. Child Depression Inventory (Kovacs, 1982)
     2. Revised Children's Manifest Anxiety Scale (Reynolds and Richmond, 1985)

grams. Structured interviews for mental disorders designed to be administered by the primary care clinician have been developed for adults (e.g., PRIME-MD), and are undergoing testing for use with adolescents. Further work is needed on these instruments before they can be used with children in primary care settings.

JOHNNY (CONTINUED) *In Johnny's case, you choose two questionnaires to augment the evaluation: the Child Behavior Checklist (CBCL) and the Conners Scales. There are parent and teacher versions for each of these instruments, and it is important to have both sets completed. Computerized scoring is available for the CBCL. The Conners Scales are formatted for easy hand scoring.*

UNDERSTAND THE FAMILY'S PERSPECTIVE It is important to ascertain the family's perspective in more detail. What does the behavior problem mean to the family, why do they think it is occurring, and who is most affected by it? Essential background family information is included in Table 3-5. If you have been providing ongoing care, this information about the family ideally will have been obtained previously and will need only to be updated.

Ask what, if anything, has changed recently in the family that may be a precipitating factor for the child's behavior. Make sure to find out who, outside the members of the household, is involved in the care of the child and will, therefore, have important opinions about the behavior problem. While doing this observe how family members discuss the child. Many families are naturally upset about their child's behavior, but some may also be very angry. It may be important to remove the child from the interview if this is the case. Additionally, family members may disagree about the nature of the behavior problem, and its origin, severity, and treatment. It is important to determine the degree of disagreement and the level of stress in the family.

ASSESSMENT OF AVAILABLE RESOURCES An assessment of family and community resources also provides important insight for the development of a treatment plan. Families may have extended supports, relations, or friends who can assist in either the evaluation or management of a child. Ask to whom the families turn for help or advice,

Table 3-5

What to Include in a Family Assessment

1. Family composition
   - Who lives in the home and how are they related to the child?
   - Is the child adopted?
   - Has the child been in foster care? Is there a caseworker? Foster parent?
   - Mother's name, age, education, occupation
   - Father's name, age, education, occupation
   - If child lives in more than one household, what is his schedule?
2. Family medical history, including mental health history
3. Family supports
   - Primary caregivers (who helps the parents with…?)
   - Extended family relationships
   - Family roles and interactions:
     - How do adults get along?
     - How do siblings and others in the family get along? Any violence?
   - Community activities and supports
   - Religious affiliation and role of religion in family
   - Extended social relationships
4. Coping and problem solving issues
   - Daily routine
   - What does family do for fun? How often?
   - Stressful activities and times
   - Ways family deals with stress
5. Family pressures
   - Marriages, divorces, separations
   - Deaths or illness
   - Births, other additions to the household
   - Financial problems or worries
   - Concern about neighborhood safety
   - Use of alcohol or drugs
6. Parenting style
   - Who disciplines children and how?
   - Agreement on discipline methods
   - Consistency of discipline

SOURCE: Adapted from National Center for Family-Centered Care, Association for the Care of Children's Health: *Physician Education Forum Report*. Bethesda, MD, 1990.

who they call in an emergency, and what community groups or agencies they belong to and the extent of their involvement in such groups. The clinician will become aware of how much families adapt and cope by using outside supports. Those families who lack supports may require more intensive service from professionals.

JOHNNY (CONTINUED) *Johnny's parents are "happily married" and agree about how they interpret Johnny's behaviors and respond to him. Both parents receive support from their families, friends, and neighbors. They also attend a community church. The family has obtained information from the Internet about ADHD, and they think this may be Johnny's condition. Overall, the level of agreement in this family is high, and the level of stress is low.*

Step 3: Assess the Child's Development/Learning Status

An assessment of the child's developmental/learning status and current behavior (the "mental status" exam of the child) is next. A child with significant cognitive deficits, learning disability, or another developmental disorder, such as a pervasive developmental disorder (PDD)/autism, may also have comorbid disruptive behavior symptoms.

For the developmental assessment, refer to past notes regarding any developmental delays and review all assessments of the child from early intervention programs or schools. These programs usually provide a report containing descriptive information as well as developmental or IQ test scores, which are norm referenced and yield age equivalents. If no prior information is available, you may perform your own developmental screening, especially if the parents are concerned that the child's academic function is poor. Screening instruments available for primary care use are listed in Table 3-3. However, in most cases it will be important to obtain definitive diagnostic information about cognitive skills from a licensed school psychologist or a psychologist practicing in another setting such as a hospital, mental health facility, or private practice.

The type of behavioral or mental status assessment performed in the primary care setting depends on the child's age and willingness to participate and the individual clinician's training, comfort level, time, and personnel constraints. This is perhaps the most impractical and difficult part of an assessment for a primary care provider. However, much information can be gained from a few simple exercises. The first exercise is observation of the child. Does the child look his or her age? Is the child neatly dressed? Is there eye contact? How distressed does the child seem? What is the child's mood? Often clinicians have devised their own ways of establishing rapport with children of various ages. Do the usual methods of establishing rapport work with this child? Next, an assessment of the child's language and conversational skills is helpful. Ask the younger child to state his or her age, identify members of the family, describe pets, and list favorite play activities. It is important to ask the child about his or her understanding of the behavioral problems, although children may have difficulty talking about this at the initial assessment visit. Another technique is to make drawings with the child as a way of initiating conversation.

Adolescents should be reassured that their conversations with you will remain confidential, unless they reveal information about behaviors that may be dangerous to themselves or others. In addition to confidential discussion, older school-age children and adolescents can complete self-administered questionnaires about their psychological symptoms, such as the Youth Self Report or the Child Depression Inventory (see Table 3-4). Finally, adolescents should be active participants in their evaluation; they should decide together with their primary care clinician what information will be shared with their parents. Once an understanding of behavioral symptoms is present, an assessment of the child's resources and strengths is useful. These include internal skills and competencies of the child, family resources, and community support. Many children may have poor behavioral control but strong skills in other areas. Such skills can be used to develop a treatment plan that includes rewards and to provide some areas for positive reinforcement.

JOHNNY (CONTINUED) *Your concern about Johnny's development is triggered by the information that he seems uninterested in learning. Your past chart notes indicate that his motor development was normal, but acquisition of language was somewhat slower, with only a few words at age 2. Hearing was normal. By age 3, he was speaking in sentences but difficult to understand. His parents often mentioned difficulty getting him to eat, sleep, and follow directions. He also has had temper tantrums, which were hard for his parents to control. He did go to a preschool 2 half days per week before kindergarten, but you have no information about his performance there. Johnny's parents recall that he had "testing" at the preschool last year, and they were told that he would need further speech and language help, but the school wanted to wait.*

You converse and play with Johnny for 5 to 10 min. He is active and impulsive, talks little, preferring to play with blocks, laughs with you, makes good eye contact, and has a normal range of affect, but is unable to talk about why he was brought to the doctor. You continue to suspect that Johnny has significant language difficulties that need further evaluation.

STEP 4: REVIEW HISTORY

A review of past medical history, family history, and a physical exam of the child should be performed. Medical problems that may present with ADHD-like behaviors but are *not* ADHD include hearing loss or visual impairment, petit mal seizures, lead toxicity, and, rarely, hyperthyroidism or insensitivity to thyroid hormone. Another category of medical conditions to consider are those that coexist with ADHD or other disruptive behaviors. These include genetic or teratogenic disorders such as Williams syndrome, fragile X syndrome, fetal alcohol syndrome, and the uncommon but important Tourette's syndrome. Additionally, some medications, such as anticonvulsants, antihistamines, decongestants, steroids, and beta agonists can create behavioral changes in children that may resemble hyperactivity, although these medications more commonly cause simple agitation. Family history may also reveal other individuals with behavioral or learning problems. It is important to check the child's hearing and vision and make sure serum lead levels are screened in children under 5 years of age. The physical exam is usually normal or may show neurologic "soft signs"—motor coordination difficulties such as problems with finger tapping or balance.

JOHNNY (CONTINUED) *You review Johnny's past history. He was a term infant, born after an uncomplicated pregnancy to a gravida 1 mother, aged 31. He has had a few colds and ear infections and one laceration of the forehead from running into a coffee table corner. He also had a dog bite, which did not require suturing. Current medical issues include picky eater, difficulty getting him to fall asleep independently, and nighttime enuresis.*

You ask about the family history and discover that Johnny's father required special education classes for "speech" problems and never enjoyed school. However, he graduated from high school and now works as a machine operator. Mother is a full-time homemaker, and Johnny has a 2-year-old sister.

During the physical exam, Johnny engages in frantically pumping the blood pressure cuff and watching the mercury rise. Attempts to wrest this from him are met with clenched fists and a grin. He wants to comply and is friendly, but has difficulty attending to your requests during the exam, and he hops off the table several times. His mother assists you in placing him back on the table and uses "1, 2, 3" warnings to help the child refocus. He has particular difficulty tracking the ophthalmoscope light and with performance of rapid finger movements and balancing activities. His physical exam is otherwise entirely normal.

Steps 5 Through 8: Synthesizing the Information and Providing Feedback

Steps 1 through 4 outline the process of information gathering necessary for a comprehensive evaluation. After obtaining all of the information listed above, the primary provider should be able to focus on the next steps in the evaluation, which involve synthesizing the information gathered and providing feedback to the patient and family.

Step 5: Categorize the Behavioral Difficulty

Categorize the type of behavioral difficulty and have some idea of the degree of severity or dysfunction associated with it. The majority of children with disruptive behaviors will be able to be categorized within the Hyperactive/Impulsive Behaviors Section of DSM-IV-PC (detailed steps on use of DSM-IV-PC are outlined earlier). If the child's presentation is severe enough to cause major functional impairment at home and school, the child meets diagnostic criteria for ADHD, Hyperactive/Impulsive Subtype or Combined Subtype. For example, disruptive behaviors that include hyperactivity, impulsivity, and inattention, have been present for more than 6 months, occur before the age of 6, and cause dysfunction for the child at home and school are quite likely to meet criteria for ADHD. The purely inattentive subtype of ADHD will not present as disruptive behaviors; rather, it will be manifested as difficulty paying attention and completing tasks. The clinician may consult DSM-IV for further information.

Step 6: Consider the Role of Medical Problems or Medications

Consider medical problems or medications as possible etiologic agents in the presentation. Clues will be contained in the history and physical exam. For the vast majority of cases of disruptive behavior disorder, these issues will not be significant.

Step 7: Consider Developmental or Psychiatric Comorbidity

Comorbidity is most often the rule with ADHD. Developmental problems or learning disability are the most common types. Clues to comorbidity include any type of developmental delay or academic difficulty, as well as family history of such problems. Confirmation comes from psychological testing. Children with ADHD also have a high likelihood of having negative emotional behaviors, such as aggressive or oppositional behaviors, which are also described in the DSM-IV-PC and DSM-IV. Biederman and colleagues estimate that between 40 and 50 percent of children with ADHD also have Oppositional-Defiant Disorder. Less common, but more severe, are children who present with secretive antisocial behaviors such as lying, cheating, stealing, or fire setting, which fall into the diagnostic category of Conduct Disorder.

After considering Oppositional-Defiant Disorder and Conduct Disorder, the most common psychiatric comorbidities are anxiety and depression. Tic disorders (including Tourette's syndrome), Obsessive-Compulsive Disorder, and Post-Traumatic Stress Disorder are also possibilities, but less common. Anxiety symptoms include excessive fearfulness or worry. Depressive symptoms include depressed mood, anhedonia (not wanting to play or enjoy others), and self-injurious or suicidal behaviors or gestures. For both depression and anxiety, it may be difficult to determine if the child has enough symptoms to warrant diagnosis of a true depressive or anxiety disorder. Referring to results of screening questionnaires and criteria listed in DSM-IV-PC may be very helpful. Consultation with mental health professionals is often helpful for these cases.

Step 8: Provide Feedback and Share Information

The last step in the evaluation process is providing feedback and sharing information with families. This step is important for several reasons. After taking the time and effort to perform a rigorous evaluation, it is equally important to ensure the effectiveness of the evaluation by providing accurate, clear information to the family. The family will then be empowered to reflect upon your conclusions and to decide on and prepare for a plan of treatment.

There are two main goals one should strive for in dealing with the family: The family must understand your evaluation process and your conclusions to trust what you say and advise. The family also must understand the diagnoses given if they are to accept treatment plans. In turn, it is also important for the clinician to gain feedback from the family. Some guidelines in achieving these goals are listed below.

1. All important family members should be present. Decide, as a group, how to involve the child/adolescent in the feedback session (whether to include him or her or give separate feedback).
2. Provide feedback in a comfortable setting, with everyone seated, few distractions, and adequate time allowed for information exchange.
3. Ask the family if they feel the information gathered in the evaluation process was accurate and unbiased. This is important to establish the validity of the evaluation. If they are unhappy at this point, they will likely not accept your conclusions.
4. Explain the evaluation process and how you arrived at your conclusions.
5. State any diagnoses clearly and explain them. The family will be particularly interested in the cause of these conditions and whether anyone is at fault or to blame.
6. Describe a treatment plan and provide, if possible, a written summary of the plan at the same time. Also provide written information to families on the diagnoses and how to access further information and support.
7. Allow enough time for questions from the family.
8. Schedule a follow-up visit.

Time Management of Evaluation

A comprehensive evaluation such as this cannot be performed within the time allotted for standard primary care office visits. Fortunately, there can be wide variability in exactly how one chooses to obtain all the information. One practical approach would be to obtain the history (step 1) and send the family home to complete behavioral/developmental questionnaires. During a follow-up visit, perform the assessment of the child, including a physical exam. Further time will be required to review the medical and family history and the questionnaire information. A variety of personnel can assist in information gathering and assessments, including behavioral health support staff. Let's look at how this approach could be applied to Johnny.

JOHNNY (CONTINUED) *Johnny presents for an acute concern visit because of suspension from kindergarten. During this visit, you obtain the initial information about the problem behaviors, which include hyperactivity at home and school, inattention at school, and aggression at school. Your physical exam is normal, as are the hearing, vision, and lead screening test results.*

You ask Johnny's parents to complete further questionnaire information. You choose the CBCL and the Conners Scales to be completed by parents and teachers. You obtain consent to speak with school personnel.

A return visit is planned. You may team up with a behavioral health professional for this visit. In between visits, this professional is able to discuss Johnny's behavior with his teacher, who describes hyperactivity, inattention, and impulsivity at school. You have already reviewed the history and are concerned about a possible speech and language problem.

At the return visit, Johnny's parents bring in a screening evaluation from his preschool program, indicating age-appropriate developmental levels except in language, in which he is 6 months behind chronological age. Parents have completed forms, and your behavioral health consultant has scored them. The CBCL scores are elevated ("abnormal") for behavioral categories indicative of attention and hyperactivity problems. The Conners Scale also shows elevated scores in the categories indicative of hyperactivity and ADHD. Your behavioral health consultant conducts a play session with Johnny and confirms your suspicion about language delays. His performance on a screening test of pre-academic skills is otherwise normal.

Scores on the CBCL are high for the attention, aggression, and delinquent subscales and greater than 2 standard deviations above the mean for Hyperactivity on the Conners Scale, both for teacher and parent ratings. This supports a diagnosis of ADHD, combined subtype. You review DSM-PC criteria with the parents and make the diagnosis. You give the parents information to read.

Another problem is the language delay, for which Johnny needs speech/language therapy in school. Such language difficulties may presage a later diagnosis of learning disability. You advise the parents to have an evaluation performed at school to obtain special education services.

On a third visit, you review the data with the family. They agree that the symptoms are consistent with a diagnosis of ADHD. Additionally, you discuss behavior management resources available in the community for Johnny's parents and how to access them. Finally, you discuss the possibility of treatment with medication and give them information about stimulants. The family is generally pleased with the information and agrees to follow-up.

This vignette represents a typical presentation for a child with mild to moderate ADHD and possible learning disability. The family is intact and functioning well to support him. It is typical in approximately 50 percent of clinical cases to have a family history of ADHD, although not often formally diagnosed. Research studies by Biederman and associates document that between 10 and 35 percent of immediate family members are likely to have the disorder.

The clinician may be able to see some ADHD symptoms even in the office, but this is not always the case. Many children appear to have well-controlled behavior at the doctor's office.

A child with more severe ADHD often presents earlier, having trouble in the preschool setting and having more significant behavior problems at home. Examples of such behavioral problems are likely to include severe tantrums, oppositional-defiant behaviors (such as always saying "no" to everything well into their school-age years) and irritability. The most severely affected children may show significant aggression, with injury to others or self, fire setting, animal abuse, and carrying weapons such as knives (comorbid conduct disorder).

JULIE (CONTINUED) *At your first visit with Julie and her grandmother, you recognize that the specific problem behaviors include high activity level, oppositional/negative symptoms, crying, few friends, and stealing money. These behaviors have been present for both Julie and her sister since they came to live with their grandmother 3 years ago. These behaviors also occur at school, accompanied by learning problems. At the first visit, you explain to grandmother that methylphenidate and/or clonidine are both appropriate medications for these symptoms, but you would be happy to go over Julie's case in more detail with her. You ask her to sign a release of information for the school and the mental health agency. You request she complete the CBCL and the Conners Scale and have the schoolteacher do the same.*

A second visit is scheduled for several weeks later to give you time to obtain and review the child's records. School information indicates that Julie has been categorized as having a learning disability. In addition, the report contains descriptions of aggression and oppositional behaviors occurring at school, such as talking back to the teacher and starting fights at recess. Teacher CBCL checklist scores are high for both the externalizing scales and depression/anxiety. Teacher Conners scores are high on all subscales, including oppositional, cognitive problems, and hyperactivity. This indicates that, despite medications, Julie continues to have significant behavioral difficulties at school.

Records from the mental health center are brief, but outline the same types of behavioral difficulties as indicated by the grandmother and school. The mental health center diagnosed Julie with ADHD, Combined Subtype, learning disability, oppositional-defiant disorder, and rule outs for post-traumatic stress disorder (PTSD), depression, and bipolar disorder. The mental health center evaluation occurred 10 months ago, and medication and individual therapy were prescribed. After 6 months without much improvement, home-based school services were initiated.

These assessments indicate a diagnosis of ADHD, as well as indicating significant comorbidities such as learning disability and, possibly, depression, bipolar disorder, or PTSD. After reviewing these possibilities, it is clear that this case is complex and needs management by mental health professionals. But something has gone wrong with that system of care from the grandmother's perspective. You decide to explore with Julie's grandmother more about why she is feeling so frustrated with the treatments Julie is receiving. On the second visit, you ask Julie's grandmother to tell the story of how Julie came to be in her care and why Julie and her treatments have been so difficult. Grandmother, who was angry on the first visit, begins to cry as she tells how Julie and her siblings were neglected by their parents. Grandmother said she felt she had no choice but to take them in, but had hoped it would only be temporary. Julie's parents, however, have left the country and are not to be found. Grandmother has found herself feeling increasingly overwhelmed. She says that when Julie's father, her son, was young, his behavior was just like this, and she also took him to psychiatrists and therapists but nothing helped him. She is afraid the same thing will happen to Julie.

At the conclusion of her remarks, you ask her to talk a bit about what she likes in Julie and what activities they share that are fun. She says that Julie can be a very caring child who especially likes helping grandmother take care of her 7-month-old cousin.

After thanking grandmother for explaining the situation to you, you give helpful feedback that is supportive of her struggles. You empathize with her that trusting mental health professionals can be hard, but you are hopeful that this time things can work better for the family. You ask permission to discuss this case with the mental health professions involved in Julie's care. Ideally, a meeting could occur with them, you, and the family, with the goal being the facilitation of care back into the mental health system.

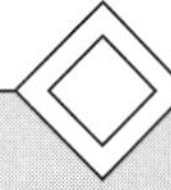

Management

Decisions about management will depend on the diagnosis of the child, the severity of the problem, the family context, the provider's level of comfort in dealing with the problem, and the availability/necessity of consultants from other disciplines and community resources. For example, a child with uncomplicated, mild ADHD can probably be managed entirely in a primary care practice unless the ability of the family to carry out your suggestions or feel supported is limited or jeopardized. For complex cases such as Julie's, management will be challenging and quite likely frustrated by the family's inability to understand how to respond to the child and support personnel. A patient like Julie is best followed within a system capable of long-term family and behavior management support, most likely involving mental health providers.

This section of the chapter will focus on management of ADHD, because the majority of children presenting with disruptive behaviors will have ADHD as a primary diagnosis, and many of these children can be treated in a primary care setting.

General Principles of Management

A multimodal approach is recommended, which includes the application of "environmental accommodations" both at home and at school, and the use of pharmacotherapy. Baumgaertel uses the analogy of treating a chronic condition such as diabetes, where medication (insulin) is necessary, but must be accompanied by behavioral modification (changes in diet and exercise) to improve outcome. Although there are limited data to show that multimodal management is better than pharmacologic treatment alone, behavioral management at home and school is necessary for children with disruptive behavior disorders because medications are not always "on board" and do not control all of the symptoms. In particular, negativity symptoms, whether oppositional or aggressive, are poorly managed with medications alone.

Environmental Accommodations

Environmental accommodations or non-pharmacologic approaches must occur at both home and school, and should ideally be coordinated so that approaches used are congruent.

Home

Home accommodations include all approaches that address those behavioral problems that most affect child-family functioning outside the school. The most important approaches involve educating parents about ADHD and how to manage it, followed by putting such knowledge into practice. Families can learn from reading books, watching videos, participating in parent support meetings, or some form of counseling. A more intense involvement with structured behavior management therapy will be useful for many families. Parents are often focused on fixing the child, however, and may have difficulty understanding that they must do significant work as well.

Child-oriented approaches alone have little proven benefit. Social skills training for children with ADHD has intuitive benefit, but no studies have documented its efficacy. Individual play therapy and psychotherapy have not been shown to improve outcomes for children with ADHD. Newer treatments such as biofeedback may be beneficial but have not undergone randomized clinical trials. The primary care clinician plays an important role in educating families about which type of "therapy" will work, helping them acknowledge the need for treatment, and accessing such treatment.

School

Because virtually all children with ADHD manifest some form of difficulty at school, modifications in the school environment are usually important. Working cooperatively with schools to optimize the child' s academic achievements and social adjustment should be the goal. For the primary care provider, effective communication with school personnel about individual cases is important. Additionally, consider expanding your role to become a school consultant or resource for behavioral health care information for the school. This puts you in a position of alliance with school personnel, who often feel distanced from health care providers.

The clinician's role should be supportive to the parents in their efforts to advocate for their child. However, the clinician may also provide specific advice about the type of services needed, such as providing written prescriptions for speech or occupational therapies or assisting parents in writing a letter to request special education services. For further information regarding schools and special education services see Martin Baren's article "Managing ADHD."[1] In addition to discussion of the stimulants, other issues relating to management of the ADHD and coexisting conditions should be discussed at regular follow-up visits. These are listed in Table 3-6.

Pharmacotherapy

The mainstay of pharmacologic treatment for ADHD has been the stimulants, including methylphenidate, dextroamphetamine, and pemoline. Secondary choices include tricyclic antidepressants, atypical antidepressants, and alpha adrenergic agonists.

Stimulants

Stimulants are the first-line medications for ADHD. They have been used for over 25 years, and over 100 studies have proven their efficacy in reducing the symptoms of inattention hyperactivity, and impulsivity. Hinshaw and colleagues found that for some children stimulants also seem partially beneficial for oppositional-defiant disorder or conduct disorder symptoms. The NIMH Collaborative Multisite, Multimodal Treatment Study of Children with ADHD (sponsored by the U.S. Depart-

[1]Baren M: Managing ADHD. *Contemporary Pediatrics* 11:29, 1994.

Table 3-6

Key Elements of ADHD Follow-Up and Monitoring

A. Medication related
- Monitor for continued efficacy of current dose
- Review current side effects and how they are handled
- Discuss 4 PM/weekend/holiday/summertime dosing

B. General issues
- Discuss behavior and academic performance at school; review of school information
- Discuss behavior and family function at home, including progress in learning about the disorder, applying behavior management strategies, child's insight into the problem, and sibling adjustments
- Decide what medication to use on weekends/holidays/summertime
- Discuss social skills issues and ways families can foster them
- Review household habits, such as chores, TV viewing and safety, presence of guns in household
- Consider comorbidity: is child becoming anxious or depressed?
- Consider new issues as children enter adolescence:
  - Decreasing symptoms with eventual tapering of medication
  - Increasing symptoms of conduct problems—substance abuse
  - Increasing symptoms of depression, academic failure, etc.

ment of Education) was undertaken with the goal of examining the long-term effectiveness of randomly assigned treatments for ADHD. The study provides the most definitive data regarding treatment recommendations, based on a large population of patients. The following guidelines incorporate some of the recommendations from the study, adapting them for clinical practice.

INDICATIONS/CONTRAINDICATIONS Any child with a diagnosis of ADHD is eligible for a stimulant trial with few exceptions. For children with severe Tourette's symptoms, stimulants are not recommended; they may worsen symptoms. Additionally, some families are too disorganized to dose medication appropriately or may have family members who might abuse the medication. When families are in disagreement about the use of medications, the trial often will fail. This is particularly true when initiating medication for an adolescent who is unwilling.

Finally, there is controversy regarding the minimum age at which a child can be placed on these medications. Children with ADHD usually have symptoms beginning in early childhood, so many will present as early as age 3 for treatment. The use of stimulants for preschool children remains controversial, and a consultation from a behavioral/developmental pediatrician or child psychiatrist is recommended when children under age 4 are considered for medication.

INITIATION OF TREATMENT The three stimulant medications currently available are methylphenidate, dextroamphetamine, and pemoline. Methylphenidate and dexedrine have both short- and long-acting or slow-release forms. Short-acting methylphenidate has peak behavioral effects within 1 to 2 h and wears off in 3 to 5 h. The slow-release form has a half-life of 4 to 6 h, with peak effects beginning within approximately 2 h and lasting 6 to 8 h. Short-acting dextroamphetamine peaks within 1 to 2 h but may last 4 to 6 h. The slow-release dexedrine spansules last between 6 and 10 h. The advantage of slow-release forms are a smoother effect, no need for mid-day dosing at school, and longer coverage. The disadvantages include generally lower efficacy and longer time to become active in the morning, often requiring a short-acting tablet after breakfast to supplement.

Typical treatment recommendations are to begin with the short-acting form of methylphenidate and use the caveat "start low and go slow." The starting dose should approximate 0.3 mg/kg, and increases in each dose should be in 2.5 to 5 mg increments. The maximum effective dose for methylphenidate is usually 0.6 to 1.0 mg/kg. Dosages above that level produce side effects without added benefit. The maximum daily dosage recommended by the *Physician's Desk Reference* is 60 mg/day, although some adults take 70 to 80 mg/day. An algorithm is included in Figure 3-1.

Carefully explain all possible side effects to families and let them know that evaluating the trial is a matter of balancing positive effects against side effects (Table 3-7). Families, along with school personnel, are the most important part of the trial and must be carefully informed. Both families and teachers should provide subjective or descriptive reporting to the clinician about the effects of the medication. Additionally, have them use objective rating forms, such as the Conner's rating scale, to determine the effect of treatment. If they see predominately positive effects with few side effects, continue the starting dose and discuss adding a third daily dose, weekend use, and drug holidays. If families report positive effects but the effects wear off quickly or

Figure 3-1

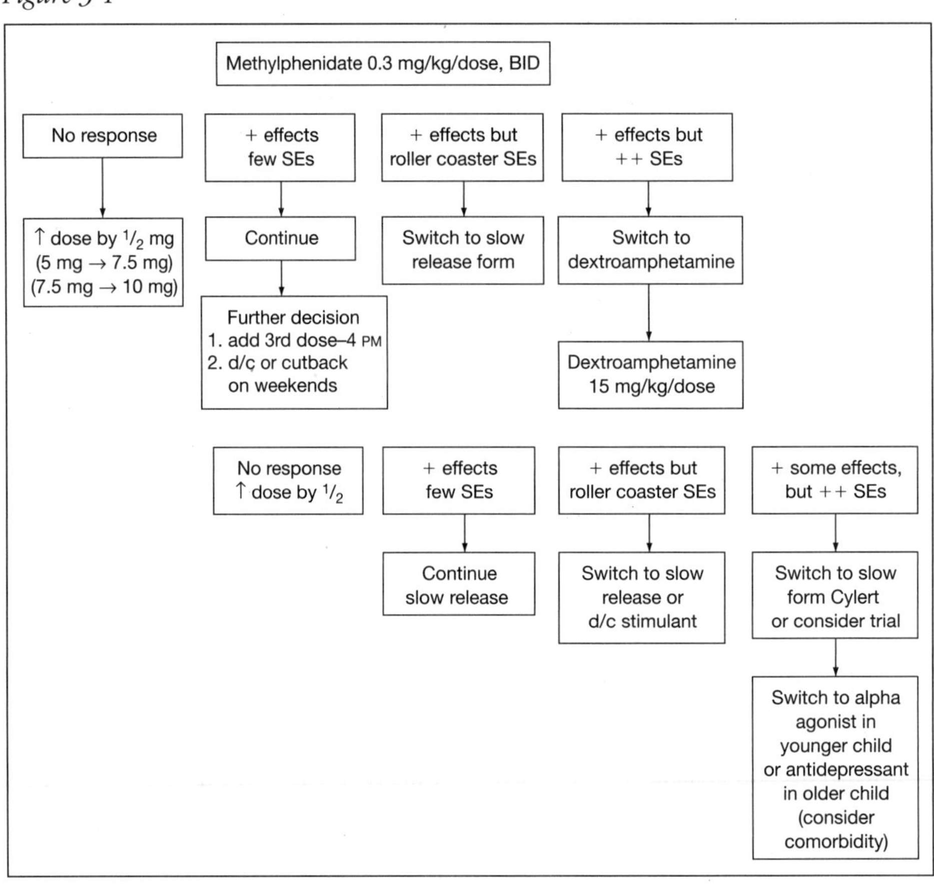

Medication algorithm for ADHD.

Table 3-7
Side Effects of Stimulants

Side Effect	Action
1. GI upset/discomfort	1. Take medication *after* a snack or a meal.
2. Appetite suppression	2. Increase meals/snacks at times when medications are not on board (i.e., evenings, nights, weekends). Monitor weight gain every 3 months.
3. Irritability	3. Ascertain relationship of irritability to medication dosing: for wear-off irritability, change from short-acting to slow-release forms; for continuous irritability, change stimulant type and consider comorbid anxiety or depression.
4. Difficulty falling asleep	4. Carefully compare pre- and postmedication changes in sleep patterns. If worsening, discontinue or decrease afternoon dosing. Use behavior management or relaxation techniques as adjuncts.
5. Lightheadedness, dizziness, spaciness	5. May indicate too high dose. Decrease dose of short-acting or change to slow-release forms.
6. Tics	6. Monitor frequency and severity of tics. If increasing, may change to second stimulant, slow release, or discontinue.
7. Increased hyperactivity	7. If occurring immediately after medication is given, consider decreasing dose or discontinuing. If occurring after medication wears off in the evening, consider slow-release forms.

NOTE: Side effects are often worse for the first few weeks of therapy.

wear off creates significant irritability (a "roller coaster" effect), consider the slow-release form, adding the two daily short-acting dosages to approximate the slow-release single dose. If the child experiences few positive effects and predominantly negative side effects, switch to dextroamphetamine and follow the same guidelines (see Fig. 3-1).

Approximately 80 to 90 percent of children and adolescents respond to methylphenidate. Of those who have too many side effects to continue methylphenidate, about 70 percent will respond to dextroamphetamine. Consider pemoline as the last choice for a stimulant trial, because there is the rare possibility (1 to 3 per 100,000 patients) of severe and sometimes fatal hepatotoxicity. However, pemoline has a lower abuse potential and longer half-life, so it may be beneficial for some adolescents.

MONITORING TREATMENT Ongoing monitoring of stimulant treatment should occur regularly. During the medication initiation phase, plan a follow-up telephone call weekly until the correct dosage regimen is established. Monitoring heart rate, blood pressure, and weight should occur initially within 4 to 6 weeks and then every 3 to 4 months. For pemoline, liver function studies should be performed at least every 6 months. No laboratory studies are required for methylphenidate or dextroamphetamine.

Issues regarding medication monitoring that are specific to the stimulants include making sure the dosage continues to be efficacious. For some children, after 2 to 3 months of good response to an initial dose, efficacy decreases, and they require an increase in dose. Generally, subsequent dosage increases are made once per year as the child gains weight.

You should continue to monitor current side effects, such as appetite suppression and sleep difficulties, and discuss how the family is managing those issues. For children who eat poorly at lunch, a common strategy is to increase amounts of food at dinner and bedtime snack.

There should also be ongoing discussion of how the family decides when to use a 4 PM or weekend dosage and when to have medication holidays. For young children who have high activity levels year round, discontinuing medication in the summer or vacation may be difficult and ill advised. As children grow older, however, they may be able to have medication holidays that are more frequent and of longer duration. Children may also be taken off medication during the school year as they get older if their symptoms decrease. Medication should not be stopped at the beginning of the school year. Instead, wait until the child has adjusted to the new class and teacher.

ANTIDEPRESSANTS

TRICYCLIC ANTIDEPRESSANTS Tricyclic antidepressants, particularly nortryptiline, have been considered the second-line treatment choice for ADHD for many years. Their efficacy is documented in well-controlled, randomized trials by Biederman and associates. Advantages include their long duration of action, minimal abuse potential, and flexible dosing. Disadvantages are considerable, however, and include cardiac conduction abnormalities requiring frequent ECG monitoring, and cardiac toxicity with overdose. Wherry and colleagues reported a series of four deaths in children treated with desipramine creating caution regarding its use.

NEWER ANTIDEPRESSANTS New antidepressants that are being studied and show some potential for efficacy include buproprion, buspirone, and venlafaxine. Data on these compounds are quite preliminary. The selective serotonin reuptake inhibitor (SSRI) compounds have yet to show efficacy in the treatment of ADHD or any disruptive behavior disorder.

ALPHA ADRENERGICS

Despite few studies documenting their safety or efficacy, the alpha agonists clonidine and guanfacine are increasingly used to treat ADHD symptoms and appear to have positive effects on enhancing mood and reducing activity level and aggression. They are not useful, however, for the primarily inattentive subtype of ADHD. They are particularly useful for preschoolers and school-age children with very high activity levels, frequent aggressive outbursts, and poor sleep regulation. They are also indicated for children and adolescents with ADHD and Tourette's syndrome for whom stimulants are not appropriate.

Adverse drug reactions for alpha adrenergics include heart rate and blood pressure abnormalities. Logsdon and associates report three deaths in children taking clonidine and methylphenidate together. Because of these concerns, use of these medications should not occur without consultation from a behavioral/developmental pediatrician or a child psychiatrist.

Management of Other Disruptive Behavior Disorders

Negative emotional behaviors, aggression, and oppositional-defiant disorder may exist in isolation but frequently accompany ADHD behaviors. Medications for ADHD may have a slight effect on the oppositional child, but these are often the behaviors that remain problematic even after medications for ADHD have proven effective. One common mistake families and professionals make is expecting these behaviors to be "treatable" with medications, thereby increasing the dosages of stimulants to try to eradicate these symptoms, only to have the child develop significant side effects. It must be explained to families that these symptoms may not go away with medications used to treat the ADHD. The most effective treatment for oppositional behaviors is behavior management strategies, applied both at home and at school.

Secretive antisocial behaviors or conduct disorder symptoms often indicate serious psychological distress in children, and often are seen in families struggling with significant difficulties themselves, either in the form of mental health problems, significant socioeconomic problems, substance use, or some combination of these. Children who steal repetitively, set fires, or carry weapons must be referred for psychiatric evaluation and treatment in a comprehensive mental health services program.

Learning disability occurs in approximately 40 to 60 percent of children with disruptive behavior disorders. Learning problems are primarily "managed" by finding the appropriate school placement or program for the child and educating families about how they can support the child's self-esteem and help with alternative learning strategies. Some school districts are very supportive of children and families, and others are not. The primary care clinician can also play a supportive role with the school by providing information for all parents. There is no medication or medical treatment available for these children at this time. However, the early identification of learning problems is extremely important, and clinicians should be very alert for such issues, especially in early school-age children.

Psychiatric comorbidity may occur as anxiety, depression, PTSD, or Tourette's syndrome. These conditions can be complex to manage, because they may not respond well to stimulant treatment, and usually require different medications or combinations of medications. Primary care clinicians should have a high index of suspicion for these conditions when seeing a child with disruptive behaviors, especially when evaluating adolescents. Clinicians should consider referral to a developmental/behavioral pediatrician, child psychiatrist, or child neurologist. If you decide a referral is indicated, be aware that the majority of persons referred to child behavior specialists do not complete the referral. Suggestions to facilitate a successful referral include the following.

- Know who is the most appropriate referral and make the appointment with the family in your office.
- Be very clear with the family about why they need the referral and how important you think it is.
- Coordinate follow-up from your office. Make sure a call is made to the family or a visit is scheduled in your office after their referral appointment.
- Send a letter to the referral specialist outlining your questions and the family's issues. Also send a copy to the family. A sample letter is shown in Table 3-8.

Follow-Up

After the initial assessment and implementation of a treatment plan, primary care clinicians should continue in their essential role of support and coordination of service. This includes monitoring medication responses both at home and at school, monitoring how well the child and family are implementing behavioral changes, deciding whether referrals to behavioral health specialists are necessary, ensuring that referrals are coordinated, and evaluating family satisfaction with treatment and with school placements. Table 3-5 lists important elements that we review with families at each follow-up visit. Most of our patients are seen on an every 3- to 4-month basis. An example of how follow-up might look for the patients in the sample vignettes follows.

JOHNNY (CONTINUED) *Johnny began treatment at age 5 years. He is placed on 5 mg methylphenidate after breakfast and lunch. His parents also give a dose at 4:00 PM for social events like sports and*

Table 3-8

Sample Physician Referral Letter

Date: ______________________________

Child's name: ______________________________

Parent(s) name(s): ______________________________

Child's birth date: ______________ UN: ______________

Type of insurance: ______________________________

Physician concerns regarding the child and family:

A. ______________________________

B. ______________________________

C. ______________________________

Parents' concerns:

A. ______________________________

B. ______________________________

C. ______________________________

Are there medical concerns in the family?

____

Recommendation for a specific therapist:

____

Name: ______________________________

Reason: ______________________________

I am referring this child for further evaluation and possible treatment.

____

Referring Specialist / Date / Phone Number

Cub Scouts and usually 1 to 2 doses on weekends. In addition, his parents worked with a behavioral management consultant for six initial sessions and have returned for "booster" sessions periodically.

As Johnny has grown, his methylphenidate dosage was gradually increased. He continued to take methylphenidate over the summer until age 8. By age 12, he was taking medication for school and only occasionally at 4:00 PM. His dose was switched to methylphenidate 20 mg slow release, supplemented with short-acting methylphenidate 10 mg in the morning. He has been enrolled in special education services since kindergarten. For high school he is planning to try a new vocational program geared toward learning computer skills. His grades have been As, Bs, and Cs.

Johnny has benefited from participation in sports activities. He is participating in the soccer, swimming, and track teams. His friends are mostly other boys on the teams. Johnny's parents continue to have a stable relationship and have received support from extended family members and friends. They have read extensively about ADHD and are members of a local ADHD support group.

You have seen Johnny at least three to four times per year to focus on his ADHD symptoms and perform sports physicals. He has remained healthy. During fifth grade, Johnny had increased behavior problems at school in the form of arguments with his teacher. During that time he expressed wishes he were dead. You requested a psychiatric evaluation to further investigate, but no significant symptoms of depression were detected. Johnny was placed in a different class with a new teacher, and his problems abated.

JULIE (CONTINUED) *Julie's grandmother agreed to work with the mental health agency. The family was given a new therapist at the center. Grandmother was diagnosed with depression and began individual treatment. Julie's medication was changed to slow-release dextroamphetamine during the day and clonidine at night for sleep. This improved the situation at home and school.*

You continued to see Julie two to three times per year to monitor her ADHD and serve as a family support. When Julie's parents resurfaced briefly and tried to obtain custody, her behavior problems worsened until custody issues were resolved. She was placed permanently into her Grandmother's care.

Julie continued her medications year round. In adolescence, she was switched by the psychiatrist to an antidepressant. At her 12-year checkup, she was relatively healthy but admitted to trying cigarettes and alcohol. With her grandmothers' permission, you spent extra time with her to go over sex education and substance abuse issues. You have a plan to see her every 6 months during adolescence, because she is still at high risk for substance abuse and early sexual experimentation.

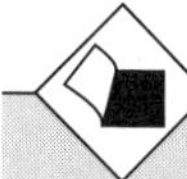

Summary

This chapter focused on the assessment and management of behavioral problems in children and adolescents, with particular emphasis on disruptive behavior problems such as ADHD. We have attempted to provide a primary care perspective and have outlined a practical, family-centered approach to these disorders. We hope this information will prove a useful guide in the evaluation and management of the many children and adolescents who present with behavioral difficulties in primary care settings.

The management of these problems can be greatly enhanced with a proactive approach that includes some or all of the following.

1. Careful attention to family and child concerns.
2. Standardized assessments and evaluations in the office.
3. Identification and communication with local mental health and education resources to support parents and families.
4. Step-wise introduction of treatment in primary care.
5. Enhancement of specialist/referral linkages.
6. Use of behaviorally trained staff support.

The necessary resources for many of these steps need to be developed before patients are seen to minimize disruption for the patients, the patient's family, and your practice. Clinicians should expect that improvements in patients will be gradual, and that they will need to help families and patients appreciate the "small" victories that occur over time.

The successful management of child behavior problems will not only increase patient and family satisfaction with care, but will also diminish provider frustration in managing these common symptoms. Moreover, participation in the multidisciplinary management of these problems will lead clinicians to better relationships with schools, mental health providers, and community resources.

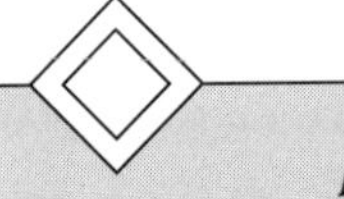

Acknowledgment

This work is supported in part by the Staunton Farm Foundation of Pittsburgh, Pittsburgh, Pennsylvania.

Suggested Reading

Parker S, Zuckerman B (eds): *Behavioral & Developmental Pediatrics: A Handbook for Primary Care*. Boston: Little, Brown; 1995.

This book has several concise but very useful chapters on office practices relating to behavioral and developmental pediatrics such as "talking with children," "helping families deal with bad news," and behavioral and developmental screening. Additionally, it contains numerous chapters that give brief overviews of relevant presenting problems such as hyperactivity, school failure, or bedwetting. An excellent quick resource.

Wolraich ML (ed): *A Practical Guide to Assessment & Management,* 2nd ed. St. Louis: Mosby-Year Book, 1996.

This text contains an excellent, detailed chapter on ADHD evaluation and management. It is also a very useful reference for those who wish to understand disorders of motor and language development, learning disabilities, and mental retardation. Additionally, there is an excellent chapter on measures of development and developmental screening.

Barkley RA (ed): *Attention Deficit Hyperactivity Disorder: A Handbook for Diagnosis and Treatment,* 2nd ed. New York: The Guilford Press; 1998.

This is one of the most comprehensive texts on ADHD available. This book is highly recommended as an authoritative, up-to-date, comprehensive text. It represents an important resource for those professionals who take care of individuals with ADHD on a regular basis.

Barkley RA, Murphy KR (eds): *Attention Deficit Hyperactivity Disorder: A Clinical Workbook,* 2nd ed. New York: The Guildford Press, 1998.

This is a workbook that accompanies Barkley's Handbook and contains a series of handouts, ratings scales, and evaluation forms for every use in the clinical assessment and management of ADHD.

Diagnosis & Treatment of Attention Deficit Hyperactivity Disorder. NIH Consensus Development Conference Statement, November 16–18, 1998.

A recent consensus statement on ADHD.

Bibliography

American Psychiatric Association. *Diagnostic and Statistical Manual of Mental Disorders: DSM-IV.* Washington, DC: American Psychiatric Association, 1994.

American Psychiatric Association. *Diagnostic and Statistical Manual of Mental Disorders, 4th ed.* Primary care version (DSM-IV-PC). Washington, DC: American Psychiatric Association, 1995.

Baumgaertel A, Copeland L, Wolraich ML: Attention deficit hyperactivity disorder. In: Wolraich ML (ed): *Disorders of Development and Learning: A Practical Guide to Assessment and Management.* St. Louis: Mosby; 1996, 437.

Biederman J, Baldessarini RJ, Wright V, et al: A double-blind placebo controlled study of desipramine in the treatment ADD: II. Serum drug levels and cardiovascular findings. *J Am Acad Child Adolesc Psychiatry* 28:903, 1989.

Biederman J, Faraone SV, Keenan K, et al: Further evidence for family-genetic risk factors in attention deficit hyperactivity disorder: Patterns of comorbidity in probands and relatives in psychiatrically and pediatrically referred samples. *Arch Gen Psychiatry* 49:728, 1992.

Biederman J, Newcorn J, Sprich S: Comorbidity of attention deficit disorders with conduct, depression, anxiety, and other disorders. *Am J Psychiatry* 148:564, 1991.

Chappell PB, Riddle MA, Scahill L, et al: Guanfacine treatment of comorbid attention-deficit hyperactivity disorder and Tourette's syndrome: Preliminary clinical experience. *J Am Acad Child Adolesc Psychiatry* 34:1140, 1995.

Cohen WI, Milberg L: The behavioral pediatrics consultation: Teaching residents to think systemically in managing behavioral pediatrics problems. *Family Sys Med* 10:169, 1992.

Department of Health and Human Services: Mental Health: A Report of the Surgeon General. Rockville, MD: U.S. Department of Health and Human Services, Substance Abuse and Mental Health Services Administration, Center for Mental Health Services, National Institutes of Health, National Institute of Mental Health; 1999.

Dulcan M: Practice parameters for the assessment and treatment of children adolescents, and adults with attention-deficit/hyperactivity disorder. American Academy of Child and Adolescent Psychiatry. *J Am Acad Child Adolesc Psychiatry* 36(Suppl 10): 85S, 1997.

Gardner W, Kelleher K, Wasserman R, et al: Primary care treatment of pediatric psychosocial problems: A study from Pediatric Research in Office Settings and Ambulatory Sentinel Practice Network. *Pediatrics* 106(4):E44, 2000.

Green M: Bright Futures: *Guidelines for Health Supervision of Infants, Children and Adolescents.* McLean, VA: National Center for Education in Maternal and Child Health; 1994.

Greenhill L: Pharmacotherapy: Stimulants in child and adolescents. *Psychiatr Clin North Am* 1:411, 1992.

Greenhill LL: Attention-deficit/hyperactivity disorder. In: Walsh BT, (ed): *Child Psychopharmacology.* Washington, DC: American Psychiatric Press; 1998.

Greenhill L, Abikoff H, Arnold L: *Psychopharmacological treatment manual, NIMH multimodal treatment study of children with attention deficit hyperactivity disorder (MTA Study).* New York: Prepared by the Psychopharmacology Subcommittee of the MTA Steering Committee; 1998.

Hinshaw SP, Heller T, McHale JP: Covert antisocial behavior in boys with attention-deficit hyperactivity disorder: External validation and effects of methylphenidate. *J Consult Clin Psychol* 60:274, 1992.

Hinshaw SP, Henker B, Whalen CK, et al: Aggressive, prosocial, and nonsocial behavior in hyperactive boys: Dose effects of methylphenidate in naturalistic settings. *J Consult Clin Psychol* 57:636, 1989.

Hoagwood K: Outcomes of Mental Health Care for Children and Adolescents: I. Comprehensive Conceptual Model. *J Am Acad Child Adolesc Psychiatry* 35:1055, 1996.

Hunt R, Arnstan A, Asbell M: An open trial of guanfacine in the treatment of attention-deficit hyperactivity disorder. *J Am Acad Child Adolesc Psychiatry* 34:41, 1995.

Hunt R, Minderaa R, Cohen D: Clonidine benefits children with attention deficit disorder and hyperactivity: Report of a double-blind placebo-crossover therapeutic trial. *J Am Acad Child Adolesc Psychiatry* 24:617, 1985.

Jellinek MS, Murphy JM, Burns BJ: Brief psychosocial screening in outpatient pediatric practice. *J Pediatr* 109:371, 1986.

Jellinek MS, Murphy JM, Little M, et al: Use of the Pediatric Symptom Checklist (PSC) to screen for psychosocial problems in pediatric primary care: A national feasibility study. *Arch Pediatr Adolesc Med* 153:254, 1994.

Jellinek M, Patel B: *Bright Futures in Practice: Mental Health Promotion.* Arlington, VA: National Center for Education in Maternal and Child Health. (In press, Fall 2001).

Kelleher KJ, Childs GE: Health care costs for children with ADHD. (Submitted).

Kelleher K, Childs G, Wasserman R, et al: Insurance status and recognition of psychosocial problems: A report from PROS and ASPN. *Arch Pediatr Adolesc Med* 151:1109, 1997.

Kelleher KJ, Hohmann A, Larson D: Prescription of psychotropic drugs in office-based practices. *Am J Dis Childhood* 143:855, 1989.

Logsdon B, Kelley L, Barrett F: Clonidine and sudden death. *Pediatrics* 96:1176, 1995.

Newacheck PW: Adolescents with special health needs: Prevalence, severity, and access to health services. *Pediatrics* 84:699, 1995.

Regier DA, Narrow WE, Rae SD, et al: The de facto U.S. mental and addictive disorders service system. *Arch Gen Psychiatry* 50:85, 1993.

Rost K, Smith GR, Matthews D, et al: The deliberate misdiagnosis of major depression in primary care. *Arch Fam Med* 3:333, 1994.

Wasserman R, Kelleher K, Bocian A, et al: Identification of attentional and hyperactivity problems in primary care: A report from pediatric research in office settings and the ambulatory sentinel practice network. *Pediatrics* 103:E38, 1999.

Wender E: Hyperactivity. In: Parker S, Zuckerman B, (eds): *Behavioral and Developmental Pediatrics: A Handbook for Primary Care.* Boston: Little, Brown and Company; 1995.

Wherry JS, Biederman J, Thisted R, et al: Resolved: Cardiac arrhythmias make desipramine an unacceptable choice in children. *J Am Acad Child Adolesc Psychiatry* 34:1239, 1995.

Deborah J. Seymour
Kirsten Black

Stress in Primary Care Patients

Introduction

Whatever happens in the mind of man, is always reflected in the diseases of his body.

Rene Dubos

Ubiquitous in modern society, stress is a contributing factor in many illnesses. It is estimated that over 70 percent of visits to primary health care providers are for stress-induced problems such as fatigue, back pain, headache, and abdominal pain. The mechanisms by which stress causes and exacerbates illness are complex. They are characterized by bidirectional interactions between external events and behaviors, subjective interpretation of those events and behaviors, and the effect of the events on physiologic systems, including the immune and neuroendocrine systems. The effects of stress can also result in the adoption of unhealthy coping strategies such as smoking, drinking, and drug use. These, in turn, have direct and indirect negative effects on health.

Given the large number of office visits in which stress is a contributing factor, clinicians who are able to identify and intervene with patients experiencing high levels of stress can ameliorate a considerable amount of unnecessary suffering and fiscal burden. It is estimated that businesses lose up to $150 billion per year owing to stress-related absenteeism. Treating stress is cost effective, leading to reductions in patient office visits and diagnostic tests, as well as increasing worker productivity.

Stress is a relevant topic for primary care practitioners not only because of the large number of patients experiencing stress-related illness, but also because of the attention given to this topic by the popular media. Patients today are aware of the impact that stress can have on health, and they are looking for practitioners whose approach to health care goes beyond simply diagnosing medical disease.

The magnitude of the effect of stress on health is reflected in the sheer volume written about it in both popular and scientific publications. In 1997 alone, there were over 3000 new scientific articles on stress listed by the *Social Sciences Citations Index*. Although this testifies to expanding knowledge in this field, keeping up with the literature can be overwhelming. Consequently, many clinicians, while recognizing that stress can influence health, are uncomfortable treating stress and are unsure of how to account for it within a differential diagnosis. The reasons for this vary, though three important factors can be identified. First, there is confusion caused by the lack of a clear definition for the word *stress.* Second, stress is a highly subjective experience, and its effects are moderated by a multitude of interacting variables. Finally, there is an inherent difficulty in integrating the psychosocial concept of stress within a biomedical model of illness and disease.

The main objective of this chapter is to provide a theoretical and practical understanding of the relationship between stress and illness to enable primary care clinicians to better recognize and respond to the needs of patients who are experiencing stress in their lives. The chapter begins by describing a theoretical framework for understanding stress, followed by a brief summary of current research linking stress to specific health outcomes. The final section is devoted to practical approaches for intervention.

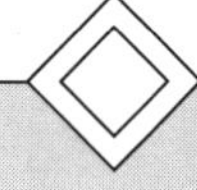

History of the Concept of Stress

With every affliction of the mind that is attended with either pain or pleasure, hope or fear, is the cause of an agitation whose influence extends to the heart.

William Harvey, 1698

Although we tend to think of stress and stress-related illnesses as modern phenomena, writings from early physicians and philosophers reveal profound insight concerning the relationship between stress and illness. With the dominance of the biomedical model in the evolution of modern medicine, however, theories about the relationship between stress and illness were largely ignored for many years. It was not until the early twentieth century that Walter Cannon undertook the first serious study of stress. Researching the physiologic changes involved in the *fight or flight* response, Cannon described stress as a disruption of the body's normal balance and the stress response as an attempt to regain physiologic homeostasis. Building on Cannon's work, Hans Selye introduced three concepts that have been foundational in the study of stress. These concepts are (1) the body's stress response is a defensive response that is unrelated to the type of stressor, (2) there are three stages of response—alarm, resistance, and exhaustion, and (3) prolonged stress can cause disease.

The next major development in the field of stress involved a shift from examining physiologic responses to measuring external stressors. Holmes and Rahe initiated work in this area by developing screening tools to quantify stressors. Although popular during the 1970s, studies later showed the tools had poor predictive value (4 to 6 percent) for illness.

Drawing on concepts from these earlier models, Lazarus and Folkman developed the transactional model that dominates our current understanding of stress. According to the transactional model, stress is a complex, dynamic interaction between individual perceptions and external demands. Whereas the previous models focused on single factors—physiologic changes and external events—the transactional model is broad and allows inclusion of a variety of interrelating factors.

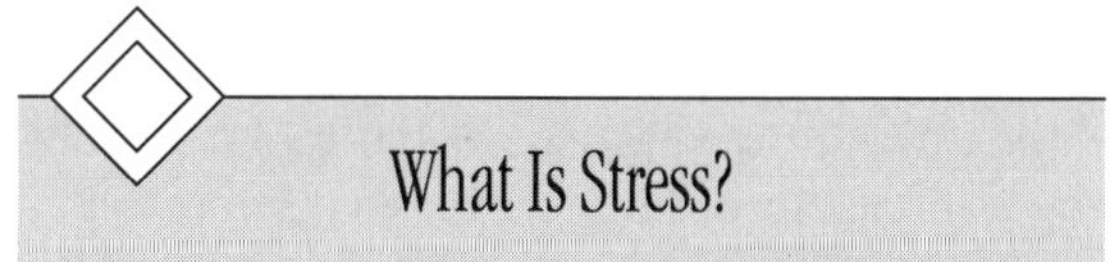

What Is Stress?

At one level, the term *stress* is well understood and seems to need no formal definition, yet at a more critical level, we find a term whose meaning is ambiguous. Although we have all experienced stress, probably few of us have given much thought to exactly what we mean when we use this term. The following section highlights some of the confusion surrounding the word *stress* and provides a useful framework for understanding the abstract concept of "stress."

Defining Stress

Since the first application of the term *stress* to the field of medicine, its meaning has been variously rendered. Selye defines stress as a response, whereas for Holmes and Rahe it is a stimulus. Lazarus and Folkman combine elements of these two views in their transactional model, yet do not attempt to define the word *stress* except to say that their model is a rubric for understanding the complex interactions associated with it. The confusion apparent in academic writing is mirrored by vernacular usage. Take for instance the common phrase "I'm stressed." This simple phrase can be interpreted in at least three ways: (1) a feeling, (2) an assessment of the demands one faces, or (3) as some combination of these two. Another source of confusion is the use of the word *stress* interchangeably with *anxiety*.

Although its meaning is commonly understood, the lack of a precise definition of stress is a problem for researchers and those attempting to make sense of the vast literature on this subject. Some have even argued that the term is worthless and should be discarded. Regardless of how one feels about the utility of the term, the reality of "stress" still exists, and primary care clinicians need to be able to recognize and discuss "stress" with their patients.

The Stress Continuum

For primary care purposes, stress can be thought of as occurring along a continuum ranging from normative stress to traumatic stress. From Fig. 4-1

Figure 4-1

Normative stress	Increasing stress	Traumatic stress
Pregnancy	Marital difficulties (chronic), Loss of job (acute)	Rape/torture (acute/chronic)

Stress can be beneficial and motivating (normative stress), but as it increases it begins to inhibit performance. Levels of stress approaching traumatic stress become oppressive.

we see that although stress is often viewed as a negative experience, some forms of stress are beneficial and motivating (i.e., pregnancy). In fact, many people report that a certain amount of stress motivates them to do their best, while the absence of stress fosters low productivity. At the other extreme, too much stress can be oppressive and inhibit performance. Stress can also be categorized as either chronic or acute. Primary care clinicians often see patients following acute stress. The provision of appropriate care in response to acute stress can prevent long-term negative sequelae.

Where along the spectrum a particular stressor for a specific individual falls is determined by the nature of the stressor, the individual's subjective interpretation of the stressor, and other factors that influence the way the stressor is experienced. For example, in Figure 4-1, pregnancy is listed as a normative stress, but it can be perceived as a severe stress by an impoverished teen mother whose dreams for scientific accomplishment in her life may be greatly challenged by having become pregnant.

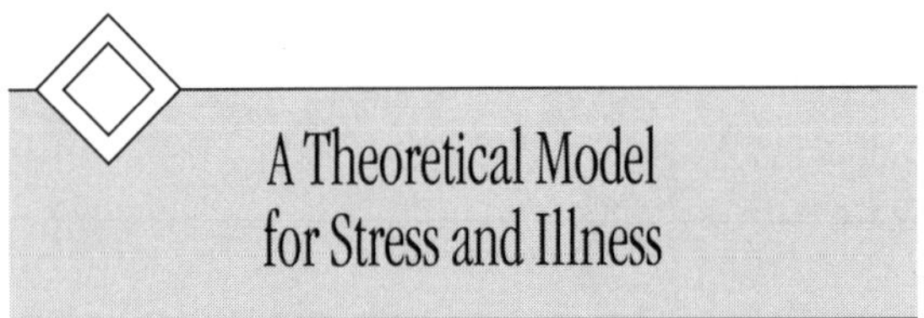

A Theoretical Model for Stress and Illness

There are a variety of models that explain the mechanism(s) by which stress affects health. Although models can be helpful for providing a general framework, they are nevertheless limited in their ability to provide a comprehensive picture of such complex interactions. For the purpose of providing a picture of stress, we have chosen to use a diagram developed by Olff (Fig. 4-2). The diagram illustrates that the health consequences of stress result from interactions between environmental events (stressors) and physical and cognitive responses. Olff's model is deceptively simple. It highlights the interconnection between environmental, psychological, and physiologic components, but does not account for the numerous intervening variables that can mediate the influence of stress. Intervening variables are highly subjective and therefore beyond the scope of this chapter. We will discuss some of them in the following sections as we review the elements in the Olff model.

Stressors

In the model, the stressor evokes a stress reaction. Stressors can be grouped as physical, environmental, life events, and positive stresses (Table 4-1). Although some have sought to quantify the experience of stress and establish a direct link between certain levels of stress and illness, we are unaware of any validated or reliable tool for assessing the effects of external stress *in primary care settings.*

One of the reasons that it is difficult, if not impossible, to develop a reliable tool for profiling patients according to stressful events is that the relationship between the individual and the stressor(s) is subjective and bidirectional. Many factors influence how a stressor affects a particular person. Characteristics of the stressor that tend

Figure 4-2

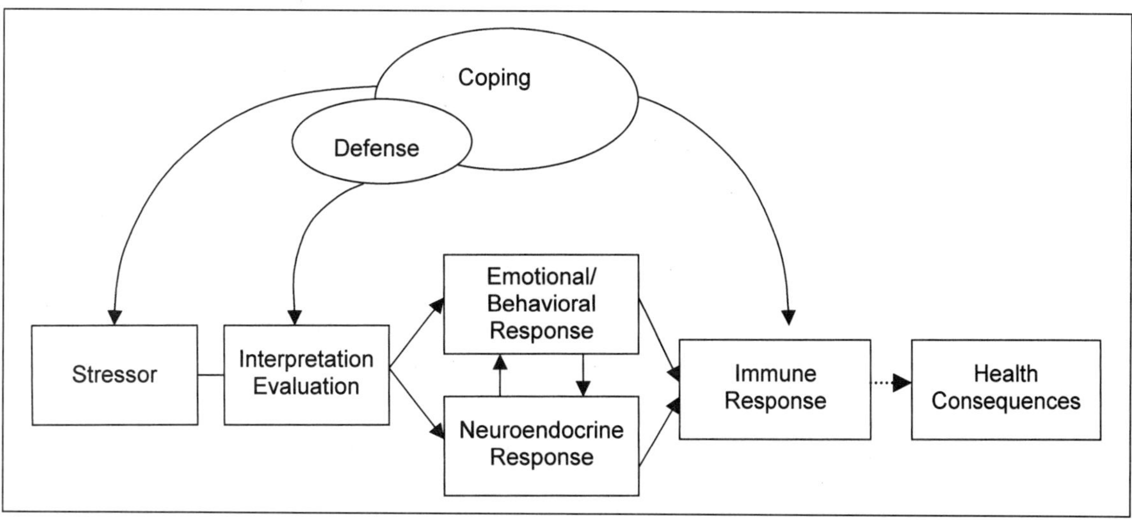

The health consequences of stress result from interactions between environmental, psychological, and physiologic components. Note that this model does not account for the numerous intervening variables that can mediate the influence of stress. *(Reproduced with permission from Olff M: Stress, depression and immunity: The role of defense and coping styles. Psychiatry Res 85:7. © 1999 Elsevier Science, Inc.)*

to increase the stress response include high intensity, chronic occurrence, complexity, and novelty. Individual interpretations often mediate the effect of stressors. For example, the stress response is generally lessened when the stressor is considered predictable and when the individual feels that it is controllable. Other mediating factors, such as the duration of stress, are discussed in the following sections.

Duration of Stressor

The duration of stress is an important independent factor in the influence of the stressor on an individual's health. Stress may be described as acute (minutes/hours), short term (days/weeks), or chronic (months/years). Differentiating the length of time that a person is exposed to stress is important because the physiologic response is dif-

Table 4-1

Common Stressors

Physical Stress	Environmental Stress	Life Events	Positive Stress
Injury	Air/noise pollution	Birth	Achievements
Illness	Overcrowding	Death	Athletic performance
Surgery	Occupational	Marriage	Personal relationships
	Traffic	Moving	
		Financial change	

ferent for acute versus long-term stress. Although there is a very profound response to acute stress, generally, the body is able to recover homeostasis without serious effects. In contrast, stress-related health concerns are commonly seen with long-term and chronic exposure to stress. Occupational and long-term caregiver stress are two areas that have been studied extensively; it has been shown that although acute stress causes a rapid increase in many immune parameters, repeated stress over time leads to a suppression of immune function.

Interpretation and Evaluation

The second stage in the stress response involves individual interpretation and evaluation of the stressor. Individual perception and interpretation is extremely variable and depends on personality and other individual factors such as optimism and introversion/extroversion. For example, public speaking may be stressful for one person, but exciting for another.

Although a number of factors have been identified that influence an individual's perception of a stressor, two of the most significant are social support and the individual's assessment of resources. When faced with a stressor, people assess whether they have sufficient resources (personal, emotional, financial, etc.) to meet the threat of the stressor. Individuals who believe they have few resources for coping with stress will experience more stress in a given situation than individuals who believe they have sufficient resources for coping with the same stress. Although the resources required to overcome any given situation vary, studies have highlighted the importance of social support. People who experience stress and have strong social support have better health outcomes than those who have less social support.

Emotional and Behavioral Responses

Activation of the stress response results in physical and emotional arousal. An individual may experience a variety of different emotions during excessive stress, such as anxiety, anger, excitement, apprehension, hopelessness, apathy, alienation, and depression. Other cognitive manifestations of excessive stress include distractibility, poor concentration, lower levels of performance, and changes in thought content. Acute physiologic responses to stress help to increase alertness and vigilance; prolonged excessive stress can cause different behaviors and emotions to develop. For instance, thinking may become rigid and less productive, there may be more irrational and self-defeating patterns of thought, and the person may adopt a passive attitude.

COPING

Coping is the individual's way of dealing with the arousal caused by stress. Although there is extensive literature on coping with stress, for our purposes it is sufficient to point out that there are different types of coping responses, and some are better adapted to particular situations than others. It is also important to recognize that individual coping mechanisms both shape and are shaped by perception and developmental influences.

DEFENSES When presented with stress, most individuals initiate a process of decreasing the negative effect of the stress on themselves. Olff calls this defense process coping; putting up a psychological barrier to prevent the stressor from overwhelming one's personal resources. For example, intellectualization is a defense mechanism in which the individual faces a stressful situation by emphasizing a thoughtful approach to the problem rather than an emotional response. This mechanism can be useful, for example, in complicated work situations where emotional responses to stress may not be considered appropriate.

Although a defensive reaction can be a useful way of dealing with some situations, in other situations the defenses can serve to further complicate a stressful situation. For example, if the same individual who use intellectualization to deal with conflict at work attempts to use intellectualization in dealing with the death of a loved one, the mourning process may become more difficult and grief may be prolonged.

COPING STRATEGIES Lazurus and Folkman describe two types of coping, problem-focused coping and emotion-focused coping. In problem-focused coping, individuals direct their action outward to alter some aspect of the stressor. By contrast, emotion-focused coping involves an attempt to change some aspect of an individual's perception or response to the stressor. The distinction between these two is illustrated in the following case scenario.

JOHN BUTLER, NORA PETERSON, AND FRANK DAVIS *One afternoon, John Butler, a supervisor who is under a lot of stress himself, marches into a work area and lectures a group of employees about their lack of productivity. The group has been working very hard, putting in long hours to meet a particular deadline, but has had little support and consequently is not going to complete the project on time. After the lecture, John leaves and the employees talk. Nora Peterson says that she has had enough of this type of treatment and plans to start looking for another job. Frank Davis says that he is lucky to have this job, all companies like theirs have this type of "lecture" from time to time, and in the grand scheme of things this is "no big deal."*

Nora exhibits an action-orientated approach to the problem; she wants to change the circumstance. Frank uses an emotion-focused approach—choosing to view the circumstances in a more positive light. Both approaches have strengths and liabilities. Most individuals employ a combination of these approaches and consciously or unconsciously select the most advantageous. However, over-reliance on a particular strategy can have negative health consequences. By drawing a patient's attention to the type of coping strategy employed, primary care providers may assist patients in making more adaptive choices.

Stress and Unhealthy Behaviors

High levels of stress increase emotional arousal. To lessen the effect of this arousal, people may turn to behaviors such as drinking, smoking, and doing drugs. These habits are unhealthy and can significantly multiply the negative effects of stress. Maladaptive, emotion-focused coping is often an underlying factor driving unhealthy habits, because this pattern of coping requires the individual to find a way to adapt to continuing stress. Unfortunately, because these habits are addictive and can be impairing, they frequently lessen the ability to make effective responses to stress.

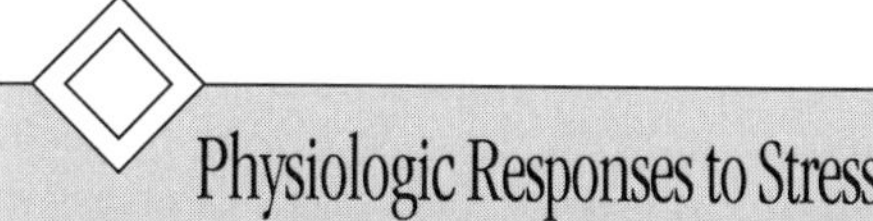

Physiologic Responses to Stress

Stressful experiences are manifested in physiologic responses involving the autonomic nervous system, the immune system, and the neuroendocrine system. Research shows that there is considerable interaction between these systems and that the body's physiologic responses to stress are extremely complex.

The most well-studied physiologic response to stress is part of the autonomic nervous system: the fight or flight response. This rapid, central nervous system (CNS)-mediated response occurs through activation of the parasympathetic (PNS) and sympathetic (SNS) nervous systems. The effects of sympathetic activation result in physiologic changes, including increased heart rate, elevated blood pressure, increased stroke volume, bronchial dilatation, changes in metabolism of glucose, and constriction of blood vessels in the stomach, skin, kidneys, and reproductive organs. These changes help to shunt blood flow away from the skin and intestines so that it can be used to supply energy necessary for an immediate physical challenge.

In addition to the autonomic nervous system response, there are various neuroendocrine responses that occur. The neuroendocrine response is slower acting and has a longer effect compared with CNS activities. Chemicals in the neuroendocrine system are involved with regulating the immune system. In response to stress, the psychoimmune response is rapid—within minutes there can be a 25 to 40 percent increase in the number of circulating natural killer cells. After cessation, natural killer cell levels return to baseline within 15 min. For more information on the complex physiologic responses to stressful experiences, the reader is referred to the suggested reading list at the end of this chapter.

Individual Susceptibility

The concept of individual susceptibility helps to explain why some people have a lot of stress in their lives and seem to have no stress-related illness while others have much less stress and a great deal of stress-related illness. The two primary factors that influence the effect of stress on the body are coping mechanisms and biological susceptibility. Strong and appropriate coping mechanisms help to lessen the physical affects of stress, but biological susceptibility determines the threshold for stress-induced illness. A person with a low threshold for stress-induced illness (i.e., greater susceptibility) will experience physical effects from stress at a lower level of stress than someone with a higher threshold.

Individual susceptibility is determined by the interactions of genetic, developmental, and environmental/behavioral factors. For example, research shows that people who have a family history of hypertension experience elevated blood pressure as a consequence of stress to a greater extent than those who have no family history of hypertension. Environmental, developmental, and behavioral factors moderate genetic predisposition. Unhealthy behaviors, such as smoking, drinking, and lack of exercise, lower the threshold for stress-induced illness while healthy behaviors can reduce health risk.

Individual differences in handling stress can set into motion any of a number of different physiologic responses. This, coupled with differences in individual susceptibility, helps to explain why one person experiences gastrointestinal (GI) upset when stressed, while another experiences low back pain.

Individual differences make researching the link between stress and illness difficult. There is considerable individual variability in how stress is perceived and dealt with as well as how it influences health. Despite the complexity of this subject, researchers have identified a number of disease states that they believe are either caused or exacerbated by stress. A brief summary of this research is presented in the following section.

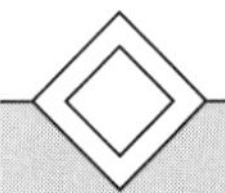

Physical Effects of Stress

People feel the physical effects of stress in a variety of ways. Stress can cause dizziness, tension headaches, muscle pain, stomach aches, heart palpitations, fatigue, and respiratory problems. Patients who experience one or more of these symptoms over a prolonged period of time may become concerned that they have an underlying disease process. This belief contributes to the development of somatoform disorders. The following section briefly outlines some of the effects that stress can have on various organ systems. For more information on this subject, the reader is referred to the chapter on somatization (Chap. 15) and the suggested reading list at the end of this chapter.

Cardiovascular Disease

Stress is an important risk factor for cardiovascular disease, which is the leading cause of death in the United States. Stress can affect the heart through a number of different mechanisms. It can cause physiologic changes leading to high blood pressure, dysfunction of the cardiac endothelium, thickening of the left ventricle, cardiac arrhythmia, metabolic changes, coagulation problems, ischemia, and cardiotoxic effects. Stress may also increase vulnerability to atherosclerosis. In patients with atherosclerosis, stress can increase susceptibility to clinical events such as myocardial ischemia, coronary thrombosis, and myocardial infarction.

Although considerable progress was been made in the 1990s in diagnosis and treatment of heart disease, up to one third of sudden cardiac deaths cannot be explained by standard risk factors. Stress is believed to be a contributing factor in up to 20 percent of these deaths. Mental stress is believed to lower the threshold for ventricular fibrillation and cause malignant ventricular arrhythmias, especially in people with underlying heart disease. The types of stress that are most often related to sudden cardiac death include bereavement, unemployment, social class, dislocation, education, mental stress, and social isolation.

Muscle Pain

Stressful events, especially those of high intensity and long duration, are closely associated with chronic pain, and patients who are exposed to stress often present with neck, shoulder, or low back pain. The pain these patients feel may be due to constant tension in their muscles; prolonged muscle contraction causes muscle fibers to be unable to relax. Workers who have high stress jobs with little control experience greater muscle pain compared to workers who perform repetitious tasks but have little stress. This difference in pain has been attributed to the fact that psychological stress remains with the person even after work, resulting in continuous muscle tensing.

Gastrointestinal Disorders

Although stress is generally thought to be a contributing factor in GI disorders, the mechanisms of the relationship are largely speculative. Gastroesophageal reflux (GERD), peptic ulcer disease (PUD), and irritable bowel syndrome (IBS) are three common GI disorders that are frequently referred to as being stress induced. Current research has shown that although stress is likely to be a factor in these disorders, its role may be less (or at least different) from what was previously thought. This does not mean that stress is not a potential factor in these diseases; rather, it points out that the causality is complex and multifactorial.

Perhaps the most widely studied stress-related GI disorder is IBS. It is estimated that over 15 percent of the adult population of the United States has reported symptoms of IBS, and that IBS accounts for between 2.5 and 3.5 million office visits per year. Research in IBS has shown that stress produces changes in gastric motility and that people with IBS have different patterns of motility than those who do not have IBS. Stress reduction treatments have been shown to be effective in reducing symptoms of IBS.

Reproductive Effects

Stress inhibits the reproductive system at many levels, through suppression of gonadotropin releasing hormone and inhibitory effects of both glucorticoids and cytokines. Stress can be a factor in dysmenorrhea, dyspareunia, endometriosis, decreased fertility, and impotence.

Pulmonary Effects

Acute stress increases respiratory rate and minute respiratory volume, alters tidal volume, and decreases blood and alveolar carbon dioxide levels. Stress can exacerbate symptoms of both asthma and chronic obstructive pulmonary disease (COPD) in certain subgroups of individuals. A number of different stress reduction techniques have been shown to be beneficial for patients who have asthma.

Stress and Immunity

Stress results in a number of important changes in the immune system, and the effects of stress on immunity have been studied extensively. Although many studies show trends that point in the direction of lower immunity, interpreting the implications of the studies for clinical practice is difficult because there is not a sufficient understanding of the levels of these factors that are necessary to maintain a healthy immune response.

Herbert and Cohen address this issue when discussing the results of their meta-analysis of immune research. They found that stress was significantly related to decreases in functional immune measures. Although changes in parameters are observed, the health consequences of these relatively small changes are unknown. They also found that duration of stress had a significant association with some outcomes. Many have wondered whether the body adapts to long-term stress to minimize its effect, but these authors found no evidence to support this view.

Some of the most clinically relevant findings regarding stress and immunity come from prospective studies conducted on individuals who were experiencing life stress. There is a vast literature on this subject, with the two groups of people studied most extensively being spousal caregivers and medical students during examination periods. Although these two populations differ considerably in age, health, and duration and type of stress, the effects of stress on certain immunologic parameters are very similar. In the student studies, researchers compared immunity during stressful examination periods to other nonstressful times such as summer vacation. Both groups had decreased response to vaccinations and delayed wound healing of up to 40 percent during periods of stress. There was also an increase in self-reported illness symptoms, enhanced susceptibility to viruses, and greater proliferation of latent viruses such as herpes. It is noteworthy that in both groups these factors were mitigated by good social support systems.

In the previous sections, we discussed the history of our understanding of the concept of stress. We defined stress as occurring along a continuum from normative stress to traumatic stress. We discussed the relationship of the stressor and an individual's response to it, including the individual's interpretation of the stressor and mechanisms for defense and coping. Finally, we discussed the physiologic and physical effects of stress on health. The rest of this chapter examines what a clinician can do while caring for patients with life stress.

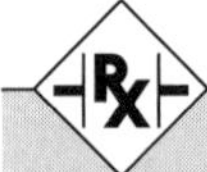

Caring for Patients With Life Stress

By discussing life stress during medical visits, primary care clinicians have a unique opportunity to assist patients with their health. Refined and empathic communication skills are essential in primary care practice and are particularly helpful when talking with patients about stress. There are three main aspects to helping your patients with stress: detecting it, discussing it, and coaching the patient about managing it. This section will highlight ways of talking with patients about stress and outline several stress reduction techniques appropriate for use in primary care settings.

Detection and Discussion of Stress

Whether a patient's stress presents to the clinician with direct effects on the patient's health or presents simply as a normal part of an individual's life context, it is well within the role of the primary care clinician to identify the stress and discuss it with the patient as a health issue. Because all people have stress, the matter of detection is not about *if* stress is present, but rather *how* stress is present. *How* stress is present is assessed simply by talking with your patients about the stress in their lives. In other words, clinicians may assume that stress is present and jump right to the business of discussing it.

Parameters for listening to and describing patient stress include type (acute, temporary, or chronic), intensity, duration, and most importantly patient interpretation of stress. Patients differ in their awareness of stress and their willingness to discuss it. Some patients are conscious of the stress that they have and will tell clinicians about it with lengthy descriptions of events and people, whereas others are more reticent about speaking of the stress in their lives. Clinicians also differ in their willingness to address stress during patient visits. Some clinicians avoid discussions about stress, fearing that they will open a Pandora's box of issues for which they have no time and no "cure." Other clinicians ask about stress at every health maintenance visit. Still others address stress only in the context of acute or chronic illness.

Some primary care clinicians report not knowing how to converse with patients about stress. Although it can be challenging, there are many ways to facilitate a frank and supportive discussion about stress and health. Marion Stewart and Joseph A. Lieberman, in their book *The Fifteen Minute Hour: Applied Psychotherapy for the Primary Care Physician*, suggest using a structured interview style. These authors describe the BATHE technique: BATHE is an acronym for interviewing about psychosocial aspects of patient's lives. Clinicians can use BATHE either during history taking as a means to gather information or during treatment planning to aid in the development of a mutually agreeable care plan. The interview is structured as follows:

Background—"What is going on in your life other than your illness?" Or "Tell me about the stresses in your life."
Affect—"How do you feel about it?"
Trouble—"What troubles you most about this?"
Handling—"How are you handling or coping with it?"
Empathy—The clinician makes an empathic statement of understanding the patient's experience. "That must be very difficult."

Many clinicians respond to a patient's report of stress by feeling a need to do something or tell the patient to *do* something to "take care of the stress." The BATHE model is especially helpful when you feel pressure to *do* something to help your patients with stress. It is important to remember that what you are *doing* is allowing your patient to speak freely and express concerns. Talking with patients about their stress and applying empathy are powerful interventions in and of themselves. Many clinicians report feeling that they have not done anything when they use talking as an intervention; however, simply talking about stress with your patients will help them to better recognize and manage their stress.

Regardless of the approach taken, it is important to be able to understand the multiple facets of stress from the patient's subjective point of view. Once you have detected and understood your patient's stress, you have the option of addressing that stress with your patient as either a normative process that may be helped with anticipatory guidance or as a particular direct or indirect health concern.

Life Cycle Stress and Anticipatory Guidance

A secret weapon in helping patients with stress is to discuss with them that stress is ubiquitous, normative, and even predictable from a life cycle perspective. Transition times (such as having a first baby) and developmental challenges (such as learning how to walk) in the family or individual life cycle are predictable times of stress. Life cycle challenges may be viewed as a part of the backdrop or context in which acute or chronic stress occurs. Table 4-2 describes the general stages of the life cycle and common developmental tasks that occur. The list in Table 4-2 may be used as a guide to providing anticipatory guidance to individuals about the added stress that is expected during times of change. See Chap. 2, Developmental and Parenting Issues in Childhood, for more information on life cycle challenges of children.

MARY AND JIM DOUGLAS *Mary Douglas, a 44-year-old healthy woman, comes in for a well-woman visit and a PAP smear. During the visit she asks you if you do vasectomies in the office. She and her husband Jim have decided to stop trying for a second child. She also tells you that their one son is up for a debate scholarship and has started to look*

Table 4-2

Major Individual Developmental Stages and Tasks

1. Infancy (approximate ages 0–2)
- Talk, communicate frustration and happiness
- Learn to make needs known and get them met
- Coordination, sit, stand, walk, run, manipulate objects
- Recognize self as separate person
- Trust others, primarily caretakers
- Overcome fears of new situations

2. Early childhood (approximate ages 2–4)
- Speech, language development, ability to relate and communicate
- Coordination, motor skills, eye–hand coordination
- Ability to control one's bodily functions, bowels and urine
- Understand self in relation to the world around oneself, awareness of others in terms of gender, race, and disability
- Cooperative play, ability to share
- Ability to obey rules
- Ability to delay gratification
- Development of trusting relationships
- Ability to form peer relationships
- Fantasy play and dramatization to master behavior and control anxieties

3. Middle childhood (approximate ages 5–12)
- Increased physical coordination and motor skills
- Ability to play team games
- Skill in reading, writing, math
- Knowledge about nature
- Understanding self in relation to family, peers, community; awareness of "otherness" in terms of gender, race, sexual orientation, culture, class, and disability
- Increased ability to conduct relationships with peers and authorities
- Ability to be intimate; to express anger, fear, and pain in nondestructive ways; to develop tolerance for difference

4. Adolescence (approximate ages 13–19)
- Bodily changes of puberty
- Development of sexual identity
- Increased physical coordination and physical skills
- Increased ability to read, write, think conceptually and mathematically
- Increased understanding of self in relation to peers, family, and community
- Development of a philosophy of life and moral identity
- Ability to handle intimate physical and social relationships as well as increased ability to judge and handle complex social situations
- Ability to work collaboratively and individually

5. Young adulthood (approximate ages 20–40)
- Ability to care for self and one's own needs
- Discipline for physical and intellectual work, sleep, sex, social relationships
- Ability to care for one's partner, children, and other family members
- More complex understanding of self in relation to peers, family, community
- Ability to support self and any children one may have
- Focus on life goals, ability to work independently and collaboratively
- Ability to negotiate evolving relationships to one's parents, peers, children, and community, including work relationships
- Ability to nurture others
- Ability to tolerate delaying gratification
- Further evolution of one's ability to promote respect for those who are dependent

6. Middle adulthood (approximate ages 40–60)
- Handle work, family, community, and social relationships and be accountable for one's responsibilities
- Some waning of physical abilities

Table 4-2

Major Individual Developmental Stages and Tasks (*continued*)

Accept that one cannot do it all and focus on mentoring others Recognition of one's accomplishments and acceptance of one's limitations Balance of multiple caretaking responsibilities for those above and below **7. Late middle age (approximate ages 60s and 70s)** Acceptance of declining physical abilities; handle work, family, community, and social relationships and be accountable for one's responsibilities Adapting to some loss of intellectual abilities, increasing one's perspective on life	Attend to one's connections with those who come after Recognizing one's triumphs and accepting one's limitations and losses **8. Aging (approximate ages 80s+)** Acceptance of declining of physical abilities and diminishing control over one's life Some loss of intellectual abilities, while maintaining wisdom Affirming and working out one's legacy to newer generation Acceptance of one's life and death

SOURCE: Reprinted with permission from "Individual and Family Life Cycle" by Eliana C. Korin, Marlene F. Watson, and Monica McGoldrick, which appears in *Fundamentals of Clinical Practice: A Textbook on the Patient, Doctor, and Society* by Mark B. Mengel and Warren L. Holleman, Plenum Publishers, 1997.

at colleges. You anticipate, from a life cycle point of view, that this is a period of potentially stressful family transition. The couple has decided to be a one-child family and that child is leaving home. You opt to bring that possibility into the discussion.

Clinician: Your health looks great, and we'll get your PAP results to you by the end of the week. Anything else that you would like to discuss today?

Mary: No, I'm just glad to hear that all is well.

Clinician: It seems to me that maybe you and your husband are moving into a new stage of your marriage in some ways. Does that seem right to you? How are you doing with that and the other normal stresses of life.

Mary: I hadn't thought of it that way, but now that you mention it we are going through a bit of a change. Jim has taken up woodworking and is very involved with that, and for some reason it makes me angry. I seem to have some of the extra time I have always wanted and would like to do more together as a couple, but I'm not sure what. I guess we are each trying to figure out, you know, what next?

Clinician: Don't underestimate how much transitions and suddenly having extra time can actually be a bit stressful. Maybe you and Jim could discuss this directly and plan for it a bit.

Mary: Interesting thought . . .

In this scenario, the clinician has tentatively predicted stress from a life cycle perspective. She then offered Mary some anticipatory guidance regarding the expectable stress. The provider also chose to point out the normative aspects of family functioning without suggesting pathology or marital problems.

Discussing Direct and Indirect Effects of Stress on Health

As described, excessive stress has both direct and indirect health effects. Primary care clinicians may address the direct and indirect health effects of stress in a variety of ways. As mentioned, the first step is always to talk with patients about their subjective experience of stress. The following section will discuss some specific strategies to employ in helping people manage their stress.

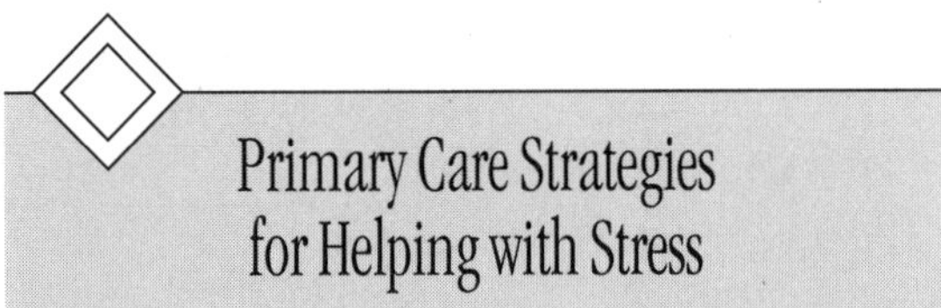

Primary Care Strategies for Helping with Stress

With the reams of existing evidence that stress affects people's health, it seems quite clear that medical clinicians should be in a position to help people with stress. Although the literature describes many effective approaches to stress management, there are few, if any, studies of their efficacy when delivered by primary care clinicians in primary care settings. Most literature about stress in primary care settings has assumed that what works in psychotherapy or stress management classes will also work in primary care offices, but that assumption is vulnerable to many variables. These variables include patient issues, the training of the clinician, the frequency of visits, and time constraints.

The next section describes cognitive behavioral and physiologic stress management techniques for use in short clinic visits. These approaches are differentiated in that the cognitive behavioral techniques intervene with stress on a mental level, whereas stress management intervenes on a physical or bodily level. We will also make recommendations for services that patients may obtain after referral to behavioral health and other providers.

Cognitive Behavioral Approaches

Cognitive behavioral approaches to stress and mental health have been used in the mental health field for decades. These techniques are just now beginning to be empirically validated for primary care use and may only partially translate effectively to primary care settings. Even so, the popularity and knowledge of these approaches is growing among primary care clinicians. In disciplines such as nursing and family medicine, basic training in cognitive behavioral techniques is becoming standard. We will describe enhancing coping strategies, enhancing stress mediation, educational approaches, and writing exercises.

Enhancing Coping Strategies

Often a person's coping responses are shaped by numerous developmental and psychosocial factors. Culture, religion, and gender, as well as family values, habits, and traditions shape the coping strategies people employ. Given the many important factors that contribute to the development of coping strategies, helping patients change their coping strategies can be difficult. Health care clinicians are largely trained to detect pathology and treat it, to identify stress and unhealthy behaviors and stop them. Paradoxically, identifying problems is often quite the opposite of what is actually helpful to most individuals who seek help with stress. Stressed people often know all too well what is wrong! What may be more helpful is identifying what is right, what is working, the strengths in individuals, and harnessing those coping strategies to enhance happiness and health. The suggestion here is that primary care clinicians become as good at diagnosing human health and strength as they are at diagnosing disease and weakness.

Lazurus and Folkman outlined six main areas from which one's capacity to cope is derived. These are health and energy, positive beliefs, material resources, problem solving skills, social skills, and social support. These areas may be used as a guide to the diagnosis of positive strengths and coping abilities. Primary care clinicians may help patients by identifying and reminding them of their coping strengths. It may be helpful to recommend that patients focus on the areas where individuals have well-developed coping skills. Once patients and their clinicians have identified preexisting strengths, clinicians may *prescribe* the use of those strengths as a means of decreasing stress and discomfort.

LUISA TAFT *Luisa comes to see you for fatigue that she's experienced over the past several weeks. You discover that she recently left her job due to job dissatisfaction and limited ability to increase her work responsibilities. She has found it more difficult to find a new job than she anticipated, and she has had car trouble that taxed her financial resources. As her primary care provider of the past 5 years, you know that Luisa is ambitious and persistent, and that she typically exercises and eats well. You both decide that the fatigue is related to the stress. You recommend increased exercise and paying special attention to her diet as a means of helping her to manage her stress. You say, "You know, one thing I know about you is that you have tremendous persistence. That strength will carry you through this. In the past you used exercise and diet to help you overcome the stress at work. Maybe it is a good time to refocus on those positive aspects of your life. I am sure you'll find a job soon, but until then why not use the extra time to renew your exercise program?"*

ENHANCING STRESS MEDIATION

Social support is a powerful mediator of the effects of stress, and social isolation is associated with higher rates of morbidity and mortality. The issue of defining social support is a complicated one; however, by any definition it is clear that having positive involvement with others, having at least one strong nurturing connection with another person, or being involved with social networks enhances one's ability to modulate stress and its effects.

Primary care clinicians should be aware of the social resources their patients have and assist them through coaching and discussion to utilize social supports more frequently during times of stress.

THERESA MADDEN *A physician assistant (PA) notices that Theresa has been to the office each week for 5 consecutive weeks. During each visit, she manages to discuss the stress in her life and seems upset about her circumstances. The conversation goes as follows:*

Theresa: I don't know what to do about it. My kids seem upset and bothered by their dad's new girl friend, but I am in no position to say anything . . .

PA: You know this has been bothering you for weeks now, and it seems like you are really needing to talk about it. It is fine to come in and talk with me, and I think it might help even more if you let a friend or your brother in on what is happening. The more support you get during this transition, the better your health will be. Then you'll be able to be there for your kids while they adjust.

EDUCATIONAL INTERVENTIONS

Educating patients about the role of stress in health and illness can motivate patients to avoid excessive stress or to engage in more healthy behaviors to combat the effects of cumulative stress. For example, there is evidence that chronic stress, lasting longer than 1 month, is associated with increased susceptibility to rhinovirus-induced colds. A clinician might reference this body of research after a patient presents with his second cold in a month, when encouraging that patient to decrease the amount of stress in his life. Such education might give a patient the intellectual motivation necessary to induce behavioral change. Of course, inducing excessive fear in a patient is neither recommended nor helpful, but with some patients it may be helpful to highlight a specific mechanism of stress-related disease.

CARLA LEONARD *Carla, 37, presents to her clinician complaining of severe back pain and muscle spasms in her shoulders. She indicates that she is desperate for relief because her job is presently requiring a lot of computer work. The interaction proceeds as follows:*

Carla: You know, I just can't deal with this right now. My shoulders and neck hurt so much. I have to finish writing a chapter by the end of next week, and I can barely sit up straight in my chair.

Clinician: You've never had back pain like this before. Is there something different going on in your life that may be causing the pain?

Carla: Well, I've had to spend all of my time at the computer and reading. I haven't been able to do the stuff I usually do, like my walking. I haven't even cleaned the house in 2 weeks. I think the posture for typing is getting to me.

Clinician: You know it sounds like you are under a lot of stress at work right now and that time is very precious. I know how that can be, but I think your back pain might be helped by walking, even though it feels like there's no time. There is research to suggest that exercise will decrease muscle tension and maybe even help your cognitive processes. In turn, that could help you get your work done.

Carla: I hadn't thought of it that way. I should probably do stretches too.

Finally, patients who experience the direct physiologic effects of stress such as rapid breathing, dizziness, and palpitations often mistake these normal stress reactions for symptoms of illness. This misinterpretation leads patients to increased stress and to seek medical care. Clinicians can educate patients about the physiologic responses to stress and thereby decrease their worries about their health, as well as increase the likelihood that they will not seek medical care unnecessarily.

Writing Exercises

There is mounting evidence that writing about stressful events and circumstances has significant power to mitigate the physiologic effects of the stress. Smyth found that patients with mild to moderately severe asthma or rheumatoid arthritis who wrote about stressful life events had clinically relevant changes in health status after 4 months as compared to a control group that wrote about emotionally less relevant matters. The instructions to patients were to write for 20 min on 3 consecutive days. Those asthmatic individuals who completed this task as instructed showed increased forced expiratory volume and those with rheumatoid arthritis showed decreased overall disease activity. Although this research has not been extended into primary care settings, this evidence suggests that primary care clinicians may prescribe writing about life traumas and/or stress and worries as an intervention for stress-related illness. Even coaching a patient to list life stresses and rank them in terms of their severity and degree to which they are under the patient's control may help some to feel a sense of mastery and control. Other innovative uses of writing to decrease the impact of stress have been developed. Clinicians should explore such techniques further to establish their potential usefulness in primary care settings.

Physiologic Approaches

Unlike cognitive behavioral approaches to stress management, physiologic approaches require little mental effort. Rather, physiologic approaches focus on the bodily symptoms of stress and act to mitigate those effects by directly interrupting the physiologic effects of stress. Stress has been shown to increase muscle tension, breathing rate, blood pressure, and more subtle measures such as body temperature regulation. If stressed individuals make conscious efforts to attend to and change these effects, they can stop the effect of stress in its somatic tracks. By teaching patients methods for interrupting certain somatic reactions to stress, primary care clinicians can provide their patients with very effective means of stress management. Below we describe progressive muscle relaxation, diaphragmatic breathing, and physical exercise.

Progressive Muscle Relaxation

Patients trained in muscle relaxation techniques can self-induce a physiologic and psychological relaxation response. Physiologic relaxation functions as a form of stress reduction and management. Jacobson introduced the technique of progressive relaxation in 1938. His technique involves developing the capacity to control given sets of muscles by tensing or contracting them. Patients first contract muscles and become aware of the muscle tension, then they release the particular muscle, which gives rise to a more relaxed state in that muscle. Patients progressively contract and release all of the striated muscle groups.

In primary care settings, clinicians may instruct patients in progressive muscle relaxation technique. Minimal instructions should include those shown in Table 4-3. Just as it is important to watch patients for proper technique for use of inhaled medicines, it is important to watch the patient practice tensing some muscle groups, such as the face, stomach, and feet, to give feedback that they are doing well. These exercises are more likely to be successful if you have time to run through each muscle group with the patient. A complete exercise requires 20 to 30 min.

After patients have mastered the basic technique, they may adapt the technique to fit their personal schedules. For example, they may use a shorter exercise with fewer muscle groups while they are at work or when time is an issue. Primary care clinicians should follow up on their recommendations for progressive muscle relaxation by discussing the patient how it went and if it was useful. If the patient finds progressive muscle relaxation useful, recheck his or her technique and reinforce its proper use. If not, attempt to ascertain why and use that information in making other recommendations.

Table 4-3

Instructions for Progressive Muscle Relaxation

1. Find a quiet, private, and comfortable place to perform the exercises.
2. Tense your muscles as hard as you can starting with your feet and moving upward
3. Hold your muscle tightness for a brief time (3–5 seconds) making sure to feel the tension before releasing. This may be repeated several times for each muscle group if time allows.
4. Make funny, tight faces when contracting the face, head, and neck muscles.
5. Breathe normally while practicing the technique.

SOURCE: Adapted from Everly GS: *A Clinical Guide to the Treatment of Human Stress Response*. New York: Plenum; 185–201.

Diaphragmatic Breathing

Another very effective way to decrease the effects of the stress response is to teach patients how to perform diaphragmatic breathing. Use of the diaphragm in breathing has been shown to induce a physiologic state associated with relaxation. This approach is particularly helpful for patients who primarily respond to stress with anxiety or panic attacks. Diaphragmatic or stomach breathing involves teaching a patient to engage in controlled breathing exercises that emphasize the use of the diaphragm. This may be both taught and practiced in a brief office visit.

In our experience, patients learn diaphragmatic breathing technique best by lying down on the exam table and having the provider place their medical chart on their abdomen. The clinician instructs the patient to "breathe slowly or at your normal rate and deeply so as to make your chart rise up and fall down." Encourage the patient to practice at home with a book or magazine. The visual aid allows the patient to monitor their technique. Clinicians should warn patients that this type of breathing can be difficult at first but that it becomes easier as muscles strengthen with practice. Patients should be instructed to practice twice per day for short periods of time for 7 days and then to practice as needed (for a detailed summary of breathing techniques see Barlow and Craske, or Fried, in Mostofsky and Barlow).

Physical Exercise

Physical exercise, in addition to being a healthy behavior, is widely believed to act as a buffer against the stress response. There are a variety of proposed mechanisms for this effect. In primary care settings it is often helpful for primary care clinicians to recommend exercise as a stress management tool, but there is large variation in the extent to which this suggestion is successfully delivered. Some patients find it helpful or more motivating to hear from their clinicians the specific positive effects that exercise has for stress rather than general statements to that end. Other patients will respond well to the suggestion of hiring an exercise coach or personal trainer or entering an exercise program with a friend as a partner. Still others will indicate that the suggestion that they should exercise adds to their level of stress.

Referral Services

Primary care clinicians should also be aware of the vast number of treatments for stress available by referral. Biofeedback, relaxation training, assertiveness training, programmed exercise, psychotherapy, hypnotherapy, tai chi, engagement in spiritually fulfilling activity, and many other interventions have been shown to have efficacy in reducing stress. Many primary care clinicians find that their patients are resistant to such recommendations. It is important that a clinician referring a patient for stress reduction or management *normalize* the patient's stress prior to making the referral. This reduces the feeling of being stigmatized or told that "it is all in your head." An example of normalization is as follows:

TOM GOLDBERG *Tom: I don't know what to do. I can't keep up with the demands at work. I believe that I am about as good at my work as anyone, but what they are asking is too much for anyone. It is like they want me to do the work of two people.*

Clinician: This is your third visit this month. I'm worried that the stress is affecting your health. Have you talked to your boss about this?

Tom: I've never been good at that sort of thing. Anyway I am sure that she would say that if I can't do the job she'll find someone who can, and I need the money that this position brings in. I'm not going to quit but I need something to help me handle it all.

Normalizing statement. . . .

Clinician: Just about everyone goes through times where work stress gets to them. I've suggested assertiveness training for a number of folks, and they have all come back reporting that it was helpful. Might you be interested in something like that?

Or empathize and normalize. . . .

Clinician: Wow, that really sounds stressful, and given that you've got the stress of two teenagers at home too, I am guessing that this stress is affecting you. In fact, I think it would affect anyone in your shoes. There is some evidence that talking about stress can help during times of high stress. Some of my patients go to a stress support group at the hospital. It's free and meets Tuesday evenings at 7:30. If you are interested, check it out. I'd be interested to know what you think of it.

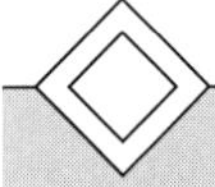

Special Cases

There are a number of special types of stress that deserve focused attention from primary care providers. These include caregiver stress, stress with comorbid psychiatric disorders, stress with comorbid physical illness, stress disorders, and stress and somatization. The following section will briefly discuss some of the issues relevant to caring for these populations.

Caregiver Stress

Because of the recent increase in life expectancy, more people are requiring care from others as they age. Caregiver stress is defined as the emotional, psychological, and physical effects of caring for another human being who is dependent or partially dependent. It is estimated that in the United States, more than 15 million adults currently provide care to dependent relatives. Primary care clinicians should pay particular attention to caregiver stress, because it affects the lives of many apparently healthy individuals.

Studies of individuals who care for spouses with Alzheimer's disease show that chronic stress can cause immunologic dysregulation that continues even after the stressor is removed. Many studies have shown that caregivers may have demonstrable changes in health measures including less response to vaccinations, greater susceptibility to viruses, slower wound healing, more expression of latent viruses, lower rates of preventive health behaviors, and greater cardiovascular reactivity. In fact, the effect of caregiver stress is powerful enough to be an independent risk factor for mortality in elderly caregivers who live with the spouse for whom they provide care.

Primary care clinicians are in a unique position to intervene in this type of stressful situation. Ways to help include evaluating the caregiving demands that exist in the home environment, discussing the stress of caregiving with patients, educating caregivers about the health risks of caregiving, and prescribing for these individuals self-care and periods of respite from caregiving responsibilities. Assistance may also be provided by coaching the caregiver on what to expect over the course of the caregiving period. Coaching about simple techniques to make life easier at home will also provide some relief from stress. Finally, primary care clinicians may be of help with caregiver stress by raising questions that caregivers may not have thought of and by being aware of local resources for dependent adults and their caregivers.

Stress and Comorbid Psychiatric Disorders

Stress has high rates of comorbidity with both physical and psychiatric disorders. In fact, it is widely accepted that stress is a factor that causes patients to bring many psychiatric illnesses to a clinician's attention. It is important, however, to remember that there are many factors that contribute to the development of illness, and stress is but one of them. Most people who suffer from psychiatric disorders report experiencing stress both as a response to the illness and as a causal factor in the development of the illness.

Primary care clinicians often believe that if patients change the stress in their lives, they will recover from the psychiatric illness. This is not always true, and changing stress is often not possible for patients who suffer from both stress and a psychiatric disorder. In cases where a formal psychiatric illness is present, diagnosis and treatment of the psychiatric disorder should usually be provided in tandem with attempts to assist the patient in dealing with the relevant stress. In many cases, when psychiatric conditions are treated, the existing level of stress becomes acceptable or less overwhelming to the individual, who then returns to a prior level of functioning with the cessation of the psychiatric problem. In other cases, patients may have trouble following through with stress reduction and other therapies until the psychiatric disorder is treated. Providers often will be able to identify a recent stress as the trigger for a patient's psychiatric condition. Where this is the case, simply eliminating or discussing the stressor may be enough to change the response that the patient has had to that stress.

A classic example is that of domestic violence. Here a clinician finds his female patient to be suffering from major depression. The clinician believes the woman's depression is related to the fact that her husband is controlling and at times physically abusive. The provider has on numerous occasions counseled the patient to leave her husband or go into couple's therapy. These suggestions are met with passive agreement and inaction on the part of the patient. The provider is hesitant to prescribe medications for depression because he fears he will be "covering up the pain instead of stopping the unjust cause of it." He fears "blaming the victim" by giving her the message that there is something wrong with her. However, this is an example of a case where treating the patient's depression might actually make it easier for the patient to change the circumstance causing the stress. For more information on domestic violence, see Chap. 6, Violence and Abuse as Primary Care Problems.

Other Comorbidity

Stress co-occurring with a physical illness, whether chronic or acute, is important for the primary care clinician to address. Certainly we know that illness, itself, causes stress due to changes that people with illnesses must make in their daily routines to accommodate the illness. This type of stress may best be handled with acknowledgement and empathy provided by the clinician. For example, the clinician might say, "It really isn't fair that you have diabetes and have to take insulin and check your sugars while other kids just get up and go to school. It must be hard that those other kids don't really understand all that you go through just to get to school. It is really unfair."

Stress that exacerbates an existing illness must be addressed in a more active manner so that the trouble the stress causes may be decreased. For example, stress may occur when an illness requires an individual to take special measures to maintain health. The same child with diabetes described above may be teased for being allowed to go to lunch early to check blood sugars and take insulin. To avoid being teased, the child may not check blood sugars or take insulin. In this scenario the clinician might actively discuss the stress caused by checking sugars at school and help the child to find ways to eliminate or modify that stress. Similarly, an air traffic controller with diabetes might be encouraged to work less stressful shifts to avoid high levels of stress, which might affect his glucose metabolism.

Stress Disorders

Post-traumatic stress disorder (PTSD), acute stress disorder, and other formal stress disorders are discussed in Chap. 19. It is important to point out that acute stress, whether traumatic or not, may be prevented from becoming a formal anxiety disorder with intense early intervention. A primary care clinician seeing a patient who has undergone a recent stressful event should encourage the patient to discuss the event and recall it in some detail while allowing associated emotions to emerge. This simple (though sometimes time-consuming) intervention may be very helpful in preventing the event from having long-term negative health sequelae. The primary care clinician may also refer the patient for professional counseling about critical incidents (so-called "critical incident debriefing").

Stress and Somatization

The presentation of medically unexplained symptoms is often attributed to stress (see Chap. 15, Unexplained Physical Symptoms and Somatoform Disorders). When stress is involved in somatization, one may view somatization as a developmentally primitive way of attempting to use coping mechanisms. Specifically, somatization allows for the enlisting of social support from a physician when other social supports are not available. Developmentally, children learn that when they present physical discomfort to their parents, it arouses a heightened sense of attention and protectiveness. This is the most basic form of social support, that between parent and child. Typically, as people mature they develop multiple and reciprocal types of mature social support to serve the role that the parent once did. Should a child grow up with illness in the context of minimally responsive parents or experience other disruptions in social development, the child may learn to overly rely on somatic symptoms as a primary means of mobilizing human contact and social support. In such cases the primary care clinician may serve to buffer symptom expression simply by being a social support and by helping the patient to attain increased and more mature forms of social support.

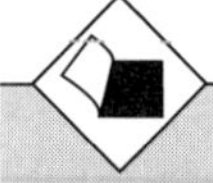

Summary

For 90 years "stress" has been an exciting but complicated area of research and clinical application. The recent findings of stress-related immune changes and neuroendocrine effects are building a fertile ground for the development of interventions that may help to increase quality and even quantity of life. In fact, the development of empirical evidence concerning the effect of stress on health is ahead of the development of practical applications of these findings, particularly in primary care settings.

Healthy People 2000 recognizes the significant health implications of our stressful society, and recommends that stress be reduced in the general population. It also suggests that primary care clinicians have a key role in affecting societal stress reduction. Our review of the literature suggests that there are many pathways to helping patients with stress, and all of them rely heavily on the attainment of good communication skills. Primary care education should provide time for the teaching and practice of talking with patients about stress. Time-efficient techniques that may be used by primary care clinicians exist, but we know little about their true effectiveness. Future research should focus on the effectiveness of brief, office-based interventions for stress as they are performed by primary care clinicians.

Suggested Reading

Mostofsky DI, Barlow DH (eds): *The Management of Stress and Anxiety in Medical Disorders*. Needham Heights, MA: Allyn and Bacon; 2000.

This book details theoretical, physiologic, and psychological knowledge about anxiety. It provides complete discussions of treatment approaches including biofeedback, cognitive behavioral intervention, hypnosis, and breathing techniques.

Mace NL, Rabins PV: *The 36-Hour Day*. Baltimore: The Johns Hopkins University Press; 1991.

This book is an excellent source of information and support for individuals who care for family members with dementia. Primary care providers can gain valuable insight into the lives and experience of their caregiving patients.

Cooper CL (ed): *Handbook of Stress Medicine, and Health*. Boca Raton, FL: CRC Press; 1996.

This book integrates medical and psychological research to provide a comprehensive overview of the relationship between stress and health. Sections explore everyday factors, such as life events, personality, social support, and families, that mediate life stress. There is also a section on prevention.

Kenny DT, Carlson JG, McGuigan FJ, et al (eds): *Stress and Health: Research and Clinical Application*. Amsterdam, The Netherlands: Harwood Academic Publishers; 2000.

This book provides an exhaustive 446-page discussion of stress and health. Subjects include health consequences of stress and management of stress and stress-related disorders. It also provides an excellent overview of recent international research on stress and health.

Hubbard JR, Workman EA (eds): *Handbook of Stress Medicine: An Organ System Approach*. Boca Raton, FL: CRC Press; 1998.

This volume, arranged according to organ systems, explores current research and theories explaining the effects of stress on the physiology and pathology of the body. Other topics include AIDS, cancer, substance abuse, anxiety disorders, and treatment of stress and anxiety disorders.

Bibliography

Barlow DH, Craske MG: *Mastery of Your Anxiety and Panic II*. Albany, NY: Graywind Publications, Inc.; 1994.

Bartlett D: *Stress Perspectives and Processes*. Buckingham, UK: Open University Press; 1998, p 1.

Begany T: Caring for the caregiver. *Patient Care* 30:108, 1996.

Boone JL, Christensen JF: In: Feldman MD, Christensen JF, (eds): *Behavioral Medicine in Primary Care*. Stamford, CT: Apppleton & Lange; 1997, p 265.

Borkovec T, Grayson J, Cooper K: Treatment of general tension: Subjective and physiological effects of progressive relaxation. *J Consult Clin Psychol* 46:518, 1978.

Brosschot F, Godaert GL, Benschop RJ, et al: Experimental stress and immunological reactivity: A closer look at perceived uncontrollability. *Psychosom Med* 60:359, 1998.

Cohen S, Frank E, Doyle WJ, et al: Types of stressors that increase susceptibility to the common cold in health adults. *Health Psychol* 17:214, 1998.

DeCarteret JC: Occupational stress claims: Effects on workers' compensation. *Am Assoc Occupa Health Nurs J* 42:494, 1994. Cited by: Lyon B: Stress, coping and health—A conceptional view. In: Rice VH (ed):

Handbook of Stress, Coping and Health—Implications for Nursing Research, Theory, and Practice. Thousand Oaks, CA: Sage; 2000, p 23.

Department of Health, Education and Welfare: *Healthy People: The Surgeon General's Report on Health Promotion and Disease Prevention.* Public Health Service Publication No. 79-55071, 1979.

Eriksen HR, Olff M, Murison R, et al: The time dimension in stress responses: Relevance for survival and health. *Psychiatry Res* 85:39, 1999.

Fried R: Breathing as a clinical tool. In: Mostofsky DI, Barlow DH (eds): *The Management of Stress and Anxiety in Medical Disorders.* Needham Heights, MA: Allyn and Bacon; 2000.

Gervirtz R: The physiology of stress. In: Kenny DT, Carlson JG, McGuigan FJ, et al (eds): *Stress and Health—Research and Clinical Applications.* Amsterdam, Netherlands: Harwood Academic Press; 2000, p 53.

Glaser R, Rabin B, Chesney M, et al: Stress-induced immunomodulation—Implications for infectious diseases? *JAMA* 281:2268, 1999.

Herbert TB, Cohen S: Stress and immunity in humans: A meta-analytic review. *Psychosom Med.* 55:364, 1993.

Holmes T, Rahe R: The social readjustment rating scale. *J Psychosom Res* 12:213, 1967.

Jacobson E: *Progressive Relaxation.* Chicago: The University of Chicago Press; 1938.

Kemeny ME, Laudenslager ML: Beyond stress: The role of individual difference factors in psychoneuroimmunology. *Brain Behav Immun* 13:73, 1999.

Kenny DT: Psychological foundations of stress and coping: A developmental perspective. In: Kenny DT, Carlson JG, McGuigan FJ, et al (eds): *Stress and Health: Research and Clinical Application.* Amsterdam, The Netherlands: Harwood Academic Publishers; 2000, p 73.

Kiecolt-Glaser JK: Stress, personal relationships and immune function: Health implications. *Brain Behav Immun* 13:61, 1999.

Krantz DS, Sheps DS, Carney RM, et al: Effects of mental stress in patients with coronary artery disease. *JAMA* 283:1800, 2000.

Lampe A, Sollner W, Krismer M, et al: The impact of stressful life events on exacerbation of chronic low-back pain. *J Psychosom Res* 44:555, 1998.

Lazarus RS, Folkman S: *Stress, Appraisal and Coping.* New York: Springer; 1984.

Lieberman JA: BATHE: An approach to the interview process in the primary care setting. *J Clin Psychiatry* 58(Suppl 3):3, 1997.

Lemack GE, Uzzo RG, Poppas DP: Effects of stress on male reproductive function. In: Hubbard JR, Workman EA (eds): *Handbook of Stress Medicine: An Organ System Approach.* Boca Raton, FL: CRC Press; 1998, p 141.

Lundberg U: Stress responses in low-status jobs and their relationship to health risks: Musculoskeletal disorders. *Ann NY Acad Sci* 896:162, 1999.

Lyon B: Stress, coping and health—A conceptional view. In: Rice VH (ed): *Handbook of Stress, Coping and Health—Implications for Nursing Research, Theory, and Practice.* Thousand Oaks, CA: Sage; 2000, p 3.

Mace NL, Rabins PV: *The 36-Hour Day.* Baltimore, MD: The Johns Hopkins University Press; 1991.

Olden K: Stress and the gastrointestinal tract. In: Hubbard JR, Workman EA (eds): *Handbook of Stress Medicine: An Organ System Approach.* Boca Raton, FL: CRC Press; 1998, p 87.

Olff M: Stress, depression and immunity: The role of defense and coping styles. *Psychiatry Res* 85:7, 1999.

Petruzzello SJ: Recent advances in mind-body understandings. In: Rippe JM (ed): *Lifestyle Medicine.* Malden, MA: Blackwell Science; 1999, p 947.

Seligman ME, Csikszentmihalyi M: Positive psychology. *Am Psychol* 55:1, 2000.

Selye H: *The Stress of Life.* New York: McGraw-Hill; 1956.

Shultz R, Beach SR: Caregiving as a risk factor for mortality. *JAMA* 282:2215, 1999.

Smyth JM, Stone AA, Hurewitz A, et al: Effects of writing about stressful experiences on symptom reduction in patients with asthma or rheumatoid arthritis: A randomized trial. *JAMA* 128:1304, 2000.

Sriram TG, Silverman JL: The effects of stress on the respiratory system. In: Hubbard JR, Workman EA (eds): *Handbook of Stress Medicine: An Organ System Approach.* Boca Raton, FL: CRC Press; 1998, p 45.

Steptoe A: The links between stress and illness. *J Psychosom Res* 35:633, 1991.

Stone AA, Bovbjerg DH, Neale JM, et al: Development of common cold symptoms following experimental rhinovirus infection is related to prior stressful life events. *Behav Med* 18:115, 1992.

Stuart MR, Lieberman JA III: *The Fifteen Minute Hour: Applied Psychotherapy for the Primary Care Physician,* 2nd ed. Westport, CT: Praeger, 1993.

Taylor SE, Kemeny ME, Bower JE, et al: Psychological resources, positive illusions and health. *Am Psychol* 55:99, 2000.

Vieweg WV, Hubbard JR: Mental stress and the cardiovascular system. In: Hubbard JR, Workman EA (eds): *Handbook of Stress Medicine: An Organ System Approach*. Boca Raton, FL: CRC Press; 1998, p 17.

Veldhuis JD, Yoshida K, Iranmanesh A: The effects of mental and metabolic stress on the female reproductive system and female reproductive hormones. In: Hubbard JR, Workman EA (eds): *Handbook of Stress Medicine: An Organ System Approach*. Boca Raton, FL: CRC Press; 1998, p 115.

Weine SM, Kulenovic AD, Pavkovic I, et al: Testimony psychotherapy in Bosnian refugees: A pilot study. *Am J Psychiatry* 155:1720, 1998.

Williams GO, Gjerde CL, Hauglandd S, et al: Patients with dementia and their caregivers 3 years after diagnosis. *Arch Fam Med* 4:512, 1995.

Clydette Stulp deGroot
Elizabeth W. Staton

Reactions to Illness

Introduction

Why does one patient with a cold come to see a clinician when another person with the same symptoms does not? For the person who comes into your office, the runny nose, sneezing, and sore throat may not be a big deal; however, the fact that last year the same symptoms turned into pneumonia and a 3-day hospitalization may make the illness seem more urgent and cause the patient to present for care. Or perhaps the patient is a former smoker and wants reassurance that the symptoms are not cancer. Maybe the patient is going out of town and wants to know how to feel better quickly. The symptoms could also be an "anniversary reaction" to the death of a child, and the patient comes in because he or she needs some emotional support. The cold symptoms in each of these situations may be routine cold symptoms, but the reaction the person has to the symptoms is subjective and variable.

However impressive the technologic advances of medical sciences, a person's experience of illness and medical care is at the heart of the first purpose of clinical medicine: the relief of human suffering. Suffering is the subjective experience that may or may not respond to therapeutic regimens directed toward the pathologic processes of disease, even when those regimens are technically effective. According to Mechanic, people's reactions to their illness and what they think about the experience of illness, as much as the technical quality of care, will determine how they benefit from and use the health care system.

Illness and particularly chronic illness is not only an individual, subjective experience, but it is also interpersonal and social. Chronic conditions shape the physical, social, psychological, vocational, cultural, familial, and financial functioning of those affected. Consider the following examples.

ALAN AND DIANE REED *Alan Reed was stunned when he suffered a major heart attack at his office desk one morning. He was the 52-year-old chief executive officer of a company he had started 20 years earlier. At 6' 1", Alan was slender, exercised three times a week, had never smoked, and was an enthusiastic, respected leader. He became a great patient; sailing through a double bypass, attending cardiac rehabilitation with the support of his wife Diane, and seeing his primary care clinician for regular follow-up. However, his life gradually changed in other ways. He became less interested in his business, his marital relationship, and sex, and he eventually withdrew into inactivity. His physical findings got better and his stress tests looked great, but something in him had died.*

CAROL CULLEN *Carol's first symptoms began when she was 34. She would wake with aches in her hands, elbows, and knees. Sometimes she noticed swelling. Until the development of these problems, she felt she was doing a great job of handling multiple demands, including her job as an accountant, her marriage, the children, and a home. After many months of attributing her malaise to the stress of raising two small children, she went to her primary care clinician. Her clinician knew her well because she had seen Carol each time she brought the children for well-child check ups, the croup, coughs, and colds. As Carol's symptoms worsened, her clinician concluded she was suffering from early stages of rheumatoid arthritis.*

Carol is now 42. Her two oldest children are in junior high and high school, and she has a 3-year old at home. Her arthritis flare ups come and go, but the pain has worsened. She finds it frustrating and depressing to not be able to do things with her children. The bicycle rides, hikes, and roller blading they shared are a thing of the past. She cut back at her job to 2 days a week and notices she can no longer grip the vacuum cleaner. Her husband tries to understand, but feels the loss resulting from his wife's limited energy and increasing frustration. Carol works hard to stay upbeat. She has taken antidepressants during the worst periods of depression resulting from her illness, and she tries to reassure her friends she is "fine." Her women friends notice, however, that she is not the same person she used to be.

JOYCE, ANGELA, AND ZACH RUIZ *Joyce Ruiz had not wanted to be a single parent, but the death of her husband due to colon cancer 6 years earlier left her no choice. Her daughter Angela is now 17, and Zach just turned 12. Joyce teaches in a public school and works as a freelance tutor in the evenings and during the summer to make ends meet. Being able to drive, Angela has been a great help to her mom. Two weeks ago, Angela suffered a broken leg in a gymnastics accident at school. Typically a good-natured and competent teen, she now is frustrated by the slightest inconvenience, yells at Zach, is demanding, and, in the words of her mother, acts like she is in the "terrible twos" again.*

With few exceptions, illness and injury generate emotional reactions. As demonstrated by the Reed, Cullen, and Ruiz families, people react in highly individualized and emotional ways to physical symptoms and diagnoses. When Angela broke her leg, she was no longer the independent teenager she once was. She was frustrated, angry, and irritable. Alan Reed had always handled multiple responsibilities in his life, but now he struggles to deal with his physical vulnerability and is uncertain about making decisions. Carol recognizes that her condition is worsening and feels she is being robbed of parts of her life.

A person's illness creates a state of disequilibrium for those with whom they are close. Angela was not the only one who suffered; the entire family responded to Angela's injury. Her mother, Joyce, scaled back her work obligations to help her daughter learn to walk on crutches and care for herself. The family felt the tension and financial pressure of Angela's limited mobility. In this family, the equilibrium will likely return once the cast comes off. Alan's and Diane's lives changed permanently, and Carol works hard to hang on to a sense of normalcy despite her long-term limitations.

When caring for people with illness, whether short-term, chronic, or disabling, clinicians must understand the subjective experience of illness. Illness often leads to numerous negative reactions as people endure the challenges of coping with something that they had not expected. The patient's subjective experience is intrinsically important in determining the quality of care, and clinicians who recognize this are more likely to help patients with not just the physical, but also the social, familial, and emotional aspects of illnesses. Although the medical system is geared to address the physical problems, the persons suffering are dealing with the effect of these physical problems on their lives. As a primary care clinician, you will be addressing both the physical problems and their effects on your patients' lives.

This chapter is not about examining psychosocial pathology. Rather, we will be looking at the everyday, normal human reactions to suffering, physical compromise, reduced mobility, and unexpected medical diagnoses—that is, reactions to illness. Illness is a broad concept and needs to be defined in terms of the patient, rather than an impersonal part of the body. Illness includes the response and reaction of the patient to the problem, including how the problem affects the person's behavior or relationships, the person's past experiences of illness, and the meaning he or she gives to the experience. Throughout this chapter, we use the collective term "illness" to refer to acute and chronic disease, traumatic injury, and disability.

The purpose of this chapter is to describe a range of possible reactions to illness that your patients may experience. First, we discuss the concept of illness in terms that may help clinicians understand their patients' experiences. Next, we discuss the characteristics of patients, families, and illnesses that affect their reactions to illnesses. We then focus on strategies that clinicians can use to understand their patients' reactions and respond compassionately and effectively. We begin by exploring in the next section how patients' experiences of and reactions to illness are related to the care giving process.

Illness Takes Many Forms Across the Life Cycle

Illness can take many forms, from acute, minor physical symptoms to severe and debilitating chronic conditions. No single factor determines who gets sick, how serious the illness will be, or how people will cope. Due to medical advances, the first attack of a serious illness (e.g., heart attack, cancer, AIDS) rarely ends in death. People can live for a long time with the diagnosis of cancer, diabetes, AIDS, and others. Children often live with illnesses such as asthma, diabetes, and cancers for their whole lives.

Throughout life, illness, and particularly chronic illness, may interfere with the developmental stages of life. The ill person may not be able to maintain a long-term relationship, have children, or successfully navigate a satisfying career. When illness begins in midlife, it can disrupt the family, work life, and finances, all of which affects partners and children. Illness late in life is common, especially chronic illness. Estimates are that 85 percent of the elderly have a chronic condition, and half of these chronic health problems cause serious physical limitations.

Getting sick usually happens over time, but a diagnosis is given in a moment. Although Alan Reed had ignored minor chest pains and shortness of breath, his heart attack was acute. His family suddenly had to adapt to a life-threatening condition. Over time, everyone had to learn to adjust to the chronicity of the situation and to adapt to new roles of care giving and an altered life style.

In contrast, a diagnosis of rheumatoid arthritis follows a gradual onset of symptoms, typified by progressive deterioration of joint function and increasing discomfort. Adjustment to this gradual onset of a chronic condition may be punctuated by periods of acutely increased symptoms. The person who is suffering and the person's family will adjust over time as they become familiar with each stage and degree of incapacitation.

Throughout the varying courses an illness can take, people will wonder about certain issues. Rarely will they directly ask questions, but they nonetheless would like some answers. The next section describes some of the questions that people have when they become ill.

Questions Most People Worry About—But Often Do Not Ask

ALAN AND DIANE REED (CONTINUED) *Alan was alarmed each time he felt the slightest twinge in his left arm. Like most people would, he kept looking for psychological or circumstantial causes for his symptoms. He wanted to make his symptoms disappear by changing habits and behaviors. Sometimes those changes added stress. When the dietician at cardiac rehabilitation told him he should eliminate ice cream from his diet, he felt even more angst. A highlight of his month was making homemade ice cream with his grandchildren the last Sunday of each month. He also felt strain in his relationships, particularly with his wife, and he knew his personality had changed.*

Internally, Alan, like most people suffering from illness or injury, replayed a number of questions in his mind:

- *What is happening to me?*
- *Why has it happened?*
- *Why is it happening to me?*
- *Why now?*
- *What should I be doing?*

Helman suggests that people's ideas and models about their illness are based on their desires to answer key questions with reference to a particular problem. These questions are the ones most people ask themselves when they realize they are sick, but people may never address these questions with their clinician. Helman codified the questions into seven areas (Table 5-1). These seven general questions are important for the primary care clinician to keep in mind. They are the driving questions that motivate patients' reactions and behaviors about an illness.

Explanatory Model of Illness

As we discuss reactions to illness, it is important to make a distinction between disease and illness. "Disease" and "illness" are terms often used inter-

Table 5-1

Questions People Ask Themselves when They Are Sick, but May Not Address with Their Clinician

1. What has happened?
2. Why has it happened?
3. Why has it happened to me?
4. Why now?
5. What would happen to me if nothing were done about it?
6. What are its likely effects on other people if nothing were done about it?
7. What should I do or to whom should I turn for help?

SOURCE: Helman CG: *Culture, Health and Illness*, 2nd ed. London: Butterworth, 1990.

changeably, but Arthur Kleinman, a well-known psychiatrist and anthropologist, and others highlight the differences. When a clinician adheres to the biomedical model, the patient's focus is on the pathology of the diseased or injured part of the body. Consequently the physician interprets the patient's *symptoms* as the "problem" or "disease." The clinician examines the history, physical, laboratory, and other findings in light of biological or disease-related theories. Measures of body temperature, blood composition, and presence or absence of infection are part of the "disease conversation." Because these terms refer to measurements, they are the "objective" findings.

Illness, on the other hand, is fundamentally different from disease. Illness, according to Kleinman, is the innately human experience of suffering. While disease is about bodily functioning, illness is about how the sick person and members of his or her family and support network perceive, live with, and adapt to the physical symptoms. Illness is about the fears, frustrations, losses, and anxiety of living in a body that is hurting. Illness complaints are what patients and their families bring to clinicians. For the patient, illness is about the physical problems, but more importantly involves what is happening to the patient's life.

According to Kleinman, "the experience of illness includes attaching meaning or significance to the sickness event."[1] Individuals attach their meaning to illness in relation to their sense of self; their cultural context of beliefs, values, learned and expected behaviors; and their relationships with parents, partners, spouses, friends, peers, coworkers, and caregivers.

One person with a new diagnosis may interpret its meaning as a death sentence, whereas another may see it as a challenge to overcome. When Carol Cullen finally realized the nature of her diagnosis, she recalls sitting alone in the exam room while her clinician went to get her some educational brochures.

CAROL CULLEN (CONTINUED) *"At first I was afraid that life as I knew it was fading away, and then I was angry at myself, thinking I had caused this by trying to do too much. But I also knew I had to make a plan. In those few moments, alone with my fear, I thought about how I got through lots of challenges in my life. As a child, my father always told me I could get through anything if I took one day at a time and worked hard. I told myself, 'Just work hard and you will get through this, too!'"*

Angela, on the other hand, has a broken leg. That is her "disease." Her illness is the isolation, loneliness, frustration, and loss of independence, particularly at a time when she was thriving in her new-found independence. And although Alan Reed has cardiac problems, his illness is about his pain, devastation, and fear about how weak he feels and what his future may bring.

The notions people have about an episode of sickness and its treatment are called their explana-

[1]Kleinman AM: Explanatory models in health care relationships: A conceptual frame for research on family-based health-care activities in relation to folk and professional forms of clinical care. In: Stoeckle J (ed): *Encounters Between Patients and Doctors*. Cambridge, MA: MIT Press; 1987.

tory model. As a clinician, learning how your patients understand their illness and making sense of their reactions to it is central to caring.

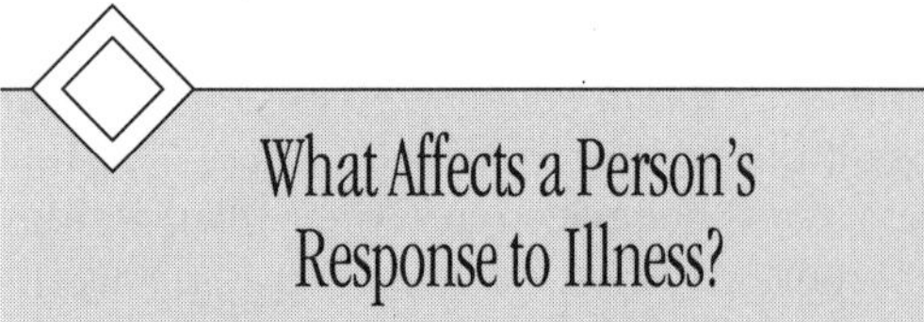

What Affects a Person's Response to Illness?

The psychological reactions to an illness depend on a number of factors, including the nature and severity of the physical symptoms, the person's cultural and family context, how the illness affects functioning, and past experiences with illnesses, clinicians, and the health care system.

The Nature and Severity of the Physical Symptoms or Diagnosis

Clearly, the more debilitating and life-threatening an illness, the more marked a person's psychological reactions. The more someone perceives an illness as altering his or her body image, self-esteem, life roles, or identity, the more intense the reactions. Roles and identity develop and change throughout a lifetime. Severe and disabling illnesses of sudden onset are more likely to initially be viewed as crises. Both Carol Cullen and Alan Reed will face long-term consequences from their illnesses and these consequences may weigh on their minds. On the other hand, Angela's recovery will be nearly over by the time her cast comes off. The severity of the illness is only one issue that affects people's response to illness. Culture and family also influence these responses.

The Patient's Cultural and Family Context

A key characteristic of cultures and families is the manner in which they approach pain and suffering. Although ethnicity is often considered the core of culture, our image of the world, learned cognitive world view, religious orientation, heritage, community, family system, and beliefs about health and medical treatment all contribute to those things we call "culture." To understand individual reactions to illness—especially chronic illness—it is essential to comprehend the personal context each person has for suffering.

Everyone has developed (or will develop at the moment of an illness) a theory about suffering, even if the person has never consciously articulated this theory. In the example of the Reed family, Alan has embodied his family's positive Puritan attitude, so he approaches his cardiac illness as he does other parts of his life: he works hard and responds well to clear direction. On the other hand, Joyce Ruiz still struggles with the loss of her husband in a system "that could not help him." She reads prolifically before a meeting with her clinician and frequently brings information to her medical visits. She is not ready to trust where she feels she has been let down.

Illness does not just happen to the person who is experiencing it. Illness also happens for others in that person's life. The necessary day-to-day and psychological adaptations to illness, the changing family roles provoked by the illness, and the stresses of caring for the ill person are some of the challenges families face. Acute, chronic, and disabling conditions are powerful forces that disrupt the structure of families and the actions and reactions of family members. Illness can effect sweeping changes in family roles and isolate family members from each other and outside connections. Chronic illness, in particular, often finds the weak links in the family and exaggerates them. Of course, no two families are ever the same. Under stress some people, like families, are strengthened, whereas others are weakened. Either way, they all change.

There are some typical patterns of how illness changes a family. When a child is sick or injured, the mother often takes on the role of primary care provider. She may become the "designated nurturer and worrier." She seeks to gather knowledge about the child's problems and makes sure things are handled. Consequently, the family system shifts as the mother develops a closer relationship with the ill child and begins to identify with her role as caregiver. If there are other children, they may feel distance and begin to shift their ideas about how to get the nurturing they need. Siblings may react to the loss of parental attention or may over-identify with the ill person, worry about their own health, and even develop somatic symptoms. Joyce's second child, Zach, began to regress after his sister's accident.

ZACH RUIZ (CONTINUED) *Zach had been an excellent student and liked school. Two weeks after Angela's accident, things changed. He got into trouble at school and stopped doing homework. His teacher reported that he "pouted when asked to do something in class and complained about feeling sick." As he regressed in reaction to feeling abandoned by his mother's attention to Angela, he unconsciously sought more help and recognition.*

When there is a father figure present in the family, his role shifts also. If a father has been the primary provider and handled challenges by taking control, illness in the family is particularly difficult. The problem becomes "how do I take control of something I do not seem to be able to control?" The mother's primary alliance has now shifted to the ill child, while the father is trying to figure out how he fits.

Spousal relationships are universally influenced by illness. Alan and Diane Reed both "tried" to keep things "normal," which meant that they could function as usual, but both worried about the other one. Diane watched Alan like a hawk, not wanting him out of her sight for even a moment. Alan, also worried about his life and future, began to feel suffocated by Diane's vigilance.

When a parent is in poor health, the children react. Some move immediately into the care giving role, and others act out. Some teenagers may act as if health problems in a parent were a personal inconvenience. Some teenagers report that once their parent became ill, they felt like they were suffering from decreased "receiving." Consequently, ill parents can feel like their children are punishing them.

As patients learn to act as the "person who is ill," family members and caregivers learn to treat patients in ways that perpetuate this view. Frequently, family members feel even greater anxiety and stress than the person who has the special health needs. The resulting anger and guilt can shift a normally functioning family into an anxious, frustrated, and guilty group of people. Illness changes the psychological and familial balance, often forever. The longer the illness is present, the longer it takes to regain a sense of balance in the family.

The Illness' Effect on the Person's Daily and Future Functioning

In addition to the nature of the illness and patient's cultural context, worries about future functioning can significantly affect the way patients react to illness. Symptoms that do not go away, fear of serious illness, or diagnosis of major illness require people to adjust to a state of compromised well-being or "disease."

Although Alan Reed had a heart attack and survived with a prognosis for a good recovery, he became withdrawn and afraid. As much as he tried to pay attention to his business and colleagues, he was distracted and turned inward. He relinquished work responsibilities over to his company vice presidents. He was functioning physically but knew he was not the same emotionally. Angela regressed, and was passive, angry, and pessimistic, even though her leg injury was temporary. Carol's arthritis left her feeling like her body was betraying her with the pain and decreased energy. Daily she lived quietly with her fear that her body was falling apart. As these patients demonstrate, illness can have a dramatic influence on one's functioning—physical as well as interpersonal and psychological.

Understanding disease progression may help clinicians comprehend a patient's level of functioning; however, understanding how well the patient *thinks* he or she is functioning is essential. Research by Berkanovic and colleagues and Clark and colleagues suggests that patients' self-reports, combined with clinicians' examination, are better indicators of physical limitation than biologically based indicators of disease progression.

Angela is a teenager with a broken leg. Her functional impairment affects her life, but to a limited degree and for perhaps only a few weeks. Contrast this with Richard, a 39-year-old single parent. He tripped, bracing the fall with his right hand, and suffered serious structural damage to the hand. His work life suffered along with his home life. He struggled to manage the basics, he could not pick his 8-year-old son up from school or do the grocery shopping unless he got a ride or took a taxi.

Illness is typically an unplanned event in someone's life and increases the sense of dependency, discomfort, powerlessness, loss of energy, loss of mobility, and concern over physical symptoms. Some of the common limitations and feelings people associate with being ill, contrasted with what most people experience when they feel healthy, are summarized in Table 5-2. This overview, developed by Shontz and Heinman, is useful for clinicians to consider when working with patients.

The role that individuals usually play in life are central to how they function. When individuals are ill, they develop an altered identity. This identity may take on new labels such as *patient, tired, restricted, unpredictable, inadequate, dependent, worried,* and *searching*. Family members and friends may also adopt these labels as part of the sick person's identity. A person who has become the primary support person faces role changes too, and may feel overprotective, tireless, selfless, worried, and burdened. Ironically, these shifted identities function in concert: the tireless wife taking care of the exhausted husband, the overprotective mother caring for the restricted daughter, and the codependent friend taking care of the patient. Depending on the nature of the illness,

Table 5-2

Common Experiences Associated with Illness and Health

Healthy People Are Likely to Experience	When Sick, People Are More Likely to Experience
Independence	Dependence
Energy	Low energy
Sense of well-being (physical and psychological)	Physical pain or psychological discomfort, which affect sense of well-being
Mobility	Limited mobility
Normal bodily functioning	Inability to depend on their body to function normally
Ability to control events over which control can be ordinarily exercised	Inability to control ordinary events
Ability to fulfill life roles (mother, father, worker, lover, etc.)	Compromised ability to fulfill roles and unsure of new role during illness
Little contact with health care world	Frequent contact with health care world
The ability to give attention to others	Withdrawing from others to conserve inner resources
Personal focus on others	Tendency to focus on self and symptoms
Ability to contemplate a future	Fear of the future
Optimism	Pessimism
Assertiveness	Passivity

Source: Shontz FC: *The Psychological Aspects of Physical Illness and Disability.* New York: MacMillan, 1975, p. 112.

these unconscious role shifts may become permanent. The relationship begins to depend on the new roles, and there is no return to healthy relationship functioning.

The Person's Past Experiences with Illnesses, Clinicians, and the Health Care System

As a primary care clinician, you will want to know about the patient's prior experience with illness, clinicians, and the health care system. Patients' past experiences form the beliefs and attitudes that influence how they approach the current illness. When Carol Cullen learned she had rheumatoid arthritis, she did not question anything her primary care clinician told her. She outwardly approached her illness with stoicism. She had learned to be matter of fact about pain and discomfort as a child. Joyce Ruiz, on the other hand, had a difficult time during her late husband's chronic illness and ultimate death. She partially blames herself for his death and still thinks he may have survived had she have taken an assertive role and demanded more aggressive care for him. Consequently, she is proactive and demanding to make sure she and her children get the care they need.

When people become patients, they may also have reactions to the clinicians caring for them. These reactions evolve from experiences of being cared for in their families and from prior treatment by clinicians. Typically, if children have confidence and trust in their parents, they are more likely to trust medical clinicians as adults. Likewise, if they could not depend on their parents and felt neglected, they will be hesitant to trust even the best of clinicians.

The Ill Person Faces the Threat of Loss, Separation, and Pain

One of the more complex issues that affects patients' reactions to their illnesses is a series of threats they face. The onset of illness brings a number of threats to people's sense of self, and this affects the way they act and the emotions they display. Either consciously or subconsciously, we are challenged to maintain some emotional balance, keep our relationships functioning, cope with the unknown, and deal with the process of seeking care.

Illness is an instant threat to a person's sense of competency and general well-being. Strain and Grossman, in their work with chronically ill patients, describe common threats experienced by people with an illness, including (1) loss of efficacy, (2) loss of love, (3) loss of functioning or body parts, (4) loss of control and rationality, and (5) pain and suffering. The magnitude and subsequent reactions to these five areas of threat depend on the nature and severity of the illness.

Threat of Loss of Self-Efficacy

Self-efficacy is defined as one's belief in his or her own ability to carry out a particular behavior. When individuals are sick, they notice that they do not function as they did before and may begin to believe they *cannot* function like before. Their self-esteem is challenged because the illness may interfere with their ability to perform a job, function at home, or enjoy leisure time. The threat of job interference, job changes, or job loss because of an illness can be overwhelming.

Alan Reed (continued) *At work, Alan began to doubt himself. He was not sure if he was really tired or just being overly cautious. He felt he was worrying more about how to do his job than actually doing it. At home, he was confronted with his limitations when he realized that he could not lift his granddaughter, because he was not supposed to lift anything over 20 lb. He could no longer hold and play with her, as he loved to do.*

Joyce and Angela Ruiz (continued) *One morning Joyce found Angela sobbing in her bedroom. "I just can't do anything anymore—I can't drive, I can't stand, and I can hardly walk. How am I supposed to get decent grades or have any friends when I am like this?"*

Threat of Loss of Love

Early in the course of an illness, most people find themselves turning inward. The newfound preoccupation with the body, functioning, and the future can be overwhelming. Soon there is an evident feeling of being disconnected from others. Inevitably, the quality of an ill person's relationships is affected because of the constraints produced by illness. Those who are ill may perceive that they have changed the unspoken "contracts" of their key relationships, and they therefore fear the loss of those relationships. The effect appears to be more substantial with degenerative or unpredictable illness, especially those involving pain or impaired cognitive functioning.

Not only are individuals confronted with the potential loss of relationships, but sometimes they also face the prospect of being alone. People who fear the loss of a relationship may engage in medically contraindicated behaviors. For example, the person suffering from diabetes conceals the need for support and engages in behaviors that exacerbate the condition, such as eating the family's traditional Sunday dinners of high-fat foods.

Depending on the nature of the illness, people may fear a loss of intimacy. Alan Reed admits that he does not want his wife to see him becoming weaker, so he tries to do all the things he was previously doing. When she is at work, he naps to hide the extent of his weakness from her. She has attended all of his appointments and seems to enjoy the caregiving role. He is worried and says he does not want her to get tired of caring for him. Sex is the furthest thing from his mind and when he does think about it, he is afraid he could not function as he once did anyway.

Patients also commonly feel that friendships are threatened by the changes associated with an illness. After Angela's accident, Joyce felt like her world became smaller. She explains, "One of the things I had to learn to do was pare down my friends. I was running out of energy. Sometimes it's ironic that relationships change right when you could really use more support." When there is an ongoing illness in the family, everyone adjusts the way they connect to each other.

The process of illness, especially chronic illness can force dependency on others. For some, this dependency rekindles early childhood fears of being apart from those who comfort us. Illness generates a powerful vulnerability, even in the strongest person. Being vulnerable and dependent are uncomfortable for those who have previously been in charge of their own lives.

Threat of Loss of Functioning

Any compromise of physical functioning is frightening. As people get sick, their bodies can begin to feel like prisons. Fear of loss of strength, stamina, continence, and mobility are just a few of the challenges ill people face. When individuals lose their health, and particularly the ability to function, they lose part of themselves as a whole person.

JOE MARTINEZ *Joe Martinez had become the patriarch of his rural community. As his diabetes progressed, he was unable to leave the house except in a wheelchair. He was embarrassed and feared humiliation if anyone saw him unable to walk. He stayed in his home and invited friends to visit. His wife would greet visitors at the door and bring them into the sitting area so they would not realize Joe could not walk. When he had to leave the house to go to his medical appointments, he would leave early in the morning, before anyone was up and would wait hours before returning home, just so no one would see him. How could he be the pillar of strength in his community if he could not get around? For Joe, losing his ability to function physically was also a loss to his sense of identity.*

For Joe and thousands of others, it is difficult to accept the limitations imposed by an illness. Even worse, there is the embarrassment, shame, and stress of trying to communicate the limitations to others.

Threat of Loss of Control and Rationality

Illness can compromise cognitive functioning and rational thinking. This loss of familiar rationality may be due to the illness, medication, or a combination of factors. Taking medications, being in pain, and being unable to do the things one was used to doing all contribute to forgetfulness, loss of previous mental functioning, and difficulty concentrating. People fear they are losing "control," which can be terrifying when people are not expecting it and do not realize it may be associated with the illness or the treatment. The threat of loss of control is then compounded by the anxiety of becoming dependent on strangers. For many people, the health care system is unfamiliar and intimidating, especially for those who have not developed relationships with their clinicians.

Threat of Pain and Suffering

No one wants to hurt, and we all fear suffering. Pain is one of the most feared and debilitating aspects of illness. Studies reported by Walker show that many people, when sick, live with a lot of pain.

The fact that pain is subjective and that individuals have different responses to pain and pain thresholds makes assessment and management difficult. In a 1989 study, 58 percent of randomly selected medical and surgical patients reported having "horrible" or "excruciating" pain at some point, and only one-third reported experiencing relief at any time.

CAROL CULLEN (CONTINUED) *Carol has never known the kind of pain she is in now. More and more she cries when she is in the shower. She wants to keep handling her responsibilities for her family, her job, and her marriage, but finds it harder and harder. She is learning to be more open and tell her clinician how bad the pain really is. Consequently, she is getting different medication and more relief. But she continues to worry that her pain may get worse.*

As clinicians, sensitivity to our patients' fears and psychological reactions to pain is a step toward alleviating as much potential suffering as possible.

Summary of Threats Ill People Face

As we have discussed, people facing illness may feel threatened by many aspects of their changed lives. These threats give rise to the adaptive tasks we must all face when we get sick. The next section describes the adaptations that ill people make so they can continue to function on some level.

The Ill Person Must Adapt to Being Ill—The Challenges People Face

During the course of an illness, patients experience life changes that disrupt the way they perceive their life and world. This disruption demands that the patient adapt psychologically to their changed word. Rarely does someone change easily or without some struggle. Researchers agree that adaptation is a process of change in reactions that is triggered by functional limitations associated with injury or illness.

Alan Reed, Angela Ruiz, Carol Cullen, and most other people suffering from illness have to cope with personal emotional ups and downs, adjust to changes in relationships, deal with the unknown, and learn to adapt to the health care system. They may not be conscious that they are adapting; they just know life is changing around them. As a clinician, being aware of common adaptive processes helps to deal with the disease as well as the spirit of the person experiencing it. The following sections highlight a number of common ways people adapt to illness.

Maintaining Emotional Balance

The stresses of illness challenge each person's internal emotional equilibrium. When a person becomes a patient, "weathering" the emotional challenges can have significant implications for quality of life and the care received. Common emotional reactions are described in more detail in the section titled, "The Ill Person Will Display Normal Emotional Reactions."

As described, Alan Reed was alarmed at his frustration and lethargy. He saw his marriage changing and felt like he was riding a roller coaster of feelings. His wife, on the other hand, said as times she felt like a boiling teapot with the holes plugged. Life gets more difficult in the face of illness, and being able to find suitable coping strategies that help gain some emotional balance is central to the process of care.

Preserving Relationships

Relationships change when someone is ill. Some people withdraw because of lack of energy and other people become demanding. Each relationship dynamic is affected.

GAYLE AND JACK *Gayle had always been physically affectionate during her 33-year marriage. When her husband Jack returned home from the hospital after a 5-day stay for a complicated gallbladder surgery, Gayle had "moved" into the guest bedroom. Weak and feeling vulnerable, Jack did not say anything. However, the sadness and loneliness of not being touched was overwhelming. Even he was aware of his increasing dependency behaviors as a way of connecting with her. Some months later, she "moved" back into their bedroom. When they did talk about it, she said she was very scared about his recovery and had not wanted to accidentally bump or hurt him. Jack still worries that she will "move away" if he gets sick again.*

Coping with the Changes and the Unknown

Illness can potentially disrupt all that grounds us to stability in our life. Our connection with certainty and other people and sense of our own identity are strained.

ALAN REED (CONTINUED) *Alan does not know what is going to happen to him next, how much he should do, or how his colleagues, wife, and children are perceiving him. He feels "shaky," like his world is quaking around him.*

ANGELA RUIZ (CONTINUED) *Angela felt like she had finally gained control of her world once she could drive. Not surprisingly, when she became injured she felt like a "kid" again.*

The future is more precarious when someone is ill. Dealing with new circumstances and the unfamiliar faces of the health care system can be daunting.

Adapting to Health Care Providers

Patients react to their illness, their clinicians, and the health care system. Learning to navigate appointments, clinics, laboratories, receptionists, and health insurance companies is challenging even to those who are well. When we get sick, we suddenly enter an unfamiliar world with new faces. It takes energy to develop new relationships and to adapt to a sometimes overwhelming system. Building new relationships with clinicians and the health care system is a challenging but necessary part of adapting to life's unexpected circumstance.

The Ill Person Will Display Normal Emotional Reactions

In the course of a lifetime, most people will experience a number of personally traumatic incidents, such as the loss of an important relationship, a serious conflict with family or friends, failure, being victimized, the death of someone close, or a serious health problem. When such traumatic or difficult life events occur, there are associated physical, cognitive, and emotional reactions. Common physical responses can include fatigue, insomnia, hypersomnia, underactivity, headaches, nightmares, hyperactivity, startle reactions, and exhaustion. Cognitively, people often experience difficulty concentrating, solving problems, and making decisions. They may notice some memory disturbance, have flashbacks, or be unable to give importance to anything other than the illness. Emotional responses to illness, particularly life-threatening illness, include shock, fear, oversensitivity, emotional numbing, frustration, anger, feelings of helplessness or powerlessness, and depression. Although illness offers no uniform course of emotional responses, a number of emotions will be experienced by nearly all people at some time during the course of their illness.

There is no right way to feel or react in response to challenging life events. A normal reaction to a challenging life event should not be perceived as a problem by the patient or by the clinician. However, if you understand that these reactions are normal and will occur, you can react positively in a number of ways. First, you can help your patients appreciate that what they are experiencing is a natural and common experience. Second, you can be empathetic about their pain and frustration and allow them to talk about it. Third, you can help people access support when their reactions become overwhelming.

Kubler-Ross and others have proposed models of adaptation to crises, illness, and loss. Each of these models describes mourning and adaptation phases to grief and bereavement following personal crises. Common to each mode of adaptation to chronic illness and disability are the specific emotional reactions of shock, anxiety, denial, depression, internalized anger, externalized hostility, acknowledgment, and adjustment. The common thread in the work of all of these authors is that there are stages each person traverses, the order of which may vary from person to person.

Although the degree and intensity of emotional reactions will differ from person to person and illness to illness, there are common and predictable emotional states that are helpful for the patient as well as for the clinician to recognize. Fear, regression, denial, anxiety, powerlessness, anger, sadness, and depression are some of the most common feelings associated with illness according to Moos and Schaefer. Table 5-3 highlights these reactions common to the process of adapting to an illness.

The following section discusses these common emotional reactions to illness. The intensity and depth of the affective response can be related to the nature and severity of the illness, as well as the nature and severity of perception of the illness on the part of the person who is suffering.

Table 5-3

Common Reactions During the Process of Adapting to Illness

STAGE OF REACTION	EMOTIONAL REACTION
Immediate	Shock Anxiery Fear
Short-term	Denial Anger Frustration Regression
Longer-term	Powerlessness Depression

SHOCK, ANXIETY, AND FEAR

Fear or shock is an individual's initial reaction to a sudden or severe physical injury or psychological trauma, such as the diagnosis of a perceived life-threatening disease. These primal feelings are common to all when our life or well-being is threatened. Almost any illness is sure to generate anxiety or fear.

Anxiety is sometimes seen as the panic reaction upon the initial sensing of the magnitude of the illness. This reaction can be characterized by confused thinking, overactivity, rapid pulse, fast breathing, and other physiologic changes. Even the calmest of patients can become anxious while waiting for test results and definitive diagnoses, anticipating invasive procedures, and experiencing life style and relationship changes in reaction to the illness. Anxiety and fear vary in intensity and form throughout the course of an illness. These feelings can cause autonomic nervous system reactions such as sweating, palpitations, gastrointestinal symptoms, and insomnia. When anxiety is not addressed and the patient does not experience some relief, it can adversely affect the disease process.

Denial

Denial is a common defense against the painful realization of the potential of an illness event. This powerful adaptive strategy counters the stress, anxiety, and other distressing emotions generated by life crises. This negation or minimization gives someone permission not to have to cope immediately with the challenge ahead. Shortly after Alan Reed returned to his office following his heart attack, he wanted to get back to all the things he was used to doing. When asked if they could help, he told colleagues he was back to normal. Denial was helping Alan protect himself from confronting and being overwhelmed by the threat of losing his ability to be strong. Initially, the idea that he might be sick was inconvenient, especially in his rapid-paced culture where individuals are encouraged to be strong and independent. His denial allowed him to gradually assimilate how his life was changing while holding on to his sense of self.

Denial helps us process threatening information. Breznitz and others suggest there are a number of things we deny in the face of a chronic or disabling illness, including denial of personal relevance, urgency, vulnerability, our emotions, emotional reactions in others around us, threatening information, or even all information. Sometimes this is expressed by wishful or unrealistic expectations of recovery, or the person may seem indifferent and unaffected by the reality. Denial helps the ill person to avoid the difficult task of coming to terms with reality. In the early stages, this can be helpful, unless immediate decision making and action are necessary.

In Joyce Ruiz's situation, her extended family was generally in denial that things had changed. They believed everything was "just fine." If they had accompanied Angela to her treatments, they may have had to acknowledge that Joyce was having a problem coping with everything.

The depth of denial depends on the person and the circumstances. Some may deny their vulnerability and fears, whereas others deny the urgency or threat of a situation. As an adaptive strategy, denial is important to survival when it counters the stress and anxiety brought about by illness.

Anger and Frustration

Fear is a precursor to anger. To say, "I am afraid" is uncomfortable, and people often do not say it. Soon the repressed fear is expressed as anger, either as internalized anger or externalized hostility. Internalized anger refers to feelings associated with self-blame. The self-blame may be related to guilt from not engaging in preventive behavior or can result from a lack of clinical improvement.

When externalized, anger appears as hostility. The hostility is directed at other persons, objects, or aspects believed to be associated with onset of the disease and its subsequent disability. Aggressive acts, such as verbalizing blame toward others, feelings of antagonism, demanding and critical behavior, abusive accusations, and passive-aggressive modes of interaction, can lead to obstruction of medical treatment as well as a frustrated clinician. Openly addressing a patient's frustration and anger can help alleviate some of the angst for the patient and make the clinician's work easier.

Regression

A return to earlier patterns of adaptation and behavior is regression. We often rely on childlike states of emotional functioning in response to the threat of an illness. When someone gets sick, the universal response to that sickness encourages an increased emotional and physical dependency. The ill person feels more vulnerable. If you see a clinician, you are relying on the clinician to do something that will help you. Your normal day-to-day functioning can be compromised. While one patient may become demanding and aggressive, another may be withdrawn and weepy. Limited regression can be adaptive by permitting needed rest and recovery from acute illnesses and during exacerbations of chronic illnesses.

Powerlessness and Depression

Powerlessness and depression are common responses to the loss, helplessness, isolation, and distress caused by illness. Illness sometimes strips even the strongest of their ability to control their world. Working harder and trying more can be met with the discouraging reminders of limitations and weakness. This powerlessness leads to depression and, in the most difficult situations, "giving up."

Rodin and colleagues report that people with a family or personal history of depression are more likely to become depressed as a reaction to damaged self-esteem and other losses associated with illness. Furthermore, depression can be caused or exacerbated by biological and neurochemical changes associated with some diseases and disabilities.

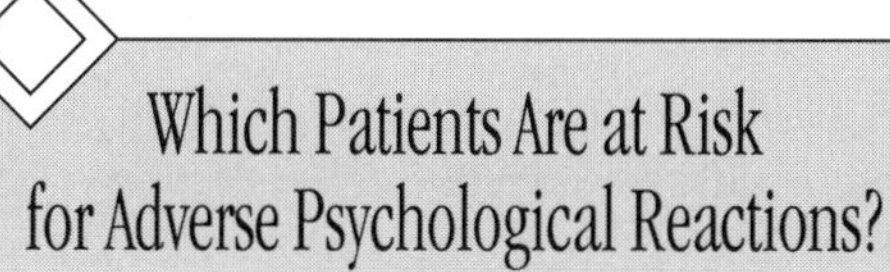

Which Patients Are at Risk for Adverse Psychological Reactions?

For the most part, people who are ill respond to their illness in common and generally adaptive ways. Coping with physical illness and disability often reflects the patient' habitual modes of dealing with threatening and hard situations. When someone has successfully adjusted to a serious illness or disability, they will demonstrate the following: (1) psychosocial equilibrium; (2) awareness of resources and functional limitations; (3) positive self-concept, self-esteem, and sense of control; (4) an ability to negotiate their environment; and (5) participation in appropriate social and vocational activities. Additionally, those who use more active, directive, problem-focused, information seeking and social-support seeking ways of coping report more successful adaptation to illness according to Livneh.

Adaptation to chronic illness or disability is complicated by a number of mediating and intervening factors, including cognitive impairment associated with the illness, chronicity of the illness, coping skills prior to the onset of illness, severity of functional limitations, accessibility of family or other supportive people, and availability of resources. Other risk factors for difficult adaptation include a previous history of psychiatric illness, unrealistic expectations, and fantasies about the illness.

Those whose coping mode is passive, nondirective, self-blaming, or avoidance-escape-resignation are more likely to have an unsuccessful course of adaptation to a serious illness. Additionally, those at greater risk for difficulty in adapting typically have lower self-esteem, withdraw socially, and are prone to denying their limitations.

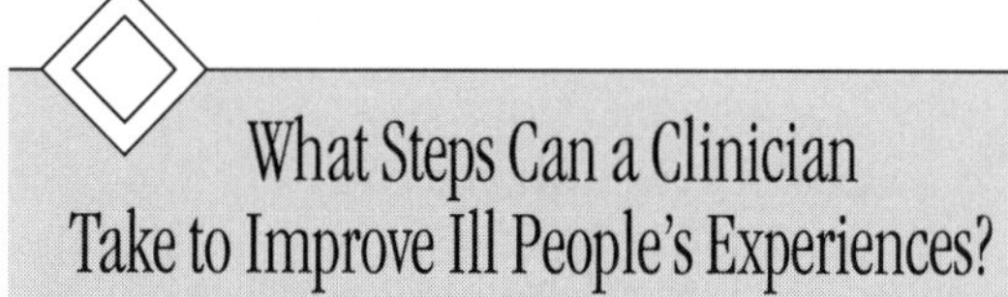

What Steps Can a Clinician Take to Improve Ill People's Experiences?

In the previous sections of this chapter, we described specific characteristics of the illness and the person that can affect the way patients react to their illnesses. We outlined the steps that patients go through when they find out they have an illness (threats–adaptation–emotional reactions). Finally, we summarized characteristics of patients who are at increased risk of having adverse psychological responses to illness.

Now we turn to describing what you, the clinician, can do to help patients deal with the enormity of being ill (even when you think the situation does not appear serious). Remember the point of the first sections of the chapter: patients' reactions to illness are subjective and affect the way the patient and his family manage when faced with what they perceive is a crisis. The first step toward effectively addressing the issue of reactions to illness is to understand your relationship with the patient and family.

Recognize the Nature of Your Relationship

When your patients are suffering from a chronic illness and you see them over months or even years, the relationship you build is at the heart of what you do as a primary care clinician. As you engage your patient as an ally, you begin to develop a partnership that supports you both in being effective. This section discusses three key issues to consider as you develop an effective alliance with the patient and the patient's family:

1. Who else in this patient's life is involved in the illness?
2. What is your role when working with this patient/family?
3. What phase of relationship are you in with the patient?

Who Else in This Patient's Life Is Involved in His Illness?

What other relationships are central to the person's care? Given that family members, extended family, and friends will have an influence on the patient's course of recovery and well-being, learning about some of these relationships allows you to include others in the care process. Long after the ill person is well, others close to him will still be dealing with changes in their lives resulting from their caregiving. Just as patients have ideas about their illness, they also have ideas about who else in their lives may be helpful to their healing and recovery process. Because illness occurs in the context of the patient's life, find out early who is significant to the patient and how they are significant. When appropriate, include family members and significant others in visits and treatment planning.

What Is Your Role When Working with This Patient/Family?

Many theorists have examined how clinicians and patients interact depending on the nature and course of an illness. Fig. 5-1 summarizes three basic models of the clinician–patient relationship. During the course of working with a patient, you will engage in each of the three roles: activity-passivity, guidance-cooperation, and mutual participation.

With the activity-passivity relationship model, the clinician is in control and takes responsibility for the functioning of the patient. This role is probably least used in primary care. The guidance-cooperation model underlies much of medical practice and is an interaction where the patient, troubled with symptoms such as fever or acute infection, actively seeks help from a clinician. The clinician makes recommendations to the patient, and the patient is expected to cooperate. In the mutual participation or partnership model, the clinician and patient have an alliance and share in

Figure 5-1

Model	Clincian's Role	Patient's Role
Activity-passivity	Does something to the patient	Passive recipient
Guidance-cooperation	Tells patient what to do	Cooperator (obeys)
Mutual participation	Helps patient help himself or herself	Participant in "partnership" (uses expert help)

Three basic models of the clinician–patient relationship. *(Adapted from Szasz PS, Hollander MH: A contribution to the philosophy of medicine: The basic models of the doctor-patient relationship.* Arch Intern Med *97:585, 1956.)*

decision making; the clinician helps patients to help themselves. The clinician and patient work together over time in a dynamic process of negotiation, reinforcement, and efficacy building. When patients are actively involved in their care, their outcomes are better.

Throughout the course of working with someone, notice the role you take. Whether you are the active decision-maker, providing guidance, or collaborating as partners, be aware that you have choices and flexibility in how you think about the relationship. Not all patients will respond the same way to being in a partnership role; however, as they gain strength and a sense of control over their situation, you both will be glad the patient is engaged in the process.

WHAT IS THE PHASE OF YOUR RELATIONSHIP WITH THIS PATIENT?

The British physician Michael Balint introduced the idea of phases in the clinician–patient relationship. His ideas about the patient and clinician interaction have influenced primary care education and practice for nearly 40 years. Balint suggests that the clinician–patient interaction is a four-phase process that takes place over time.

First, the patient brings an illness, in the form of symptoms or complaints, to the clinician. Patients usually have a tentative explanation of what they think is going on, as well as unexpressed fears about potential outcomes. The task of this first phase is to learn as much about what patients know about their symptoms as possible.

Second, the clinician has a view of the patient's situation. The clinician quickly develops ideas about the patient's complaints and symptoms and brings to the interaction core beliefs and feelings (based on medical knowledge and personal experience) about the nature of the patient's medical complaints.

As a result of the first two phases, the goal of the third phase of the relationship is to reach some common ground of understanding. This transpires when patients feel their physical and affective concerns have been addressed and the clinician is confident that the patient's problems have been dealt with appropriately. When this happens, the clinician–patient relationship proceeds smoothly.

The fourth phase is the consequence of what occurred in the first three phases. Successful navigation of this phase requires integrating the patient's view of the world with that of the clinician. Agreement between clinician and patient often leads to improved satisfaction, medical care, adherence to diagnostic or treatment recommendations, and medical outcomes. Expressed or unexpressed disagreement between patient and clinician can lead to dissatisfaction, poor diagnostic and treatment plans, and less than desired outcomes. Fleming found that when both the patient's and clinician's beliefs are incorporated into the negotiated treatment plan, compliance, acceptance of the plan, and outcomes improve.

When working with a person with an illness, it is paramount to know how the patient understands her condition. Ultimately, taking the time to unravel the patient's explanatory model of illness in the first phase offers essential information, sets the stage for the rest of the phases to go smoothly, and saves time over the course of the clinician–patient relationship.

Involve the Patient and the Patient's Family in the Process

Family members, significant others, and close friends may have a greater influence than the clinician on a patient's experience of illness. Patients depend on families to help make decisions and advocate for them. The single largest provider of most people's care is a family member, according to Griffith and Griffith. Families, however, do not necessarily always know what to do and may need to learn from the clinician about what the patient needs. Tansella found that involving the family and supportive others early can improve the caregiver's knowledge and the family's overall functioning around the illness. Engage family members when possible in the discussions about dealing with the illness. Families often want and need the same things the patient needs: someone to know they are concerned, that they need information, and that they have questions about what to do. Give them a chance to talk.

While the patient is focusing on the immediate physical symptoms, it may be the family members that are worried about the long-term process of recovery. Alan's wife, Diane, was involved in his care, attending all visits with him. As Alan's strength and energy returned and he was feeling "back to his regular self" again, it was Diane who was still worried. She asked the clinician more questions than Alan did about the exercise, diet, and prevention program and expressed more concerns about Alan's overall well-being.

Learn as Much as You Can about the Patient and Family's View of the Illness

As Lewis Barnett suggests in *Essentials of Family Medicine,* "The commonplace experience of the clinician often deals with life-shaping issues for the patient."[2] Similarly, someone once said that the science of medicine has to do with the ways in which all people are alike, and the art of medicine has to do with the ways in which all people are different. When we are talking about our patients' individual stories, we are talking about the art. The good clinician, when conversing with patients, will draw upon learning and experience to provide an informed and humane response, an enlightened interest in the person, and a willingness to try to understand the events and circumstances of that individual.

Patient's stories about their symptoms, how their lives are changing, their fears, and their concerns are their "illness" experience. This story will help both you and the patient make sense of the patient's medical challenge. In the following section, we discuss specific ways that you can learn about your patients' view of their illnesses. You should begin by simply having a discussion.

Be Willing to Have the Illness Conversation

When individuals are sick, what happens to their body happens to their *life.* Lab results and medical data are important to the sick person, but equally vital are the fears, anxieties, suffering, and disappointments that go along with them. As the primary clinician caring for a person with a life-threatening illness, you need to hear the "disease talk" regarding the patient's problem, and he needs to have the "illness conversation," telling the story about what is happening. As individuals become patients, they learn to talk "disease talk." Patients will model this conversation after what they learn from their clinicians, and share the disease conversation with their family and friends. When one of Alan Reed's colleagues asked him how he was doing, he responded, "I think pretty good. My cardiac tests are stable, my last EKG was normal, and the treadmill looked good." Alan had learned to speak of his illness as though it was separate from him as a person.

However, internally Alan was worried about his life, his marriage, his future, and whether or not he could play with his grandchildren. The illness was the experience of living with the disease, and was potentially a lonely experience for him. Even the briefest "illness conversation" can alleviate some of patients' stress, fear, and frustration of being in a body that is breaking down. The following section offers specific ideas to help you quickly learn about the patient's explanatory model of illness and give the patient the opportunity to talk about their experience with the illness.

Ask Quality Questions to Uncover the Patient's Explanatory Model of Their Illness

Effective questions are one of your most powerful tools as a clinician. Questions communicate interest and concern and help you to learn about the patient. To learn about a person's disease, it is essential to ask information-gathering questions

[2]Barnett LB: From cradle to rocker: Providing care across the human life cycle. In: Sloane PD, Slatt LM, Curtis P, et al (eds): *Essentials of Family Medicine*, 3rd ed. New York: Lippincott Williams & Wilkins; 1998.

such as, "When did this start?" "Where is the pain?" and "When are you most uncomfortable?" These clinically driven questions are important, because the answers help you to reach a possible diagnosis and decide the next course of action; however, they are not the whole picture.

Patients come to a clinician with a lot of other information about their symptoms. They naturally bring four other pieces of essential information.

1. Their own ideas about the nature of the problem, its causes, its importance, and its possible outcome
2. Concerns about what is happening to their life because of these symptoms
3. Expectations about the visit
4. Experiences of successful coping (self-efficacy)

These ideas, concerns, and expectations originate from the patient's previous experiences with medical care. Occasionally these ideas, concerns, and expectations agree with those of the clinician; however, when they differ, it is useful information for the clinician to understand. Use the questions described in this section (Table 5-4) to help you learn about your patients' ideas, concerns, and expectations while creating the partnership relationship paramount to working effectively over time. More immediately, using the questions will help both you and your patients make sense out of what they need. Thinking about these questions also helps patients understand their care and begin to address their underlying concerns. As the clinician, you will have access to your patient's explanatory model of her illness—important information to help you work well with the person with the illness.

The questions presented here presuppose that individuals have thought about their illness, have ideas about what is going on, and have attempted to remedy the situation. Understanding the role that patients have already played in their own illnesses and the role they want in the future is fundamental to effective care. In addition to being

Table 5-4

Questions to Elicit Patient's Ideas, Concerns, and Self-Efficacy

Ideas	1. What ideas do you have about what has caused (or is causing) this problem (or injury)? 2. What ideas do you have about why this is happening now? 3. What ideas do you have about what your illness (or injury) does to your body?
Concerns	1. What concerns you most about your illness? *or* 2. What are your main concerns about your illness?
Expectations	1. When you came in today, what is the one thing you hoped would happen? 2. What do you think would be most helpful to you now? 3. What kind of treatment do you think you need now? 4. What kind of results do you hope to receive from this treatment?
Self efficacy	1. What have you done so far that have been helpful to you? 2. What are some of the ways you are effectively managing your symptoms? 3. What have others done that has been helpful? 4. What resources (people, services, etc.) are likely to be the most helpful to you?

helpful to the patient, these questions, which focus on the four central areas of patients' ideas, concerns, expectations, and successful coping (self-efficacy), will aid your assessment process and can be helpful to ongoing monitoring during the course of care.

Ideas: Eliciting the Patient's Ideas about the Illness

WHAT *IDEAS* DO YOU HAVE ABOUT WHAT HAS CAUSED THIS PROBLEM (OR INJURY)? This question helps discover the potential etiology of the problem, at least the one the patient is concerned about. You will learn information about the patient's history that is not likely to be revealed otherwise. In one of Alan's follow-up visits to his primary care clinician, he was asked what ideas he had about what contributed to his heart attack. Alan talked about recently returning to the mountains of Colorado after 6 months of living at sea level. He was worried that he had developed a reaction to the altitude. Also, he was worried about selling his company and thought he was "pretty stressed."

A more vivid example of the utility of asking the patient about her ideas is the example of 34-year-old Lisa.

LISA *This was the third time Lisa had seen her clinician in the past 2 weeks. Again, she complained of a sore throat. Lab tests had been done at the prior visits, and the results were negative. When her clinician said she was at a loss and asked Lisa about her ideas regarding what was causing this "soreness," Lisa broke down in tears and talked about an incident with her boyfriend where he tried to choke her. She had had a "sore throat" since.*

WHAT *IDEAS* DO YOU HAVE ABOUT WHY THIS IS HAPPENING NOW? This question reaches the patient's ideas about the onset of the problem and about the significance (if there is any) of the symptoms occurring now. When Alan Reed's clinician asked him what ideas he had about why this was happening now, Alan talked about his transition out of his business. He also mentioned his sadness of not hearing from his daughter for the past year and realizing he was not going to see her again this holiday season.

WHAT *IDEAS* DO YOU HAVE ABOUT WHAT YOUR SICKNESS (OR INJURY) DOES TO YOU AND YOUR BODY? It is difficult to appreciate all the contextual and cultural nuances playing a part in someone's reaction to symptoms. However, these questions open the door to essential information about how patients think about what is happening in their body and their perception of severity.

When Angela Ruiz's clinician asked her what ideas she had about what her broken leg was doing to her body, she replied, "I'm afraid I am never going to walk without limping again, let alone drive or dance, or have friends . . . (starts to sob) . . . I'll be a geek . . . and my mom acts like its all really no big deal."

Concerns: Eliciting the Patient's Concerns about the Illness

Questions about concerns and worries provide valuable information about patients' emotional reactions and can help the clinician generate ideas about prognosis.

WHAT *CONCERNS* YOU MOST ABOUT YOUR SICKNESS? WHAT ARE YOUR MAIN *CONCERNS* ABOUT THIS ILLNESS? These questions elicit the core threat and subsequent fears a patient is experiencing, giving the clinician an opportunity to respond with empathy, validate the emotional reactions, and help the patient reconcile those threats and fears with medical reality. Often, patients' fears are more severe than the reality of what is happening. As addressed earlier in this chapter, the person who comes in because of cold symptoms may actually be afraid of dying from pneumonia, because that is what happened to a relative. If this fear is not acknowledged during the meeting, the patient feels only minimal relief, and the symptoms may even escalate. Because we know that beliefs can be a predictor of illness outcomes, asking well-designed questions can sometimes reach the root of a health-influencing belief rather quickly. As clinicians, you then can play a role in influencing that belief.

Expectations: Eliciting the Patient's Expectations about Her Care

1. When you came in today, what is the one thing you hoped would happen?
2. What do you think would be most helpful to you now?
3. What kind of treatment do you think you need now?
4. What kind of results do you hope to receive from this treatment?

Asking these questions uncovers the patient's unspoken expectation(s) about the visit and treatment. This information helps you appreciate what kinds of treatment are most likely to be effective for this patient. Many times people are at a loss and will give minimal responses to questions about treatment. When Carol Cullen's clinician asked what she thought would be most helpful, Carol said it would be to tell her what to expect over the next few years, so that she could prepare. "I know this is not likely to get better, but I want to know what to do to make sure it doesn't get any worse than it has to."

Coping and Self-Efficacy: Eliciting Information about Successful Coping and Self-Efficacy

In addition to asking patients about their ideas, concerns, and expectations, inquiring about coping and self-efficacy helps mobilize positive self-care behaviors.

1. What have you done so far that has been helpful to you?
2. What have your family or others done that has been helpful?
3. What are some of the ways that you are effectively managing your symptoms?
4. What resources (people, services, etc.) could be helpful to you?

These questions assume that patients have done something so far to help themselves. These questions also presuppose competency on the part of the patient. Notice the difference if you ask the patient, "Have you done anything that was helpful?" They might say "no," and you feel like you have hit a barrier. The patient's sense of self-efficacy and options for coping can increase as she talks about the things she has done to help herself. By responding to the question, patients remind themselves about some of their options and where they might access support in their life. You and the patient stay in a partnership role, and this ultimately reinforces helpful behaviors.

Angela Ruiz (continued) *When Angela's clinician asked her what she had done so far to help her to get around and take care of herself since she broke her leg, Angela looked at him in some disbelief and asked, "What have I done?" She then went on to say, "Well, I have been practicing with my crutches, and I did put my school stuff in a backpack so I could carry it myself." He and Angela then discussed other ideas she had for staying active while her leg was healing.*

Of course, it is not feasible to ask all the ideas, concerns, expectations, self-efficacy questions in any one meeting with a patient. The key is to notice how the patient responds and use these questions to gain a deeper understanding of the illness process. With attention and practice, these questions can become part of your practice repertoire.

When clinicians and patients enter a dialogue that includes these issues, they begin to jointly answer the universal questions patients bring but often do not ask. Remember that earlier we discussed that many people who are ill wonder (1) What has happened? (2) Why has it happened? (3) Why is this happening to me? (4) Why now? (5) What would happen is nothing was done about it? (6) What are the likely effects on other people if nothing is done? (7) What should I do, or whom should I turn to for help? Patient-focused questions about cause, possible diagnosis, treatment ideas, prognosis, and coping can help the patient become more comfortable with the understanding of his illness. It can guide your partnership with the patient, help you discover what is relevant to the patient, and direct your interventions.

Provide Emotional Support

When people are free to express the natural emotional reactions associated with illness, they are more likely to gain control over what is happening to them. People are less overwhelmed when they can share their fear, self-doubt, frustration, anger, and sorrow with someone. In addition to good medical treatment, your patients want to know that you understand their struggle. The goal in empathic listening is to lessen the person's distress and enhance support. Emotional support conveys a sense of sincere concern and caring for someone. Being supportive of someone evokes images of gentle reassurance, addressing the unspoken feelings behind the words, or simply acknowledging the patient's efforts. In his work on emotional and social support, Wortman developed a taxonomy that defines support (emotional and social) as the following:

- Encouraging a patient to express beliefs and feelings openly;
- Acknowledging a patient's feelings, beliefs, or interpretations;
- Expressing positive affect, including the sense that the sick person is cared for or esteemed;
- Providing appropriate advice and needed information; and
- Giving the patient a sense of belonging to a network or support system of mutual obligation or reciprocal help.

We cannot overstate the therapeutic value of allowing patients to express illness-related affect. Noticing how the person is feeling, asking questions to elicit concerns, and empathically reflecting those back to the patient acknowledges and validates their experience. Acknowledging someone's emotional reaction reassures the individual that you understand.

Sometimes clinicians have mentioned that they are afraid to acknowledge a patient's affect, for fear the patient will never stop expressing, crying, or talking about the fears, anxieties, and so on. This is rarely the case. Once a patient feels that you understand, the patient is often ready to move on. The goal is acknowledgement and emotional support, not to "fix" the feelings. However, not addressing the struggle diminishes trust in the relationship and can causes the feelings to escalate. Notice the difference in the examples below.

CAROL CULLEN (CONTINUED) *Carol saw her clinician after a tough weekend of arthritic pain. She sat in the exam room, hunched over, looking ashen and tired. When her clinician saw her, he said, "You look pretty tough. This is a crummy way to feel, isn't it?"*

Carol sat up, sighed and said, "Yes . . . I am having trouble picking up my baby because of the pain and that breaks my heart."

"That must hurt almost more than the pain," he replied.

Muffling her words a bit, she responded, "You're right . . . it does."

He then went on to discuss an agenda for the visit that day, keeping Carol engaged in the process. "It sounds like this is a big concern for you today . . . shall we see what we can figure out to deal with the pain?"

Later Carol mentioned how relieved she was that her clinician understood her misery. Note that what the clinician did was give her a chance to express how she was reacting to her situation and acknowledged her "hurt." As a result, Carol felt the validation of his empathy. Now they were both ready to move on.

The opposite of empathy in communication terms is invalidation. This is what happens when you express feelings and the person to whom you are speaking contradicts or rejects your feelings. When the feeling happens to be anxiety, sorrow, or fear, the rejection can be especially painful.

CAROL CULLEN (CONTINUED) *During her weekend of agony, Carol called a friend. Well-meaning, her friend assured her, "Oh, don't worry, I'm sure you will be better in a few days. Maybe if you just relaxed a little you would feel better. A hot bath always helps."*

Carol's friend, trying to be supportive, ended up minimizing Carol's experience. This produced more pain for Carol and prevented a possible supportive interaction from occurring.

Another example illustrates the effect of emotional support. Alan Reed is having a follow-up appointment with his primary care clinician.

ALAN REED (CONTINUED) *The clinician walks into the exam room, and, looking at Alan's chart, says "So, it looks like you're doing great . . . the tests are back to normal, your last treadmill was good, and cardiac rehab says you have been coming weekly."*

Alan responds, "I have been going to rehab, but, man, I just don't have any energy and can't get motivated to do much."

The clinician then says, "That will come with time, you've just got to hang in there . . . everything is looking good."

As contrasted with this reply:

The clinician then says, "You seemed pretty discouraged about the lack of energy and motivation. This has to be concerning."

As a result of that more facilitative response from the clinician, Alan says, "You know, it really is . . . I'm worried that something else is wrong that I need to be paying attention to. I've always been able to do anything, and now I'm even afraid to go to sleep at night for fear of not waking up."

There is now a greater likelihood that Alan and his clinician can have a more productive visit, where Alan's real concerns can be addressed.

In summary, providing emotional support is really about acknowledging the affect associated with illness. However, it is a lot to expect a primary care clinician to be the sole emotional support for all patients when necessary; therefore, it is appropriate to seek collaboration, particularly with mental health professionals.

Provide Information to the Patient and the Patient's Family/Support System

Individualization, feedback, reinforcement, and involvement of the family in the patient education process increase the effectiveness of information. Information is important to patients. The absence of information about the illness leads to misunderstanding and anxiety for both the patient and the family. They need information and they need to understand how to incorporate the information into their situations. Additionally, the more the patient and the family are involved in the care, the more they are able to use information effectively.

Earlier we discussed the comfort people often feel when they have "enough" information about what is happening to them. When the clinician carefully tells the patient about what is going to happen, common things they might expect, and common emotional reactions that can occur, the patient often feels more secure and less anxious when those things actually do happen. The reactions are expected and, therefore, feel "normal."

Typically, patients value information about their prognosis, diagnosis, and cause of illness according to Kindelan and Kent. However, each patient and his family respond best to information tailored to them. Some patients mange the stress of their illness by focusing on detailed information. They can feel in control when they know everything they can about their illness, the tests, the treatments, and the expected outcomes. Others become overwhelmed when given too much information, and may not need such detailed information.

As a clinician, monitor the situation by asking people what information is helpful and if they need more. Also check to see whether they need help in processing the information that you give them. When you recognize that a patient needs a lot of information, answer the patient's questions as fully as possible and ask what other information would be helpful.

Help Strengthen Patient and Family Adaptive Responses

What you see in your office is only the tip of the iceberg of what is really going on in a person's life as the individual deals with health problems and readjusts her world around those problems. Such patients need support, and so do their families. Patients affect families and families affect patients. Constant stress resulting from inadequate functioning can also adversely affect the health of another family member. Even though the primary focus is the health and development of an individual, the family's role is paramount to coping with illness, particularly chronic illness.

Being connected to a support system outside the family can make the future more manageable for patients and families. There are local and national organizations that offer assistance for almost every major chronic illness. These organizations sponsor support and educational groups, have Internet sites, and send out educational materials or newsletters. Support groups often offer education about all aspects of a condition, practical advice from people struggling with the same issue, a chance to express feelings without guilt or fear, and separate support for friends and family members who may be dealing with different issues.

ALAN AND DIANE REED (CONTINUED) *Helping her husband cope with his illness, life style, and recent professional changes were just some of the challenges Diane faced as the primary family caregiver for her husband. She was not only dealing with the medical concerns and changes in their eating habits, but also Alan's emotional adjustment to his potentially progressive problem. Alan's primary care clinician encouraged her to participate in a support group for spouses of cardiac patients. She learned a lot there. She was most grateful, however, to realize that Alan's outbursts of frustration and sometimes anger were not attacks on her but a result of his own frustration about losing strength and independence. Over time, and the with help of peer support, both Alan and Diane have learned more effective ways of interacting.*

CAROL CULLEN (CONTINUED) *Carol feels her arthritis support group has saved her life and her family. She and her husband attend together. Her husband says that for a long time he tried to protect the children from Carol's disease, by making excuses and denying that it existed. Now, he is comfortable being honest with them and lets them know that their mom cannot go backpacking and will not be playing tennis with them. However, she does a lot of other things with them. Carol's husband says he also learned that Carol's illness is teaching their children about life . . . sometimes it is hard, and you learn to cope, anyway.*

When illness strikes a family, everyone needs to be able to talk in a safe environment. Become aware of professional organizations and illness-related support groups in your area. Encourage your patients to participate. Then, follow-up and see what they are learning.

People with chronic illnesses often become more passive and dependent in their health care. They may decrease their physical and social activity, while depending on others to make decisions. Increased involvement will help people and their families feel they are more in charge of the illness and their lives.

Stay Involved over Time

As the primary clinician, you often become the consistent anchor in the rough seas of illness. For many patients, perhaps you will be their only health care clinician. For those whose illness is more complex, you may be the coordinator of their care with a number of specialists. However, you will be the one familiar relationship in your patient's journey through the health care system.

CAROL CULLEN (CONTINUED) *In a support group for young arthritis sufferers, Carol talked about the comfort and sense of security she felt because she had known her family physician for a few years* *and appreciated that he understood her long and painful journey. "I used to be afraid that as my condition worsened, I would be referred to specialists and then not be able to go back to my family doctor. But he always says, 'I want to see you again in a few months, or sooner if necessary.' My children and my husband know him, and he has helped them understand what is happening to me . . . and that is important"*

As Carol, points out, the family needs your help with their caregiving. You have been not only the anchor for the patient, but also for the family. As they take over more of the caregiving responsibility, your role becomes one of periodic consultation, listening, encouraging, and affirming.

Be Aware of Your Own Reactions

It is not always easy to care for sick people. Just as your patients will have reactions to you, you will have reactions to them. Throughout your practice, experiences with patients will extend across many phases of the life cycle, and your own life will become interwoven with that of your patients. Your personal history of health, illness, and suffering naturally influences your perceptions of others. The way your family of origin perceived, reacted to, and ultimately handled illness colors how you perceive and care for others.

As you notice the effects of your own behavior on the patient, be aware of your reactions to them. The key is to be able to choose strategies and processes that are appropriate to you, the patient, and the problem. Notice when your responses may be negatively influencing the care you give. Seek consultation to help with the care and sort through your reactions as necessary. See Chap. 12, Caring for Patients Experienced as Difficult, for more information.

Recognize Your Limits

Illness exaggerates emotion and challenges the best of coping skills. Your patients and their families' needs will often extend beyond your professional limits and competency. You do not have to be alone when working with challenging situations. Seek collaboration with other caregivers and mental health professionals when appropriate.

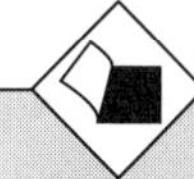

Summary

People who are ill face many challenges—physical, emotional, psychological, and social. They need the support of an understanding and caring clinician. In this chapter we sought to provide primary care clinicians with a theoretical foundation that helps explain some of your patients' varied reactions to their illnesses. More importantly, we tried to suggest concrete ways of communicating with, supporting, and caring for your patients so that they have the resources they need to navigate the difficult situations they encounter.

Suggested Reading

Kleinman AM: *The illness narratives: Suffering, healing, and the human condition.* New York: Basic Books; 1988.

Harvard professor, Arthur Kleinman, has prepared and presented an excellent collection of case studies and analysis on the topic of suffering and dealing with chronic pain. This book is perfect for clinicians who want to understand their patients or a patient who is trying to deal with a life of pain. Either way, the book is a fascinating study of how to live life in the face of illness.

McDaniel S, Hepworth J, Doherty W (eds): *Medical family therapy: A biopsychosocial approach to families with health problems.* New York: Basic Books; 1992.

An essential primer for primary care clinicians who wish to understand the influence of the family context on health and illness behaviors.

Register C: *The chronic illness experience: Essential support and inspiration for people with chronic illness and those who love them.* Center City, MN: Hazelden; 1999.

An insightful exploration, from the patient's point of view, of the physical, psychological, and emotional realities of living with chronic illness.

Rolland JS: Chronic illness and the life cycle: A conceptual framework. *Fam Process* 26:201, 1987.

John Rolland offers a powerful and practical systems framework for all clinicians to consider when working with patients with chronic illness at the various stages of life.

Tansella CZ: Illness and family functioning: Theoretical and practical consideration from the primary care point of view. *Fam Pract* 12:214, 1995.

This article offers primary care clinicians practical ideas about how to think about illness and family functioning.

Bibliography

Balint M: *The Doctor, His Patient and the Illness.* New York: International Universities Press; 1972.

Baron RJ: An introduction to medical phenomenology: I can't hear you while I'm listening. *Ann Intern Med* 93:718, 1980.

Bandura A: *Self-Efficacy: The Exercise of Control.* New York: Freeman; 1997.

Barnett LB: From cradle to rocker: Providing care across the human life cycle. In: Sloane PD, Slatt LM, Curtis P, et al (eds): *Essentials of Family Medicine,* 3rd ed. New York: Lippincott Williams & Wilkins; 1998.

Berkanovic E, Hurwicz, M, Lachenbruch PA: Concordant and discrepant views of patient's physical functioning. *Arthritis Care Res* 8:94, 1995.

Bowlby J: *Attachment and Loss: Volume 2. Separation and Anger.* New York: Basic Books; 1973.

Bowlby J: *Attachment and Loss: Volume 3. Loss, Sadness and Depression.* New York: Basic Books; 1980.

Breznitz S: The seven kinds of denial. In: Breznitz S (ed): *The Denial of Stress.* New York: International Universities Press; 1983, p 257.

Burman B, Margolin G: Analysis of the association between marital relationships: An interactional perspective. *Psychol Bull* 112:39, 1992.

Campbell TL: Family's impact on health: A critical review and annotated bibliography. *Family Sys Med* 4:135, 1986.

Cassel EJ: The nature of suffering and the goals of medicine. *N Engl J Med* 306:639, 1982.

Cassel EJ: *The Nature of Suffering and the Goals of Medicine.* New York: Oxford University Press; 1991.

Clarke AE, Fries JF: Health status instruments and physical examination techniques in clinical measurement methodologies. *Curr Opin Rheumatol* 4:45, 1992.

Dimou N: Illness and culture: Learning differences. *Patient Educ Couns* 26:153, 1995.

Fleitas J: When Jack fell down . . . Jill came tumbling after. Siblings in the web of illness and disability. *Am J Matern Child Nurs* 25:267, 2000.

Fleming S: Supporting the family's role in patient recovery, rehabilitation. *Promoting Health* 8(Suppl):1, 1987.

Frank AW: Just listening: Narrative and deep illness. *Families Sys Health* 16:197, 1986.

Frank AW: *At the Will of the Body.* Boston, MA: Houghton Mifflin; 1991.

Germain C: Cultural care: A bridge between sickness, illness and disease. *Holist Nurs Pract* 6:1, 1992.

Glantz K, Mullis RM: Environmental interventions to promote healthy eating: A review of models, programs, and evidence. *Health Educ Quart* 15:395, 1988.

Griffith JL, Griffith ME: Structural family therapy in chronic illness. *Psychosomatics* 28:202, 1987.

Helman CG: Diseases versus illness in general practice. *J R Coll Gen Pract* 31:548, 1981.

Helman CG: *Culture, Health and Illness,* 2nd ed. London, UK: Butterworth; 1990.

Horowitz MJ: *Stress Response Syndromes,* 2nd ed. New York: Jason Aronson; 1986.

Jacobson JL, Morse JM: Regaining control: The process of adjustment after myocardial infarction. *Heart Lung* 19:126, 1990.

Kindelan K, Kent G: Concordance between patients' information preferences and general practitioners' perceptions. *Psychol Health* 1:399, 1987.

Kleinman A, Eisenberg L, Good B: Culture, illness, and care: Lessons from anthropologic and cross-cultural research. *Ann Intern Med* 88:251, 1978.

Kleinman AM: *The Illness Narratives: Suffering, Healing, and the Human Condition.* New York: Basic Books; 1988.

Kubler-Ross E: *On Death and Dying.* New York: MacMillan; 1969.

Livneh H, Antonak RF: *Psychosocial Adaptation to Illness.* Gaithersburg, MD: Aspen; 1997, p 1.

Lewis KS: Emotional adjustment to a chronic illness. *Prim Care Pract* 2:38.

Lyons R: The effects of acquired illness and disability of friendships. In: Perlman D (ed): *Advances in Personal Relationships.* London, UK: Kingsley; 1991, p 223.

Marple RL, Kroenke K, Lucey CR, et al: Concerns and expectations in patients presenting with physical complaints. *Arch Intern Med* 157:1482, 1997.

McDaniel S, Hepworth J, Doherty W (eds): *Medical Family Therapy: A Biopsychosocial Approach to Families with Health Problems.* New York: Basic Books; 1992.

McWhinney IR: *A Textbook of Family Medicine*, 2nd ed. New York: Oxford Press; 1997.

Mechanic D: Health and illness behavior and patient-practitioner relationships. *Soc Sci Med* 34:1345, 1992.

Moos RH, Schaefer JA: The crises of physical illness. In: Moos RH (ed): *Coping with Physical Illness, volume 2. New Perspectives.* New York: Plenum; 1984, p 3.

Mullen PD, Green LW, Persinger GS: Clinical trials of patient education for chronic conditions: A comparative meta-analysis of intervention types. *Prev Med* 14:753, 1985.

Pendeton D, Schofield T, Tate P, et al: *The Consultation.* New York: Oxford University Press; 1997.

Robinson DL: Family stress theory: Implications for family health. *J Am Acad Nurse Pract* 9:17, 1997.

Rodin G, Crave J, Littlefield C: *Depression in the Medically Ill: An Integrated Approach.* New York: Brunner/Mazel; 1991.

Rolland JS: Chronic illness and the life cycle: A conceptual framework. *Fam Process* 26:203, 1987.

Rolland JS: Anticipatory loss: A family systems developmental framework. *Fam Process* 29:229, 1990.

Shontz FC: *The Psychological Aspects of Physical Illness and Disability.* New York: MacMillan, 1975; p 112.

Strain JJ, Grossman S: *Psychological Care of the Medically Ill: A Primer in Liaison Psychiatry.* New York: Appleton-Century-Crofts; 1975.

Szasz PS, Hollander MH: A contribution to the philosophy of medicine: The basic models of the doctor–patient relationship. *Arch Intern Med* 97:585, 1956.

Tansella CZ: Illness and family functioning: Theoretical and practical considerations from the primary care point of view. *Fam Pract* 12:214, 1995.

Thompson DR, Webster RA, Cordle DJ, et al: Specific courses and patterns in male patients with first myocardial infarction. *Br J Med Psychol* 60:343, 1987.

Walker JD: Enhancing physical comfort. In: *Through the Patient's Eyes.* San Francisco: Jossey-Bass; 1993, p 119.

Wortman CB: Social Support and the cancer patient. *Cancer* 54(Suppl):2339, 1984.

W. Perry Dickinson
L. Miriam Dickinson

Chapter 6

Violence and Abuse as Primary Care Problems

Introduction

"Violence is the leading public health problem in America, and we're doing virtually nothing about it," states Harold Eist, MD, past president of the American Psychiatric Association. Evidence suggests that over half of all primary care patients have been personally affected by violence or abuse at some time in their lives, yet the magnitude of these problems and their potential long-term effects on mental and physical health have generally been underestimated or have gone completely unrecognized by most health care professionals.

Violence and abuse can take many forms, including child abuse and neglect, domestic violence, intimate partner abuse, sexual assault, elder abuse and neglect, criminal victimization, and school violence. The problem affects children and adults, males and females, educated and uneducated, rich and poor, black, Hispanic, white, and any other ethnic group: none are immune from the "disease" of violence and abuse. It can affect individuals and families at any time during their lives, and in some cases it is part of an ongoing pattern.

In this chapter, we will focus on several particular types of abuse that are common in primary care practice and that have a major effect on health: childhood sexual and physical abuse, adults with a past history of abuse, domestic violence, and adult sexual assault. We will look at the risk of exposure for these types of abuse and describe the patterns of abuse and violence, the adverse effects on physical and mental health, and associated features. We will address diagnosis, management, and treatment options.

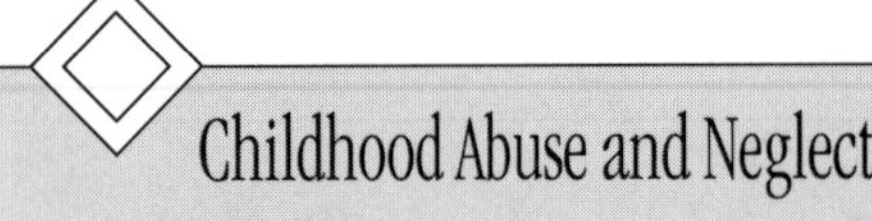

Childhood Abuse and Neglect

Child abuse and neglect have been recognized and openly addressed in recent years, but this has not always been the case. For over a century, there has been an ongoing struggle between accepting and denying of the reality of child abuse and violence against children. Freud initially dealt with patients' stories of childhood abuse through a model that included such abuse as an important factor in patients' subsequent mental health. However, in developing his psychoanalytic model, he questioned the reality of memories of abuse, attributing the symptoms and stories of childhood abuse to fantasy and unresolved conflicts. The psychoanalytic model dominated psychiatry and psychology for many years, so that abuse was not dealt with as a serious factor in the development of mental health problems. Later, concurrent with the growth of the feminist movement, most mental health professionals began to acknowledge the reality of child abuse and to investigate its relationship to mental health problems.

Children may be subjected to multiple kinds of abuse or violence, inflicted both by family members and by people outside of the family. In some families, patterns of abuse may be pervasive or even intergenerational. Forms of maltreatment in childhood include sexual abuse, physical and emotional abuse, and neglect. We will first address the sexual abuse of children.

Sexual Abuse

Studies have repeatedly shown that child sexual abuse occurs in all racial, cultural, and socioeconomic groups. Clinicians who believe that sexual abuse does not occur in their patient populations are just not looking for it. Primary care clinicians see children who have been sexually abused when examining children coming in for routine physical exams or for unrelated medical illnesses. Such children may be brought to the clinic by a family member who does or does not suspect abuse.

Definitions of child sexual abuse vary. The American Medical Association (AMA) diagnostic and treatment guidelines define child sexual abuse as "the engagement of the child in sexual activities for which the child is developmentally unprepared and cannot give informed consent." This may include "genital or anal contact by or to the child, or non-touching abuses, such as exhibitionism, voyeurism, or using the child in the production of pornography."[1] The effect of sexual abuse depends on multiple characteristics of the abuse, although even a level of abuse that might ordinarily be considered minimal can result in considerable psychological problems. In general, the effect tends to be higher when

- there is a higher level of physical contact,
- the abuse is intrafamilial,
- the perpetrator is in a position of power,
- there are multiple incidents, and
- there is violence associated with the sexual abuse.

Estimates of the prevalence of childhood sexual abuse vary depending on the criteria used to define abuse. Such estimates are often obtained from studies in which adults are asked about a history of sexual abuse during childhood, and there may be marked differences in methods and definitions from study to study. Reported prevalence rates for a history of childhood sexual abuse range from about 16 to 40 percent for women seen in primary care settings. Few studies include males,.but recent estimates suggest that the risk of sexual abuse for male children may be in the range of 12 to 15 percent, which is higher than previously thought.

Early warnings of sexual abuse may be subtle behavior changes, indirect statements made by the child, or sexual acting out during play. Behavioral changes are common, although there is no single symptom or symptom complex that is diagnostic of sexual abuse. Specific and nonspecific symptoms possibly associated with sexual abuse in children are shown in Table 6-1.

The perpetrator of sexual abuse is often either a family member or someone outside the family who is known to the child. In such cases the abuse can persist for months or years. Suspected perpetrators commonly deny the abuse, and the child may be attached to or even protective of the perpetrator. The perpetrator often uses a seductive approach over time rather than force. Secrecy is often used as a defense of the perpetrator, and the perpetrator may tell children that they will be hurt or blamed if anyone finds out about the abuse.

Table 6-1

Symptoms of Childhood Sexual Abuse

Specific Symptoms	Nonspecific Symptoms
Rectal or genital pain or bleeding	Shame or guilt
Sexually transmissible diseases	Poor self-esteem
Sexually precocious behavior	Depression
Pregnancy	Distorted body image
	Regressive or pseudo-mature behavior
	Sleep disturbance
	Eating disorders
	Enuresis or encopresis
	Fears and phobias, particularly of adults
	Anger and/or temper tantrums
	Deterioration in academic performance
	Sexually provocative or promiscuous behavior
	Indirect or direct statements about sexual acts
	Compulsive masturbation
	Running away
	Conduct problems
	Extremes of activity
	Attempted suicide

Source: American Medical Association: *Diagnostic and Treatment Guidelines on Child Sexual Abuse*. Chicago: American Medical Association; 1992.

ROBERT AND SARAH *Robert is a 4-year-old boy brought in by his mother, Sarah, for a physical exam, with a history of a normal health maintenance exam 6 months ago. After initially denying any specific problems, Sarah states that Robert has been complaining of dysuria and penile irritation.*

[1]American Medical Association: *Diagnostic and Treatment Guidelines on Child Sexual Abuse*. Chicago, IL: American Medical Association; 1992.

Upon further questioning, Sarah says that the symptoms started after she started leaving Robert for day care for 2 days a week. After an initial period of seeming to enjoy the day care situation, Robert began to cry for no apparent reason when she left him. Sarah admits that she has worried that someone in the day care center (based in an individual's home) might be abusing him. Robert denies that anyone has been touching or playing with his genitals, but shows a lot of embarrassment and discomfort at the questions. He also denies anyone hitting or otherwise physically abusing him. The physical exam was completely normal. Because of your suspicion about possible abuse, referral is made to the local human resources office for further investigation, and you schedule a return visit in 2 weeks to determine the results of the evaluation and to assess the need for additional intervention.

Assessment

Clinicians need to take extra care on a number of levels when evaluating a child for possible sexual abuse. Time and care should be taken to establish a sense of trust with the child. Often, clinicians spend much of the initial portion of a usual clinic visit interacting with the adult accompanying the child, getting the appropriate historical information. The clinician tends to ignore the child, who becomes progressively bored and often gets into things around the office as a way of trying to attract attention and get into the interaction. Then the child is suddenly swept up, placed on an exam table, and probed and prodded in an invasive and uncomfortable manner. This scenario is inappropriate under the best of circumstances, but when the child has been sexually or physically abused, this can be harmful and counterproductive.

As early as possible in the visit, the clinician should try to engage the child in some form of interaction appropriate for the age of the child. Talking or playing with the child at intervals, even when the primary data gathering involves the accompanying adult, will engage the child in the interaction and help increase the child's level of comfort and trust in the clinician. If children are old enough to provide information themselves, it is important that the clinician encourage them to talk to their level of comfort about what happened. Children often are hesitant and reluctant to talk about their abuse, but generally will come around with gentle encouragement and explicit permission to talk about things that may be uncomfortable or "secret."

The level of the history that the clinician needs to take will vary according to whether the abuse is an acute event versus something that happened in the past, and whether this abuse has been previously disclosed versus the initial identification of the abuse. When the episode is acute or when the abuse is initially identified, the facts surrounding the abuse should be ascertained and recorded as fully as possible. In more chronic, previously identified situations, a more general understanding of what happened is usually sufficient. Most children who have been victimized blame themselves for what happened, and perpetrators often reinforce that feeling by telling their victims that it was their fault. Therefore, it is extremely important that the clinician assure these children that what happened never should have occurred and was not their fault.

Physical Examination

When the clinician has spent an appropriate amount of time making the child comfortable, the physical exam is much easier. The transition to the physical exam should be handled carefully, so that the child is not frightened or further traumatized. A supportive parent or other accompanying adult can help the child in undressing and preparing for the exam. The clinician should explain to the child what will happen at each stage of the examination.

Examining a small child on a parent's lap can often help, although older children should be examined on the exam table, with the parent nearby if appropriate. A good light source is vital. Clinicians should carefully document the exam, noting specific details regarding any injuries. A body map can be useful in creating a pictorial record of injuries, and color photographs can be very helpful in cases where legal proceedings are or may be involved.

A general physical exam, looking for any signs of physical trauma, is an appropriate first step, followed by examination of the genitals and anus. The anus can be examined in the lateral decubitus position, looking for tears, scars, dilatation, abrasions, or bleeding. Poor anal tone can also be a sign of abuse. For the genital exam, the child should be place in a frog-leg position. In girls, the labia should be examined for bruising, tears, or abrasions, the vestibule for discharge or bleeding, the posterior forchette for scarring or vascular changes, and the hymen for shape and trauma. In boys, the penis should be examined for swelling, erythema, or other signs of trauma, and the urethra for inflammation and bleeding. In both girls and boys, condylomata or herpetic lesions should be carefully noted. Colposcopy can be a useful adjunct for the genital and anal examination, providing magnified views and photographs.

Lab tests largely depend on the history and the physical exam findings. A rape kit should be used in situations where abuse has occurred within the past 72 h. Materials in the kit should facilitate the gathering of cultures for gonorrhea, *Chlamydia,* and/or herpes simplex, and HIV testing, along with specimens for detecting other potentially useful medical evidence. A wet prep and KOH smears of vaginal discharge looking for *Gardnerella* or *Trichomonas* should be performed if there is any clinical indication.

After the examination, the clinician should reassure the child that there are no major problems. The clinician should tell supportive family members what the examination revealed, formulating management plans based on the findings. If sexual or physical abuse is suspected, immediate intervention is indicated, even if the evidence is equivocal. Legally and ethically, this intervention must include reporting the suspicion of abuse to the appropriate legal authorities so that the case can be carefully investigated. The child should also be referred for counseling, both to deal with the acute situation and to attempt to prevent long-term psychological consequences.

Physical Abuse and Neglect

Professional understanding of physical abuse and neglect of children has somewhat paralleled that of sexual abuse, but with physical abuse, there is less outright denial of the extent of the problem. Although clinicians began noticing patterns of injury in children consistent with abuse around mid-century, the appearance of Kempe's landmark article, "The Battered Child Syndrome" in the *Journal of the American Medical Association* in 1962, led to increased awareness of and legislation to tackle this problem.

The reported prevalence of childhood physical abuse in primary care practices varies, but most studies report that about one of every five males and one of every four females has been the victim of physical abuse. Some children are at increased risk for abuse or neglect, especially children who were born prematurely or have physical or mental disabilities or abnormalities. Children in families where there is other abuse or violence are also at higher risk of abuse or neglect. Furthermore, when a parent was abused as a child, either sexually or physically, the child may be at increased risk of abuse, either by that parent directly or by the parent's failure to provide adequate protection for the child. Similarly, some parents are more likely to abuse or neglect their children. Parents who are not sufficiently mature to care for a child, who have substance abuse problems or mental illness, who are under extreme stress, or who have unrealistically high expectations of the child are more likely to abuse or fail to provide adequate care for their children. Low socioeconomic status has been associated with higher risks of physical abuse or neglect in some studies, but like sexual abuse, child physical abuse and neglect occurs throughout society in all socioeconomic groups.

Identification of Child Abuse

To identify cases of child abuse, clinicians must have a high index of suspicion and explore any situation in which there is possibility of abuse. Signs and symptoms of child physical abuse and neglect include any of the full range of injuries that are seen in children, such as bruises, erythema, bullae, burns (especially cigarette burns, immersion burns, or burns shaped like an object), lacerations, abrasions, fractures, abdominal injuries, and central nervous system injuries, especially shaken child syndrome. Persistent failure to thrive also can be indicative of abuse or neglect. The level of suspicion should increase when a clinician notices multiple minor injuries or identifies old injuries.

Most of the nonspecific symptoms of sexual abuse listed in Table 6-1 also apply to physical abuse. These include deterioration in school performance, poor self-esteem, running away, conduct issues, regressive behavior, sleep disorders, enuresis, encopresis, fears and phobias, and depression.

Assessment

Gathering an adequate history is critical for identifying abuse and neglect. Any injury without an adequate explanation should raise concern about the possibility of abuse. Anyone who has parented a toddler can testify to the endless variety of injuries that they inflict upon themselves in their aggressive exploration of their environment. However, in many cases of abuse, the injuries could not have occurred in the manner described. Conflicting and changing stories about the injury can be an indication of potential problems. Additionally, unreasonable delays in seeking treatment should raise suspicions that the injuries may have occurred as the result of abuse.

The history and physical exam of the child should follow the general format discussed for sexual abuse as described, above. A primary issue is the establishment of a comfortable and trusting therapeutic environment. Clinicians should use direct, straightforward, and nonleading questions to try to ascertain the facts, documenting the responses in detail.

Physical Examination

Clinicians should conduct a complete physical exam when they suspect physical abuse. A dermatologic exam is especially important, as injuries to the skin and subcutaneous tissues are very common. In particular, multiple injuries in various stages of healing commonly indicate abuse. The clinician should record the precise appearance of the injury, using narrative descriptions, drawings on body charts, and/or photographs. The dating of the injuries is often very important and can be estimated by the color of bruises and the apparent age of fractures.

The patterns of bruises can sometimes indicate the method of injury. For example, slaps may leave the outline of fingers or hands, beating with belts leave linear marks about belt width, and tying with rope or cords leaves circumferential bruising around the wrists or ankles. Bite injuries commonly leave characteristic injury patterns from teeth marks. Cigarette burns are generally circular and about a centimeter in diameter. Other contact burns may show the pattern of the instrument used to inflict them, such as a steam iron, stove burner, or curling iron. Immersion burns, such as from sticking a hand into hot water, are common. Finally, an examination of the scalp may reveal hematomas or traumatic alopecia.

Blunt trauma to the trunk may result in deep injury to thoracic or abdominal viscera. Rib fractures, pulmonary contusion, pneumothorax, and injury to the liver, spleen, or kidneys can result from blows to the thoracic cage. Respiratory difficulty or bruising may or may not be present. Old rib fractures are especially common in children with a long history of abuse. Abdominal injury is more common in young victims and is commonly missed by clinicians because bruising is often absent, even with very significant abdominal injury. Any of the abdominal organs may rupture in response to blunt trauma, with resultant hemorrhage, peritonitis, or shock.

Head injuries are an especially significant cause of mortality and morbidity in abused children. Blows to the head or severe shaking of the child can result in severe injury, including subdural hematoma, skull fracture, subarachnoid hemorrhage, or retinal hemorrhage.

Skeletal injuries are also very common in physical abuse, especially in younger children. Clinicians may detect old fractures through radiographs for unrelated problems or through skeletal surveys. Types of skeletal injuries that should particularly raise suspicions for abuse include multiple fractures at different stages of healing, fractures out of proportion to the suggested mechanism of injury, metaphyseal injury of a long bone, and chip or bucket-handle fractures.

LAB AND X-RAYS

Clinicians may use diagnostic imaging to detect abuse injuries, including plain radiographs of the area of injury, skeletal surveys to document both old and current skeletal injuries, and CT or MRI for trauma to the head, abdomen, or chest, or for other injuries. If bruising is a prominent part of the clinical picture, laboratory tests should include a screen for bleeding disorders.

MANAGEMENT

As with sexual abuse, clinicians should immediately report any form of suspected child physical abuse or neglect to the appropriate governmental child protection agency. If severe acute injury is involved or if the clinician thinks the child is in danger by returning to the home, the clinician should undertake an emergency hospitalization. Long-term management of previous abuse should include counseling by a mental health professional skilled in dealing with abuse issues.

Adult Survivors of Previous Abuse

The adult survivor of previous child abuse is commonly seen, but not recognized, in primary care. Childhood abuse not only affects children during and soon after the abuse, but also can have adverse consequences on an individual's health and functioning throughout life. Long-term effects of childhood sexual abuse among general medical patients include more medical problems and physical symptoms, lower health status, more surgeries, somatization, and high-risk behaviors. Survivors of previous abuse commonly display a pattern of social and psychiatric problems, including attempted or completed suicide, panic, dissociation, anxiety, depression, sleep problems, and long-term sexual problems. Other forms of abuse and trauma that occur during adulthood can also have long-term effects similar to those seen after childhood abuse.

Childhood abuse has an effect on adult health that appears to be equal to or greater than the effect of current adulthood abuse or other major psychological trauma. For example, a large-scale study of over 1900 women in primary care practices revealed that those physically or sexually abused only as children had adult health problems at about the same levels as those who were in currently abusive situations, with both groups experiencing significantly more problems than those with no abuse histories. Results from the DSM-IV field trials on post-traumatic stress disorder (PTSD), which included both men and women in a combined community and treatment-seeking sample, suggest that those who experience early-onset interpersonal abuse have significantly higher rates of several psychological problems and unexplained physical symptoms than those exposed to natural disasters.

Much of the research on long-term effects of abuse has focused on women. There are multiple indications that childhood abuse causes a different pattern of long-term problems in men than in women. In response to early abuse, women tend to internalize, resulting in depression, somatization, and other related mental health issues. Although some men also display this type of reaction, many more men abused in childhood externalize and act out the emotional effect of the abuse, resulting in violent and sociopathic behavior. Although the nature of childhood abuse tends to differ somewhat by gender, the overall rates are similar, with almost 40 percent of both men and women reporting childhood physical or sexual abuse. Because of the sex differences in the sequelae of childhood abuse, women abused during childhood are seen in clinical settings much more frequently than men, presenting with somatized, unexplained physical symptoms, depression, anxiety, and multiple other problems.

TERRY *Terry, a divorced female, age 40, presents for care with multiple pain symptoms (chest, abdominal, neck, back, arm, headache), indigestion, palpitations, feelings of dyspnea and suffocation, and dizziness. You learn that her past history includes a previous hysterectomy and diagnoses of mitral valve prolapse, mild hyperlipidemia, hiatal hernia, TMJ syndrome, and anxiety. As part of your history you ask about abuse and learn that Terry was sexually molested by a grandfather beginning when she was a small child and raped by her stepfather at age 12. You also note that she seems to be under a great deal of stress and that some of her symptoms are related to that. Psychiatric evaluation later reveals that this patient qualifies for diagnoses of major depressive disorder, dysthymia, generalized anxiety disorder, panic disorder, PTSD, and somatization disorder.*

Identification of Past Abuse

Clinicians rarely question adults about previous abuse. This absence of questioning would be reasonable if previous abuse had little long-term effect on health; however, the persistent negative effects of abuse on mental and physical health indicate that it is important for clinicians to inquire about abuse among both male and female patients. The trauma that abused people have lived through has exacted a toll, and to understand the effects on their health, clinicians need to know about the abuse.

The nature of the diagnostic process for detecting previous abuse is different than that for detecting current abuse in children or adults, where legal reasons require verifying the abuse and detailing the facts. With victims of past abuse, the point is to understand their pain and suffering and to view their symptoms and health risks in this context.

Victims of childhood abuse very seldom volunteer information about the abuse without being directly questioned. In fact, many of them have never shared their story with anyone. As discussed, the perpetrators of the abuse often tell the victims that it is their fault. Developmentally, children often take on responsibility for even random events that do not involve them whatsoever, so it is easy for them to blame themselves for events in which they are involved that are confusing and emotional. Even if the survivors of abuse try to tell family members, friends, or others about the abuse, their attempts often fail or are not received well, and sometimes even meet with an angry response from those close to them. The violation of trust that the abuse represents also decreases the likelihood that the victim will discuss what happened with anyone. Thus, the stories of the abuse are very often kept hidden—unprocessed, not well understood, and surrounded by a sense of shame and guilt.

Paradoxically, most victims of abuse are ready and willing to talk about their experiences when presented with the right opportunity. Clinicians can set the stage for this opportunity by providing a supportive, trusting, therapeutic relationship, giving the patient permission to talk about matters of concern. Within this context, direct questions regarding past (or present) experiences of abuse will generally meet with a positive response. Vague, general questions about "how things are going" in the patient's life will almost never result in the patient revealing a history of abuse.

Compared with current abuse, past abuse produces even fewer cues that victimization may be playing a role in patients' symptoms. As with other forms of abuse, clinicians tend to only ask about abuse when they suspect it—and they rarely suspect it. Because of the important health consequences of past and present abuse, clinicians should ask *every* patient about experiences of abuse.

Questions about current abuse described in the section on domestic violence, later in this chapter, should be supplemented by inquiry about past abuse. Using a genogram interview can assist clinicians with the entire process of inquiry into this area, providing a natural, fact-based way of entering into a discussion of current and past family and personal events. Transitional statements can help in preparing the patient for the questions, such as "We are increasingly discovering that past abuse has long-term effects on people's health, and it is so common that I now ask every patient about their history of abuse." Then the clinician should ask a series of direct questions, along the lines of the following.

- Have you ever had anything really bad happen to you?
- Have you ever been abused, physically, sexually, or emotionally?
- Have you ever been forced to have sex against your wishes?

The manner in which the clinician deals with the emerging stories of victimization is extremely important in determining the outcome. If patients perceive any sense of rejection or retreat on the part of the clinician, they often will close down and not share the complete story. Facilitating responses, such as "That must have been really difficult for you" or "I am really sorry that happened to you" can encourage patients to keep going with this story. Some of the stories can be very disturbing to listen to. Clinicians may find themselves reacting negatively to what they are hearing and, through this reaction, communicating revulsion or rejection to the patient. In such situations, clinicians should briefly explain what they are experiencing so that the patient does not misinterpret their reactions, using single statements like: "That must have been terrible. It is painful just hearing about it. However, it is really important for you to talk about it."

After the patient has finished telling the story, it is important for the clinician to deal with the guilt and shame surrounding the memories of abuse. Statements such as the following are appropriate. "Many people who have been abused feel guilty about the abuse, as if somehow they caused their abuse to happen. It is important for you to know that this was not your fault. This never should have happened to you, and I am really sorry that it did."

Clinicians willing to incorporate this line of inquiry into their standard practices will discover an astonishing number of patients with remarkable histories of trauma and maltreatment. They also will start to develop a completely new and fuller understanding of the problems and behaviors of many of their patients.

The experience of telling a primary care clinician about past abuse can start the patient on a path to healing. Research has indicated that telling and processing stories of traumatic experiences can have an extremely positive effect on health. This telling will often need to be supplemented with additional counseling by a mental health professional skilled in this area, to further process and understand the experiences. The effect can be substantial for abuse victims who are able to tell their stories to supportive primary care clinicians who then use the contextual information in the patient's subsequent health care.

Management

There are a number of ways in which knowledge of past abuse can and should influence care. For many abuse victims, the health care system in general and the primary care office specifically can be a very scary place. We regularly poke, prod, and traumatize patients through our physical exams, diagnostic tests, and treatments. Simply being touched by an authority figure may be uncomfortable for some survivors of abuse. Thus, in caring for an abuse victim, the clinician must be willing to go much more slowly than usual, telling the patient what is involved at each step, asking the patient's permission to proceed, and giving the patient full permission to stop things that are uncomfortable. Patients who have learned to dissociate in response to stress as part of coping with their abuse may actually not be able to respond well to information or questions during physical exams or procedures and may need a support person present to assist them. The clinician should give the patient full control over what happens, which is often a very different and empowering situation for an abuse survivor to experience.

Another important aspect of managing patients with a history of abuse involves assisting the patient in understanding physical symptoms, especially when somatization is a prominent effect of the abuse. There are multiple reasons for abuse survivors to have increased physical symptoms and to have difficulty in interpreting and responding to their symptoms. Patients who have experienced multiple episodes of abuse and trauma may be hypervigilant, always having a heightened sense of watchfulness and sensitivity to what is going on around them. This hypervigilance may result in an increased sensitivity to physical symptoms and may also more directly produce symptoms through the effects of tense muscles, increased catecholamine levels, and other physiologic processes. Multiple past traumas also may make victims' bodies more sensitive to subsequent stresses. A subset of abuse victims learn to dissociate in response to painful stimuli as a way of dealing with the pain of their abuse, and these people may have much trouble recognizing their symptoms and seeking care appropriately. They actually get into trouble by not being able to tell when their bodies are having difficulty, and therefore do not seek care in a timely fashion. In either case, clinicians can assist a patient who has a disturbed experience of physical symptoms due to previous abuse by entering into a partnership for the management of those symptoms.

The first step in establishing a clinician–patient partnership is to assist the patient in developing an understanding of the connection between past experiences and current physical symptoms. For a patient with somatization, the clinician should communicate an understanding that the symptoms experienced by the patient are very real and uncomfortable, but also explain that they are not necessarily indicative of a serious medical process. For a patient who dissociates in response to discomfort, the clinician may need to actually encourage the patient to come in or call at the earliest sign that something is wrong, so that together the patient and clinician can decide whether evaluation is needed. This type of approach should result in the patients using fewer health care resources and having less impairment from unexplained symptoms. Somatizing patients should experience fewer iatrogenic complications, and dissociating patients should experience fewer serious complications of unrecognized medical problems. Both somatizing and dissociating patients should feel increased comfort and satisfaction with the health care system.

Another important aspect of the management of patients with previous abuse is related to screening. Clinicians should screen for mental health issues, including depression, post-traumatic stress, panic, anxiety, and other syndromes, both at subthreshold levels and at levels meeting the DSM-IV criteria for full disorders. Although many abuse survivors go through their lives with only minimal mental health problems, others may have complex combinations of mental health symptoms with severe impairment. Factors associated with increased levels of mental health symptoms include those shown in Table 6-2. In situations in which there are mental health issues associated with previous abuse, referral to a mental health professional skilled in dealing with abuse issues, along with appropriate pharmacotherapy for specific disorders, can be very helpful.

Table 6-2

Factors Associated with Higher Levels of Mental Health Symptoms in Victims of Abuse

Increased levels of abuse
More episodes
Abuse in both childhood and adulthood
Combined physical and sexual abuse
Family dysfunction
Family violence and sociopathy, especially in the family of origin

SOURCE: Dickinson LM, deGruy FV, Dickinson WP, et al: Health-related quality of life and symptom profiles of female survivors of sexual abuse in primary care. *Arch Fam Med* 8:35–43, 1999.

Probably the most important aspect of caring for abuse victims is recognizing the privilege of taking care of people who have managed to survive and often flourish despite suffering through some of the worst trauma that people can inflict on one another. Their stories can be extremely difficult to hear, but they were tremendously more difficult to experience. Suddenly, some of the patients that may have been very difficult to understand and take care of can be seen for the incredible people that they really are, and their symptoms and problems start making sense when seen in this new context. It can be challenging but vastly rewarding work for caring clinicians.

Table 6-3

Behavior Seen in Domestic Abuse

Behavior Seen in Domestic Abuse
Physical attacks
Isolation of the victim from friends and family
Threats
Emotional abuse
Control of financial resources
Destruction of the victim's personal belongings
Threats or actual harm to children in the family

SOURCE: Ganley AL: Understanding domestic violence. In: Warshaw C, Ganley AL (eds): *Improving the Health Care Response to Violence: A Resource Manual for Health Care Providers,* 2nd ed. San Francisco, CA: Family Violence Prevention Fund; 1998.

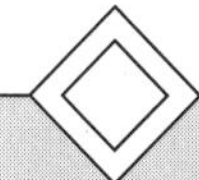

Domestic Violence

Domestic violence has increasingly been identified as a common and destructive public health problem in the United States. The data regarding domestic violence are shocking: Straus and colleagues report that close to 4 million women in the U.S. are physically abused each year. Many of these women are seen in the health care system, most commonly in primary care settings or the emergency room. Studies in primary care settings have indicated lifetime prevalence rates for domestic violence ranging from 28 to 39 percent, with 14 to 23 percent of patients currently or recently experiencing abuse. Domestic violence can include physical, sexual, and emotional abuse, and it occurs between intimate partners who may or may not be married, in gay or lesbian relationships, and in adolescents' dating relationships. The dynamics of intimate partner abuse are different than in situations where the victim is a child, although in families where there is domestic violence there may be child abuse as well.

Domestic violence has been defined as "a pattern of assaultive and coercive behaviors, including physical, sexual, and psychological attacks, as well as economic coercion, that adults or adolescents use against their intimate partners."[2] Domestic violence occurs over time; it is not typically an isolated event. The relationship between perpetrator and victim is characterized by a long-term pattern of abusive behaviors engaged in purposefully by the perpetrator to exercise control over the victim, with physical violence or the threat of physical violence at the root of the perpetrator's power. These behaviors include but are not limited to those shown in Table 6-3. Physical attacks on the victim may include hitting, punching, slapping, choking, kicking, assault with a weapon, or any of the myriad other types of interpersonal violent behavior that can result in injury or death.

Sometimes both partners engage in abusive or violent behavior. In some situations both sides are verbally aggressive, with one partner (usually the male) physically assaulting the other. However, there is generally a power differential between women and men, even when there is violent behavior in both. In most cases, the woman's violent behavior represents self-defense or resistance, whereas the man uses force and violence to exert control.

[2]Ganley AL: Understanding domestic violence. In: Warshaw C, Ganley AL (eds): *Improving the Health Care Response to Violence: A Resource Manual for Health Care Providers,* 2nd ed. San Francisco, CA: Family Violence Prevention Fund; 1998.

An important fact to keep in mind when dealing with domestic violence is that the intentional and long-term use of power and control tactics by the perpetrator is *not caused* by outbursts of anger or loss of control due to alcohol or drugs, although these may be contributing factors. Neither is domestic violence caused by genetic factors or illness. Rather, domestic violence is *learned behavior*. The perpetrators have observed the use of physical force to exert control in their family of origin, school, community, and other settings. The violent behavior is reinforced over a period of time as the perpetrator finds this approach works with few adverse consequences. Unfortunately, certain cultural norms may lend support to a perpetrator's sense of entitlement and control while encouraging the victim to be submissive and keep the family together at all costs. Several researchers have found no distinguishing personality or demographic characteristics of female victims that predict battering. There have, however, been consistent risk markers for male perpetrators, including witnessing violence between parents as a child or adolescent and sexual aggression toward their partners, according to Hotaling and Sugarman.

Children as Victims of Domestic Violence

Adults are seen as the primary victims of domestic violence, but children are often victims as well. Children are commonly used as tools in domestic violence situations. They may be abused or threatened as a way of controlling the victim. They sometimes are made to watch the abuse and occasionally are even forced to become involved in the abuse. They are also sometimes injured as innocent bystanders drawn into the violence. Children often feel responsible for the episodes of violence, and sometimes the perpetrator actually says that this is the case. Children then feel guilt and anger that may cause mental health issues and erode their self-esteem.

The effects of domestic violence on children vary according to the age and developmental stage at which the violence occurs. The consequences can be both short and long term, and include eating, sleeping, and mood disorders; suicidal ideation; emotional clinging or withdrawal; acting out; school problems; and somatic complaints. Experiencing domestic violence during childhood also can establish patterns of behavior that can come out in subsequent adult relationships, with violence begetting violence.

Response of the Health Care Community to Domestic Violence

Various health care organizations have recognized the seriousness of domestic violence as a health problem and called for clinicians to take deliberate action. The Council on Ethical and Judicial Affairs of the American Medical Association recommends that physicians "routinely inquire about abuse as part of the medical history."[3] The American Academy of Family Physicians, in its policy statement on violence, stated that "family physicians must be able to recognize family violence and must know how to intervene."[4] The policy statement recognized that "family physicians are in an ideal position to take on this challenge" and urged physicians to screen for, recognize, and treat domestic abuse." Objectives of *Healthy People 2000* include "[extending] protocols for routinely identifying and properly referring . . . victims of sexual assault and spouse abuse."[5]

Barriers to Identification

Even with such statements by national health care groups, studies indicate that physicians and other clinicians fail to recognize most cases of domestic

---

[3]American Medical Association Council on Ethical and Judicial Affairs: Physicians and domestic violence: Ethical considerations. *JAMA* 267:3190–3193, 1992.

[4]American Academy of Family Physicians: Family violence: An AAFP white paper. *Am Fam Physician* 50:1636, 1644, 1994.

[5]U.S. Public Health Service: *Healthy People 2000: National Health Promotion and Disease Prevention Objectives.* Washington, DC: U.S. Department of Health and Human Services, Public Health Service; 1991.

abuse. It is difficult to understand the reasons for this failure, although a number of barriers to the identification of domestic violence have been cited. Burge reports that because domestic violence does not have a biomedical etiology, clinicians may not perceive it as a problem that they should deal with. This explanation is not adequate, however, because clinicians regularly deal with other conditions that do not have a biomedical etiology. An example of this is cigarette smoking, which is not in itself a biomedical problem but has serious health consequences that cause clinicians to deal with it as a medical concern.

Certainly, the training of medical students and primary care residents in domestic violence has been deficient, although their training appears to be improving over the past few years. As a result, most physicians currently in practice may feel inadequately trained to deal with this difficult and complex problem. Some clinicians may not ask about domestic violence because they view it as a private matter between husband and wife. However, there are numerous examples of very private issues that are discussed in medical encounters. Candib, in a wonderful discussion of the failure of family practice to face and deal effectively with domestic violence, lists a number of additional issues that would appear to influence this dilemma. Among other issues, she argues that the use of family systems theory as part of a basic approach to this type of family issue may contribute to the problem. Application of family systems concepts may lead family physicians to believe that they should avoid blame and maintain a neutral stance, that the violence is all just part of the homeostasis of the family, and that battered women actually contribute to their own abuse. She recommends a feminist perspective, providing a supportive relationship and making safety of the victim a priority in treatment.

Barriers to Intervention

Clinicians who have seen battered women repeatedly return to their batterers may develop a sense of hopelessness and helplessness about the possibility of successfully intervening in domestic violence situations. For clinicians who are otherwise sensitive to issues around domestic violence, the feeling of ineffectiveness can be a major barrier to screening and intervention efforts. Primary care clinicians need to understand the dynamics that lead some victims of domestic violence to stay with or return to the perpetrator.

Fear of escalated violence is one very potent reason for a battered woman to return to an abusive situation. Perpetrators commonly threaten increased violence against the victim or the children if the victim attempts to leave the relationship. The fear is realistic; research has shown that the lethality of the violence often increases when the victim leaves or prepares to leave. Most of the homicides associated with domestic violence occur during the time when the victim is getting ready to leave. Other very important reasons for staying in an abusive relationship may include those in Table 6-4.

It is much easier for a clinician to encourage a victim to leave an abusive relationship than it is for the victim to leave. Staying in or returning to the relationship is often perceived as being much safer than the alternatives. The victims often feel that they have no refuge. They may believe that the perpetrator will find and punish them and their children wherever they go. In extreme situations, they may believe that to completely escape, they would have to abandon their previous lives, leaving family and friends behind and starting over in a new area. This situation is incredibly difficult, both financially and emotionally. Even those victims who eventually are successful at leaving often go through a number of false starts.

Clinicians need to learn patience and compassion rather than becoming offended and fatalistic when victims fail to successfully follow the clinicians' suggestions. A recent study of physicians who were skilled at intervening with domestic violence indicated that small victories and gradual shifts by victims should be taken as positive feedback for physician efforts.

Table 6-4

Reasons Why Victims Stay in Abusive Relationships

Continued contact with the perpetrator because of his [or her] access to the children
Dependence on the perpetrator for health insurance
Immobilization by the accumulated physical and emotional trauma
Cultural, religious, or family values that encourage holding the family together at all costs
Continual hope and belief that the perpetrator will change and stop being violent
Insufficient community resources to help with transition out of the abusive relationship
Lack of alternatives for employment and financial assistance
Lack of affordable legal assistance
Lack of affordable housing
Being told by the perpetrator, counselors, family members, ministers, friends, and others that the violence is the victim's fault

SOURCE: Ganley AL: Understanding domestic violence. In: Warshaw C, Ganley AL (eds): *Improving the Health Care Response to Violence: A Resource Manual for Health Care Providers,* 2nd ed. San Francisco, CA: Family Violence Prevention Fund; 1998.

Health Problems Associated with Domestic Violence

Clinicians regularly treat victims and perpetrators of domestic violence, often without knowing that their patients are in or have been in a violent relationship. "Silent" consequences of domestic violence may be treated by clinicians who have no knowledge of their cause.

INJURY

Almost any type of injury can be a result of domestic violence, including burns, broken bones, internal injuries, vaginal injuries, miscarriages, head injuries, dental injuries, knife or gunshot wounds, cuts, injuries to the eyes or ears, and back strains. The most common sites of injury are the head, face, and areas that are usually covered by clothing, with extremity injuries possible but less common.

UNEXPLAINED PHYSICAL SYMPTOMS

Although the acute injuries are the outcomes that are most directly linked to domestic violence, the long-term medical and psychosocial consequences of the violence are very damaging and debilitating. Pain is one of the most common presenting symptoms, both as a direct result of battering and secondary to the stress of the ongoing abuse. Somatization is also a common result of domestic violence, especially when it occurs in the context of previous childhood abuse. Thus, battered women frequently present to primary care clinicians with vague, medically unexplained symptoms, including pain, sleep disturbances, fatigue, dyspnea, nausea, dizziness, and a variety of others. If clinicians do not uncover and understand the connection to a background of abuse, they may subject abused women to a variety of diagnostic tests and procedures, some unnecessary, some invasive, and all costly.

MENTAL HEALTH PROBLEMS

Battered women commonly present with the psychiatric consequences of abuse. Studies of battered women indicate a high prevalence of psychiatric diagnosis, especially depression, generalized anxiety, panic disorder, PTSD, alcohol and drug abuse, and somatization. In addition, many battered women present with complex syndromes consisting of multiple psychiatric symptoms, some of which may not meet the threshold for DSM-IV diagnoses but still produce significant impairment. Although domestic violence may produce new psychiatric symptoms or aggravate existing psychiatric symptoms, these symptoms may also represent a response to a very dysfunctional and dangerous situation and remit once the violence is gone. Basically, psychiatric symptoms should serve as a red flag to probe for both ongoing and past victimization. Treatment of the psychiatric problems can sometimes help the victim to mobilize and problem solve more effectively to overcome the abusive situation. Both pharmacotherapy and psychotherapy can be helpful, depending on the situation.

Interaction with Other Chronic Health Problems

The stress resulting from domestic violence can exacerbate chronic conditions such as lupus, asthma, diabetes, multiple sclerosis, or cardiac disease. An additional problem for victims of domestic violence with chronic diseases concerns the long-term management of their disease: victims of domestic violence may not able to get needed health care because the perpetrator may not allow the victim to visit the doctor, have prescriptions filled, or follow their clinician's instructions. Unfortunately, a clinician who is unaware of the ongoing domestic abuse may view their patients' inaction as noncompliance. When clinicians encounter situations in which a patient is not responding to treatment as anticipated or in which they suspect nonadherence, the clinician should think about and screen for domestic violence.

Battering during Pregnancy

Battering during pregnancy represents a serious risk for a woman and her unborn child. Women who are battered during pregnancy have higher abortion and miscarriage rates, as well as other health problems. In a study of postpartum women, Campbell found that about 7 percent had been battered by a partner during the pregnancy. Women who are in abusive relationships prior to pregnancy are more likely to be battered during pregnancy, and often the battering escalates during pregnancy, according to Helton and colleagues. However, in some abusive situations the battering may actually decrease or disappear during pregnancy. Campbell reports that women who are battered during pregnancy tend to have more housing problems, less social support, more depression and anxiety, more substance abuse, and less adequate prenatal care than nonbattered women. Although the relationships are unclear at this point, these characteristics are speculated to be consequences of battering. For example, abusers may limit their partner's social interactions and access to medical care, putting the woman in a position of isolation with few resources.

SUSAN *Susan is a 24-year-old woman presenting with multiple contusions. She says that her boyfriend beat her and threatened to kill her. Susan says she has been to the ER several times and has required stitches. She and her partner have a daughter who was removed from the house by child protective services, and she is trying to meet requirements to get her child back, including taking a parenting class, working on her GED, and looking for a job. Susan had a positive home pregnancy test 2 weeks ago. The current violent episode with her partner may have been precipitated when she told him about the pregnancy. Because there was a short period of time when they were separated after a previous battering episode, the boyfriend accused her of being pregnant by someone else. Susan's pregnancy test was positive, and her urinalysis revealed that she has a urinary tract infection.*

Possible Warning Signs of Abuse during Pregnancy

Clinicians should have a heightened awareness of signs of potential abuse during pregnancy. When a woman delays initiating prenatal care, the clinician should ask about domestic violence. McFarlane and associates found that abused women are twice as likely as nonabused women to delay prenatal care until the third trimester. Furthermore, although the presence of the husband at prenatal visits is often perceived as a positive indication of the husband's support and involvement, it could also be a sign to clinicians that they should inquire about domestic violence. The husband may actually be accompanying the wife to the prenatal visits to exercise control and prevent identification of the abuse. The clinician should make an effort to find a reason to separate the woman from her husband and inquire about domestic violence.

Screening for Domestic Violence

Appropriate intervention and assistance for domestic violence victims hinge on clinicians identifying these women. All of the descriptions of possible consequences of domestic violence detailed above serve to identify clinical situations in which domestic violence is more likely to be present. However, inquiring about violence only in situations where the clinician suspects domestic violence is not adequate. The clinical manifestations and presentations of abuse victims are extremely varied, and most clinicians do not consider the possibility of domestic violence even for patients with very typical presentations. Rodriguez and colleagues found that despite increased attention to the importance of routine screening, relatively few physicians report screening all women for abuse. Basically, every woman presenting for care should be screened for domestic violence as part of her routine health assessment.

Most abused women are willing to talk about their experiences, especially if they feel safe and supported. An appropriate transition to this topic area can be very useful. Clinicians can say something like "Domestic violence is a very common problem for women and can cause a number of health problems. I have started asking all the women in my practice whether they are being mistreated in some way." This can be followed by a series of direct and specific questions regarding the woman's experience of violence. Useful questions (modified according to the woman's marital status) include those listed in Table 6-5.

Table 6-5

Useful Questions for Identifying Victims of Domestic Violence

Has your partner ever physically hurt you or threatened to hurt you?
Does your partner try to control you?
Are you afraid of your partner?
Do you feel safe at home?

In situations in which the clinician does not believe that a trustful and safe relationship has been established with the patient, indirect questions may be appropriate, such as giving the patient permission to talk about psychosocial problems. However, patients rarely provide their history of current or past abuse in response to vague, indirect questions. Indirect questions should always be followed by more direct questions such as those described in Table 6-5.

Brief screening instruments, such as the Woman Abuse Screening Tool, the Partner Violence Scale, and the HITS scale, have been developed and validated to detect cases of domestic violence. Clinicians can incorporate these instruments into practice in a variety of ways. Some clinicians administer them to ascertain the presence of abuse in specific cases when they suspect it. Others have used them as a more general screening tool for all female patients, either alone or as part of a larger health history assessment.

SARAH AND ROBERT (CONTINUED) *Sarah comes in today needing refills on asthma medication and complaining of pain from cigarette burns inflicted by her husband. Sarah says she has been under a lot of stress and feels anxious and depressed. She also has difficulty sleeping and has tried unsuccessfully to stop smoking. She has had several severe asthma attacks and visits to the ER recently, one of which resulted in admission. Sarah says the anxiety attacks bring on her asthma. Upon further questioning, Sarah revealed that she had been physically and sexually abused as a child and grew up in a violent family. She is attempting to leave an abusive relationship and to take care of an 8-month-old daughter and 4-year-old son, and she recently had to testify in court against her husband. After a careful safety assessment and plan, you start her on an SSRI for her panic attacks and refer her to a counselor for cognitive behavioral therapy and anxiety management techniques.*

Assessment

Once domestic violence is identified as a problem, the clinician should carefully assess the situation to determine the best management strategy. The assessment will vary depending on whether the visit is related to an acute battering episode or the domestic violence is identified as an ongoing, chronic situation without acute injury.

Establishment of a Therapeutic Relationship

One of the most important initial tasks is to make sure that the clinical relationship is safe, supportive, and therapeutic for the victim. This both helps with the assessment process and begins the intervention process. Validation of the victim's worth as a person, that he or she does not deserve the abuse, and that he or she is not alone in the process are extremely important parts of the healing process. In one study by Hamberger and associates, battered women rated compassion and validation from their physicians as some of the most desirable and positive interventions they could receive. Validating statements that should be communicated during the first interaction as well as throughout the ongoing care, include each of those in Table 6-6.

Table 6-6

Important Statements to Include in Discussions with Victims of Domestic Violence

A statement of concern for the victim's safety
An indication that the situation is not the victim's fault
A further statement that the victim does not "deserve" the abuse and that there is no excuse for this type of treatment
A clear statement that the victim is not alone in dealing with this problem
Reassurance that there are resources that are available to help, and that the clinician is an important part of those resources and is available to assist the victim in accessing those resources.

Source: Warshaw C: Identification, assessment, and intervention with victims of domestic violence. In: Warshaw C, Ganley A (eds): *Improving the Health Care Response to Violence: A Resource Manual for Health Care Providers.* San Francisco, CA: Family Violence Prevention Fund; 1998.

Table 6-7

Risk Factors for Serious Injury to Victims of Domestic Violence

Violence toward the children
Violence outside of the home
Homicidal or suicidal threats
Escalating violence and threats
Alcohol or drug abuse
Abuse during pregnancy
Attempted or planned separation or divorce
Sexual assault included in the abuse
Perpetrator displaying obsessed behavior
Weapons readily available
Threats to friends or family members
Indications that the victim is fearful for her life

Source: Warshaw C: Identification, assessment, and intervention with victims of domestic violence. In: Warshaw C, Ganley A (eds): *Improving the Health Care Response to Violence: A Resource Manual for Health Care Providers.* San Francisco, CA: Family Violence Prevention Fund; 1998.

Assessing Safety Issues

In some situations safety may be an immediate concern, such as when the abuser is present in the office. If the clinician determines the situation has potential for harm of the victim or office personnel, the clinician should immediately contact the police or security agency. Beyond the acute situation, the clinician should assess the victim's level of concern regarding his or her safety and that of the children or others in the household. This can lead to the development of a safety plan, as outlined further in the intervention section below. Risk factors for serious injury from domestic violence situations include those in Table 6-7.

Assessment of Mental Health

It is important to screen for mental health symptoms because of the high prevalence of associated mental health problems that are seen in domestic abuse victims. At a minimum, screening questions regarding depression, post-traumatic stress, and panic attacks can be especially useful. Such problems can interfere with a victim's ability to deal with the ongoing abusive situation, and treatment for the underlying mental health conditions may be an important part of the therapeutic intervention for domestic violence. In some circumstances, the mental health issues may be largely alleviated through resolution of the domestic violence. Referral to a mental health professional skilled in dealing with abuse and violence situations can sometimes assist with treatment of both the domestic violence and the mental health symptoms; however, patients may be resistant to referrals for counseling or may fear that their abuser will not allow them to pursue counseling. In addition to counseling, pharmacotherapy can also be a very viable treatment option.

Suicide and Homicide Assessment

Victimization is a risk factor for suicide, especially when the victim feels trapped in a situation with no way out. Thus, it is very important that clinicians conduct an assessment of suicide risk. Similarly, victims of domestic violence may contemplate killing the perpetrator as a way of protecting themselves and their children. The assessment process is similar for suicidal and homicidal ideation. First, the clinician should determine the presence of suicidal or homicidal ideation though a question such as "Have you considered killing yourself or your abuser?" If suicidal or homicidal ideation is present, then the clinician should assess the level of risk that the victim will act on the ideation. Serial questions can be asked to ascertain the seriousness, potential lethality of plans for the suicide/homicide, and whether the victim has actually acted toward the accomplishment of the plans. It is important to protect the victim who has serious plans to commit suicide or homicide, as well as the perpetrator who may be a potential homicide victim. Difficult ethical and legal issues may arise regarding such things as warning the perpetrator of the potential for harm or committing the victim to psychiatric hospitalization. The best resolution of situations in which serious homicide or suicide risk exists is often voluntary psychiatric hospitalization, which can accomplish the protection of both parties. In situations where there is some suicidal ideation but lower risk, a suicide contract may be helpful.

Assessment of Injury

In situations where there has been recent battering, the clinician should thoroughly assess and document the victim's injuries. Obtain and record specific descriptions of the abuse, including the time and location of the abuse, what happened, the identity of the abuser, who else was present, and the extent of the injuries. A careful and thorough physical exam should then be performed. The clinician should take extra care to inform the patient of what will be done at each stage of the physical exam, especially for anything that might be uncomfortable or invasive, thereby keeping the exam from being a traumatic experience for the victim. The clinician should carefully evaluate and describe in specific terms any injuries. Drawings, such as a body map, can be very useful for documenting injuries. Photographs of the injuries can also be included in the medical record. Polaroid photographs may be particularly effective as legal evidence of the abuse, because 35 mm or digital photographs can sometimes be manipulated. Torn clothing and other physical evidence of abuse should also be documented and may be retained as evidence with written permission from the victim. The evidence should be placed in a sealed paper bag, with documentation of the circumstances and the time of collection of the evidence.

Intervention Strategies for Domestic Violence

This section describes several intervention strategies that are useful for domestic violence situations, beginning with developing a therapeutic relationship.

Therapeutic Relationship

As related in the assessment section, establishing a trusting and supportive therapeutic relationship is one of the most important issues for both assessment and treatment of victims of domestic violence. Support, the provision of validating messages, nonjudgmental listening, dealing with confidentiality issues, and the establishment of trust all are key components of a positive, healing relationship. One of the key issues involves empowering the victim to take the steps that she thinks are important. The clinician can provide information and suggestions regarding resources and possible interventions, but the patient has to make the final decisions and take action.

It is inappropriate for the clinician to take charge and prescribe the next steps for the patient. When that occurs, the message to the patient is that she really is not able to make her own decisions or take care of herself, reinforcing one of the messages that her abuser may be using to control her behavior. The patient needs to hear that the clinician understands the difficulty of the situation, but has confidence in her ability to do the right thing and to eventually overcome the problem. The clinician then is responsible for providing ongoing support for the patient, through the false starts, successes, and failures that may occur, without blaming or becoming frustrated.

Patient Education

Victims of abuse often feel isolated and shamed by their experiences. Information regarding the high prevalence of domestic violence and other forms of abuse can sometimes help victims to recognize that their experiences are not unique or something to be ashamed of. A description of the patterns of abusive behavior can also help victims in understanding what has happened to them and to anticipate possible future problems.

Perhaps the most important information for victims of ongoing domestic violence is that the violence usually continues over time and tends to increase in intensity. A description of the "cycle of violence" can help victims understand aspects of perpetrators' behavior that often are very confusing and disturbing. This conceptual framework models the cycle through which tension builds up in the perpetrator, leading up to violent explosions. After violent episodes, tension is reduced and the perpetrator is often contrite and apologetic, claiming that the violence will never happen again. However, tension gradually builds up again, leading to further violent episodes. Over time, the periods between violent episodes tend to shorten, the violence escalates, and the contriteness decreases.

Information about resources available in the community and legal options can be very valuable. Written materials can be very helpful. Small, laminated cards with important phone numbers for emergency assistance can be especially helpful and can often be hidden more effectively than more extensive materials. Posters with information on domestic abuse resources can be placed in office bathrooms, with a supply of the cards with emergency numbers that patients can take anonymously. Unfortunately, if such materials are discovered by the perpetrators, it can lead to confrontations and further violence. One useful tactic is for the victim to hide such a card in a shoe for future reference.

Safety Planning

One of the top priorities in managing domestic violence situations is the development of a safety plan for the victim. A thorough knowledge of community resources for domestic violence is essential for this process.

Emergency housing issues often are especially difficult and pressing. Battered women's shelters can provide emergency shelter for battered women and their children. Although shelters are often full and may even have waiting lists, many can provide hotel vouchers even when they do not have room in the shelter. Many shelters also provide a variety of other services, including crisis lines, counseling services, support groups, assistance with developing management plans, legal counseling, job training, literacy programs, and many other special programs. Although many women may be resistant to using shelters for housing, clinicians should certainly encourage them to use shelters for other types of services. As a last resort, a short emergency hospitalization, under an assumed name if necessary, can provide safety while a better plan is developed.

In many situations, the clinician may discover the domestic violence during a period between violent episodes, or the victim may elect to return to the abuser despite an acute episode. In these situations, a careful plan for the safety of the victim and other members of the household should be developed, to be implemented if there are further violent episodes. Clinicians and victims should develop plans for how to best use the victim's support network in case of an emergency. They should discuss the basic legal options for calling the police, having the perpetrator arrested, and obtaining a restraining order against the perpetrator. The clinician should ask the victim whether she can tell when the tension is mounting and leading to an episode of violence, and what precautions she could take for protection in those circumstances. An escape plan, including what to take and where to go, can help in getting the victim away before the situation gets completely out of hand. This can include keeping a bag packed with items that might be needed if she needs to make a quick exit, including such things as clothing and toiletries for several days, birth certificates, medications, important papers, a checkbook, keys, emergency phone numbers, and money.

In situations in which the victim is already separated from the abuser, there are somewhat different safety concerns. If the perpetrator is still harassing, threatening, or abusing the victim, safety measures such as changing locks, installing outdoor lighting, asking neighbors for help in monitoring the safety of the home, and other such measures can help to provide additional barriers for the abuser. Children should be taught how to use the phone, including how and when to call 911 when their mother may not be able to do so. Schools or day care facilities should be carefully instructed about who has permission to pick the children up.

Office Organization and Team Approach

An effective strategy for dealing with domestic violence can and should involve other members of the clinician's office staff. For example, the front office staff often observes family interactions that may raise concerns for the presence of domestic violence. The nursing staff can be incorporated into an office-wide screening strategy. A member of the staff with a special interest in these issues can be encouraged to develop a thorough understanding of the available community resources so that she can give clinicians and patients information when it is needed. Other staff members can be used as sources for patient education. The primary care offices that do the best in dealing with domestic violence have this as an area of emphasis for the entire practice, with an office-wide, interdisciplinary plan.

In summary, primary care clinicians have an incredibly important role in identifying and intervening in cases of domestic violence. They often can be extremely important resources for victims of abuse, providing a therapeutic relationship and safe, supportive refuge. The process of change can be very slow and frustrating for abuse victims, but patience and support from sympathetic clinicians can help to see them through the difficult times.

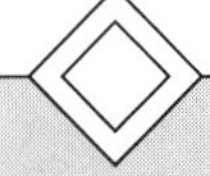

Sexual Assault of Women

Sexual assault is a serious violent crime that often goes unreported. According to Beebe and colleagues, fewer than one in four women who are victims of rape or attempted rape report the crime to the police, although this number is somewhat higher for stranger rape. The perpetrator of sexual assault may be a stranger or someone known to the victim. Sexual assault can also occur in the context of domestic violence, including date rape. Reported rates of sexual assault vary, with definitions ranging from any unwanted sexual activity to completed rape (forced intercourse). Completed rape has been reported by 13 to 24 percent of community samples and 15 percent of a sample of family practice patients. In addition, many women experience attempted rape or other forced sexual activity that does not result in a completed rape. Walker reported that 29 percent of women in a primary care setting had been victimized by adult rape or attempted rape. Many victims of sexual assault are adolescents. It is estimated that approximately 12 percent of adolescent girls up to age 18 have been victims of rape or attempted rape.

As with childhood sexual abuse, sexual assault is associated with numerous short- and long-term health consequences, including depression, anxiety, sexual dysfunction, PTSD, rape trauma syndrome, and an increased number of medical problems. The psychological consequences of rape are often persistent and long lasting. These effects are compounded when someone who has a prior history of sexual abuse in childhood is raped. Threats and intimidation by the perpetrator are very common and often result in intense fear and worse consequences for the victim.

Medical Treatment and Counseling

When caring for the victims of sexual assault, clinicians' primary concerns should be maintaining the safety and comfort of the victim and detecting and treating injuries, sexually transmitted infections, and pregnancy. In the case of a recent assault, clinicians should also gather and preserve evidence for any legal proceedings that might result. Clinicians should carefully give the victim a sense of control over what happens throughout the interview and examination. A record of the assault should include the information in Table 6-8.

Table 6-8

Important Information to Obtain When Taking a History from a Rape Victim

Site and time of the assault
Identifying characteristics of the assailant(s)
Nature of the contact
Any physical injuries that may have resulted
Any activities by the victim since the assault that might have affected the evidence of the assault

A careful gynecologic history should also be recorded, along with the general medical history. If the assault is recent and the preservation of physical evidence important, the clinician should use a rape kit for the examination. Rape kits are available in most emergency departments, and in the emergency department setting, it is probably much easier to both secure the necessary evidence and to maintain the chain of evidence. If clinicians are going to conduct rape examinations in the clinician's office, they should maintain rape kits and carefully go over the necessary procedures with the involved staff. More detailed information regarding the medical evaluation of sexual assault victims will not be covered here, but is included in various articles and the review by Hampton cited in the reference list of this chapter.

Rape and other forms of sexual assault can have profound effects on the victims and their families, and careful follow-up and attention to their emotional and mental health needs is very important. Acutely, the patient may be numb and may not be able to either voice her feelings and concerns or to absorb much of what she is told. She should, however, be given the phone number for a local rape crisis center, if there is one available, and urged to contact it as soon as practical. The clinician should provide a referral to a mental health counselor, as well, with an appointment in 1 to 2 weeks unless there appears to be a more acute need.

The victim should make a return appointment with the primary care clinician, generally in about 2 weeks. At that time, the clinician should follow-up on the various lab tests, check for any medical problems, provide support, and screen for mental health issues. In particular, close monitoring for PTSD and depression are very important, with treatment as indicated by the clinical course. Decisions about continued monitoring will depend on the clinical situation with the patient, but in many cases multiple follow-up visits may be needed, especially to address the mental health effects of the assault. This may be especially true for patients who were previously victimized. Refer to the section on adult victims of previous abuse, which deals with some of the chronic issues that commonly persist after victimization.

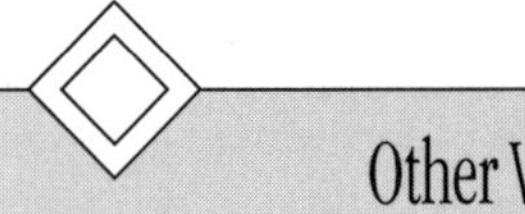

Other Violence

In addition to the forms of victimization addressed in the sections above, there are multiple ways in which abuse and violence affect the lives of our patients. Unfortunately, many of these are worthy of chapters to themselves, but only three will be mentioned briefly here: elder abuse and neglect, criminal victimization, and youth violence.

Elder Abuse and Neglect

Elder abuse involves the mistreatment of vulnerable older people by those responsible for their care or otherwise in positions of power over them. As with other forms of victimization, elder abuse can involve physical violence, sexual or psychological abuse, as well as theft of property and resources. Neglect can also be an issue in situations where elderly patients become incapable of taking care of themselves due to dementia or other medical problems. In such situations, family members may not come forward to take adequate care of the elder's needs because of inattention, disinterest, denial, distance from the situation, or concern about resources.

Estimated rates of elder abuse and neglect in various community samples range from 4 to 10 percent. Elder abuse can be very difficult to detect unless there are signs of physical injury, and even that can often be explained away by falls or other accidents. It takes a high index of suspicion on the part of the primary care clinician to uncover cases of elder abuse. In various studies, poverty, functional disability, cognitive impairment, a history of violence, recent stressful events, and depression all have been shown to be risk factors for elder abuse and neglect. Adult protective services agencies can be very helpful in investigating suspected cases of abuse, and many states mandate the reporting of suspected elder abuse.

Criminal Victimization

In a population-based survey in four southeastern cities, Norris found that 21 percent of the sample had experienced a violent event (robbery, physical assault, sexual assault) in the past year alone, with men more likely to experience physical assault (18.7 percent). The subjects of this study demonstrated significantly higher levels of global and traumatic stress than unexposed subjects or subjects exposed to natural disasters. Any form of criminal victimization can be a very significant traumatic event and produce post-traumatic stress reactions that can cause patients to present to their primary care clinicians.

Youth Violence and Exposure to Violence

Exposure to violence is disturbingly high among adolescents, especially in urban settings. In a survey by Singer and colleagues of students attending six public high schools in urban, small city, and suburban settings, a substantial proportion of students had experienced or witnessed violence within the past year, with rates differing by site. Among males,

3 to 22 percent reported being beaten or mugged in their own neighborhoods, 3 to 33 percent reported being shot or shot at, and 6 to 16 percent reported being attacked or stabbed with a knife. Much higher rates were reported for witnessing violence. Rates for females were somewhat lower for physical assault, but 12 to 17 percent reported being sexually abused or assaulted within the previous year.

Exposure to violence through television, movies, video games, and music is extensive and appears to be increasing. Schools are increasingly viewed as sources of potential danger for children rather than the safe havens that many expect they should be. It is unclear whether violent acts in schools have actually increased or not, but there have been notable instances where violent outbursts have resulted in tragic outcomes. Youth violence needs and deserves our attention as a major public health issue in this country.

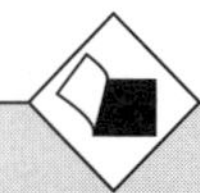

Summary

Violence and abuse are extremely common issues in our patients' lives. Clinicians often bury their heads in the sand and almost seem to adopt a "don't ask, don't tell" strategy for dealing with these issues. However, they will not go away, and neither will the patients who continue to present to their primary care clinicians with problems related to victimization and exposure to violence. This is a problem that primary care clinicians must be prepared to deal with efficiently and effectively.

Suggested Reading

Warshaw C, Ganley AL (eds): *Improving the Health Care Response to Violence: A Resource Manual for Health Care Providers*, 2nd ed. San Francisco: Family Violence Prevention Fund; 1998.

This is an outstanding resource and reference for anyone interested in dealing with domestic violence, but especially for primary care clinicians. It is comprehensive and contains a number of very useful tools. Family Violence Prevention Fund can be reached at 1.800.313.1310.

Various authors: *Diagnostic and Treatment Guidelines on Family Violence.* Chicago, IL: American Medical Association, various dates.

The AMA has published a series of guidelines on family violence, including separate publications on child abuse and neglect, child sexual abuse, domestic violence, elder abuse and neglect, sexual assault, mental health effects of family violence, media violence, and firearm safety. These are extremely valuable and helpful resources and can be obtained from the AMA. Ordering information can be found on their website or call 1.312.464.5563. The AMA also supports the Coalition of Physicians Against Family Violence, begun in 1992. Members receive the diagnostic and treatment guidelines as they are issued, along with other resources. Membership is open to physicians and other providers and is free for AMA members.

AMA Council on Scientific Affairs: Violence against women: Relevance for medical practitioners. *JAMA* 267:3184, 1992.

This excellent article was published in one of the first of a series of special issues dealing with violence published by JAMA. While the data are beginning to be a little outdated, this article still is one of the best available compilations of basic data regarding violence toward women.

Candib LM: Naming the contradiction: Family medicine's failure to face violence against women. *Family Community Health* 13:47, 1990.

Dr. Candib writes eloquently and provocatively about a number of topics, but especially violence against women. This is an excellent discussion of the failure of family medicine to deal with this issue, although most of it applies to any primary care discipline. To supplement this article, look for anything published by Lucy Candib, as virtually everything that she writes is worth reading.

Bibliography

American Academy of Family Physicians: Family violence: An AAFP white paper. *Am Fam Physician* 50:1636/1644, 1994.

American Medical Association: *Diagnostic and Treatment Guidelines on Child Sexual Abuse.* Chicago, IL: American Medical Association; 1992.

American Medical Association: *Diagnostic and Treatment Guidelines on Child Physical Abuse and Neglect.* Chicago, IL: American Medical Association; 1992.

American Medical Association Council on Ethical and Judicial Affairs: Physicians and domestic violence: Ethical considerations. *JAMA* 267:3190, 1992.

Beebe DK, Gulledge KM, Lee CM, et al: Prevalence of sexual assault among women patients seen in family practice clinics. *Family Prac Res J* 4:223, 1994.

Briere J, Runtz M: The trauma symptom checklist (TSC-33) Early data on a new scale. *J Interpersonal Violence* 4:151, 1989.

Burge SK: Violence against women as a health care issue. *Fam Med* 21:368,1989.

Brown JB, Lent B, Brett P, et al: Development of the women abuse-screening tool for use in family practice. *Fam Med* 28:422, 1996.

Brown JB, Lent B, Schmidt G, et al: Application of the women abuse screening tool (WAST) and WAST-short in the family practice setting. *J Fam Pract* 49:896, 2000.

Campbell JC, Poland ML, Waller JB, et al: Correlates of battering during pregnancy. *Res Nurs Health* 15:219, 1992.

Candib LM: Naming the contradiction: Family medicine's failure to face violence against women. *Family Community Health* 13:47, 1990.

Clark CB: Geriatric abuse: Out of the closet. *J Tennessee Med Assoc* 77:470, 1984.

Comijs HC, Pot AM, Smit JH, et al: Elder abuse in the community: Prevalence and consequences. *J Am Geriatr Soc* 46:885, 1998.

Dickinson LM, deGruy FV, Dickinson WP, et al: Health-related quality of life and symptom profiles of female survivors of sexual abuse in primary care. *Arch Fam Med* 8:35, 1999.

Dickinson WP, Dickinson LM, Adams M, et al: Abuse and violence in primary care patients. Presented at the annual meeting of the Society for Teachers of Family Medicine. Chicago, IL: April 1998.

Drossman DA, Leserman J, Nachman G, et al: Sexual and physical abuse in women with functional or organic gastrointestinal disorders. *Ann Intern Med* 113:828, 1990.

Dumas CA, Katerndahl DA, Burge SK: Familial patterns in patients with infrequent panic attacks. *Arch Fam Med* 4:863, 1995.

Dyer CB, Pavlik VN, Murphy KP, et al: The high prevalence of depression and dementia in elder abuse or neglect. *J Am Geriatr Soc* 48:205, 2000.

Feldhaus KM, Koziol-McLain J, Amsbury HL, et al: Accuracy of 3 brief screening questions for detecting partner violence in the emergency department. *JAMA* 277:1357, 1997.

Ganley AL: Understanding domestic violence. In: Warshaw C, Ganley AL (eds): *Improving the Health Care Response to Violence: A Resource Manual for Health Care Providers*, 2nd ed. San Francisco, CA: Family Violence Prevention Fund; 1998.

Gerbert B, Caspers N, Milliken N, et al: Interventions that help victims of domestic violence. *J Fam Pract* 49:889, 2000.

Gould DA, Stevens NG, Ward NG, et al: Self-reported childhood abuse in an adult population in a primary care setting. *Arch Fam Med* 3:252, 1994.

Gremillion DH, Kanof EP: Overcoming barriers to physician involvement in identifying and referring victims of domestic violence. *Ann Emerg Med* 27:760, 1996.

Hamberger K, Ambuel B, Marbella A, et al: Physician interaction with battered women. *Arch Fam Med* 7:575, 1998.

Hamberger LK, Potente T: Counseling heterosexual women arrested for domestic violence: Implications for theory and practice. *Violence Vict* 9:125, 1994.

Hamberger LK, Saunders DG, Hovey M: Prevalence of domestic violence in community practice and rate of physician inquiry. *Fam Med* 24:283, 1992.

Hampton HL: Current concepts: Care of the woman who has been raped. *N Engl J Med* 332:234, 1995.

Helton AS, McFarlane J, Anderson ET: Battered and pregnant: A prevalence study. *Am J Public Health* 77:1337, 1987.

Hotaling GT, Sugarman DB: An analysis of risk markers in husband to wife violence: The current state of knowledge. *Violence Vict* 1:101, 1986.

Jacobson N, Gottman J, Waltz J, et al: Affect, verbal content, and psychophysiology in the arguments of couples with a violent husband. *J Consult Clin Psychol* 62:982, 1994.

Jaffe P, Wolfe D, Wilson S: *Children of Battered Women.* Newbury Park, CA: Sage; 1990.

Kempe C, Silverman F, Steele B: The battered child syndrome. *JAMA* 181:17, 1962.

Koss MP, Woodruff WJ, Dos PG: Criminal victimization among primary care medical patients: Prevalence, incidence, and physician usage. *Behav Sci Law* 9:85, 1991.

Krueger P, Patterson C: Detecting and managing elder abuse: Challenges in primary care. *CMAJ* 157:1095, 1997.

Lachs MS, Williams C, O'Brien S, et al: Risk factors for reported elder abuse and neglect: A nine-year observational cohort study. *Gerontologist* 37:469, 1997.

Lamberg L: Preventing school violence: No easy answers. *JAMA* 280:404, 1998.

Lechner ME, Vogel M, Garcia-Shelton LM, et al: Self-reported medical problems of adult female survivors of childhood sexual abuse. *J Fam Pract* 36:633, 1993.

Mazza D, Dennerstein L, Ryan V: Physical, sexual and emotional violence against women: A general practice-based prevalence study. *Med J Aust* 164:14, 1996.

McCauley J, Kern D, Kolodner K, et al: Clinical characteristics of women with a history of childhood abuse: Unhealed wounds. *JAMA* 277:1362, 1997.

McFarlane J, Parker B, Soeken K, et al: Assessing for abuse during pregnancy: Severity and frequency of injuries and associated entry into prenatal care. *JAMA* 267:3176, 1992.

McLeer SV, Anwar R: A study of battered women presenting in an emergency department. *Am J Public Health* 79:65, 1989.

Norris FH: Epidemiology of trauma: Frequency and impact of different potentially traumatic events on different demographic groups. *J Consult Clin Psychol* 60:409, 1992.

Pelcovitz D: Development of a criteria set and a structured interview for disorders of extreme stress. *J Trauma Stress* 10:3, 1997.

Pennebaker JW: Putting stress into words: Health, linguistic, and therapeutic implications. *Behav Res Ther* 31:539, 1993.

Radomsky NA: The association of parental alcoholism and rigidity with chronic illness and abuse among women. *J Fam Pract* 35:54, 1992.

Resnick HS, Kilpatrick DG, Dansky BS, et al: Prevalence of civilian trauma and posttraumatic stress disorder in a representative national sample of women. *J Consult Clin Psychol* 61:984, 1993.

Rodriguez MA, Bauer HM, McLoughlin E, et al: Screening and intervention for intimate partner abuse. *JAMA* 282:468, 1999.

Russell D: *Sexual Exploitation: Rape, Child Sexual Abuse, and Workplace Harassment.* Newbury Park, CA: Sage; 1984.

Saunders D: When battered women use violence: Husband-abuse or self-defense? *Violence Vict* 1:47, 1986.

Sherin KM, Sinacore JM, Li X-Q, et al: HITS: A short domestic violence screening tool for use in a family practice setting. *Fam Med* 30:508, 1998.

Singer MI, Anglin TM, Song Ly, et al: Adolescents' exposure to violence and associated symptoms of psychological trauma. *JAMA* 273:477, 1995.

Smyth JM, Stone AA, Hurewitz A, et al: Effects of writing about stressful experiences on symptom reduction in patients with asthma or rheumatoid arthritis. *JAMA* 281:1304, 1999.

Springs FE, Friedrich WN: Health risk behaviors and medical sequelae of childhood sexual abuse. *Mayo Clin Proc* 67:527, 1992.

Straus M, Gelles R, Steinmetz S: *Behind Closed Doors: A Survey of Family Violence in America.* New York: Doubleday; 1980.

U.S. Public Health Service: *Healthy People 2000: National Health Promotion and Disease Prevention Objectives.* Washington, DC: U.S. Department of Health and Human Services, Public Health Service; 1991.

Wagner PJ, Mongan P, Hamrick D, et al: Experience of abuse in primary care patients: Racial and rural differences. *Arch Fam Med* 4:956, 1995.

Walch AG, Broadhead WE: Prevalence of lifetime sexual victimization among female patients. *J Fam Pract* 35:511, 1992.

Walker EA, Torkelson N, Katon WJ, et al: The prevalence rate of sexual abuse in a primary care clinic. *J Am Board Fam Pract* 6:465, 1993.

Warshaw C: Identification, assessment, and intervention with victims of domestic violence. In: Warshaw C, Ganley A (eds): *Improving the Health Care Response to Violence: A Resource Manual for Health Care Providers.* San Francisco, CA: Family Violence Prevention Fund; 1998.

Sharon J. Parish
William H. Salazar

Sexual Problems

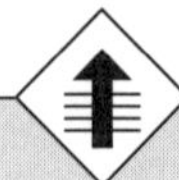

Introduction

Sexuality is the quintessential biopsychosocial phenomenon. It is an integration of biological, emotional, somatic, intellectual, and social aspects of an individual. Sexual practices encompass a wide range of activities, from missionary style heterosexual intercourse to fetishism. Sexual intimacy may be central to the maintenance of long-term relationships, or it may occur in one-time, anonymous encounters. Sexuality involves the relationship between the individual and society, and it is influenced by social and religious views. Sexual functioning may be integral to one's identity, self-esteem, and sense of personal efficacy. Sexual behavior requires the acquisition of skills that involve the complex integration of physical and emotional behaviors.

Given the complexity of these interfacing domains, it is not surprising that when people develop sexual problems, the problems can have a significant effect on social functioning and emotional well-being. Primary care clinicians can play an important role in managing sexual disorders and thus have a favorable influence on the quality of their patients' lives, but they must be willing and able to broach the topic.

The Clinical Spectrum of Sexual Problems

While sexual disorders have unifying features, their presentation in the primary care setting can be multifaceted and diverse. Consider the etiology, appropriate history and evaluation, and treatment for the following cases.

MIKE TAYLOR *Mike Taylor is a 58-year-old married man. His medical history includes hypertension (he is taking an antihypertensive medication), hyperlipidemia, and an extensive smoking history. He presents with a several month history of episodic erectile dysfunction.*

MARIA CARLOS *A 64-year-old widow, Maria Carlos has controlled type 2 diabetes and mild osteoporosis. She has recently become sexually active with a new partner, and comes to your office complaining of pain with intercourse.*

BRIAN DILLER *Brian Diller is 26 years old. He presents with a complaint of "coming too soon."*

OLGA MARTIN *Mrs. Martin, a 44-year-old married woman on effective antidepressant medication, expresses concern about diminished interest in sex and difficulty reaching orgasm.*

LISA BARON *A 35-year-old married woman, Lisa wonders if her husband's "weird sexual fantasies" are "normal."*

In this chapter, we will discuss the rationale and approach to screening, detecting, evaluating, and treating common sexual disorders. We will describe an eight-step model for approaching sexual disorders that includes sexual history taking; the sexual response cycle; the biological, psychological, and social causes; physical exam;

laboratory and diagnostic testing; the classification of the sexual dysfunction; treatment, including pharmacologic and office-based sex therapy; and indications for referral.

The content of this chapter reflects the frequency with which patients with sexual dysfunction present to primary care clinicians. We will offer the most practical clinical approach for detecting and treating sexual dysfunction. We also will present the scientific evidence available regarding the accuracy and efficacy of the various diagnostic approaches and therapies. Although female sexual disorders have been studied far less extensively than male sexual disorders, disorders in both sexes will be given equal attention, based on available knowledge.

Epidemiology and Rationale

Sexual concerns and problems are common. Spector and Carey reviewed several community studies and found that the prevalence of sexual dysfunction ranges from 10 to 52 percent in men and 20 to 63 percent in women. Frank and colleagues studied heterosexual couples with a high degree of marital satisfaction and report that 63 percent of women and 40 percent of men had sexual dysfunctions, and 77 percent of women and 50 percent of men had self-defined sexual "difficulties." A recent survey of adults' (ages 18 to 59) sexual behavior revealed that 43 percent of women and 31 percent of men have sexual dysfunctions that are associated with poor quality of life. Women with any sexual disorder experience feelings of unhappiness and diminished physical and emotional satisfaction, as do men with certain sexual disorders such as erectile dysfunction and low sexual desire. Sexual activity and overall health are related, as are sexual activity and happiness.

Despite the high frequency and effect of sexual problems, Laumann and associates found that only 10 percent of men and 20 percent of women who have sexual disorders seek medical consultation. Medical practitioners rarely take sexual histories and patients are reluctant to spontaneously complain about sexual problems, so detection rates are low. However, improving clinicians' sexual history skills does improve detection. In one study by Ende and colleagues, clinicians who were trained to take screening sexual histories detected sexual problems in 53 percent of patients. Almost all of the patients interviewed said they considered questions about sexuality an appropriate part of the interview. In 50 percent of the encounters clinicians said they elicited medically relevant information.

Although more than 50 percent of patients may have sexual problems, not all patients want treatment. Nonetheless, detecting a problem is critical to discerning which circumstances require further inquiry and which patients might benefit from treating problems that would not otherwise be discussed.

Barriers to Addressing Sexual Problems

Why don't clinicians routinely address sexual problems? The most common reason is not knowing what to ask or what to do after opening "Pandora's box." Other reasons clinicians do not address sexual problems include their unfamiliarity with treatment options, fear of sexual misconduct charges, unfamiliarity with certain sexual practices, personal discomfort with sexuality, and personal history of sexual trauma. Patients may not bring up their sexual problems because they are uncertain about clinicians' comfort, feel shame, or are unaware of potential treatments. Despite these barriers, primary care clinicians can learn to initiate discussions that are acceptable and desirable, conduct sexual evaluations, and manage common sexual disorders.

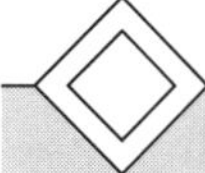

Normal Sexual Function

Evaluation and management of sexual disorders requires knowledge of normal sexual function including the sexual response cycle, the physiology of the sexual response, and the spectrum of normal sexual behavior.

The Sexual Response Cycle

The human sexual response was described by Masters and Johnson and revised by Kaplan, creating a synthesized model consisting of four phases:

1. *Desire:* fantasies about and the desire for sexual activity.
2. *Excitement and plateau:* a subjective sense of sexual pleasure and accompanying physiologic changes of vasocongestion. The major physiologic changes in women are vaginal lubrication and expansion and swelling of the external genitalia. In men, the major physiologic change is erection.
3. *Orgasm:* a peaking of sexual pleasure with release of sexual tension and rhythmic contractions of the perineal muscles, reproductive organs, anal sphincter, and in women the outer third of the vagina. Men have both an emission and ejaculation phase. Women do not have an emission phase but may have an analogous perception of orgasmic inevitability.
4. *Resolution:* a sense of muscular relaxation and general well-being. During this phase males are refractory, while females may be able to respond to additional stimulation almost immediately.

Sexual dysfunctions are classified in the *Diagnostic and Statistical Manual of Mental Disorders* (DSM-IV) according to the desire, excitement/plateau, and orgasm phases. There are no described sexual dysfunctions in the resolution phase.

Although the conceptual model of the sexual response cycle has been widely adopted as the basis for evaluating sexual dysfunctions, this approach has faced some criticism. The first concern is that the sexual response does not always proceed in a sequential fashion. For example, women may reach orgasm without any preceding desire. The second criticism championed by Tiefer and others is that classifying sexual dysfunctions in terms of the sexual response cycle may be too physiologically oriented and "genitally focused." This approach may promote heterosexual intercourse as the normative sexual activity by "defining dysfunctions as failures in coitus."[1] It may overlook the "human relations" aspect of the sexual experience and the wide range of sexual practices and preferences, as well as underrepresent the perspective of women, who may value intimacy and communication over orgasm in a sexual relationship. In this chapter, we will classify the sexual dysfunction according to the sexual response cycle, but we will also include a variety of perspectives in our discussion. In the next section, we describe normal physiology, another key component of sexuality.

Normal Physiology

The central nervous system (CNS), neurologic, vascular, and hormonal mechanisms all control sexual response. The CNS behavioral mechanisms in the hypothalamic, limbic, and other systems orchestrate libido. Hormones, particularly androgens, maintain sexual desire when they are present in normal levels.

In women, estrogen acts locally to maintain clitoral and vaginal blood flow and mucosal lubrication. During arousal, genital vasocongestion is achieved via a local reflex pathway involving the pudendal sensory nerve fibers and parasympathetic fibers from S2–S4 ganglia and by cortical influences initiated by psychic stimuli. The blood supply is derived from the internal iliac arteries via the internal pudendal artery. Increased blood flow results in clitoral and labial engorgement, as well as vaginal wall relaxation and increased lubrication.

In men, neural signals are transmitted down the spinal cord via peripheral pathways to the neuromuscular junctions in the corpus cavernosa.

[1]Tiefer L: *Sex Is Not a Natural Act and Other Essays*. Boulder, CO: Westview Press; 1995.

Here the synthesis and release of the neurotransmitter nitric oxide causes dilatation of the penile sinuses, increased penile blood flow, and venous outflow constriction, resulting in erection. Penile erection is similar to clitoral engorgement; however, the clitoris does not have sinusoidal lacunae and therefore does not have a veno-occlusive mechanism.

In men and women, orgasm is achieved by skeletal muscle contractions via the pudendal nerve. Sympathetic fibers are involved in emission and ejaculation in men and play a role in the female orgasm, including the perception of orgasmic inevitability. The subjective pleasurable sensation is purely cortical.

Sexual Normalcy and Sexual Concerns

Although sexual performance is a subjective experience with wide variation in interpretation, definitions of normal do exist. Sexual "normalcy" as defined by the World Health Organization has biological, psychological, and social aspects. Biological facets include the usual sequence of developing secondary sexual characteristics and the capacity to experience the physiologic sexual response cycle, including vaginal lubrication or the development of an erection in response to stimulation. Psychological normalcy involves psychosexual development and cultivation of the various skills required for intimate personal relationships. Social normalcy relates to cultural norms of behavior and sexual mores as they compare with an individual's sexual practices.

The classic sexual dysfunctions are important, but primary care clinicians will more often see patients with concerns about "normalcy." Patients have concerns about timing, frequency, techniques to reach orgasm, masturbation, and fantasy. Concerns may arise because sexual partners have disparate needs, different attitudes or values, problems with communication, unrealistic performance expectations, or lack of knowledge about sexual functioning. Any of these sexual concerns may evolve into sexual problems if they create conflict between partners or affect sexual functioning.

Common Misconceptions about Normalcy

Patients may have a variety of misconceptions about sexual normalcy that may lead to sexual concerns and even dysfunctions. Among the most common misconceptions about sex according to Bullard and Caplan are the following.

Masturbation: From a medical standpoint masturbation is considered a normal and universal behavior, physically safe, and a marker of sexual self-esteem. It can create a problem when it is associated with excessive guilt or used compulsively to avoid healthy sexual interactions.

Frequency: The normal range for sexual frequency is widely varied, from near abstinence to several times a day. Individuals and couples must determine what is appropriate for them.

Fantasy: Sexual fantasies are normal as long as they do not result in disturbing or intrusive thoughts, which may be a sign of deeper psychosexual conflict.

Life Cycle Issues: Sexuality and Aging

Clinicians should examine their own beliefs and attitudes to ensure that misconceptions about sexuality during the life cycle do not create barriers to effective care. For example, clinicians must make sure that they do not assume that older patients are not concerned with sexuality.

Sexual issues span the three phases of the adult life cycle (adolescence and early adulthood, middle adulthood, and late middle age and old age). Patients in each life stage have specific concerns. Understanding their issues as the normal sexual changes of that stage of life will help clinicians focus the history and interpret the patient's symptoms.

Sexual Changes as Women Age

Physiologic changes in sexual function occur in women as they age. Estrogen levels decline with menopause, and some women experience problems because of atrophic changes. However, in women, desire and orgasm functions are typically maintained with age. In fact, orgasmic capacity seems to improve with age and increasing sexual experience; older women who remain sexually active have fewer sexual disorders than younger women. One study evaluating sexual functioning of postmenopausal women age 45 to 64 demonstrated that 64 percent of the women remained sexually active and 73 percent were satisfied with their activity. The PEPI trial found that most common causes of inactivity are the lack of an available primary partner and the partner's physical problems.

Sexual Changes as Men Age

In men, normal sexual changes with aging include decreased penile sensitivity to tactile stimulation, increased latency period between sexual stimulation and erection, less rigid erections, decreased urge to ejaculate, less forceful ejaculation, decreased ejaculatory volume, and longer refractory periods between ejaculation and subsequent erection. Because older men experience higher rates of sexual problems than younger men do, clinicians need to distinguish the normal changes of aging from actual dysfunctions.

Homosexuality

Homosexuality involves both sexual preference and life-style choices. Gay, lesbian, and bisexual men and women constitute approximately 3 to 8 percent of the adult population. Their choices regarding sexual activity can include celibacy, sex exclusively with men or women, or sex with both men and women. Their patterns of intimacy are similar to those of heterosexuals, including monogamy, serial monogamy, and multiple partners. Most individuals do not wish to have their sexual orientation questioned or changed. During the "coming out process" (the formation and evolution of sexual identity into a homosexual life style), these individuals may experience internal conflict and suffer the consequences of social stigmatization and "internalized homophobia," including depression and self-esteem problems. Their sexual concerns and dysfunctions are also comparable to those of heterosexuals. To guide evaluation of sexual problems in gay, lesbian, or bisexual patients, clinicians should become comfortable discussing sexual practices that both heterosexuals and homosexuals may engage in, such as anal and oral sex. In summary, clinicians should avoid generalizations and biases, and assess the effect of sexual orientation on an individual basis.

Up to one-fifth of adults, who may not identify themselves as homosexual, have had at least one same-sex encounter. Interestingly, Laumann found that women reporting same-sex activity are not at higher risk of having a sexual disorder, whereas men who have engaged in same-sex activity are twice as likely to experience premature ejaculation and low desire.

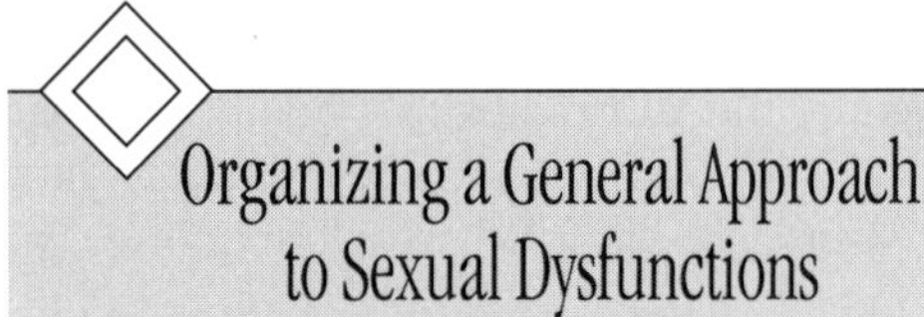

Organizing a General Approach to Sexual Dysfunctions

Sexual dysfunctions can best be understood by using a model that combines the phase(s) of the sexual response cycle affected: the biological, psychological, and social causes; and the roles played by those causal factors over time in predisposing, precipitating, and maintaining the sexual dysfunction. Although these dimensions are not absolutely discrete, the three-dimensional model (Fig. 7-1) can serve as a guide to formulating an explanatory model for a patient's problem. In their efforts to understand and manage sexual dysfunction using this three-dimensional model, clinicians can follow an eight-step approach (Table 7-1). This approach will integrate the information presented in the following section on general considerations in sexual problems and the subsequent section on specific dysfunctions.

Figure 7-1

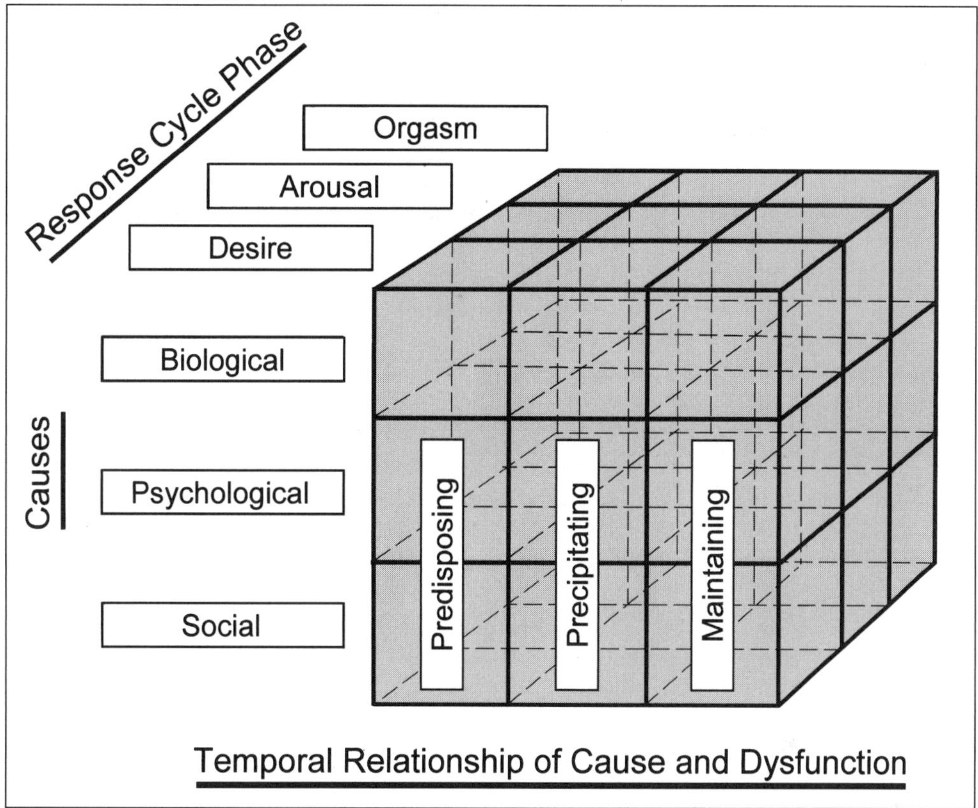

This three-dimensional model depicts the temporal relationship between sexual response cycle phase and causes of dysfunction. The model, which integrates with the eight-step approach outlined in Table 7-1, can guide clinicians as they formulate an explanatory model for a patient's problem.

Biopsychosocial Factors in Sexual Dysfunction

The causes and pathogenesis of sexual dysfunction encompass a continuum from organic to psychogenic and often include a mosaic of factors. The following sections cover biological, psychological, and social causes, as well as cultural factors.

Biological Causes

Organic (biological) problems affect all phases of the sexual response cycle. The predominant causes are impairment of the neurologic, vascular, or hormonal systems; local tissue damage; drug or medication effects; and systemic medical illness. Each of these factors will be discussed in more depth in the context of the specific sexual dysfunctions.

Medical illnesses with direct influence on the neurovascular system include high blood pressure, diabetes, and multiple sclerosis. Other conditions that affect sexuality include reproductive problems, sexually transmitted diseases (STDs), and chronic medical illnesses, such as arthritis, chronic renal failure, and congestive heart failure. Table 7-2 lists organic medical problems that can affect sexual function.

Table 7-1

An Eight-Step Approach to Evaluating and Managing of Sexual Problems

Step	Selected Elements
1. Take the sexual history.	Obtain a description of a typical sexual experience using the sexual response cycle as a guide.
2. Assess causal factors.	Assess the biological, psychological, and social factors. Assess predisposing, precipitating, and maintaining factors. Create a preliminary explanatory model for the interaction of causal factors. Assess opportunities to intervene.
3. Assess life-cycle issues.	
4. Perform targeted physical exam.	
5. Order appropriate diagnostic tests.	
6. Label the sexual dysfunction.	Assess comorbid sexual dysfunction(s), perhaps in different phases of the sexual response.
7. Initiate appropriate therapy.	Educate the patient. Suggest behavioral therapies. Initiate pharmacologic treatments, if appropriate.
8. Refer to specialists.	Determine if medical specialty consultation is needed, and refer. Utilize psychiatric and counseling resources as appropriate.

Clinicians should always consider medications and other substances that might cause impairment in these biological categories. Smoking, drinking alcohol, doing drugs, and taking certain prescription and over-the-counter medications can all influence sexual function. Clinicians should also consider the relationship of sexual symptoms to the institution, dosing, or cessation of a medication or substance. Table 7-3 lists medications that affect sexual function.

Psychological Causes

Whether or not an organic cause is identified, there are often contributing psychological and social factors. Some problems are primarily psychogenic in origin. Medical illnesses that do not have a direct effect on sexual function but that have symbolic implications may affect sexuality. For example, after a mastectomy, as a result of the perceived disfigurement, women may experience shame or fear of rejection, which can decrease sexual desire. After a myocardial infarction, sexual frequency decreases 40 to 70 percent in men and women, regardless of the actual risk that sexual activity poses. Schorer and Jensen found that in women who have had cardiovascular events, sexual impairment depends most on the woman's premorbid sexual functioning, the quality of her nonsexual relationship with her partner(s), her view of the importance of continuing sexuality in her life, and the presence and effectiveness of post-event counseling. The clinician, however, should avoid assumptions about symbolic significance. For example, recent data by Kjerulff suggest that sexual functioning after hysterectomy actually improves in some women, probably as a result of pain relief and diminished medical concern.

Table 7-2

Organic Factors That May Affect Sexual Function

Medical illnesses
- Angina pectoris, recent myocardial infarction
- Atherosclerosis
- Chronic systemic disease (anemia, uremia, cirrhosis)
- Chronic obstructive pulmonary disease
- Degenerative arthritis
- Diabetes mellitus
- Hyperlipidemia
- Hypertension
- Sickle cell disease

Endocrine disorders (generally affect the desire phase)
- Adrenal insufficiency (Addison's disease, adrenalectomy)
- Cushing's disease
- Hyperprolactinemia
- Hypo- and hyperthyroidism
- Hypogonadism (testicular, ovarian, and liver disease)
- Hypopituitarism

Neurologic disorders (generally affect the arousal and orgasm phases)
- Cord lesions: low and high
- Disc disease of lumbosacral spine
- Multiple sclerosis
- Neurogenic bladder
- Neuromuscular disease
- Peripheral neuropathy (alcohol, diabetes)
- Temporal or cortical lobe lesions

Vascular disease (generally affect the arousal phase)
- Large artery vessel (Leriche's syndrome)
- Small artery vessel (pelvic vascular insufficiency)
- Venous insufficiency

Miscellaneous disorders
- Pelvic fracture
- Pelvic radiation
- Radical abdominal, pelvic, or urologic surgery

SOURCE: Adapted with permission from Schmidt CW: Sexual disorders. In: Barker LR, Burton RB, Zieve PD (eds): *Ambulatory Medicine,* 4th ed. Baltimore, MD: Williams & Wilkins; 1991, 188.

Table 7-3

Medications and Substances That May Affect Sexual Function

Antihypertensives
- ACE inhibitors
- Beta blockers
- Calcium channel blockers
- Centrally acting: clonidine, methyldopa
- Diuretics
- Spironolactone

Substances of abuse
- Alcohol (high dose)
- Amphetamines
- Cocaine
- Marijuana (high dose)
- Narcotics
- Stimulants (high dose)
- Tobacco

Psychiatric
- Antidepressants: serotonin uptake inhibitors, tricyclic antidepressants
- Antipyschotics
- Benzodiazepines
- Lithium
- Sedatives (high dose)

Other CNS
- Antihistamines
- Bromocryptine
- L-Dopa
- Phenytoin

Hormonal
- Androgens
- Anti-androgens
- Estrogens
- Progesterone

Miscellaneous
- Cimetidine
- Digoxin
- Disulfiram
- Neurotoxic chemotherapy agents (vincristine)

The relationship between psychological functioning and sexual functioning is very complex. Although sexual dysfunction may be a primary presenting symptom of psychiatric illnesses, such as depression, anxiety, substance abuse, and somatoform disorders, the treatments of these disorders may also cause sexual symptoms. For example, schizophrenia affects all three phases of the sexual response cycle independent of the dose of neuroleptic medication, which also may affect sexual response. Additionally, psychiatric symptoms and sexual problems may be the result of an underlying medical condition. For example, a patient can have both depression and decreased libido as a consequence of hypothyroidism. Sexual disorders such as organic erectile dysfunction can cause psychological reactions, such as performance anxiety. Similarly, the psychological impact of sexual trauma often has a long-term detrimental effect on sexual functioning in men and women.

SOCIAL CAUSES

Social factors may have intrapsychic and interpersonal effects on sexuality. For example, childrearing and work stress may diminish the time for and attention to sexual intimacy. Homosexual individuals may be stigmatized or suffer the consequences of internalized homophobia, with deleterious effect on sexual functioning. In general, those who experience emotional or stress-related problems are more likely to have difficulties in all phases of the sexual response cycle. Research by Laumann and associates has shown that declining economic status is associated with sexual disorders in women and erectile dysfunction in men, whereas married status and higher educational attainment are associated with lower rates of sexual symptoms.

CULTURAL, ETHNIC, AND RACIAL FACTORS

Cultural, religious, and ethnic factors may influence sexual desire, expectations, and attitudes about performance. In some cultures there are mixed messages about sex, which often originate with parents' education, religious instruction, and societal mores. For example, in Western culture, young people are praised for appearing sexually attractive but chastised for behaving sexually. This can lead to guilt about sex and result in future sexual dysfunction. Racial and ethnic differences in sexual problems are modest in women and present to a lesser extent in men. Specific disorders may have variable prevalences in specific ethnic or racial groups. For example, Laumann and colleagues report that white women have the highest rates of sexual pain disorders.

ORGANIC VERSUS PSYCHOGENIC

In some patients, the sexual problem may be clearly due to either an organic or a psychogenic cause, especially in younger, healthier individuals. Psychogenic problems usually begin abruptly, are situational or episodic, and are temporally related to specific events or stressors. Except for those problems caused by physical trauma, organic problems are usually gradual in onset and persistent, progressing from partial to absolute, and correlating with the progression of medical disease.

However, as suggested by the three-dimensional model (see Fig. 7-1), most sexual problems are multifactorial. This is especially true in older patients with comorbid medical illnesses, where biological, psychological, and social factors can affect all three phases of the sexual response cycle, often simultaneously (see Fig. 7-1 and Table 7-2). Given these complex interactions, the best approach, guided by the steps outlined in Table 7-1, is to consider the relative importance of each identified factor and address those factors that are amenable to intervention. The following vignette demonstrates the level of complexity that can be found in some clinical cases.

SALLY HARPER *Sally Harper is 42 years old, and a former intravenous drug user on methadone maintenance. She has symptomatic AIDS, recurrent genital herpes lesions, depression, and takes* *multiple medications. She complains of decreased libido and pain with intercourse worsened by condom use. On further history she describes low self-esteem, feelings of being "dirty," and interpersonal difficulties with her male partner, who continues to use intravenous drugs.*

Conceptualizing Sexual Problems

The development of a sexual dysfunction is conceptualized by Wincze and Carey as having "predisposing," "precipitating," and "maintaining" factors (see Fig. 7-1 and Table 7-1). Predisposing factors, such as prior life experiences (e.g., childhood trauma) and medical conditions (e.g., diabetes), place an individual at risk. Patients must have a predisposing factor, but these factors alone are often insufficient to cause sexual dysfunction. Precipitating causes are those reactions, feelings, and organic factors that immediately impinge on sexual responsiveness. Examples include medication side effects, performance anxiety, and "spectatoring" (obsessive self-observation during sex). Precipitating factors translate predisposing factors into real sexual dysfunctions. Maintaining factors are those ongoing life circumstances or physical ailments that contribute to the persistence of a sexual problem.

Historically, sexual conflicts were understood in terms of the traditional psychoanalytic view of deep-seated conflicts and developmental problems. It is now recognized that the sexual response is a learned phenomenon that is subject to behavioral conditioning. Therefore, sexual function and dysfunction can be learned and unlearned. This premise is the theoretical foundation of most forms of sex therapy.

HAROLD LOCKWOOD *Mr. Lockwood is 52 years old. He is* ***predisposed*** *to erectile problems by use of a calcium channel blocker and hypertension. Erectile dysfunction is* ***precipitated*** *by an argument with his wife just prior to sex. His problem persists even after the medication is stopped, probably* ***maintained*** *in part by learned inhibition.*

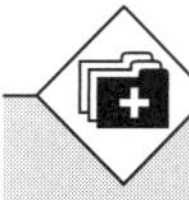

The Sexual History

Clinicians do not regularly ask about sexual problems, nor do patients initiate discussions about such problems. Schorer and Jensen found that only 23 percent of men and 56 percent of women say that they will raise sexual concerns with their clinicians, and just 10 percent of patients with chronic illness actually request help with sexual problems. Furthermore, many sexual concerns are masked as psychosomatic complaints (e.g., headaches, abdominal pain, fatigue, or sleeping problems). Clinicians need to understand that a patient's failure to mention sexual concerns does not mean that such concerns are absent.

Clinicians may be reluctant to discuss sexual issues because they do not want to offend the patient and feel awkward using sexual language. However, patients are almost always grateful and willing to discuss a problem when the clinician initiates these conversations.

Screening for Sexual Problems

The sexual history can be inserted into the medical interview where the clinician finds it appropriate and when the questions arise naturally. Good opportunities to introduce the topic include the urogenital or gynecologic systems review or when questioning about social habits such as smoking or alcohol intake. Many clinicians find it more comfortable to ask sexual questions in the context of relationship issues: "Are you having a meaningful relationship at this time?" or "Are you sexually involved in this relationship?" The clinician can begin the discussion by asking permission and universalizing the process: "May I ask you some questions about your sexual functioning that I ask all my patients?" Once the topic is introduced, the clinician should take a brief screening sexual history that covers STD risk assessment, partners, practices, and sexual satisfaction. A screening history includes the following questions:

- Do you engage in oral sex?
- Do you have vaginal or anal intercourse?
- How many partners have you had?
- Are your partners men, women, or both?
- What is your pattern of sexual activity (monogamy, multiple, or casual partners)?
- Do you use condoms?
- Do you use other forms of birth control?

Next, the clinician should ask more detailed questions about the patient's sexual functioning. The clinician may even wish to tell patients that she will now be asking more specific questions. Important specific questions include the following:

- How satisfied are you with your sexual functioning?
- Do you have any problems with sexual interest, such as too little interest?
- *For men:* Do you have problems developing or maintaining an erection?
- *For women:* Do you have problems becoming excited or with lubrication?
- Do you reach orgasm? Does it happen in the right amount of time for you?
- *For men:* Does your ejaculation happen in the wrong direction or with pain?
- Have you (or your partner) noticed any changes in your sexual experience lately?
- *When appropriate:* Does your illness interfere with sex? If so, how?
- Do you have pain with sexual activity?

Additionally, it is good policy to follow these questions with a "safety net" of questions such as: "Do you have any other questions or concerns about sex?"

It is important not to make assumptions about the patient's sexuality based on the patient's age, marital status, gender, or appearance. A primary relationship may not be the only one that a patient is having. Individuals may be having extramarital relationships, some of which may be with same-sex partners. An elderly patient assumed to be sexually inactive may in fact be engaging in high-risk sexual behavior. Clinicians should also avoid framing questions by heterosexual standards; for example, instead of asking about a boyfriend or girlfriend, ask about a partner.

Communications Issues in Taking a Patient's Sexual History

When taking a sexual history, it is most useful to start with a closed-ended question instead of the open-ended questions usually recommended in the general medical interview. This reversal of the open to closed sequence assists patients in overcoming barriers to discussing difficult topics and models the desired level of explicitness. Examples of such closed-ended questions are "Do you experience any troubles with orgasm?" or "Have you had any homosexual experiences?" Positive answers should be followed up with open-ended questions such as "Can you tell me more about that?"

Responding to Emotions

Skillful and careful attention to emotions promotes the therapeutic alliance, comforts and supports the patient, encourages patients to bring up difficult or embarrassing issues, and facilitates information gathering. The interviewer may initially experience discomfort, but, as with many other areas of interviewing that are difficult, the discomfort will diminish with persistence and practice. Clinicians should be aware that they might be the only individuals that have ever inquired about the patient's sexual history.

The emotional content can sometimes be extreme by any measure. For example, a patient who has been sexually abused may disclose the abuse in a very emotional manner. Therefore, the clinician should be prepared to listen and respond with problem-specific interventions such as referral to a trained mental health specialist.

LANGUAGE

Clinicians should use language that is clear and explicit. Following a patient's lead is a good way to start. The following guidelines by Williams may be helpful.

- Avoid euphemisms (e.g., "losing one's nature") and clarify any terms that patients use.
- Avoid both over-medicalized terms ("anorgasmia") and excessive informality ("can't get it up").
- Use terminology appropriate to the patient's level of understanding and comfort.
- If unsure, start with more formal terms and progress to colloquial terms as needed.
- Use language that is comfortable for you as well as for the patient.

The interviewer may also use interventions such as: "Let me know if you are not sure what I am asking," or "Use your own words and I will tell you if I do not understand." The interviewer should avoid words that are demeaning or appear judgmental. "Impotence" or "adultery" may be replaced with objective, descriptive phrases such as: "Do you have difficulty maintaining erections" or "Do you have sex outside your marriage?"

Sexual Problem History

After discovering a sexual concern, the practitioner's next step is to conduct a sexual problem interview. The following steps can serve as a guide.

First, ask for a detailed description of the symptom or problem using the closed to open questioning approach. Lead the patient through a typical sexual experience, going through each step of the sexual response cycle. Have the patient characterize a problem as it develops over time from its onset. The presenting complaint may actually be the result of a dysfunction in another phase. For example, a patient presenting with erectile dysfunction (an arousal disorder) may actually have premature ejaculation (an orgasm phase disorder) as the primary problem. Determine in what situations the problem occurs. Does it occur with all partners and under all circumstances, including masturbation?

Explore the biopsychosocial context, including the circumstances at the onset. Inquire about the patient's and partner's reactions and responses to the problem. Discuss the nature of the relationship with the partner(s). Ask about nonsexual characteristics of the relationship such as affection and communication. Review prior sexual functioning and traumatic events, such as embarrassing sexual episodes, previous sexual abuse, or same-sex encounters. Assess the patient's motivation for treatment, especially if the problem is not a chief complaint.

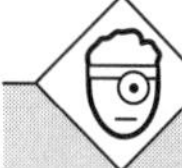

Physical Examination

The clinical evaluation should include a general physical and mental status examination. The clinician should assess the overall effect of chronic medical illnesses and screen for conditions such diabetes and hypertension. More extensive physical examination should be tailored to the individual situation, focusing on the anatomy and physiology related to the sexual response phase of the presenting problem.

The endocrine evaluation is particularly important for evaluation of desire phase disorders. This evaluation should include secondary sex characteristics, and thyroid, adrenal, and pituitary function, including a check for galactorrhea in men and women. Particularly important for arousal disorders, the vascular system assessment should consist of blood pressure, pulses, bruits, and evidence of peripheral vascular disease (skin temperature and color changes, hair growth, ulceration). The nervous system exam involves checking spinal cord function (motor strength and reflexes), distal and saddle sensation, anal sphincter tone and the bulbocavernosus reflex, as well as looking for surgical scars from a procedure that might have affected nerve supply to the genitals.

The male exam, as clinically indicated, should look for evidence of gynecomastia and assess hair pattern (beard, balding, axillary and pubic hair). It should include examination of the testes and scrotum (for evidence of varicocele, atrophy, mass, hernia), penis (to look for curvature, phimosis, paraphimosis, ulcerations, scars, and discharge), anus (especially checking for loss of sphincter tone), and prostate.

The female exam, guided by the clinical situation, should include a thorough genital exam. The vulvar exam should include looking for clitoral enlargement, infections, ulcers, lesions, and scars. The woman can use a mirror to indicate painful areas, and a Q-tip can be used to check for areas of tenderness. The vaginal exam may reveal atrophy, discharge, vaginal atresia, or a defective vaginal repair (including female circumcision). During the speculum and bimanual exam, the clinician should evaluate perineal muscle tone and search for signs of pregnancy, pelvic inflammatory disease, masses, cystitis, urethritis, and pelvic relaxation.

Performing a physical exam can contribute to other components of assessment and treatment. For example, whether or not the exam is normal, the clinician's reassurance will help alleviate the patient's anxiety, which can often be profound. Naming genital parts can give patients further permission to bring up specific questions about their body and its functioning.

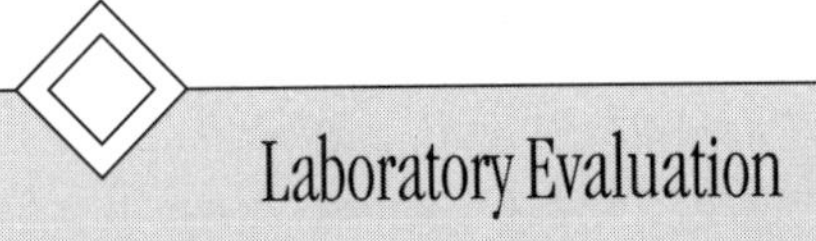

Laboratory Evaluation

There is no such thing as baseline laboratory testing for sexual dysfunctions, especially in patients with apparently psychogenic problems. Instead, laboratory testing is based on the type of disorder being examined. The general laboratory evaluation to rule out organic causes of desire and arousal disorders includes a complete blood count; profiles to evaluate thyroid, liver, and renal functions; and any work-up indicated for a suspected chronic illness. Arousal disorder testing should also include a fasting glucose, urinalysis, and serologic tests for syphilis.

In women, clinicians should focus further evaluation on suspected or identified problems (e.g., wet mount for vaginitis, pelvic ultrasound for fibroids, laparoscopy for endometriosis). In perimenopausal women, checking levels of estradiol, luteinizing hormone (LH), and follicle-stimulating hormone (FSH) may be helpful. For low sexual desire associated with galactorrhea or menstrual irregularities, tests for prolactin and androgens, such as testosterone and dehydroepiandrosterone sulfate (DHEAS), may be ordered. In all women, estradiol levels less than 35 correlate with low frequency of sexual activity.

Clinicians should check testosterone levels in men with decreased libido if there is a suspicion of hypogonadism. If the total testosterone level is below 500 ng/dL, free testosterone, FSH, LH, and prolactin should be measured. Although common clinical practice, it is controversial whether all men with erectile dysfunction should have serum prolactin and testosterone levels measured. It is probably worthwhile to order these tests in men with both desire and arousal problems if the etiology is unclear. Specific clinical concerns may warrant tests such as prostate specific antigen (PSA) for a prostate nodule, urethral culture for urethritis, and so on.

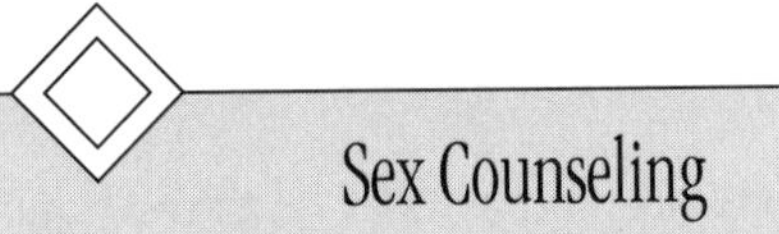

Sex Counseling

The primary care setting is often the only place where patients will have the opportunity to receive sex therapy because the accessibility to formal sex therapy is often limited by availability, cost, or managed care restrictions. Therefore, primary care clinicians should learn to incorporate the basic skills of sex therapy into clinical practice. This section describes the "P-LI-SS-IT" model, a set of general principles that clinicians can use to guide brief, office-based sex therapy.

The P-LI-SS-IT Model

The P-LI-SS-IT model, developed by Annon, is a widely accepted step-wise approach to managing sexual disorders. The primary goal of the P-LI-SS-IT intervention is to restore the individual's or the couple's mutual sexual comfort and satisfaction.

P—Permission

This critical step is designed to give patients permission to discuss, explore, and resolve sexual concerns. The clinician should model communication skills, such as reflective listening (stating what you heard the patient say) and empathic statements, which can be a form of communication skills training for the patient. By offering authoritative reassurance, the clinician can normalize and universalize sexual concerns. Other permission-giving interventions might include encouraging a patient to talk more openly with a partner or supporting the patient in saying no to undesired sexual activity.

LI—Limited Information

The clinician may also provide factual information related to the patient's specific concerns or questions. Descriptions should be focused on the concern, in language the patient understands, and possibly accompanied by diagrams of genitals or anatomic structures. Explanations might include the physiology of the sexual response, medication side effects, or the effect of inexperience or aging on sexual responsiveness. The clinician should be able to recommend several lay press publications to patients as a form of sex education.

SS—Specific Suggestions

Often, patients will be grateful for permission, reassurance, and information, but they may require further guidance in dealing with a sexual problem. The clinician can use specific suggestions aimed at improved emotional and sexual communication. Because sexual concerns are often relationship concerns, discussion about treatment should usually involve the sexual partner, if the patient has one. Inviting the patient to include the partner helps to gain the partner's perspective and begins the therapeutic process. This intervention reassures the couple that sexual problems are treatable, and immediately begins to unburden the couple, offer relief, and orient them toward the future. Below are several therapeutic options clinicians can suggest to the patients.

SENSATE FOCUS EXERCISES The sensate focus exercises help couples to improve sexual functioning by reducing performance anxiety. These exercises are designed to develop a heightened awareness of and focus on sensations rather than focusing on performance.

The clinician gives the couples explicit instructions for intimacy. The couples are advised to temporarily refrain from sexual intercourse and reapproach sexual relations in a gradual, nonthreatening manner. They are instructed to progress from pleasurable touch (initially clothed), to kissing, to genital caressing. When the couple gains confidence and perceives diminished anxiety and improved communication, intercourse is reintroduced in a controlled fashion, often with specific behavioral and technical suggestions. The clinician recommends the steps as homework and sees the couple at regular intervals to monitor their progress.

KEGEL EXERCISES Kegel exercises involve contracting the pubococcygeus muscles to intensify the sexual response. Both men and women can contract these muscles. A clinician can instruct a woman on this technique during the two-finger pelvic exam, by having the woman contract her muscles around the fingers. Men can be told to identify the muscles' location by contracting their anal sphincter. Patients practice this contraction and then incorporate it into sexual activity.

TECHNICAL ADVICE Clinicians might include specific technical suggestions such as the use of lubricants or a change in sexual positioning from the traditional missionary position. For example, some women are not aware that having the woman on top during intercourse may enhance control over timing and clitoral stimulation.

DIRECT SELF-STIMULATION (MASTURBATION TRAINING) The clinician can recommend that patients masturbate as a way of helping them explore their sexual responsiveness and sensations in a nonthreatening manner.

STIMULUS CONTROL AND SCHEDULING The clinician may recommend that the patient or couple establish a pleasant, relaxing environment that is conducive to sexual expression. Suggestions might include scheduling time for sex or arranging childcare.

COGNITIVE RESTRUCTURING This approach aims at helping patients to identify negative thought patterns and reduce interfering thoughts. For example, a woman whose prior partner was unfaithful may have difficulty trusting a new partner. The clinician can help her examine the influence of old experiences on current feelings. Many patients express concern about intruding thoughts, such as work concerns, during sex. Practitioners can suggest compartmentalizing thoughts during specific times of the day and scheduling time for pleasurable thoughts and sexual fantasies.

IT—Intensive Therapy

When the three previous levels of the P-LI-SS-IT model (permission giving, limited information, specific suggestions) have not been effective, the next step is referral for intensive therapy. It is important to clarify patients' or couples' motivation for such treatment. Sex therapy often intensifies the principles described above and employs additional modalities including psychotherapy, relaxation training, hypnosis and imagery, and group therapy. Practitioners should acquaint themselves with resources available in a practice setting. The indications for referral include the following.

- Sexual dysfunctions not responsive to primary care interventions,
- Relationship difficulties requiring counseling,
- Mental disorders requiring psychiatric referral for diagnosis and treatment,
- Intrapsychic issues requiring psychotherapy, and
- Past sexual or other trauma requiring treatment.

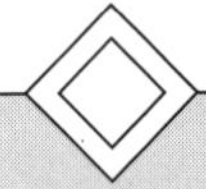

The Classic Sexual Dysfunctions

Sexual dysfunctions, as classified by the DSM-IV, are disturbances in the sexual response cycle or pain associated with sexual intercourse (Table 7-4). Sexual disorders can cause marked distress and interpersonal conflict. These dysfunctions can be classified as occurring during the desire phase, the arousal phase, and the orgasm phase. They can further be classified as primary/lifelong (no previous history of functioning) or secondary/acquired (previous normal function), and as generalized/global (all partners, activities, situations, forms of sexual expression) or situational (certain partners, circumstances, practices).

Desire Phase Disorders

Hypoactive Sexual Desire

More than 50 percent of patients presenting for treatment for sexual disorders complain of hypoactive desire, according to Laumann and colleagues. It occurs in 22 percent of women in community samples. The essential feature is a deficiency or absence of sexual fantasies and lack of desire for sexual activity. Individuals with this disorder do not usually initiate sexual activity and reluctantly agree when it is initiated by their partner. Usually the frequency of sexual activity is low. Because

Table 7-4

Sexual Dysfunctions Categorized by Phase of the Sexual Response Cycle*

PHASES	CHARACTERISTICS	DYSFUNCTION
Desire	Sexual fantasies and the desire for sex.	Hypoactive sexual desire disorder; sexual aversion disorder; substance-induced sexual dysfunction with impaired desire.
Arousal	A subjective sense of sexual pleasure and accompanying physiologic changes.	Female sexual arousal disorder and male erectile disorder (may be due to a general medical condition); substance-induced sexual dysfunction with impaired arousal.
Orgasm	A peaking of sexual pleasure, with release of sexual tension and rhythmic contraction of the perineal muscles and pelvic reproductive organs.	Female orgasmic disorder; male orgasmic disorder; premature ejaculation; male delayed, retrograde, and painful ejaculation; substance-induced sexual dysfunction with impaired orgasm.
Non–phase-specific disorder	These disorders affect various phases of the response cycle.	Sexual pain disorders; dyspareunia and vaginismus.

*DSM-IV consolidates the Masters and Johnson excitement and plateau phases into a single arousal phase. The orgasm phase remains the same as originally described by Masters and Johnson. The resolution phase is omitted because sexual problems with this phase are rare.
SOURCE: Adapted with permission from Sadock V: Normal human sexuality and sexual and gender identity disorders. In: Sadock, Kaplan (eds): *Comprehensive Textbook of Psychiatry*. Baltimore, MD: Williams & Wilkins; 1995, 1295.

there are no standards for frequency and degree of sexual desire, the diagnosis of this disorder is mainly based on clinical judgment of the individuals' characteristics, interpersonal determinants, life context, and cultural setting.

SITUATIONAL ACQUIRED HYPOACTIVE SEXUAL DESIRE DISORDER Individuals with situational hypoactive sexual desire disorder may have sustained masturbatory behavior and active fantasy but diminished interest in their partner, or they may have interest only in partners outside their primary relationship. These problems most likely reflect interpersonal difficulties or other psychogenic issues and are therefore best managed by referral for counseling.

When there are discrepancies between the sexual desire of each partner, it is important to assess both partners. Apparently low sexual desire in one partner may actually reflect an excessive need for sexual expression by the other partner. Sometimes, partners may have the same sexual desire but at different times. The most common relationship issue in hypoactive sexual disorder is unresolved conflict and disappointment that leads to subsequent anger, hidden resentment, and unconscious alienation.

Treatment of hypoactive sexual desire depends on the cause. Interventions might include facilitating communication between partners, recommending scheduled time for renewed intimacy, or brief, targeted couples therapy. Acute stress can have a transient effect on desire, and offering this explanation as well as giving permission to say no temporarily to sex can be helpful. Occasionally, clinicians may encounter patients with atypical arousal patterns, such as fetishism, that emerge only during periods of extreme stress. They require referral if the patterns are persistent or distressing to the individual.

GENERALIZED ACQUIRED HYPOACTIVE DESIRE DISORDER Generalized acquired desire disorders can be caused by illness, medications, depression, and hormonal abnormalities such as thyroid dysfunction, androgen deficiency, panhypopitituitarism, or hyperprolactinemia. They can also occur in situations in which there is an excess of endogenous beta-endorphins (e.g., in athletes) or exogenous opioids (e.g., prescription drugs) (see Tables 7-2 and 7-3). Pregnancy and premenstrual syndrome may also produce decreased desire, the latter probably due to the cyclic changes in mood rather than hormonal effects. These cases are managed by addressing the underlying condition.

Hypogonadism is discovered in 15 percent of men with decreased desire. The serum LH level can be helpful in distinguishing the cause of a low testosterone level. The LH level will be low in pituitary dysfunction and high in men with testicular failure. Testosterone levels decline with age, and older men may have signs and symptoms of hypogonadism with testosterone levels in the low-normal range. Testosterone replacement is available in injection (dose of 200 mg intramuscularly every 2 weeks), transdermal (dose of 5 to 10 mg), and gel preparations (5 g/day). Injections result in high testosterone levels initially and then have decreased efficacy, and the topical agents may cause local irritation or be difficult to apply. In young hypogonadal men, testosterone therapy has clearly been shown to improve libido, erections, and mood. HIV-infected hypogonadal men also demonstrate increased energy and body mass with testosterone treatment. In older men with low or low-normal testosterone levels, the benefits of therapy are less clear. The main adverse effects of testosterone therapy are acne, polycythemia, hepatic abnormalities, prostate enlargement, and increased growth of undiagnosed prostate cancer. Treatment is contraindicated in those with prostate cancer or bladder neck obstruction due to prostatic hypertrophy. There is also evidence that exogenous testosterone can adversely influence lipid levels and may increase the risk of developing prostate cancer. Therefore, the testosterone level, hematocrit, lipids, and PSA should be measured every 6 months, and the prostate exam should also be regularly monitored.

While there is no evidence that estrogen deficiency in women impairs sexual desire, declining estrogen levels at menopause cause decreased lubrication, which can affect arousal and, secondarily, desire. There has been some controversy about the effect of declining levels of androgens (testosterone and DHEAS) on desire in postmenopausal women. Recent information suggests that combined estrogen-androgen replacement provides greater improvement in psychologic (depression, concentration, fatigue) and sexual symptoms (desire and ability to reach orgasm) than does estrogen alone. In postmenopausal women who have decreased libido and do not respond to hormone replacement therapy alone for this problem, you may use physiologic doses of oral testosterone combined with estrogen replacement therapy in the form of Estratest or Estratest HS, which has oral methyltestosterone. It seems to help libido in some women and appears to be safe. Data are not yet available on estrogen replacement therapy longer than a few years.

In oophorectomized women there was an important study by Shifren and colleagues looking at the use of testosterone patch in women on estrogen replacement therapy for 2 months or more. With the 300 μg testosterone dose patch, women over 48 years of age had improved sexual functioning compared to placebo. This is very short-term data (12 weeks) and leaves open long-term issues of safety.

Testosterone therapy in women has the potential but undemonstrated risks of virilization, lipid, and liver function abnormalities, nonlipid negative cardiovascular effects, and unfavorable changes in body composition. The theoretical risks apply to both long term oral and transdermal testosterone therapy.

LIFELONG GENERALIZED HYPOACTIVE DESIRE DISORDERS

Lifelong generalized hypoactive sexual desire is usually a psychogenic disorder that is complicated in origin and difficult to treat. Positive sexual experiences acquired through sensate focus, masturbation training with fantasy, or the use of erotica can increase desire. However, this condition is often best managed by a sex therapy specialist. Patients with a history of sexual abuse may have a lifelong pattern of chronic intermittent libido problems and may require extremely high levels of intimacy and safety to experience sexual desire. Such patients should also be referred for specialized treatment.

ANDREA NELSON *Andrea Nelson is a 33-year-old woman who has migraine headaches that are controlled with beta-blocker prophylactic therapy. On screening sexual history performed during a visit for a Pap smear, she reports that she has had difficulty finding a steady partner, primarily because she has very little sexual interest and has not felt pleasure with most of her partners. Her most satisfying sexual relationship was with a very close female co-worker. Primary care management for Andrea includes changing her medication, recommending masturbation, and referring her for psychotherapy to resolve her expressed concerns about sexual orientation and intimacy.*

SEXUAL AVERSION DISORDER

The essential feature of this rare desire disorder is the aversion to and active avoidance of genital sexual contact with a sexual partner. Patients report marked anxiety and distress when confronted with an opportunity for sexual activity. The aversion to genital contact may be focused on a particular aspect of the sexual experience (e.g., genital secretion, vaginal penetration), and patients may have extreme psychological distress. Although 25 percent of afflicted individuals meet criteria for panic disorder, it is believed that the panic disorder is comorbid with rather than the cause of this sexual disorder. Sexual aversion disorder is usually rooted in developmental factors (often sexual trauma), family of origin conflicts, or serious psychopathology. Patients with sexual aversion disorder should be referred to a specialist.

Arousal Phase Disorders

In men and women, arousal phase dysfunction is defined as the recurrent and persistent inhibition of arousal in the presence of sexual stimulation that is adequate in focus, intensity, and duration. It may be associated with lack of desire, orgasm difficulties, and dyspareunia. It can be caused by an extensive list of medical conditions, medications, and psychosocial factors (see Tables 7-2 and 7-3).

MALE ERECTILE DISORDER

Much attention has been focused on male erectile disorder in the past decade due to increased recognition, improved knowledge of the pathophysiology, and dramatic improvements in therapy, all of which have led to treatment in the primary care arena. Although the estimated prevalence of erectile disorder in all age groups is 5 percent, the Massachusetts Male Aging Study and its follow-up study revealed that 52 percent of men ages 40 to 70 had some degree of erectile dysfunction, with 17 percent having minimum, 25 percent having moderate, and 10 percent having complete erectile failure. Fifteen percent of men over age 70 have complete erectile failure. An organic cause is much more likely in men over 50. However, almost all organic problems have a psychosocial component.

As men age, they may require more direct physical stimulation of the penis to achieve and maintain an erection, so it is important to determine the degree and manner of stimulation during a typical sexual experience. Men with organic erectile disorder may develop performance anxiety and premature ejaculation, which may be the presenting complaint. Therefore, it is important to review the evolution of the disorder from its onset over time.

Lifelong generalized erectile problems may result from congenital vascular problems and focal cavernosal arterial blockade secondary to trauma at a prepubescent age. The problems require referral to a urologist for evaluation. On the other hand, situational (intermittent) but lifelong erectile difficulties are usually psychogenic. They are rarely encountered in primary care settings and usually require psychiatric treatment.

ACQUIRED PSYCHOGENIC ERECTILE DYSFUNCTION These disorders are commonly seen by primary care clinicians. The most important first task for the clinician is to establish whether the problem is situational or pervasive. The presence of erectile dysfunction in sexual situations but adequate morning erections establishes normal physiologic functioning and suggests a psychogenic rather than an organic cause. The same conclusion is true for men who can perform normally in certain sexual situations and not in others. However, men with mild to moderate erectile impairment can have varying degrees of success depending on the situation and may be very sensitive to the effect of a medication or alcohol or to even the setting. Such short-lived psychogenic problems can often be managed by reassurance that physical causes are absent and that such difficulties are common and often resolve on their own. In men with psychogenic erectile disorder due to relationship issues, targeted behavioral therapy that includes the partner can have success rates as high as 70 percent, according to Seagraves and Rahman. Specific techniques may include sensate focus exercises, Kegel exercises, and enhanced direct penile stimulation during foreplay, possibly with the use of lubricants.

If office-based counseling and behavioral therapy are unsuccessful, a medication may be tried. In men with severe performance anxiety, low-dose beta-blocker treatment (e.g., propanolol 10 mg) has been effective. Yohimbine, prescribed in 5.4-mg doses three times daily for 4 to 6 weeks, may help 15 to 20 percent of men improve desire and erections. Its side effects, which may include palpitations, fine tremor, anxiety, and elevated blood pressure, may be limiting, and it is contraindicated in men with ulcer disease and hypertension. Yohimbine can be combined with 50 mg of trazadone at bedtime, although the data to support this approach are limited. Sildenafil is often effective for psychogenic disorders (discussed below). Patients whose condition is refractory to medication should be referred for urological and psychological evaluation.

ACQUIRED ERECTILE DISORDER AND DEPRESSION Generalized acquired erectile disorders are usually caused by organic problems or depression, which can be both a cause and a result of erectile difficulties. Men with erectile disorders are four times as likely to report low general happiness, and in the Massachusetts Male Aging Study the degree of depression correlated directly with erectile dysfunction. Feldman and colleagues found that severe depression is nearly 100 percent predictive of erectile disorder. At least 50 percent of men seeking help for erectile dysfunction will have some depressive symptoms. Patients with erectile disorders who remained depressed were more likely to discontinue erectile disorder treatment, demonstrating the importance of depression as barrier to treatment. On the other hand, treatment of erectile dysfunction can alleviate depression and improve quality of life.

ACQUIRED ORGANIC ERECTILE DYSFUNCTION Organic erectile dysfunction may result from neurologic, vascular, cavernosal, or hormonal causes, as well as medications and substances (see Tables 7-2 and 7-3). Neurologic dysfunction can result from any sensory disturbance of the local sacral reflex arc involved in erection. Nervous system causes include peripheral neuropathy (e.g., diabetes, multiple sclerosis, or chronic alcohol use), CNS disorders (e.g., Alzheimer's disease or strokes), and spinal cord injury. Pelvic surgery or pelvic injury can also disrupt neurologic function. For example, when Stanford and associates asked a sample of men who had had a radical prostatectomy, "how big a problem is sexual functioning?" 50 percent responded "moderate to big." Their problems improved only modestly over time.

Vascular causes include generalized arterial insufficiency due to hypertension, hyperlipidemia, or pelvic irradiation, and small vessel disease caused by diabetes or smoking. In diabetic men, vascular factors are probably more important than neurogenic factors. Vascular factors can be aggravated by cigarette smoking, which causes vascular endothelial damage and reversible local vasoconstriction due to elevated levels of carbon monoxide in the blood. Some men can improve their erectile function within 24 h of complete smoking cessation. Offering this information may be highly motivating to some patients. Other vascular factors include focal stenosis of the common penile artery due to pelvic or perineal injury and veno-occlusive dysfunction caused by diabetes, Peyronie's disease, or aging.

Many hypogonadal men experience desire-based arousal problems, even though androgens are not essential for erections. Therefore, hypogonadal men can present with an arousal phase disorder. The effect of hypogonadism on desire was discussed earlier in this chapter.

An array of medications cause erectile problems. Common culprits include antihypertensives and psychotropic drugs. Alcohol in small quantities improves erections but in large amounts causes transient dysfunction and detrimental effects on the peripheral nervous system and androgen production.

Some chronic medical illnesses cause erectile disorder through multiple mechanisms, often with devastating effects. For example, 50 percent of diabetic men have erectile disorder. Patients who have chronic renal failure experience erectile problems resulting from the combination of low testosterone levels, vascular disease, multiple medications, autonomic and peripheral neuropathy, and psychogenic factors.

Diagnosis of Erectile Dysfunction

In addition to the laboratory evaluation, studies of physiologic function may be performed. To help distinguish psychogenic from organic disorders, diagnostic testing may include an assessment of nocturnal erections with the home "postage stamp test," which can be suggested if the patient can obtain serrated stamps. The patient is instructed to wrap a ring of stamps snugly around his flaccid penis at night before going to bed, moistening the overlapping stamps to seal the ring. A positive test is finding the ring of stamps broken along the perforations when he awakens in the morning. Further diagnostic studies of tumescence require referral to a urologist. These studies include the inexpensive snap gauge, Rigiscan (a home monitoring program that is interpreted by computer software in the clinician's office), and measurement of nocturnal penile erections in a sleep laboratory. It is important to note that while the absence of tumescence strongly suggests an organic cause for erectile dysfunction, it does not conclusively rule out psychogenic causes, because diminished nocturnal erections may occur in depression.

When a vascular cause of erectile dysfunction is suspected, additional specialty testing might include duplex ultrasound of the corpus cavernosa, cavernosometry, cavernosonography, and pelvic arteriography, which are most often used in men under 40 with a history of pelvic trauma. Another useful test is to note the response to injection of a local vasodilator (prostaglandin E_1) combined with visual stimulation by erotica; this combination is used as an evaluation of arterial function and a therapeutic test in men desiring intracavernous therapy. Urologists occasionally evaluate patients with erectile disorders by using neurologic tests such as biothesiometry, bulbocavernosus latency time, evoked sacral responses, tests for autonomic neuropathy, and electromyography.

The decision to refer to a specialist for this testing depends on the patient's motivation for treatment and the complexity of the medical condition. Some conditions warranting referral include complex endocrine or gonadal disorders, brain or spinal cord injury, Peyronie's disease, and vascular conditions in men who are not candidates for oral medications like sildenafil.

Treatment of Organic Erectile Disorders

The primary care clinician can often address factors that accompany organic erectile problems using the principles of office-based therapy. The clinician can also educate the patient about lifestyle factors, such as smoking and the use of alcohol, and motivate the patient toward behavior change. The patient's desire to improve his sexual satisfaction can also be used to encourage the patient to deal with contributing medical illnesses, such as hyperlipidemia and hypertension.

The clinician may also prescribe an oral medication, such as sildenafil. Sexual stimulation releases nitric oxide, which activates cyclic guanosine monophosphate (cGMP) and causes vasodilation. Sildenafil enhances this process through selective inhibition of phosphodiesterase type 5, which inactivates cGMP. Since it was released in the United States in 1998, sildenafil has become first-line therapy for men with erectile disorder. For men without contraindications to the medication, sildenafil can be prescribed by the primary care clinician, often prior to any neurovascular work-up and without specialty referral. Over 20 clinical trials have demonstrated its efficacy in men with organic, psychogenic, and mixed causes of erectile dysfunction (including diabetes mellitus, spinal cord injury, radical prostatectomy, nonspecific psychogenic, and depression).

There has been much confusion and controversy regarding the use of sildenafil in men with cardiovascular disease. The present recommendations by Cheitlin and colleagues and published by the American Heart Association, are as follows:

1. Because the combination of sildenafil and nitrates can cause severe hypotension and death, sildenafil is absolutely contraindicated in men taking any form of nitrate medications and men who use nitrates for exercise-induced symptoms.
2. Although the risk of cardiac events caused by sildenafil in the absence of nitrates is low, treadmill testing may be indicated prior to instituting therapy in men with possible cardiac disease to assess the risk of ischemia during sexual activity.
3. Because of the hypotensive effect of sildenafil, blood pressure monitoring should be considered on initiation of treatment for men with congestive heart failure, low volume status, and complex antihypertensive regimens.

Sildenafil's main side effects, which are often transient and dose related, include headache, flushing, dyspepsia, nasal congestion, and visual changes. Because of changes to the retina, patients with retinal diseases (including diabetics) should have an ophthalmologic evaluation before they start taking sildenafil. Retinitis pigmentosa is a contraindication to treatment. The recommended starting dose is 50 mg (range 25 to 100 mg) taken 1 h before intended sexual activity, with a maximum frequency of one dose daily.

Many of the clinical trials evaluating the efficacy of sildenafil used a standardized questionnaire, the International Index of Erectile Function (IIEF). This is a 15-question survey from which the clinically applicable Sexual Health Inventory for Men was derived. This tool can be used in primary care practice to objectively track and assess a patient's response to treatment.

INTRACAVERNOUS, TRANSURETHRAL, AND MECHANICAL THERAPIES FOR ERECTILE DISORDERS Alprostadil is a synthetic of prostaglandin E_1 that is available in transurethral and intracavernous preparations. Transurethral alprostadil is effective in 43 percent of men with organic erectile disorder. It is easy to use and unlikely to cause drug interactions. The main side effects are urethral pain and burning. The ultimate dose range is 250 to 1000 μg, and the first dose (500 μg) should be given under the supervision of a clinician. Intracavernous alprostadil has higher success rates, resulting in erections in 70 percent of men. The main concerns with its use are priapism (up to 4 percent) and fibrosis, which can be minimized by administering the drug with proper technique, so the patient must be instructed by a urologist as to how to perform the injections. Up to one third of men on intracavernous alprostadil experience painful erections. Intracavernous alprostadil appears to work best in men with underlying nerve injury, although these men in particular may experience hyperalgesia. The dose range is 5 to 20 mg, and the appropriate dose provides an erection adequate for intercourse but that does not last longer than 1 h. Maximal use is two times weekly. Despite the favorable success rate, many men discontinue therapy or alternate with other treatments. The other available intracavernous therapy combines papaverine, phentolamine, and alprostadil (TRIMIX). Although alprostadil is not FDA approved, the drug combination has very high success rates and is widely used in the U. S.

Vacuum erection devices produce erections by passive suction. A tension ring is then placed at the base of the erect penis. This treatment is selected for men with organic causes who are not candidates for other therapies. Vacuum erection devices result in erection sufficient for intercourse 90 percent of the time. The main side effects are bruising, pain, and numbness. They cannot be used in men with Peyronie's disease or men who are taking anticoagulants. Some men are concerned that the device is artificial and intrusive and are disappointed with the quality of their erection.

Penile prostheses (implants) are considered when other treatments have failed or are rejected. Prostheses may be semi-rigid or inflatable. Their main risk is infection and mechanical failure, both of which require the device to be removed or replaced. Seventy-five percent of men receiving penile implants are satisfied with treatment.

Penile vascular reconstructive surgery is generally reserved for young men who have had pelvic vascular trauma. Men with large vessel abdominal aortic insufficiency, thigh claudication, and Leriche's syndrome may sometimes benefit from peripheral vascular bypass surgery.

Female Sexual Arousal Disorder

Less frequently seen in primary care is female sexual arousal disorder. Laumann and associates report the prevalence of sexual arousal disorder is 14 percent in women ages 18 to 59. It may be more common and undetected in older women. Patients present with a persistent or recurrent inability to attain or maintain an adequate lubrication-swelling response despite adequate stimulation. Usually libido is diminished. The most common causes of acquired arousal phase dysfunction are estrogen deficiency due to menopause, lactation, depression, anticholinergic medications, antihistaminic medications, or tricyclic antidepressants.

Female arousal is often maintained by psychological and physical stimulation. If decreased lubrication is associated with normal desire in premenopausal women who have no organic problem, the explanation is usually inadequate stimulation. If a woman is concerned about her decreased lubrication, psychogenic factors (e.g., anxiety resulting in self-observation) may maintain either a situational or generalized sexual dysfunction. Lifelong problems with arousal are usually psychogenic and require mental health referral.

Organic causes of female arousal disorders have not been studied as extensively as in men. Because physiologic arousal relies on vascular and neurologic systems, impairments in either domain may lead to difficulties. Studies reported by Schorer and Jensen suggest that women with type 1 diabetes are prone to arousal problems, and women with type 2 diabetes are much less sexually satisfied and have difficulties in all phases of the sexual response cycle. There is some evidence that antihypertensive medications have effects on women's sexual function that are similar to the effects seen in men.

Diagnosis of Female Arousal Dysfunction

Techniques for measuring nocturnal vaginal blood flow have shown that vaginal engorgement cycles take place during rapid eye movement (REM) sleep with the same frequency that erectile cycles occur in men. To date, the only clearly successful clinical use of monitoring nocturnal vaginal blood flow has been to show that postmenopausal women presenting with vaginal atrophy and dyspareunia lack basal levels of vaginal capillary blood flow. During arousal these women do not reach the level of engorgement that unaffected women do. Estrogen replacement therapy reverses these findings. However, in laboratory studies of women with impaired vaginal blood flow and arousal despite erotic stimulation, it is unclear whether the cause is psychological or physiologic. Presently, there are no satisfactory measurements of sensory, motor, or autonomic nerve function.

Treatment of Female Arousal Phase Disorder

In estrogen-deficient women, the treatment of choice is estrogen replacement, either in the form of systemic or topical therapy. Systemic estrogen regimens can be used either continuously or cyclically. Topical therapy is self-administered several times weekly with a vaginal applicator. Systemic absorption occurs, so topical estrogens are inappropriate for women with a history of breast cancer or other contraindications to estrogen therapy. Other options include the use of topical vaginal moisturizers (used regularly) and water soluble lubricants (used during sexual activity). These may be recommended for women who are not candidates for estrogen therapy or have other medical causes, such as vascular insufficiency. Medical factors that might be involved in the problem should also be addressed.

Office-based counseling and behavioral therapies are helpful adjuncts in the treatment of arousal problems. These include giving women permission to discover and explore what stimulation works best, educating them about the physiology of arousal and the role of anxiety, and offering technical suggestions, including genital caressing exercises and use of self-help books.

LAURA AND HANK GRANT *Mrs. Grant is 58 years old. She has well-controlled type 2 diabetes. She mentions to her clinician during a routine visit that she is concerned about her lack of interest in sex. She describes vaginal dryness and pain with intercourse, and her exam reveals atrophy. She notes that she and Hank, her husband of 32 years, have sex much less often, and he always initiates it. She wishes "things were like before." The clinician asks her to bring Hank to the next visit.*

When interviewing the couple, the clinician learns that Hank has had a gradual but progressive course of erectile dysfunction over the past 5 years. He has diabetes and hypertension and is on insulin and several antihypertensive medications. He had considered using sildenafil, but decided not to because he was uncomfortable "using an artificial substance for a natural act." Their typical sexual experience involves little foreplay prior to intercourse. They both acknowledge that they have been withdrawing from one another sexually and have very little physical intimacy. They are spending less time together overall, even though their four grown children have left home.

The clinician reflects to Hank and Laura that they still have a great deal of love for one another and both want to renew the intimate aspects of their relationship. He encourages them to talk more to one another about these feelings and to spend more nonsexual time together. He explains that many men need more direct penile stimulation with age and that many women need psychological and physical stimulation for excitement. He encourages Hank and Laura to use the sensate focus approach, including a temporary prohibition on intercourse and progression from nongenital to genital touching prior to resuming intercourse. He prescribes topical estrogen for Laura and recommends that she use vaginal lubricants with intercourse. He emphasizes the benefits of sildenafil to Hank and encourages him to reconsider using this medication if the problem does not improve. He also sets up a return visit in 2 weeks for follow-up.

Orgasm Phase Disorders

Orgasm phase disorders are common. They include premature ejaculation and other conditions in men, and delayed or absent orgasm in women. These disorders can often be treated in primary care settings.

Premature Ejaculation

Premature ejaculation is the most common problem in men presenting for sexual dysfunction treatment. The estimated prevalence is 21 to 36 percent, and the condition is predominantly seen in younger men. Terms like rapid or early ejaculation are sometimes used because they emphasize the subjective nature of the complaint, defining it as ejaculation "before the person wishes it." This approach focuses on the man's sense of control and satisfaction. It is important to consider the psychosocial context, as well as obtain a description of a sexual experience in which the problem has occurred. For example, an episode of rapid ejaculation may be normal after starting a new relationship, or a man may be unrealistic about the length of time he can maintain an erection after penetration.

Lifelong premature ejaculation is an idiopathic and psychogenic disorder. Etiologic theories include poor perception of ejaculatory inevitability, early conditioning experiences in which patients learn to masturbate rapidly, and somatic hypersensitivity, all potentially combined with performance anxiety. Acquired premature ejaculation points to a psychosocial problem, such as guilt over an extramarital affair or relationship difficulty. Over time, this disorder can create a sense of inadequacy, secondary erectile failure, and reactions in the partner.

Premature ejaculation can be easily managed in the primary care setting. Behavioral treatment requires diminishing anxiety and retraining the ejaculatory reflex. The clinician should explain that this is a common problem and that improved control can be learned. The clinician can teach patients about the consequences of early conditioning and performance anxiety. Specific suggestions include increasing the frequency of ejaculation (e.g., masturbate before an intended sexual encounter), relaxing pelvic muscles, increasing foreplay prior to penetration, changing positions during intercourse, using condoms, and reading self-help books.

The "stop-start" technique is the most commonly used behavioral therapy. It is best to include a partner, if the patient has one, although the man can modify the approach on his own. In the initial phase, the couple is told to refrain from intercourse. The partner is instructed to orally or manually stimulate the patient, who is told to signal his partner when ejaculation is inevitable, at which point stimulation is discontinued. This process is repeated three times prior to ejaculation. Some failed attempts are part of the learning process. When the man's latency time to ejaculation is between 5 and 10 min, intercourse is reintroduced. Then the stop-start pauses are used with the woman on top.

If behavioral treatment is unsuccessful, the clinician can institute pharmacologic treatment to induce ejaculatory delay. Medication may be used initially if the problem is severe or if the patient does not have a steady partner. The antidepressant clomipramine (a hybrid tricyclic and serotonin reuptake inhibitor) can be used in doses of 25 to 50 mg 6 h prior to intended intercourse. If this is unsuccessful or inconvenient, the same dose can be taken daily. The serotonin reuptake inhibitors are also effective in delaying ejaculation. Paroxetine (20 to 40 mg) and sertraline (100 to 150 mg) can be used daily. The maximal effect may take several weeks. Although randomized trial data support their use, these medications are not FDA approved for this indication. They are also ineffective in men with acquired disorders, which often require psychotherapy. Premature ejaculation will frequently occur when drugs are discontinued, so it may be best to combine medication with behavioral therapy.

Other Male Orgasm Phase Disorders

These disorders include anorgasmia, ejaculatory delay, retrograde ejaculation, and painful orgasm, which have a combined prevalence of 8 percent. By definition, they occur after a normal excitation phase. In primary care, lifelong inhibited male orgasm is rarely seen. Its origins are psychogenic and warrant mental health referral. Inhibited male orgasm disorder is usually situational.

These disorders are usually acquired as a result of medical conditions (see Tables 7-3 and 7-5). Painful ejaculation may result from medications such as tricyclic antidepressants or vacuum erection devices. Delayed ejaculation is usually caused by organic factors such as neurologic conditions,

Table 7-5

Dyspareunia in Women: Organic Factors

Superficial	Deep
Atrophic vaginitis	Adhesions
Bartholin's gland inflammation	Cervical cancer
Inadequate vaginal lubrication secondary to hormonal changes: lactation, oophorectomy	Cervicitis
Episiotomy scar	Endometriosis
Female circumcision	Hemorrhoids
Human papilloma virus infection	Intrauterine device complication
Hymen: fibrotic, imperforate	Ovarian cysts, tumors
Infections: bacterial vaginosis, *Candida albicans*, *Chlamydia*, herpes, *Trichomonas*	Pelvic tumors
Irritants: contraceptives, douches	Pelvic inflammatory disease
Postradiation vaginal changes	Uterus: prolapsed, retroverted fibroid
Sjögren's syndrome	**Miscellaneous**
Urethritis	Constipation and irritable bowel syndrome
Vaginal adhesions, scar tissue, and stenosis	Cystitis
	Cystocele
	Rectocele

medications (e.g., serotonin reuptake inhibitors), and recreational drugs. Retrograde ejaculation occurs when the muscles of the urethra do not pump properly during orgasm and sperm are forced backward into the bladder. Retrograde ejaculation can result from any medical or surgical condition that causes dysfunction of the sphincter at the junction of the urethra and the bladder neck, including transurethral prostatectomy, spinal cord injury, diabetes, and medications such as antipsychotics, antidepressants, and antihypertensives. Treatment of retrograde ejaculation involves reassurance, education, and possibly altering the medical regimen. If retrograde ejaculation causes infertility, alpha-adrenergic drugs may be helpful.

Female Orgasm Phase Disorder

Female orgasmic disorder is characterized by a persistent and recurrent delay in or absence of orgasm following a normal sexual excitement phase. Women exhibit wide variability in the type or intensity of stimulation that triggers orgasm. Many women require clitoral stimulation to reach orgasm, and approximately one third of women reach orgasm exclusively in this manner. With female orgasmic disorder, the woman's orgasmic capacity is less than would be reasonably expected for her age, sexual experience, and the adequacy of sexual stimulation.

Women with the primary disorder have never reached orgasm by any means. By contrast, in the more common lifelong and situational disorder, the woman is orgasmic in some circumstances (e.g., by masturbation or by clitoral stimulation) but not in others (e.g., intercourse).

Once a woman learns how to reach orgasm, it is uncommon for her to lose that capacity unless poor sexual communication, a relationship conflict, a traumatic experience, a mood disorder, or a medical condition intervenes. No organic causes of primary inhibited orgasm have been identified, and the disorder is assumed to be psychological. Common psychological etiologies include guilt due to a rigid moral upbringing, inability to abandon oneself to pleasure, or insufficient stimulation for orgasm. In acquired disorders, the most common organic factor is medication, particularly psychotropics. Limited research implicates neurologic damage from surgery and illnesses such as diabetes mellitus and multiple sclerosis.

Female orgasmic disorder is more prevalent in younger women. According to Laumann and colleagues, the prevalence of the primary disorder is 5 to 10 percent, and 24 percent of women report difficulty reaching orgasm in any year. Female orgasmic dysfunction can affect self-esteem, body image, and relationship satisfaction. There are no specific laboratory or diagnostic tests for this disorder. However, it is important to evaluate the partner because premature ejaculation can contribute to anorgasmia.

The prognosis for orgasm phase disorder is favorable. The treatment is behavioral therapy, which involves systematic desensitization to prohibitions on experiencing pleasure and information on reaching orgasm. The primary care clinician can educate the patients about female anatomy using diagrams; recommend self-help books, fantasy material, and vibrators to assist in masturbation; and prescribe Kegel exercises. Some patients may require referral for more intensive behavioral treatment.

Treatment of situational lifelong female orgasm phase disorders includes reassurance. For example, the clinician can explain that some women reach orgasm exclusively through clitoral stimulation. Clinicians can encourage and "normalize" a variety of methods for stimulating the clitoris during sexual activity and can also encourage the patient to incorporate the conditions under which she successfully masturbates into her sexual activity during intercourse.

Medication-Induced Orgasmic Dysfunction

The serotonin reuptake inhibitors (e.g., fluoxetine, sertraline, and paroxetine) are commonly prescribed, well-known medications that can cause decreased libido, ejaculatory delay in men, and anorgasmia in women. Only 25 percent of patients spontaneously report these side effects. However, when patients are asked directly, 54 to 65 percent (in some studies over 90 percent) admit to sexual dysfunction. Options for managing these side effects include reducing the dose and waiting for tolerance, using an antidote medication, or changing to a medication that has less of an effect on sexual function. Such medications include buproprion and nefazodone.

Sexual Pain Disorders

DYSPAREUNIA Dyspareunia is genital pain associated with sexual intercourse. It can occur before, during, or after intercourse. Although seen in both sexes, it is more common in women, present in 7 to 20 percent of women in the community. In women, the pain can be described as "superficial" during penetration or as "deep" during penile thrusting. To be labeled as dyspareunia, the disturbance cannot be due to vaginismus or lack of lubrication. Repeated pain during intercourse may result in avoidance, disruption of relationships, or limitation of new sexual relationships. Dyspareunia in women is associated with many organic and psychological factors, but an organic cause is identified in only 30 to 40 percent of patients (see Table 7-5). Even when the source of the pain is removed, the fear of pain and anxiety may inhibit further arousal and create a vicious cycle. Women with dyspareunia may experience vaginismus as a result of anticipatory pain. Psychological factors that may contribute to female dyspareunia include anxiety, fear of pain, distressing early sexual experiences, guilt about intercourse and pleasure, problems with the partner, and tension associated with new sexual situations.

Dyspareunia in men is almost always due to an organic cause, such as a structural abnormality, medication, or referred pain. Management includes a search for and treatment of these conditions (Table 7-6).

VAGINISMUS The essential feature of vaginismus is the recurrent or persistent involuntary contrac-

Table 7-6

Organic Factors That May Affect Sexual Function in Men

Dyspareunia
Abnormal penile anatomy: Peyronie's disease, urethral stricture
Penile skin infections (chancroid, herpes, syphilis)
Priapism
Prostatic infections
Testicular disease (epididymitis, orchitis, trauma, tumor)
Urethral infections (*Chlamydia, Gonorrhea,* nonspecific)
Mechanical problems
Hernia
Hydrocele
Surgical procedures
Bowel resection
Lumbar sympathectomy
Orchiectomy
Prostatectomy

SOURCE: Adapted with permission from Schmidt CW: Sexual disorders. In: Barker LR, Burton RB, Zieve PD (eds): *Ambulatory Medicine,* 4th ed. Baltimore, MD: Williams & Wilkins; 1991, 188.

tion (spasm) of the perineal muscles surrounding the outer third of the vagina when penetration with penis, finger, tampon, or speculum is attempted. Even the anticipation of vaginal insertion may result in muscle spasm. Contractions may be mild or severe enough to prevent penetration.

Vaginismus is a purely psychological disorder in which the underlying concern is fear of pain with penetration. The disorder is more common in younger women who have negative attitudes towards sex or a history of sexual abuse. The diagnosis may be made during routine pelvic examination; however, the gynecological exam may not reflect actual sexual experience.

Vaginismus is often treatable with counseling and behavioral therapy. Clinicians can demonstrate during a pelvic exam that the condition is involuntary and suggest Kegel exercises to develop a better sense of control over the pelvic muscles. Behavioral therapy consists of inserting either fingers or vaginal dilators of increasing size progressively over time, until the spasm improves and the women is able to attempt intercourse. Lubricants and relaxation exercises can help. Lifelong problems with vaginismus may require referral to a sex therapist.

CINDY PARKER *Mrs. Parker is a 38-year-old woman who comes to her primary care clinician for her first Pap smear. She recently married and is interested in starting a family. During the pelvic exam, the patient develops intense spasm of the perineal muscles, and the speculum exam and bimanual are performed with difficulty. Afterward, the clinician inquires about the patient's sexual functioning. Mrs. Parker explains that because of her cultural background she did not engage in premarital sex. She is anxious during sexual relations with her new husband, and she finds intercourse painful. She wants to enjoy sex and please her husband. The clinician explains that fear of pain is common in women who are newly sexually active and recommends a self-help book on female sexuality, the use of lubricants, and gradual desensitization using increasingly larger fingers. On follow-up the patient notes improvement in her sexual comfort and enjoyment.*

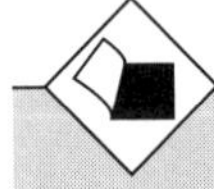

Summary

Sexual problems are among the most challenging issues a primary care clinician can face. Their management requires the use of the biopsychosocial model, excellent communication skills, an understanding of pathophysiology, medical assessment and treatment, and specialized therapeutic techniques. Happily, when these disorders are successfully addressed, patients achieve more intimate and satisfying relationships, enhanced self-esteem, and improved quality of life.

Suggested Reading

Laumann EO, Paik A, Rosen RC: Sexual dysfunction in the United States: Prevalence and predictors. *JAMA* 289:537, 1999.

A comprehensive epidemiologic survey.

Maurice W: *Sexual Medicine in Primary Care.* St. Louis, MO: Mosby; 1999.

A comprehensive manual on sexual disorders in primary care. The best single overall reference on the topic.

Williams S: The sexual history. In: Lipkin M Jr, Putnam SM, Lazare A (eds): *The Medical Interview. Clinical Care, Education, and Research.* New York: Springer-Verlag; 1995.

An excellent chapter on the sexual history.

Lue TF, Wood AJJ: Erectile dysfunction. *NEJM* 342:1802, 2000.

An up-to-date, evidence-based review of erectile disorders, including treatment algorithms.

Seagraves RT, Rahman MI: Sexual disorders. In: Goldman LS, Wise TN, Brody DS (eds): *Psychiatry for Primary Care Clinicians.* Chicago, IL: American Medical Association; 1998.

Concise and sophisticated overview of DSM-IV sexual dysfunctions.

Bibliography

Annon JS: *Behavioral Treatment of Sexual Problems.* Hagerstown, MD: Harper & Row, 1976.

Bross R, Javanbakht M, Bhasin S: *J Clin Endocrinol Metab* 84:3420, 1999.

Bullard DG, Caplan H: Sexual problems. In: Feldman MD, Christensen JF (eds): *Behavioral Medicine in Primary Care.* Stamford, CT: Appleton & Lange; 1997, p 247.

Cheitlin MD, Hutter AM Jr, Brindis RG, et al: Use of sildenafil (Viagra) in patients with cardiovascular disease. *Circulation* 99:168, 1999.

Ende J, Rockwell S, Glasgow M: The sexual history in general medicine practice. *Arch Intern Med* 144:558, 1984.

Feldman HA, Goldstein I, Hatzichristou DG, et al: Impotence and its medical and psychosocial correlates. Results of the Massachusetts Male Aging Study. *J Urol* 151:54, 1994.

Frank E, Anderson C, Rubenstein D: Frequency of sexual dysfunction in "normal" couples. *N Engl J Med* 299:111, 1978.

Greendale GA, Hogan P, Shurnaker S: Sexual functioning in postmenopausal women: The postmenopausal estrogen/progestin in interventions (PEPI) trial. *J Women's Health* 5:445, 1996.

Johannes CB, Arajou AB, Feldman HA: Incidence of erectile dysfunction in men 40–69 years old: Longitudinal results from the Massachusetts Male Aging Study. *J Urol* 163:460, 2000.

Kaplan HS: *The New Sex Therapy.* New York: Brunner/Mazel; 1974.

Klingman EW: Office evaluation of sexual function and complaints. *Clin Geriatr Med* 7:15, 1991.

Laumann EO, Gagnon JH, Michael RT, et al: *The Social Organization of Sexuality: Sexual Practices in the United States.* Chicago: The University of Chicago Press; 1994.

Laumann EO, Paik A, Rosen RC: Sexual dysfunction in the United States: Prevalence and predictors. *JAMA* 289:537, 1999.

Lue TF, Wood AJJ (ed): Erectile dysfunction. *NEJM* 342:1802, 2000.

Masters WH, Johnson VE: *The Human Sexual Response.* Boston, MA: Little, Brown; 1966.

Maurice W: *Sexual Medicine in Primary Care.* St. Louis, MO: Mosby; 1999.

Rhodes JC, Kjerulff KH, Langenberg PW, et al: Hysterectomy and sexual functioning, *JAMA* 282:1934, 1999.

Rosen RC, Cappelleri JC, Smith JD, et al: Development and evaluation of an abridged, 5-item version of the International Index of Erectile Function (IIEF-5) as a diagnostic tool for erectile dysfunction. *Int J Impot Res* 11:319, 1999.

Sadock VA: Normal human sexuality and sexual and gender identity disorders. In: Sadock BJ, Kaplan HI (eds): *Comprehensive Textbook of Psychiatry, 6th ed.* Baltimore, MD; Williams & Wilkins; 1995, p 1295.

Schmidt CW: Sexual disorders. In: Barker LR, Burton JR, Zieve PD (eds): *Ambulatory Medicine.* Baltimore, MD: Williams & Wilkins; 1995, p 188.

Schorer LR, Jensen SB: *Sexuality and Chronic Illness. A Comprehensive Approach.* New York: Guilford Press; 1988.

Seagraves RT, Rahman MI: Sexual disorders. In: Goldman LS, Wise TN, Brody DS (eds): *Psychiatry for Primary Care Clinicians.* Chicago, IL: American Medical Association; 1998, p 197.

Shifren JL, Braunstein GD, Simon JA, et al: Transdermal testosterone treatment in women with impaired sexual function after oophorectomy. *New Eng J Med* 343:682, 2000.

Spector IP, Carey MP: Incidence and prevalence of the sexual dysfunctions: A critical review of the empirical literature. *Arch Sex Behav* 19:389, 1990.

Stanford JL, Feng Z, Hamilton AS, et al: Urinary and sexual function after radical prostatectomy for clinically localized prostate cancer. *JAMA* 283:354, 2000.

Tiefer L: *Sex Is Not a Natural Act and Other Essays*. Boulder, CO: Westview Press; 1995.

Williams S: The sexual history. In: Lipkin M Jr, Putnam SM, Lazare A (eds): *The Medical Interview. Clinical Care, Education, and Research*. New York: Springer-Verlag; 1995, p 235.

Wincze JP, Carey MP: *Sexual Dysfunction. A Guide for Assessment and Treatment*. New York: Guilford Press, 1991.

Deborah S. Main
Jo Ann Rosenfeld
Elizabeth W. Staton

Identifying and Changing Health-Risk Behaviors

Introduction

A small number of behaviors contribute greatly to mortality and morbidity from cardiovascular disease, cancer, and other chronic diseases. These behaviors include tobacco use, sedentary life style, poor diet, and alcohol consumption. These behaviors are the result of a complex set of individual, social, and cultural factors that make it challenging to get individuals to change their behavior. Prevention represents the soundest approach for addressing these very complicated behaviors—don't let them happen in the first place. However, these behaviors are quite prevalent in the U.S. population. Thus, in addition to preventing these at-risk behaviors in those who have not adopted them, primary care clinicians have an important role in helping patients who have already adopted these behaviors to modify them.

The focus of the primary care clinician's efforts is clear: if we are to have any hope of changing the patterns of death and disability in our nation, we must focus on a few preventable behaviors, such as tobacco use, lack of physical activity, poor diets, and alcohol misuse. Primary care clinicians are often the point of first contact for adults and children who engage in such "risk behaviors" and can play a role in early identification and risk reduction—before these behaviors result in the development of debilitating chronic conditions. As important, primary care clinicians can help those patients with chronic disease better manage their health through changes in diet, physical activity, and tobacco and alcohol use.

This chapter reviews general approaches for identifying and intervening with patients to help them change health-risk behaviors. We describe some of the challenges in health risk reduction and present an approach for tailoring brief, office-based interventions to promote healthy behaviors in diverse patient populations.

Primary Care and Health Risk Reduction

Primary care clinicians do not focus enough attention on the issue of their patients' health habits. For example, a survey of 1349 internists found that 48 percent reported counseling all their patients about exercise, but only 15 percent reported regularly counseling inactive patients about exercise. Pinto and associates found that physicians are more likely to provide exercise counseling for high-risk patients, rather than for healthy patients during preventive care visits. Similarly, family physicians rarely counsel patients about their health habits such as injury prevention, drug use, and exposure to sunlight, according to Stange and colleagues.

Barriers to the provision of clinical prevention services include those listed in Table 8-1. These barriers are not insurmountable. Training clinicians to counsel patients about physical activity can increase patients' short-term adoption of physical activity. Marcus and colleagues report that such brief counseling is feasible and acceptable to physicians and their office staff, and can be integrated into the daily primary care office routine.

Physicians, psychologists, sociologists, and other social scientists have tackled the issue of health behavior change for decades. We now have well-developed theories on health behavior

Table 8-1

Barriers to Providing Preventive Services

Limited flexibility from the health care system and its culture for clinicians.
Lack of time.
Lack of counseling skills.
Perceived ineffectiveness and lack of confidence in counseling.
Negative or neutral physician feedback regarding preventive care efforts.
Inadequate resources.
Poor reimbursement.

and behavior change that guide the design of risk reduction interventions and reinforce current understanding that health behavior is difficult to change—and even harder to sustain.

Changing patients' behavior in primary care settings presents barriers in addition to those shown in Table 8-1. According to Glasgow and Eakin, these additional barriers include (a) delivering interventions during the short time allotted for patient visits, (b) clinicians' limited knowledge and skills in effective strategies for patient risk reduction, (c) limited reimbursement for patient counseling and screening, and (d) inadequate systems for supporting behavior changes once they occur. To have the greatest public health effect, risk reduction should specifically target those behaviors that lead to common causes of death and disability (Table 8-2) and that are amenable to change through brief, office-based interventions. For those interventions to work in primary care, they must be easy for busy clinicians to implement and must be proven effective.

Table 8-2

Leading Causes of Death in the United States–1998

Cause	Number	Percentage of All Deaths
Diseases of heart	724,859	31.0
Malignant neoplasms	541,532	23.2
Cerebrovascular diseases	158,448	6.8
Chronic obstructive pulmonary diseases	112,584	4.8
Unintentional injuries	97,835	4.2
Pneumonia and influenza	91,871	3.9
Diabetes mellitus	64,751	2.8
Suicide	30,575	1.3
Nephritis, nephrotic syndrome, and nephrosis	26,182	1.1
Chronic liver disease and cirrhosis	25,192	1.1

SOURCE: National Center for Health Statistics. *Health, United States, 2000 with Adolescent Chartbook*. Hyattsville, MD, 2000. Available online: http://www.cdc.gov/nchs/products/pubs/pubsd/hus.htm.

In this chapter, we focus on a common approach to changing patient behaviors that increase risk for chronic disease. We discuss behaviors such as physical activity, diet, and tobacco use because they are appropriate targets for brief interventions and share many common strategies for helping patients make and sustain changes. Although critically important, we will not review risk reduction related to behaviors leading to intentional and unintentional injuries or sexually transmitted disease. Such behaviors are beyond the scope of this chapter.

Getting Patients to Come in for Preventive Care

Getting patients into the office is the first step in helping them make desired changes in behavior. Many strategies have been adopted and examined to increase the likelihood of getting individuals to come for preventive care. Letters, telephone calls, outreach programs, and brochures have all been used with variable success. One study by Lee and associates showed that minority women, who often have a decreased likelihood of receiving preventive care, were more likely to respond to a letter than to a telephone call. Another showed that the only intervention that successfully increased the use of infant car seats gave parents free seats and made their use a legal requirement. Other studies showed that women, especially minority women with a medical illness, were more likely to receive preventive care, probably because they already were seeing a clinician for the illness. This literature reinforces the notion that clinicians must take advantage of any opportunities, including office visits for illness care, to promote healthy behavior. What happens during these visits often distinguishes successful from less successful office-based behavior change interventions. The following sections review a process for taking advantage of your office visits with patients to help them change health behaviors.

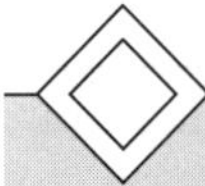

Understanding Patient Readiness to Change

Clinicians have long designed risk reduction interventions based on the erroneous assumption that people who are engaging in unhealthy behaviors want to change those behaviors. Substantial research suggests quite the opposite, and many risk reduction programs have had low participation rates, high dropout rates, and negligible effect on long-term behavior change. We now know that these interventions were not designed to reflect how people really change.

During the past two decades we have learned more about factors underlying successful behavior changes. One of those critical factors is patient motivation or "readiness to change." According to Prochaska and colleagues, people are not always ready to change and often go through a series of stages or cycles before a change can occur. These stages are shown in Table 8-3.

People do not always go through these stages in order. In fact, they commonly cycle back through the change stages multiple times. People often have to make several change attempts before a change will "stick," with each attempt a chance to learn more and enhance the likelihood of future success.

Table 8-3

Stages of Change (Prochaska Model)

Precontemplation—when patients are not even thinking about changing (*I won't*).
Contemplation—when patients are actively considering a change (*I might*).
Preparation—when patiens are thinking about and planning to make changes soon (*I will*).
Action—when patients have recently made changes (*I am*).
Maintenance—when patients are sustaining these changes over time (*I have*).

SOURCE: Reproduced from Reed GR, Velicer WF, Prochaska JO, et al: What makes a good staging algorithm: Examples from regular exercise. *Am J Health Promotion* 12:57–66, 1997.

Some individuals are more likely to be ready to make a change than others. Individuals who have suffered some harm from their hazardous or risky behaviors, and therefore are particularly open to influence from their clinicians, are more likely to change those behaviors at that point when harm occurs. For example, individuals with newly diagnosed heart disease, a myocardial infarction, or a first serious hospitalization for lung disease are more likely to change than others. Women who have had an abnormal mammogram and biopsy are more likely to undergo subsequent regular screening mammography, according to Pisano. The clinician should use the opportunity presented by such unfortunate harms to identify a time when individuals may be more likely to take action and change behavior.

Instead of or in addition to readiness to change, it may also be helpful to ask your patients about two critical dimensions that may affect their willingness and ability to make and maintain changes in health behaviors—whether they believe a change is *important* and whether they feel *confident* that they can be successful in making this change. Assessing and discussing these dimensions with your patients can be a useful tool for enhancing a collaborative, shared decision making and change process.

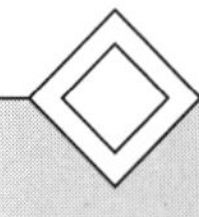

Tailoring Interventions to a Person's Readiness to Change

Tailoring an intervention is the process of appropriately matching the behavior change strategy to a patient's readiness to change. For some patients who smoke, for example, an appropriate risk reduction intervention is to increase their awareness of the detrimental health effects of smoking—to move them from precontemplation to a higher stage of change. In contrast, patients in the planning stage of smoking cessation do not need to be convinced of the need for making a change. Instead, an effective intervention would be to help them develop the appropriate skills and self-confidence to successfully carry out their plans to reduce or quit smoking.

Ask, Assess, Advise, Assist, and Arrange

The next section of the chapter describes a framework for thinking about behavior change through communicating with patients. Schorling found that the number of patient medical encounters is predictive of greater likelihood of being ready to take action in smoking cessation. Therefore, primary care clinicians should ask about health risk behaviors and offer assistance whenever possible at every office visit. Patients who need to change their behaviors will hear and need to hear different messages at different times. You will not always know the stage of change for each patient. Providing reaffirming support and advice will catch individuals when they are ready to take the step to contemplation or action. When the individual seems receptive, more in-depth counseling can occur. The following framework may help you assess readiness to change and provide risk reduction interventions.

1. *Ask* about the behavior.
2. *Assess* the patient's readiness to change.
3. *Advise* and counsel.
4. Offer to *assist* if the individual is ready to change.
5. *Arrange* follow-up.

This framework, based on the National Cancer Institute's 4 A's, is described in detail in Chap. 9. Another simple protocol, developed by Ockene and others for smoking cessation, suggests five areas of questioning which can be used with other behavioral changes. The model involves (1) motivation, (2) past experience, (3) problems, (4) resources, and (5) plan for action. Table 8-4 provides examples of how clinicians can tailor Ockene's counseling method for both smoking and weight reduction.

The key to successful intervention is consistency—patients should come to realize and expect that you care about their health and are interested in helping them reduce their risks. Although it may not seem like you make much progress with some patients, it has been determined that consistent, periodic counseling about health risk behaviors is, indeed, important. More patients report receiving too little health advice than too much health advice. Patients who appear resistant to your advice may still benefit from your sugges-

Table 8-4

Ockene's Method of Fostering Behavioral Changes

Counseling Protocol	Smoking	Dieting/Weight Reduction
Motivation	How do you feel about stopping smoking?	How do you feel about dieting?
Past experiences	Have you tried to stop before? How?	Have you dieted before? How did you do it?
Problems	What problems did you encounter when you tried to quit, or have kept you from quitting?	What problems did you have trying to lose weight?
Resources	What would help you to quit? Would gum, patches, or pills help? Support groups?	What worked for you? How have you tried to exercise?
Plan for action	How can we plan together the way you will quit smoking?	How can I help you? Shall we get you to a dietician? What exercise are you going to do?

tions. Even among those who report receiving too much advice, Taira and colleagues found that a large portion report attempting to change their health behaviors.

Many clinicians express discouragement that they repeatedly encourage individuals to quit smoking or exercise, and it does no good. This discouragement is caused partially by lack of confidence and training in how to counsel behavioral changes and relay messages, and partially by frustration at being unable to see any response or success. Even so, repetitive messages, even short ones, do have some effect. For example, Gritz and associates report that brief clinician intervention at a critical time increases abstinence from smoking significantly. Just 5 to 10 min of clinician counseling about stopping smoking can produce quit rates of up to 30 percent and long-term abstinence rates of up to 18 percent. Having a strategy will help you work with individuals who need to change their behaviors.

Although attacking multiple problem behaviors at one time may sound like a good idea, it is important *not* to expect or encourage your patients to make multiple behavior changes at once. Successful health risk reduction requires learning and relearning new patterns of thinking and acting. Each behavior change usually requires new thoughts and skills to modify perceived attitudes, reduce barriers, and enhance self-confidence—and patients may not be at the same stage of readiness for different health behaviors. When patients do decide to make more than one behavior change at a time—for example, decreasing dietary fat *and* increasing physical activity for weight loss—be sure that successfully changing one behavior does not lead to decrements in another. For example, you want to make sure that increasing physical activity does not lead to unhealthy dietary fat consumption that defeats any weight loss goals.

Brief Interventions Work

One study by Calfas and colleagues, used an intervention tailored on the stages of change model. Clinicians provided 3 to 5 min of exercise counseling tailored to the patient's level of activity and readiness to become active. A health educator called the patients 2 weeks after that visit to provide a "boost." Patients increased their exercise duration and readiness to become active. Another study by Pinto and associates adapted the "Five A" questions to exercise counseling. They found that patients who received such intervention reported significantly increased exercise duration at 1-month follow-up.

Marcus and colleagues compared brief behavioral counseling versus standard health promotion advice in primary care practice with patients at increased risk of cardiovascular disease. They found that behavioral counseling led to greater reductions in fat consumption, number of cigarettes smoked, and increases in activity at 4 and 12 months. The intervention included brief counseling about smoking cessation, physical activity, and diet. In yet another study of older smokers conducted by Morgan and associates, smoking abstinence was significantly increased by brief interventions tailored to the patient's age and integrated into routine care. Clearly, brief interventions can work in primary care settings.

Implementing Health-Risk Reduction in Primary Care Practice

Primary care clinicians are among the most trusted sources of health information for their patients, both through their objective expertise and the development of long-lasting relationships with those patients. These clinicians are thus in an excellent position to encourage patients, through brief office-based interventions, to reduce their health risks. As noted, these interventions must be useful and practical for busy medical offices. In this section, we describe the critical ingredients for implementing such health risk reduction interventions in primary care settings.

Identify Health-Risk Behaviors

An important component of any health risk reduction intervention is to identify health risks *before* they lead to disability or death. This requires the collection of concise information on a handful of health behaviors such as smoking, alcohol and other drug use, physical activity, diet, and obesity. An example of such concise information would be calculating a patient's body mass index (BMI) from the patient's weight and height, and using the data to determine health risk from obesity. Ideally, this information should be collected as a routine part of a health maintenance visit. Another example is using screening systems that systematically identify and document smoking status; such systems result in higher rates of smoking interventions by clinicians, according to Wilk and colleagues. Similarly, Adams and associates found that having a practice-wide screening routine for problem drinking doubles the frequency with which clinicians discuss alcohol.

Once you determine that a particular behavior may be placing your patient at an increased health risk, you may want to collect more comprehensive information to determine the extent of the problem. Thus, you use brief and highly sensitive screens to identify patients who may be at risk. You then follow this screening with more detailed measures or questioning to rule out false positive screens and to gather necessary additional information on true positive screens.

DETERMINE THE PATIENT'S READINESS TO CHANGE

To determine your patients' readiness to change for a particular health behavior, you can ask them to answer "Yes" or "No" to a simple question with selected response options. Be sure to specifically define each health behavior you are asking about. For example, if you are determining a patient's readiness to increase exercise, be sure to tell him or her that "exercise means three times or more per week for 20 minutes or longer." Table 8-5 provides an example of how you can stage your patients in terms of their readiness to increase physical activity.

As a screening instrument, the question and the possible responses can be printed (without mention of the patient's stage of change) and the patient can answer the question as a written survey. You can use the patient's responses to determine the patient's readiness to change and then to tailor a risk reduction intervention, as discussed below. A second, complementary approach, described by Miller and Rollnick, is to ask your patients two specific questions about a particular health behavior change—whether they think the desired change is important and how confident they feel in making a successful change. Use the following two questions to guide your assessment and determination of a patient's interest and ability to change:

1. How important is it for you to you to make a change right now?
   (0 = not important, 10 = very important)
2. If you decided to change right now, how confident do you feel about your success?
   (0 = not confident, 10 = very confident)

Table 8-5
Staging Patient's Readiness to Increase Physical Activity

PATIENT'S REPLY	PATIENT'S STAGE OF CHANGE
Question: Do you exercise three times a week for at least 20 min each time?	
Yes, I have been for more than 6 months.	Maintenance
Yes, I have been for less than 6 months.	Action
No, but I am planning to start in the next 30 days.	Preparation
No, but I am planning to start in the next 6 months.	Contemplation
No, and I don't plan to start in the next 6 months.	Precontemplation

These two questions not only give you useful information but also serve as a communication tool for beginning discussions with your patients about change.

These two assessment strategies—readiness to change and importance/confidence—can be used alone or together to gather useful information about whether your patient is interested and ready to make a change. The choice of strategy may depend on personal preference. Try either or a combination of both to determine what works best for you and your patients.

Tailor Risk Reduction Interventions

READINESS TO CHANGE You can determine the most appropriate stage-specific intervention by using information on patient readiness. Patients who are in precontemplation need to become more aware of the fact that their behaviors are increasing their risk for more serious chronic health conditions. Although most of your patients *know* that cigarettes cause lung cancer, for example, it is helpful to deliver more personalized information to help patients consider the potential consequences of *their* behavior. The more this information can be tied to health consequences that patients recognize in themselves, the more likely it is to have an effect on their behavior. Particularly with precontemplators, asking and advising about health-risk behaviors can be awkward. However, a message from you is effective. Continue asking and advising during most or all health visits.

For patients in the contemplation and planning stages, review the benefits and barriers associated with making health-related changes. The goal is to help these patients believe that the benefits of change far outweigh the barriers. Reinforce patients who have a plan; help them to figure out what they need to ensure that their plan is successful. Encourage them to identify and recruit useful sources of social support. For example, encourage a patient beginning an exercise program to begin a regular walking program with a friend.

Patients in the action and maintenance stages are making changes. Those in the action stage must develop and strengthen skills to continue working toward behavior change goals. Because they have already begun changes, they may realize just how difficult it may be to meet their behavioral goals. You may help these patients in their problem solving; for example, to identify ways of coping with "high-risk" situations (i.e., those situations that make it difficult for them to make desired changes). Those in the maintenance stage may require minimal intervention. However, continue checking in with these people, as they may encounter "slips" in their progress and need you to help with problem solving and reinforcement. Table 8-6 presents information on how to tailor risk reduction for each stage of change.

IMPORTANCE AND CONFIDENCE Based on patients' responses to questions on importance and confidence, you can determine the next steps for helping them begin or continue a program of change. Some clinicians find it useful to plot a patient's responses on a piece of paper (some put these in the patient's chart) and to use this diagram as a tool for talking with patients about desired changes (Fig. 8-1). Knowing whether a patient believes a change is important and/or feels confident about it can help you determine how to work with each patient on a change plan.

Low Importance/Low Confidence. This is a warning sign that, at this particular stage, change does not seem realistic to your patient. A realistic goal is to begin to help these patients see the value in making a change in a particular area, perhaps by expressing your personal concern for their health. You may want to ask them what it would take for this change to feel more important to them or to make them feel more confident.

High Importance/Low Confidence. These patients believe that a change is important, yet do not yet believe that they can be successful. A realistic goal is to help them begin to set small, incremental goals. They need to begin to realize that they *can*

Table 8-6

Tailoring Risk Reduction to Patient's Stage of Change

Stage	General Description	Goal	Strategies
Precontemplation	Not thinking about it; resistant or unmotivated.	Increase awareness of benefits; increase knowledge.	Ask; provide educational materials.
Contemplation	Aware of reasons to change, perceives many barriers, costs outweigh benefits.	Motivate, reduce barriers, enhance self-efficacy.	Advise, problem-solve barriers, "mini-trial" of new behavior.
Preparation	Have a plan of action; may have taken some action in past year.	Discuss, encourage and support patients to make change; identify critical issues for success.	Assist, problem-solve barriers, identify useful social support, and set gradual, realistic goals.
Action	Recently made changes, may not have yet met goals, hasn't sustained change.	Help patient continue to make changes, provide appropriate feedback and support.	Arrange; remind of benefits of change; reinforce changes to date; problem-solve anticipated struggles.
Maintenance	Less risk for relapse; high confidence in sustaining goal behavior.	Help patient sustain health risk reduction.	Reinforce; problem-solve high-risk situations (slips).

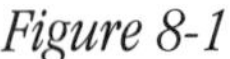

Figure 8-1

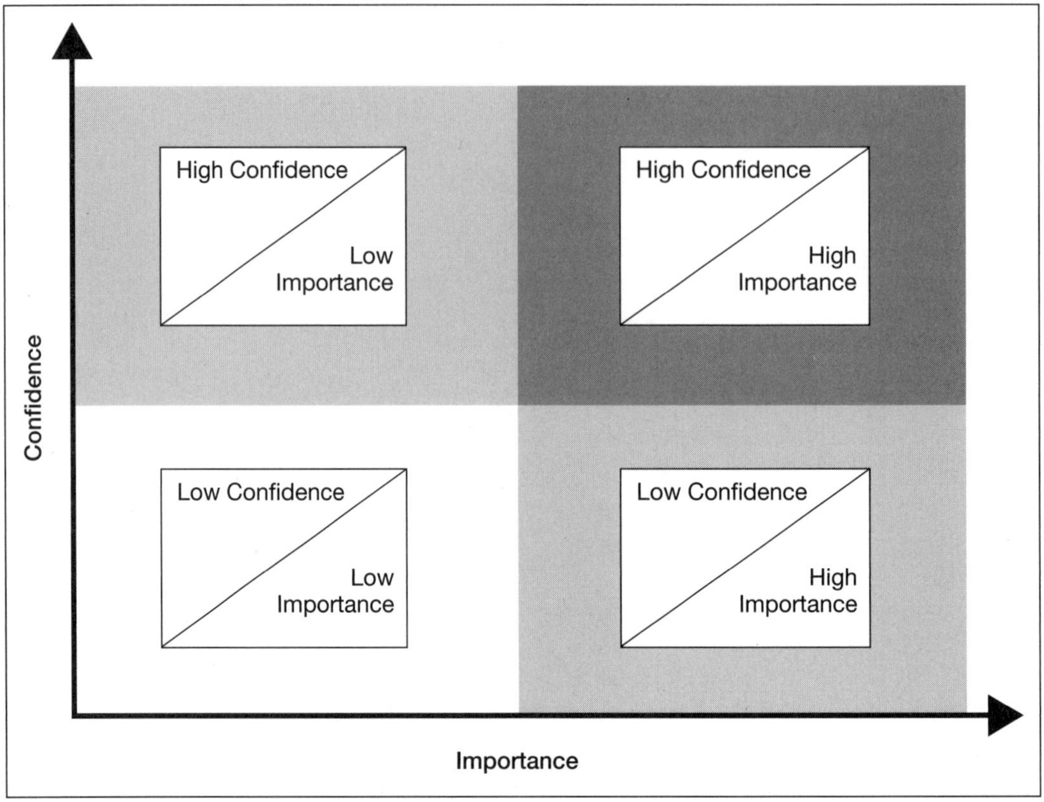

Using importance and confidence to discuss planned change.

begin to make the change, and they need to experience some success in doing so. Reinforce these small successes to help these patients become more confident in their ability to change.

Low Importance/High Confidence. These people must be convinced that a particular health behavior change is personally important. Until this happens, they will not see a need to change. If this happens (i.e., that they realize that change is important), these patients can quickly plan and make changes.

High Importance/High Confidence. These people are ready and able to make a desired change. Help these patients make a change plan and reinforce the importance of changing at this time.

Here are a few suggestions from Rollnick and colleagues for using the confidence and importance questions with your patients:

- If importance is low, focus on explaining the importance of the change to your patient.
- When importance and confidence are scored disparately, focus on the one with the lower score.
- If the patient's ratings are equal on importance and confidence, focus on importance.
- If the patient's ratings are low on both, lower your expectations.
- Use the patient's responses as a prompt for additional discussion and problem solving.
  - If importance rating is low, ask: "What would it take today for this to feel more important to you?"

Figure 8-2

Stages of Change

Precontemplation — Contemplation — Plan — Action — Maintenance

Importance more of an issue — *Confidence* more of an issue

Stages of change and importance/confidence: Conceptual overlap.

– If confidence rating is low, ask: "What would it take today for you to feel more confident about successfully making a change?"

Like stages of change, these questions will help you decide how to begin working with your patients to make successful changes. In fact, you may notice that importance/confidence questions map nicely with stages of change (Fig. 8-2).

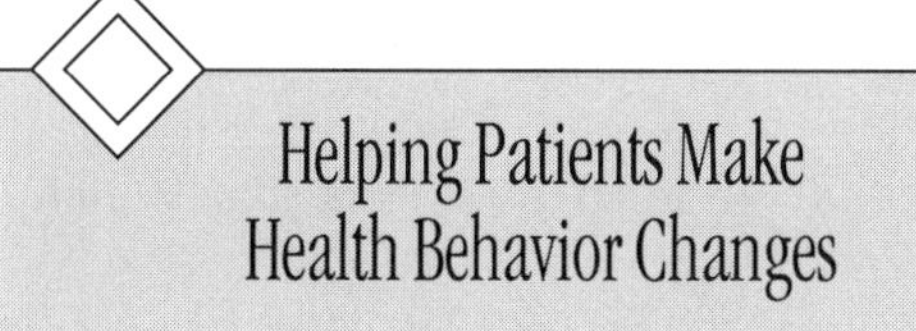

Helping Patients Make Health Behavior Changes

Helping patients make behavioral changes may be among the most challenging aspects of primary care practice. Behavior change is a process that takes time and often involves discussing sensitive information within an ongoing, supportive relationship. Patients often want and expect their clinicians to help them make and sustain health behavior changes, and clinicians can play a particularly important role in ensuring that patients make such changes using the most safe and effective strategies. The good news is that a common set of strategies can be used in primary care to help patients make health behavior changes in a variety of areas. In the following section, we lay out a series of steps to use in helping patients make and maintain health behavior changes. We illustrate this process by using the example of weight loss described in the following case example.

DON RUSSEL *Don, a 55-year-old man, comes to see you for a health maintenance visit. You have been his primary care provider for 6 years, and you care for his entire family. Don's wife, during her recent check-up, expressed concern about her husband's health, particularly the fact that he has gained over 25 pounds in the past 2 years. Don has a family history of heart disease—his older brother recently had to undergo triple-bypass surgery. You decide that today's visit provides the right opportunity to discuss with him a plan for weight loss.*

Ask and Assess: Determine the Patient's Health Risks and Motivation to Lose Weight

Through an honest discussion about the health risks of obesity and a sedentary lifestyle, you should encourage the patient to consider thinking about how he can make even small changes. You may want to calculate the patient's BMI as a way to quantify and communicate the health risks of obesity. You should then determine the patient's readiness to change to tailor discussions, educational materials, and programs to enhance the likelihood that a change program will be successful.

Remember that you may diminish your chances of helping patients if you ignore their level of motivation. Do not assume that all patients are ready to make changes immediately. Those patients who are not ready can still benefit from a frank discussion about their health risks and expressed concern that they will develop debilitating chronic diseases. For those patients who are relatively unaware of their current health behaviors (i.e., their eating or exercise patterns), it may be useful to encourage them to keep track of their diet and physical activity for 1 week and schedule a follow-up visit to review their food or activity "journals." This increased awareness through self-monitoring and follow-up discussion will help some people move toward a higher stage of readiness.

DON RUSSEL (CONTINUED) *After a series of questions, it is apparent that Don is at a stage where he may be more ready than ever to consider or even plan changes (contemplation or preparation). Although we know that fear tactics are not usually effective, Don's sense of vulnerability to heart disease is particularly high at this time. His older brother just had triple-bypass surgery, so his clinician uses this as an excellent "teachable moment" to first ask Don about his weight and other risks for heart disease and next to encourage him to make a plan for change.*

Advise and Assist: Determine the Patient's Preferences and Tailor Interventions

Once you know *whether* someone is ready to change, the next step requires a brief discussion of *how* the person would like to make and sustain such changes. It is important to know individual preferences and to understand and help individuals develop plans that fit their life styles. Be sure to incorporate the following issues in your discussions.

Consider the Patient's Preferences

People prefer to learn and change in a variety of ways. For example, some people like to learn a lot about their health problems—they use the Internet, read educational materials and books, and ask a lot of questions. Others are much more action oriented—they just want to begin, without the need to know all of the facts. Some people prefer making changes by joining groups, at least in part because of the interaction with other people. They like the social pressure that is provided within groups such as Weight Watchers, and they may also benefit from joining exercise clubs or participating in competitions. Others prefer to make changes alone, perhaps monitoring their behavior by keeping food or exercise diaries. Knowing these and other preferences will help you to help patients develop a behavior change plan that will be most effective for them.

Consider the Patient's Life Style

A key ingredient to a successful behavior change plan is that it has to fit into the patient's life style. For example, people who are frequent business travelers must learn how to exercise and eat on the road. Those juggling the many pressures of work, raising kids, and maintaining relationships must learn how to add something else to an already busy schedule. It is important that any discussion around behavior change be geared toward those particular issues or concerns that are most salient to the patient. Use the information from your brief assessment and discussion to advise the patient about next steps and determine the most appropriate, stage-specific plan.

DON RUSSEL (CONTINUED) *Don's heightened level of concern and current knowledge of his own risks for heart disease present an opportunity—he wants to make a plan. Due to frequent business travel, Don indicates that he could make a few changes almost immediately. He wants to eat healthier meals while eating out, and he vows to exercise in the workout facility located in his hotel.*

Help the Patient Set Goals and Solve Problems

Helping patients set realistic goals is among the most important steps toward long-term behavior change. It is critical that goals are reachable, because failure to reach goals can lead to frustration, lower confidence, and limited likelihood that a patient will persevere in making and sustaining desired behavior changes in the future. An important strategy for all behavior change efforts is a careful review and discussion of barriers. Patients will think of many reasons why a particular behavior change will be difficult for them. Your role is to help patients identify barriers and come up with potential solutions for overcoming those barriers. For example, for some patients, eating out in restaurants is a "high-risk" proposition that may result in failure to adhere to dietary recommendations. You can help them problem solve ways to overcome this particular barrier by talking about lower calorie menu choices, encouraging patients to bring their own salad dressing with them, and so on.

Consider the following when you are helping patients who would like to change a health habit.

- People are more likely to continue healthy activities that more easily fit into their lives. Highly structured programs are much harder to follow and therefore harder to sustain over time. Help them determine what actions will fit for them.
- Encourage patients to monitor their habits by keeping a simple journal.
- Remind patients that changing habits is a long process. It often requires changing behaviors that have developed over a lifetime.
- Emphasize the health benefits of even modest changes (instead of achieving a specific target or goal).
- Provide educational materials.

Strategies to Consider While Working with Patients to Increase Physical Activity

- Encourage low to moderate intensity activities. They are more likely to be continued than higher intensity activities.
- Remind patients that intermittent or short bouts of activity are beneficial. You do not have to exercise to exhaustion to reap the benefits. Activities such as brisk walking, gardening, and taking stairs instead of elevators are all valuable forms of activity that benefit health.

Arrange: Help Patients Identify Strategies to Enable Planned Change

Most research indicates that social support is important for change in general and weight loss programs in particular. Specific factors that increase the likelihood of successful change include having a supportive spouse who is actively involved in the program, maintaining consistent contact with counselors or health care clinicians (by mail, phone, or in person), having a peer group that meets to monitor progress and give support and praise, and identifying social support to help patients make and maintain changes. Other strategies that assist patients in carrying out change include

- establishing a follow-up plan
- linking the patient with other helpful resources such as a nutritionist, a personal trainer, and web sites
- helping patients self-monitor, particularly during "high risk" situations such as holidays and vacations (mailings, fax, e-mail)

Helping your patients plan and make changes is a challenging yet rewarding process. The key is to take advantage of medical visits at opportune times, using the most efficient yet effective strategies.

DON RUSSEL (CONTINUED) *Don indicates that he likes getting information from the Internet, which he can do even during business travel. With his work schedule, he cannot regularly attend local support group sessions, and he would like to look into the possibility of an Internet-based support group. He agrees to look into those resources and bring information back to review during his next visit in 3 weeks.*

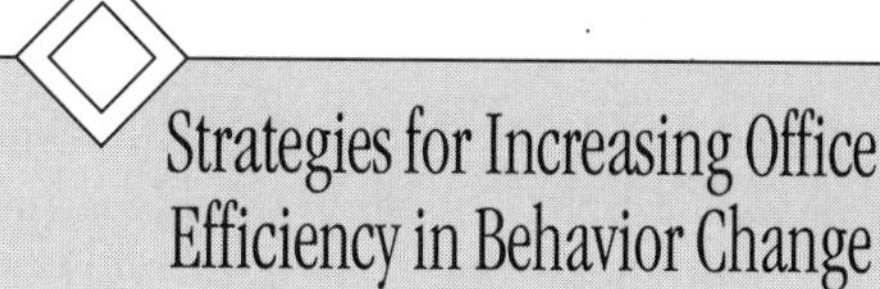

Strategies for Increasing Office Efficiency in Behavior Change

Despite best efforts to keep brief interventions brief, even "minimal" interventions can take anywhere from 20 min to over an hour of a clinician's time. Recent research has explored several strategies for increasing the efficiency and effectiveness of interventions in primary care settings. Two strategies that hold a great deal of promise are (1) using group rather than individual visits and (2) implementing collaborative care models through the more intensive use of nonphysician clinicians.

The use of drop-in group visits is one strategy used to improve care. Teams of physicians, health educators, nurses, and others meet with groups of patients who share a similar health condition, such as diabetes. This group visit often involves a combination of medical care, review of treatments, discussion of life-style issues, problem solving, encouragement, and support. These groups allow more time with patients to address the complex set of medical, psychosocial, and behavioral issues faced by those with chronic conditions. Group visits can also be used for addressing particular behavior change areas, such as tobacco use, nutrition, and physical activity.

Another approach gaining popularity is the use of nonphysician providers to help patients with chronic disease and other care management. Assigning a nurse, health educator, or medical assistant to be responsible for helping assess, plan, and counsel patients on behavior change may be a more efficient and cost-effective approach to primary and secondary prevention. Ideally, these providers collaborate closely with physicians to ensure that patients receive comprehensive and coordinated care. These "care managers" may be able to spend the time required to plan and implement a behavior change program tailored to each patient based on his readiness and preference for change and designed to ensure that patients gain the proper skills and support to sustain these behavior changes over the long term.

Some programs have used peers who role model appropriate behaviors and provide counseling. Although these outreach peer workers need their own support and education systems, this strategy can help change behavior.

Technology can also be used to further extend contacts and reminders for patients attempting behavioral change. For example, one study by Friedman showed that regular computer-linked telephone messages counseling about medication regimens and healthy diets increased the likelihood of healthy behaviors in as few as 3 months.

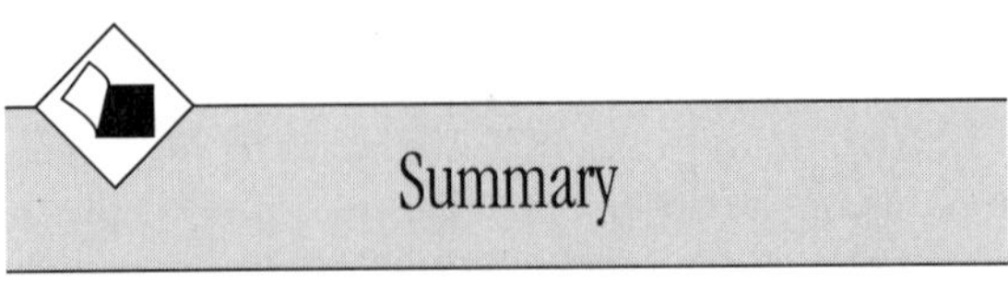

Summary

This chapter reviewed a common set of strategies for helping patients make and sustain changes in several health-related areas. Just as patients need to learn and develop new skills for changing behavior, busy clinicians can learn and adopt more efficient, effective ways of helping their patients reduce health risks. Because the busy medical practice presents many challenges in helping patients change these complex behaviors, we present suggestions for ways of increasing medical office efficiency through innovative, collaborative care models for patient risk reduction.

Suggested Reading

Glanz K, Lewis FM, Rimer BK (eds): *Health Behavior and Health Education: Theory, Research and Practice,* 2nd ed. San Francisco, CA: Jossey-Bass, 1996.

An excellent overview of the most common theories of health behavior and behavior change and their application.

Rollnick S, Mason P, Butler C: *Health Behavior Change: A Guide for Practitioners.* London, UK: Churchill Livingstone; 2000.

A very practical book on the use of motivational interviewing for helping people make and sustain health behavior changes.

Glasgow R, Eakin E: Medical office-based interventions. In: Snoek F, Skinner C (eds): *Psychology in Diabetes Care.* New York: John Wiley & Sons, Inc.; 2000.

An excellent book chapter that reviews the opportunities and challenges involved in implementing brief interventions in the busy medical office setting.

Prochaska JO, Velicer WF: The transtheoretical model of health behavior change. *Am J Health Promotion* 12:38, 1997.

An easy-to-read review article that describes the transtheoretical model of health behavior change—

more commonly known as "readiness to change." Explains both stages and processes of change and ways to help people move from one stage to the next.

Prochaska JO, Norcross JC, DiClemente CC: *Changing for Good.* New York: William Morrow & Co; 1994.

A book written for the lay public that details each stage of change, provides tools for self-assessment, and describes tips and processes people may use to move up the continuum of change.

Bibliography

Adams A, Ockene JK, Wheller EV, et al: Alcohol counseling: Physicians will do it. *J Gen Intern Med* 13:692, 1998.

Calfas KJ, Long BJ, Sallis JF, et al: A controlled trial of physician counseling to promote the adoption of physical activity. *Prev Med* 25:225, 1996.

Douketis JD: Incorporating preventive care recommendations into clinical practice: How do we bridge the gap? *CMAJ* 160:1171, 1999.

Friedman RH: Automated telephone conversations to assess health behavior and deliver behavioral interventions. *J Med Sys* 22:95, 1998.

Glanz K, Lewis FM, Rimer BK: *Health Behavior and Health Education: Theory, Research, and Practice,* 2nd ed. San Francisco: Jossey-Bass; 1996.

Glasgow R, Eakin E: Medical Office-based interventions. In: Snoek F, Skinner C (eds): *Psychology in Diabetes Care.* New York: Wiley; 2000.

Glynn TJ, Manley MW: *How to Help Your Patients Stop Smoking: A National Cancer Institute Manual for Physicians.* Bethesda: Smoking and Tobacco Control Program, Division of Cancer Prevention and Control, National Cancer Institute, U.S. Department of Health and Human Services, Public Health Service, National Institutes of Health; 1991.

Gritz ER, Kristeller JL, Burns DM: Treating nicotine addiction in high-risk groups and individuals with medical co-morbidity. In: Orleans CT, Slade J (eds): *Nicotine Addiction: Principles and Management.* New York: Oxford University Press; 1993, p 279.

Lee RE, McGinnis KA, Sallis JF, et al: Active vs. passive methods of recruiting ethnic minority women to a health promotion program. *Ann Behav Med* 19:378, 1998.

Lowry R, Kann L, Collins JL, et al: The effect of socioeconomic status on chronic disease risk behaviors among US adolescents. *JAMA* 276:792, 1996.

Marcus BH, Bock BC, Pinto BM, et al: Efficacy of an individualized, motivationally-tailored physical activity intervention. *Ann Behav Med* 20:174, 1998.

Marcus BH, Goldstein MG, Jette A, et al: Training physicians to conduct physical activity counseling. *Prev Med* 26:382, 1997.

McGinnis JM, Foege WH: Actual causes of death in the United States. *JAMA* 270:2207, 1993.

Miller WR, Rollnick S: *Motivational Interviewing: Preparing People to Change Addictive Behavior.* New York: Guilford Press, 1991.

Morgan GD, Noll EL, Orleans CT, et al: Reaching midlife and older smokers: Tailored interventions for routine medical care. *Prev Med* 25:346, 1996.

Noffsinger EB: Will drop-in group medical appointments (DIGMA) work in practice? *Permanente J* 3(3):58, 1999.

Ockene JK, Kristeller J, Goldberg R, et al: Increasing the efficacy of physician-delivered smoking interventions: A randomized clinical trial. *J Gen Intern Med* 6:1, 1991.

Ockene JK, Quirk ME, Goldberg RJ, et al: A residents' training program for the development of smoking intervention skills. *Arch Intern Med* 148:1039, 1988.

Pinto BM, Goldstein MG, Marcus BH: Activity counseling by primary care physicians. *Prev Med* 27:506, 1998.

Pisano ED, Earp J, Schell M, et al: Screening behavior of women after a false-positive mammogram. *Radiology* 208:245, 1998.

Prochaska JO, Velicer WF: The transtheoretical model of health behavior change. *Am J Health Promotion* 12:38, 1997.

Rollnick S, Mason P, Butler C: *Health Behavior Change: A Guide for Practitioners.* London, UK: Churchill Livingstone; 2000.

Schorling JB: The stages of change of rural African-American smokers. *Am J Preventive Med* 11:170, 1995.

Scott J, Gade G, McKenzie M, et al: Cooperative health care clinics: A group approach to individual care. *Geriatrics* 53:68, 76, 81, 1998.

Sherman BR, Sanders LM, Yearde J: Role-modeling healthy behavior: Peer counseling for pregnant and postpartum women in recovery. *Womens Health Issues* 8:230, 1998.

Stange KC, Flocke SA, Goodwin MA, et al: Direct observation of rates of preventive service delivery in community family practice. *Prev Med* 31:167, 2000.

Taira DA, Safran DG, Seto TB, et al: The relationship between patient income and physician discussion of health risk behaviors. *JAMA* 278:1412, 1997.

Thompson RS, Taplin SH, McAfee TA, et al: Primary and secondary prevention services in clinical practice. Twenty years' experience in development, implementation, and evaluation. *JAMA* 273:1130, 1995.

National Center for Health Statistics. Health, United States, 2000 with Adolescent Health Chartbook. Hyattsville, MD; 2000. Available at http://www.cdc.gov/nchs/products/pubs/pubd/hus/hus.htm.

Wilk AI, Jensen NM, Havighurst TC: Meta-analysis of randomized control trials addressing brief interventions in heavy alcohol drinkers. *J Gen Intern Med* 12:274, 1997.

Carlos Roberto Jaén
Daniel C. Vinson

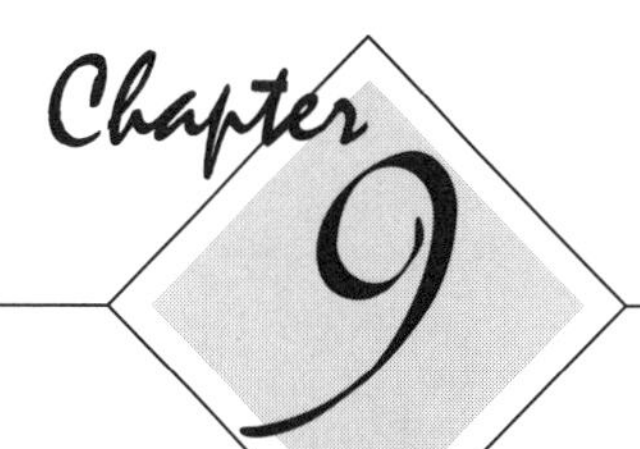

Problem Drinking and Tobacco Use

Tobacco and Alcohol Problems in Primary Care

When was the last time you spent a day in your office and no alcohol- or tobacco-related problems surfaced as you were taking care of your patients? Whether or not they realize it, primary care clinicians encounter patients with alcohol and tobacco problems on a daily basis. By virtue of their direct access to a large population of patients with these problems, credibility with patients, and availability of effective interventions, primary care clinicians have a unique and powerful opportunity to contribute to the control of the ravages of tobacco and alcohol abuse.

Tobacco and alcohol problems are common, chronic, and deadly diseases that require behavior change as part of treatment, not unlike hypertension and diabetes. Just as clinicians should not expect diabetic and hypertensive patients to immediately adopt dietary and physical activity recommendations, they should not expect immediate success from a single alcohol or tobacco intervention. The key is to incorporate appropriate interventions into each encounter with patients.

The purpose of this chapter is to discuss the most important aspects of brief smoking cessation and alcohol counseling interventions for primary care clinicians. After reading this chapter, you should understand appropriate interventions and treatment options for patients who use tobacco or who are problem drinkers. This chapter emphasizes knowledge, but ultimately your success depends on your ability to incorporate these recommendations into everyday routines.

ARNOLD RALPH *Arnold Ralph is a 40-year-old man who comes in to have a skin lesion removed from his ear. You notice that the index and middle fingers on his right hand are stained yellow, and that he has a faint smell of alcohol on his breath. You ask if he has been drinking and he admits that he has had a beer this afternoon. He says he drinks about a six-pack each evening after work, and has been doing this for almost 20 years. His wife doesn't like it, and won't take him with her to visit her family because of it, but he claims that it doesn't interfere with his work. He has smoked a pack of cigarettes a day for 25 years, since he was 15.*

Definitions

Although the definition of a smoker or a drinker may seem obvious, there are nuances that should be explained to accurately characterize these patients. In this section, we define problem and moderate drinking, and smoking and tobacco use.

Moderate and Problem Drinking

Some people should not drink at all: women who are pregnant or trying to conceive; people who plan to drive or engage in other activities that require attention or skill; people taking certain medications, including over-the-counter medications; recovering alcoholics; and people for whom drinking is illegal (e.g., people under the age of 21). These people should be *abstainers*, or persons who do not drink alcohol. For others, the National Institute on Alcohol Abuse and Alcoholism recommends limiting drinking; light drinking may be beneficial to some.

The National Institute on Alcohol Abuse and Alcoholism defines *at-risk drinking* as drinking more than 1 drink a day or 7 drinks a week for women, and more than 2 drinks a day or 14 drinks a week for men. The at-risk cutoff points are lower for women because women have a lower volume of distribution of alcohol and lower levels of gastric alcohol dehydrogenase, the enzyme that breaks down alcohol before it reaches the bloodstream. A standard drink is generally considered to be 12 ounces of beer (360 mL), 5 ounces of wine (150 mL), or 1.5 ounces of 90-proof distilled spirits (45 mL). Each of these drinks contain approximately 0.5 ounces or 12 grams of absolute alcohol.

Persons who have adverse consequences because of their drinking and who continue to drink can be diagnosed as having an *alcohol use disorder*, either alcohol abuse (also called harmful drinking) or alcohol dependence. The criteria for these disorders are listed in Table 9-1. The term *alcoholism* sometimes refers to any alcohol use disorder, sometimes to alcohol dependence, and sometimes to severely affected alcohol dependent patients. Because of the ambiguity of the term "alcoholic," and because the term often has a negative connotation, clinicians should probably avoid using this term. In this chapter, we use *problem drinking* to cover the whole spectrum from at-risk drinking to alcohol dependence.

SMOKING AND OTHER TOBACCO USE

Unlike light drinking, which may be beneficial for some people, there is no safe level of tobacco use. Cigarette smokers, cigar smokers, those who chew tobacco, and those who use snuff are all at risk for major adverse health consequences from their tobacco use. Cigarettes are the most commonly used form of tobacco and cause the largest proportion of tobacco-related deaths. We will concentrate on cigarette smoking for the remainder of the chapter with the understanding that many of the approaches used to help cigarette smokers quit are potentially helpful for individuals who use other forms of tobacco.

The American Psychiatric Association includes nicotine dependence as a type of psychoactive substance use disorder. The essential feature of substance dependence is "a cluster of cognitive, behavioral, and physiologic symptoms indicating that the individual continues use of the substance despite significant substance-related problems. There is a pattern of repeated self-administration that usually results in tolerance, withdrawal, and compulsive drug taking behavior."[1] Table 9-1 shows examples of how these criteria apply to tobacco and alcohol abuse.

In surveillance surveys, "ever smokers" are defined as persons who report they have smoked at least 100 cigarettes. "Current smokers" are ever smokers who report currently smoking every day or on some days. "Former smokers" are ever smokers who are not smoking daily or on some days.

ARNOLD RALPH (CONTINUED) *Mr. Ralph says he has never had alcohol withdrawal symptoms and claims that he could stop drinking tomorrow if he had to. He tells you that he has never attempted to cut down on his alcohol consumption, and he considers the conflicts he and his wife have over his beer drinking "her problem." You also learn that he has had two DUI citations and that he still occasionally drives after drinking. Based on his alcohol-related legal and family problems, you determine that Mr. Ralph has an alcohol use disorder, as well as nicotine dependence.*

Prevalence and Costs of Alcohol and Tobacco Problems

The direct and indirect costs of alcohol and tobacco use are high. In the United States, smoking and alcohol abuse cost more than $167 billion a year in direct and indirect costs. Smoking-attributable cost for medical care in 1993 was estimated by Herdman and associates at $50 billion and the cost from lost productivity and earnings was estimated at $47 billion a year. In 1990, Rice estimated the cost of alcohol abuse at $98 billion, including $12.6 billion for health care, $33.6 billion from premature mortality, $36.6 billion from reduced or lost productivity, and $15.8 billion from social costs including crime and its consequences. Alcohol and tobacco use in the United States are very common, as we describe in this section.

PREVALENCE OF PROBLEM DRINKING

In 1992, 44 percent of American adults were current drinkers, 22 percent were former drinkers, and 34 percent were lifetime abstainers. In the general population, the past year prevalence of alcohol abuse and dependence is 7.4 percent, higher in men (11.0 percent) than in women (4.1 percent). Additionally, at-risk drinking without alcohol abuse or dependence is common in primary care. In a 1994 survey by Frazier and col-

[1]American Psychiatric Association: *Diagnostic and Statistical Manual of Mental Disorders: DSM-IV*, 4th ed. Washington, DC: American Psychiatric Association; 1994.

Table 9-1

Criteria for Substance Dependence from DSM-IV and Examples Specific for Tobacco and Alcohol Use

Criteria	Tobacco Use Examples	Alcohol Use Examples
Need for markedly increased amounts of the substance to achieve intoxication or desired effect (tolerance)	Adolescents smoke on more days per month and smoke more cigarettes per day as they grow older; the number of cigarettes smoked daily is twice as high for adult smokers (18 to 20 per day) as for adolescent smokers (9 per day).	Those who are alcohol dependent must drink a greater amount of alcohol and/or drink in a shorter amount of time to achieve intoxication.
Markedly diminished effect with continued use of the same amount of the substance (tolerance)	After persistent use, smokers experience absence of nausea, dizziness, or other features they experienced at first use.	Those who drink experience an ability to function at higher blood alcohol levels (especially over 0.15 g/100 mL), indicating tolerance.
The characteristic withdrawal syndrome	Following daily use of nicotine for at least several weeks, those who abruptly cease using nicotine, or reduce the amount of nicotine used, experience within 24 h four (or more) of the following signs: • dysphoric or depressed mood • insomnia • irritability • frustration or anger • anxiety • difficulty concentrating • restlessness • decreased heart rate • increased appetite or weight gain Craving is also an important element in nicotine withdrawal.	Those who experience alcohol withdrawal have symptoms that vary from minor to severe. Minor symptoms, which often occur early in the course of withdrawal, include • anxiety • tremors • sweating • nausea • tachycardia • hypertension Seizures can occur at any time, and may be related more to heavy drinking than to withdrawal. Delirium tremens is a specific syndrome, that often occurs days after cessation of drinking, with agitation, hallucinations, and severe autonomic dysregulation.
The same or closely related subtance is taken to avoid withdrawal symptoms.	Many smokers report that they smoke to prevent or control symptoms such as irritability and difficulty concentrating. People who smoke after being in a situation where smoking is not permitted, such as an airplane or theater, often do so to relieve withdrawal.	Acohol-dependent patients sometimes seek benzodiazepines or other sedatives to self-medicate their withdrawal symptoms.

Table 9-1

Criteria for Substance Dependence from DSM-IV and Examples Specific for Tobacco and Alcohol Use (*continued*)

Criteria	Tobacco Use Examples	Alcohol Use Examples
The substance is often taken in larger amounts or over a longer period of time than the person intended.	Of high school seniors who were daily smokers and didn't expect to be smokers 5 years later, 73% were still smoking; 70% of adolescent smokers and 80% of adult smokers regret ever starting; few smokers can restrict their smoking to only a few occasions.	Whether controlled drinking is ever possible for an alcohol-dependent person is controversial, but a person who loses control and drinks much more than intended, on every drinking occasion, is likely alcohol dependent.
There is a persistent desire or unsuccessful efforts to cut down or control substance abuse.	About 70% of smokers want to quit; 35 million try to cut down every year, but 25 million are unable to do so; about one-third of smokers quit for a day every year, but <10% of those who do remain abstinent. Relapse rates following treatment are similar to those for alcohol and heroin. Less than 5% of self-quitters maintain abstinence.	The first of the CAGE questions ("Have you ever thought you ought to cut down on your drinking?") reflects this criterion.
A great deal of time is spent in activities necessary to obtain the substance, use the substance, or recover from its effects.	Chain smoking	Alcohol-dependent persons often plan where to buy alcohol. Time spent intoxicated and coping with withdrawal may be substantial.
Important social, occupational, or recreational activities are given up or reduced because of substance use.	This behavior becomes more evident as smoke-free indoor policies become more prevalent.	Alcohol dependence is often associated with loss of job, relationships with family, and a change in the acquaintances with whom one associates.
Substance use is continued despite knowledge of having a persistent or recurrent physical or psychological problem that is likely to have been caused or exacerbated by the subtance.	Many persons continue to smoke even though they have documented medical conditions that are made worse by their smoking: nearly half resume smoking following surgery for lung cancer; 38% returned to smoking while still hospitalized following a heart attack; 40% smoked again following a laryngectomy. Most smokers acknowledge that smoking has affected their health, but they continue to smoke.	Psychological consequences for those who are alcohol dependent include anterograde amnesia ("blackouts" in which the person can not store new information in memory), depression, and anxiety. Physical conditions include cirrhosis, alcoholic cardiomyopathy, and pancreatitis.

Source: Adapted from American Psychiatric Association: *The Diagnositc and Statistical Manual of Mental Disorders*, 4th ed. Washington, DC: American Psychiatric Association; 1994. Used with permission.

leagues, 14 percent of all adults reported drinking five or more drinks on at least one occasion in the past 30 days. The probability of heavy drinking or having been intoxicated on a weekly or more frequent basis shows no variation by race or ethnicity, but is inversely related to age, education, and income, according to Dawson and co-workers.

Prevalence of Tobacco Use

In 1994, 48 million adult Americans were current smokers: 25 million men and 23 million women, according to the Centers for Disease Control and Prevention (CDC). The overall 1994 prevalence of tobacco use among adults (18 years old or older) in the United States was 26 percent, 28 percent among males and 23 percent among females. Among males, those who were between 35 and 54 years old have the highest prevalence at 32 percent; among females, those between 25 and 44 years old have the highest prevalence at 27 percent. Prevalence is lowest in the over 65 age group (14 percent for men and 11 percent for women).

The CDC reports that among racial/ethnic minority adults, American Indians and Alaskan Natives have the highest prevalence of tobacco use (39 percent), followed by African Americans (27 percent), and Hispanics (19 percent). Asian Americans and Pacific Islanders have the lowest rate (15 percent). In all four racial/ethnic minority groups, except American Indian and Alaska Natives, men have a higher prevalence of smoking than women.

Tobacco growing states in the southeast United States had the highest rates of smoking. The CDC reports that Kentucky had the highest rate at 28 percent, more than double the rate in Utah at 13 percent. Among the 50 states, Utah is the only state to have achieved the *Healthy People 2000* objective to reduce prevalence of smoking to no more than 15 percent of the population.

Poverty appears to have an independent effect on smoking prevalence. Individuals living under the poverty threshold are about 30 percent more likely to smoke cigarettes and 20 to 30 percent less likely to quit smoking, according to Flint and Novotny. This effect is seen even after controlling for education, gender, age, race/ethnicity, employment status, marital status, and geographic region.

Giovino and colleagues report that across categories of occupation, marital status, and military status, the highest prevalences of cigarette smoking are found in the following subgroups: blue collar workers, persons separated or divorced, and active duty military personnel. Almost half of all American ever smokers quit smoking during the decades that followed the early Surgeon General's warning about the dangers of smoking. Wealthier and more educated individuals were more likely to stop smoking. For example, the World Health Organization (WHO) reports that by 1991 only 3 percent of physicians and 18 percent of nurses were smokers.

Coexistence of Substance Use Problems

Manwell and associates conducted a large epidemiologic study that included more than 20,000 adult patients cared for by 88 primary care physicians. The study found that tobacco use and alcohol problems are common: the 90-day prevalence of tobacco use was 27 percent, 40 percent were alcohol abstainers, 38 percent were moderate drinkers, 9 percent were at-risk drinkers, and 13 percent had either alcohol abuse or dependence as indicated by two or more positive responses to the CAGE questions (described later under "Step 1: Ask").

Smoking and drinking problems often coexist. Shiffman and Balabanis report that the prevalence of smoking among persons who are alcohol dependent is 80 to 95 percent. It is also estimated that 30 percent of smokers can be diagnosed as alcoholics. Adolescents who begin smoking are 3 times more likely to begin using alcohol, and smokers are 10 times more likely to develop alcoholism than are nonsmokers, according to Hughes. Miller and Gold suggest that when clinicians identify that a patient smokes, they should screen that patient for alcohol problems.

Animal studies support biological mechanisms for the coexistence of alcohol and nicotine addiction. Either drug may increase the rewarding effects of the other, or either may decrease the toxic or unpleasant effects of the other. For example, alcohol appears to induce loss of physical coordination in mice by inhibiting nicotinic receptors in the cerebellum. Administration of nicotine appears to remove the inhibition and restore coordination. Alcohol also interferes with the normal functioning of vasopressin, a neurotransmitter that may be involved in memory processes and may be associated with the development of tolerance to alcohol. Nicotine appears to normalize vasopressin function in the brain, reducing alcohol-induced impairment of memory and other intellectual functions.

Health Effects of Smoking and Drinking

Every year in the United States there are over 400,000 deaths directly attributed to cigarette smoking, including 120,000 from lung cancer and 100,000 from coronary heart disease. It is estimated that more than 10 million Americans have died prematurely from causes attributed to smoking since the Surgeon General first reported the health effects of smoking in 1964. Drinking, like smoking, increases mortality. In long-term cohort studies, drinking more than two or three drinks a day is associated with increased overall mortality. In the following section, we describe the health effects of both smoking and drinking.

Health Effects of Smoking

Since the early 1950s and 1960s, a massive body of epidemiologic evidence has accumulated demonstrating the negative consequences of smoking. In addition to lung cancer, smoking is directly related to cancers of the oral cavity, pharynx, larynx, pancreas, kidney, bladder, and cervix, according to the Surgeon General. Smoking promotes atherosclerosis and is a major risk factor for coronary artery disease, thromboembolic disease, and peripheral vascular disease. Cigarette smoke has direct toxic effects on the respiratory tissue of all smokers, resulting in paralysis of ciliary epithelia and increased difficulty clearing respiratory irritants and carcinogens. Cigarette smoke also accelerates the decline in lung function among patients with chronic obstructive pulmonary disease. Use of smokeless tobacco and cigars also have deadly consequences in terms of lung, larynx, esophageal, and oral cancer.

There are multiple effects of cigarette smoking that may not cause death but produce significant pain and suffering. Individuals who continue to smoke after their diagnoses of peptic ulcer disease have more difficulty healing despite administration of appropriate medications. Smoking is an important risk factor for the development of osteoporosis. Tobacco use is associated with gum disease and tooth decay. Less well-known effects of smoking in men include decreases in testosterone levels, decrease in percentage of sperm with normal morphology, and increased risk of impotence. There is also consistent evidence reported by Grady that cigarette smoking causes facial wrinkling that could make smokers appear unattractive and prematurely old. Though not deadly, these effects lower quality of life for smokers.

Smoking affects the health of nonsmokers. Maternal smoking during pregnancy increases the risk of perinatal death, low birth weight, preterm delivery, miscarriage, and fetal growth retardation. Environmental tobacco smoke, the most important contaminant of indoor air, is composed of both "sidestream" smoke, which comes from the smoldering cigarette, and "mainstream" smoke, which is exhaled by smokers. Exposure to environmental tobacco smoke increases the risk of middle ear effusions, bronchitis, and pneumonia. It causes 8000 to 26,000 new cases of asthma a year and contributes to increased symptoms of asthma in 200,000 to 1,000,000 children a year. The Environmental Protection Agency declared environmental tobacco smoke as a group A (known human) carcinogen, in the same group as asbestos, vinyl chloride, and radon. Exposure to environmental tobacco smoke is widespread. Traces of cotinine, a metabolite of nicotine, are detected in the blood of 88 percent of nonsmokers in the United States, according to Pirkle and co-workers. It is estimated that environmental tobacco smoke causes about 3000 yearly deaths from lung cancer and increases the risk of coronary disease in nonsmokers.

Health Effects of Drinking Alcohol

Problem drinking causes over 100,000 deaths each year in the United States. Almost half of these deaths are from injuries, both intentional (homicide and suicide) and unintentional. Injuries account for an estimated 80 percent of the years of productive life lost due to alcohol. Heavy drinking is a major cause of liver disease, cardiomyopathy, coronary artery disease, hemorrhagic stroke, dementia, and other diseases, according to Thakker.

Unlike tobacco, where no safe level of use has been established, light drinking, even as little as two drinks per *week*, appears to be associated with some health benefits including improved psychological well-being and about a 12 percent reduction in risk of coronary heart disease, according to Maclure. Baum-Baicker found that low or moderate amounts of alcohol appear to reduce stress, increase affective expression, promote conviviality, and decrease tension, anxiety, and self-consciousness. Moderate drinking in the elderly—no more than one drink per day because of the smaller volume of distribution—stimulates appetite and promotes regular bowel function, Dufour and colleagues report. When considering alcohol use in elderly patients, remember that many prescription and over-the-counter medications interact with alcohol. Alcohol and tobacco also interact with management of other common disorders, such as hypertension, diabetes, and psychiatric syndromes.

Hypertension in Those Who Smoke and Drink

Both cigarette smoking and at-risk drinking interfere with the management and control of hypertension. Smoking is a major risk factor for all cardiovascular complications associated with hypertension. Hypertensive smokers who do not stop smoking are not likely to benefit from the protection afforded by antihypertensive therapy. Each cigarette smoked produces a significant rise in blood pressure. Additionally, drinking alcohol in excess of moderate levels is an important risk factor for the development of hypertension. Drinking may cause resistance to antihypertensive medication and is a risk factor for stroke.

Diabetes in Those Who Smoke and Drink

The macrovascular complications from type 2 diabetes are associated with cigarette smoking. Trying to control diabetes without trying to help patients stop smoking will likely be unsuccessful. It is essential that smokers with diabetes stop smoking. Likewise, alcohol use can be especially detrimental to patients with diabetes, because excessive alcohol use is an important cause of hospital admissions for hypoglycemia among diabetics taking insulin.

Psychiatric Syndromes in Those Who Smoke and Drink

Results from the Epidemiologic Catchment Area, a large survey conducted by the National Institute of Mental Health, show that compared to nonalcoholics, alcoholics are 21 times more likely to be diagnosed with antisocial personality disorder, 4 times more likely to be diagnosed with drug abuse, 6 times more likely to be diagnosed with mania, and 4 times more likely to be diagnosed with schizophrenia. The association between alcoholism and depression was less strong (alcoholics were 1.7 times more likely than nonalcoholics to be diagnosed with depression). These findings, reported by Helzer and Pryzbeck, have important implications for treatment of alcoholics in primary care.

Arnold Ralph (continued) *Mr. Ralph has had three episodes of acute bronchitis in the past 2 years and has moderate hypertension controlled with a diuretic and an ACE inhibitor. He has had intermittent epigastric pain for about 5 years, but otherwise considers himself healthy.*

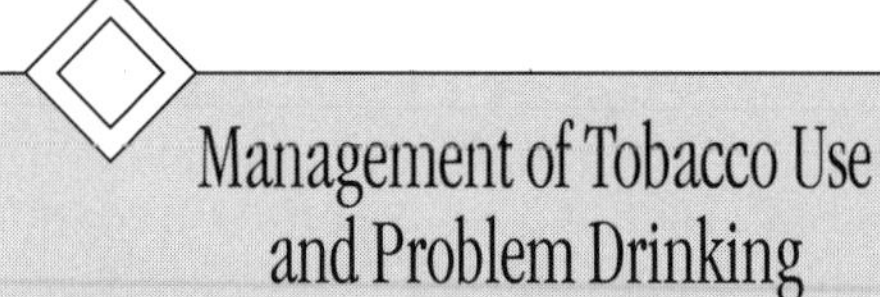

Management of Tobacco Use and Problem Drinking

Patients who use tobacco and problem drinkers can change those behaviors. A multitude of controlled clinical trials with smokers and with problem drinkers have shown that brief clinician interventions are effective in helping our patients change. The clinical practice guideline on treating tobacco use and dependence, developed by the U.S. Department of Health and Human Services (DHHS) in 2000, provides extensive guidance for the management of tobacco use. Much of this section on management is based on that guideline.

One way to approach both tobacco and alcohol issues is with the 5 A's: Ask, Assess, Advise, Assist, and Arrange.

Step 1: Ask

The first step of managing patients who use tobacco or have a problem with alcohol is to identify them. This is not as obvious as it might seem. Most clinical problems we encounter are brought to us (as symptoms or complaints) by our patients, but few patients come in with a chief complaint of smoking or problem drinking. Therefore, identifying the patients who could benefit from behavior change requires finding them, and that requires routinely screening all patients.

Because tobacco use in any amount is potentially harmful, screening for it requires only one question: "Do you use tobacco?" Because people usually begin smoking in adolescence, the Department of Health and Human Services guideline recommends that primary care clinicians should begin screening at every visit starting when patients are around age 11. A practical and effective way to document this status is to include tobacco use (current, former, or never) with other vital signs measured routinely. In view of competing demands of practice experienced by most primary care clinicians, it makes sense that this function be delegated to other members of the clinical team, such as nurses or medical office assistants, who can start counseling interventions that can then be reinforced by the primary care clinician. As documented in nine randomized clinical trials, screening systems that systematically identify and document smoking status result in higher rates of smoking interventions by clinicians. Given the large number of smokers who visit primary care clinicians every year, the potential public health impact of higher rates of intervention is substantial. When treating children, take advantage of the opportunity and screen their parents for tobacco use. If the caregivers choose not to quit smoking, advise them to smoke outside. Smoking in the basement, bathroom, or other room is not sufficiently protective in homes that are insulated and have poor ventilation patterns.

Routine screening for problem drinking also increases intervention rates. Adams and colleagues found that having a screening routine in place in a practice doubles the frequency with which clinicians discuss alcohol. Unlike screening for tobacco use, screening for problem drinking requires time for assessment of both the pattern of drinking and the severity of alcohol-related problems. Many instruments are available to screen for problem drinking, including the widely used CAGE questions:

C. Have you ever felt you should *cut* down on your drinking?
A. Have people *annoyed you* by criticizing your drinking?
G. Have you ever felt bad or *guilty* about your drinking?
E. Have you ever had a drink first thing in the morning to steady your nerves or to get rid of a hangover (*eye* opener)?

The CAGE questions are commonly recommended, but may miss at-risk drinkers.

Another technique shows that clinicians can identify at-risk drinkers and patients with alcohol use disorders by asking a single question, "When was the last time you had more than 5 (for men, 4 for women) drinks on one occasion?" Taj et al found that this technique identifies at-risk drinkers and patients with alcohol use disorders with reasonable sensitivity and specificity. More importantly, this technique is simple enough for routine use with every adolescent and adult patient.

ARNOLD RALPH (CONTINUED) *You ask Mr. Ralph "When was the last time you had more than five* *on one occasion?" and he answers with, "Last night." He answers "No" to all the CAGE questions except A—annoyance.*

Step 2: Assess

The second step in the management of problem drinking and tobacco use is assessment. In dealing with tobacco use, assessment is relatively straightforward. Essentially, everyone who uses tobacco needs to quit, and clinicians do not need to spend much time assessing how much of a problem tobacco is for their patients. Quantity and frequency are less of an issue with smoking than with drinking, and assessment of consequences is less important except in helping the patient identify the potential benefits of quitting.

For assessing alcohol use, the clinician asked in step 1, "When was the last time you had more than five drinks on one occasion?" If a patient answers "Last Saturday," the clinician needs to learn more about the pattern of the patient's drinking and its consequences: "How much did you drink then? How often do you drink that much? Have you ever had any problems because of alcohol? Any DWIs (driving while intoxicated), job problems, family problems?"

Additionally, there is a third dimension that the clinician needs to assess in dealing with these behavioral issues: Do the patients see smoking or drinking as a problem for them? How ready are they to change? Behavior change is a process rather than a discrete event. Readiness to change is a framework for thinking about the change process that includes stages of precontemplation (not even thinking about change), contemplation, preparation, action, maintenance, and relapse. This framework is described in more detail in Chap. 8, Identifying and Changing Health-Risk Behaviors.

In dealing with smokers, the term precontemplation denotes smokers who have no thoughts about quitting smoking in the (near) future. About 40 percent of smokers are in precontemplation. Smokers in the contemplation stage (another 40 percent) are those planning to quit smoking in the next 6 months but not in the next 30 days. Preparation (the last 20 percent) includes smokers who plan to stop smoking in the next 30 days.

Smokers in different stages differ in terms of expected positive outcomes from quitting and their belief in their ability to stop smoking successfully (their self-efficacy). Dijkstra and colleagues determined which stage smokers were in at baseline, then contacted them 3 and 14 months later, after they participated in a smoking cessation intervention. The results showed that the stage of readiness to change at baseline was highly predictive of quitting at both 3 and 14 months follow-up. No differences were found between different stages in terms of number of cigarettes smoked daily, the nicotine dependency score, or the number of years smoked.

Just as problem drinking covers a wide spectrum of severity, the concept of readiness to change is less easily defined when dealing with alcohol issues. In approaching problem drinkers, however, Rollnick suggests that it is helpful to picture readiness to change as having three dimensions: the patient's openness to discussing alcohol, the patient's perceptions of the severity of the problem and the importance of change, and the patient's self-confidence in his or her ability to change. For example, patients might be quite aware of their problem and quite confident (rightly or wrongly) in their own ability to change their drinking patterns, but unwilling to talk about their drinking at all. Understanding how ready patients are to change can guide clinicians' intervention efforts and help focus their time on those patients who stand to benefit most.

ARNOLD RALPH (CONTINUED) *At his first follow-up visit, Mr. Ralph tells you that he is tired of his morning cough and is thinking about quitting smoking. However, he enjoys his beers at night and has no intention of giving them up.*

Step 3: Advise

Once a clinician has identified which patients use tobacco or have problem drinking, how severe their problem is (quantity and consequences, especially for alcohol), and how ready they are to change their behavior, the clinician has an opportunity to help them change. Helping patients change behaviors really begins with the way we ask about tobacco and alcohol use and how we assess their use. Bien and co-workers report that when we assess patterns of use, consequences, and readiness to change with empathy while encouraging both self-confidence and a sense of self-responsibility, patients are more likely to change.

Once that foundation is well laid, it is time for the third step in managing problem drinking and tobacco use: advising. The process of giving advice is really one of negotiation. It is our job to give advice, but it is the patient's job to change. It does little good, and may do harm, to try to force the patient to accept advice they are not ready for. Furthermore, it is more comfortable for us if we make our efforts patient centered, skillfully negotiating changes that can help patients move toward healthier lifestyles, even if those changes are only small steps moving from precontemplation to simply thinking about changing. The advice we give must be clear, strong and personalized. Table 9-2 gives examples of phrases that may be useful.

Most smokers and problem drinkers are not ready to quit at any particular moment, and giving precontemplators and contemplators advice about *actions* to take is a waste of time. Instead, clinicians should use the approach outlined in Table 9-3. Clinicians must connect the advice message to a topic that is relevant to the patient, allowing the patient to list risks of continuing smoking or problematic drinking, roadblocks, and the rewards that would come with changing that behavior. The clinician should repeat this, briefly, at each visit.

Most primary care clinicians identify their patients who smoke and offer smoking cessation advice to selected ones, prioritizing patients seen during wellness visits and patients with established diagnoses related to tobacco use. Overall, studies show that only about 25 percent of smokers receive smoking cessation advice at every visit. Clinicians may believe that there is not sufficient time to advise every smoker during every visit. Jaén and colleagues found that on average, it takes about 1½ min per patient for smoking cessation coun-

Table 9-2

ADVISE—Strongly Urge All Smokers to Quit

Action	Strategies for Implementation
In a clear, strong and personalized manner urge every smoker to quit.	Advice should be • *Clear*—"I think it is important for you to quit smoking now and I will help you." "Cutting down while you are ill is not enough." • *Strong*—"As your clinician, I need you to know that quitting smoking is the most important thing you can do to protect your current and future health." "If you need a doctor to tell you that you need to quit, I'm it." • *Personalized*—"I know that you're concerned about your cough and the fact that your son gets so many colds. If you stop smoking, your cough should improve, and your son might get fewer colds, as well." "You asked me for help with your acne, if you stop smoking you will also get fewer wrinkles in your face."

Source: Adapted from DHHS Smoking Cessation Guidelines.

Table 9-3

Components of Clinical Interventions Designed to Enhance Motivation to Quit Smoking: "The Four Rs"

Relevance	Motivational information given to a patient has the greatest impact if it is relevant to a patient's disease status, family or social situation (e.g., having children in the home), health concerns, age, gender, and other important patient characteristics (e.g., prior quitting experience).
Risks	The clinician should ask the patient to identify the potential negative consequences of smoking. The clinician may suggest and highlight those that seem most relevant to the patient. The clinician should emphasize that smoking low-tar/low-nicotine cigarettes or use of other forms of tobacco (e.g., smokeless tobacco, cigars, pipes) will not eliminate the risks. Example of risks follow: • *Acute risks:* Shortness of breath, exacerbation of asthma, impotence, infertility, and increases in serum carbon monoxide. • *Long-term risks:* Heart attacks and strokes, lung and other cancers (larynx, oral cavity, pharynx, esophagus, pancreas, bladder, cervix, leukemia), chronic obstructive pulmonary diseases (chronic bronchitis and emphysema). • *Environmental risks:* Increased risk of lung cancer in spouse and children; higher rates of smoking by children of smokers; increased risk of SIDS, asthma, middle ear diseases, and respiratory infections in children of smokers.
Rewards	The clinician should ask the patient to identify the potential benefits of quitting smoking. The clinician may suggest and highlight those that seem most relevant to the patient. Examples of rewards follow: • Improved health • Improved sense of smell • Feel better about yourself • Can stop worrying about quitting • Have healthy babies and children • Feel better physically • Perform better in sports • Food will taste better • Save money • Home, car, breath will smell better • Set a good example for kids • Not worry about exposing others to smoke • Freedom from addiction
Repetition	The motivational intervention should be repeated every time an unmotivated patient visits the clinic setting.

SOURCE: Adapted from DHHS Smoking Cessation Guideline.

seling during primary care visits. If a clinician sees 30 patients a day and about 25 percent of them are smokers, counseling each smoker about cessation would add 11 minutes to the entire day.

ARNOLD RALPH (CONTINUED) *You strongly advise Mr. Ralph to stop smoking and drinking, and explain how his cough, hypertension, and possibly his epigastric pain will improve if he does so. You also explain that Mr. Ralph's relationship with his wife, and his wife's family, will most likely improve as well.*

Step 4: Assist

The fourth step in managing patients who use tobacco or drink too much is to assist them. Hypnosis and acupuncture are popular approaches for smoking cessation. The evidence from randomized clinical trials is too sparse to allow a judgment regarding the efficacy of hypnosis and does not show efficacy for "active" versus "control" acupuncture. Brief clinician interventions and more intensive counseling are both effective in helping patients change behaviors. Additionally, several medications can help some patients, as described later in this chapter.

Brief Clinician Interventions

TOBACCO COUNSELING Table 9-4 gives examples of brief interventions for dealing with tobacco: helping the patient with a plan for quitting, encourag-

Table 9-4

ASSIST—Aid the Patient in Quitting

Action	Strategies for Implementation
Help the patient with a quit plan.	Set a quit date—Ideally, the quite date should be within 2 weeks, taking patient preference into account. A patient's preparations for quitting: • Inform family, friends, and co-workers of quitting and request understanding and support. • Remove cigarettes from your environment. Prior to quitting, avoid smoking in places where you spend a lot of time (e.g., home, car). • Review previous quit attempts. What helped you? What led to relapse? • Anticipate challenges to planned quit attempt, particularly during the critical first weeks. These include nicotine withdrawal symptoms.
Encourage nicotine replacement therapy or other pharmacotherapies except in special circumstances.	Encourage the use of nicotine patch, nicotine gum, or sustained release buproprion therapy for smoking cessation. Give specific information regarding use, side effects, and clarify expectations.
Give key advice on quitting.	*Abstinence*—Total abstinence is essential. "Not even a single puff after the quit date." *Alcohol*—Drinking alcohol is highly associated with relapse to smoking. Those who stop smoking should review their alcohol use and consider limiting/abstaining from alcohol during the quit process. *Other smokers in the household*—The presence of other smokers in the household, particularly a spouse, is associated with lower success rates. Patients should consider quitting with their significant others and/or developing specific plans to stay quit in a household where others still smoke.
Provide supplementary materials.	*Sources*—Federal agencies, including AHRQ; nonprofit agencies (American Cancer Society, American Lung Association, American Heart Association); or local/state health departments. *Type*—Culturally/racially/educationally/age appropriate for the patient. *Location*—Readily available in every clinic office.

Source: Adapted from DHHS Smoking Cessation Guideline.

ing use of nicotine replacement or other effective pharmacologic aids, giving key advice on successful quitting, and providing supplementary materials.

In dealing with smokers, clinicians should focus the advice on problem-solving skills and on social support, as outlined in Tables 9–5 and 9–6. Effective treatments include problem solving, skill training, intra-treatment and extra-treatment social support, and aversive smoking. Aversive smoking involves sessions of guided smoking where the patient smokes intensely, often to the point of discomfort or malaise. Some aversive smoking techniques, such as rapid smoking, may present a health risk and should only be conducted under direct medical supervision and screening.

Most smokers gain weight after quitting smoking. Williamson and associates report that the average weight gain is about 10 pounds, but up to 10 percent of quitters may gain more than 30 pounds. Weight gain is likely related to a decrease in basal metabolic rate once nicotine is removed. Clinicians should advise smokers who are quitting against extreme dieting during their quit attempt and should tell patients to not attempt weight loss until they are secure about their quitting behavior.

If a patient is motivated to participate in a group or intense counseling program, clinicians need to facilitate this participation. There is strong evidence that for smoking cessation, more intervention is always better with a direct relationship between the duration and intensity of treatment and quit rates. The DHHS guideline reports that patients who participate in high-intensity (>10 min/session) counseling are twice as likely to quit; those who are in treatment for more than eight sessions are 2.3 times more likely to quit than smokers not participating in these sessions. In clinical practice, few patients are willing or able to participate in smoking cessation programs. Therefore, most offices need to offer brief smoking cessation interventions.

Table 9-5

Common Elements of Problem-Solving/Skill-Training Smoking Cessation Treatments

PROBLEM SOLVING TREATMENT COMPONENT	EXAMPLES
Recognition of danger situations Identification of events, internal states, or activities that are thought to increase the risk of smoking or relapse.	• Being around other smokers • Being under time pressure • Getting into an argument • Experiencing urges or negative moods • Drinking alcohol
Coping skills Identification and practice of coping or problem solving skills. Typically, these skills are intended to cope with danger situations.	• Learning to anticipate and avoid danger situations • Learning cognitive strategies that will reduce negative moods • Accomplishing life-style changes that reduce stress, improve quality of life, or produce pleasure • Learning cognitive and behavioral activities that distract attention from smoking urges
Basic information Provision of basic information about smoking and successful quitting.	• The nature/time course of withdrawal • The addictive nature of smoking • The fact that any smoking (even a single puff) increases the likelihood of full relapse

SOURCE: Adapted from DHHS Smoking Cessation Guideline.

Table 9-6

Common Elements of Supportive Smoking Cessation Treatments

SUPPORTIVE TREATMENT COMPONENT	EXAMPLES
Encourage the patient in the quit attempt.	• Note that effective cessation treatments are now available • Note that half of all people who have ever smoked, have now quit • Communicate belief in patient's ability to quit
Communicate caring and concern.	• Ask about how patient feels about quitting • Directly express concern and willingness to help • Be open to the patient's expression of fears of quitting, difficulties experienced, and ambivalent feelings
Encourage the patient to talk about the quitting process.	Ask about • Reasons the patient wants to quit • Difficulties encountered while quitting • Success the patient has achieved • Concerns or worries about quitting
Provide basic information about smoking and successful quitting.	• The nature/time course of withdrawal • The addictive nature of smoking • The fact that any smoking (even a single puff) increases the likelihood of full relapse

SOURCE: Adapted from DHHS Smoking Cessation Guideline.

ALCOHOL COUNSELING Unlike smoking cessation interventions, which can take as little as 1 or 2 min, brief interventions with problem drinkers require one or more office visits devoted to discussing alcohol.

Brief clinician interventions with at-risk drinkers and patients with alcohol abuse have been proven effective in over a dozen randomized clinical trials. Bien and colleagues have summarized the key elements. Table 9-7 lists them in a mnemonic fashion as FRAMES. Clinicians do not need to use all six during any one visit with a patient, but the elements can guide efforts to help a precontemplator move toward contemplation and the contemplator move toward planning and action. Among other techniques, comparing the pattern of the patient's drinking with population-based statistics and negotiating a written behavioral contract (often on an ordinary prescription form) have been part of several successful clinical trials with problem drinkers.

Although brief clinician interventions are effective with at-risk drinkers and patients with alcohol abuse, they appear to be much less effective with alcohol-dependent patients. Therefore, the goal of the brief intervention with an alcohol-dependent patient should be to get them into specialized treatment.

As with other chronic diseases, some patients with alcohol dependence respond to treatment better than others, some patients fail despite multiple attempts at treatment, and relapse is common even among those who respond. But some patients with addiction succeed very well. Unlike most other chronic diseases, the outcome can look like a total cure, with cessation of drinking and resolution of the resulting problems. Although they will often refer to themselves as being "in recovery" rather than "recovered," long-term success does occur in patients with addiction and can be facilitated by treatment.

In the treatment of alcohol dependence, several treatment approaches are available. If well

Table 9-7

Elements of Successful Brief Interventions With Problem Drinkers

ELEMENT	EXAMPLES
Feedback	Simply tell the patient what's wrong. Relate the medical problems you see to their drinking, or, even better, help them make the connection. Compare their drinking pattern to societal norms.
Responsibility	Changing the patient's drinking is the patient's job, not yours, and you tell the patient that.
Advice	Give direct, clear advice about what you think the patient should do.
Menu	Provide several options about what the patient should do, including cutting down, stopping drinking, or thinking about the problems. Negotiate a plan, and put it in writing for the patient to sign.
Empathy	Reflective listening with an understanding approach.
Self-efficacy	The other side of responsibility. Emphasize "You can change."

SOURCE: Adapted from Bien TH, Miller WR, Tonigan JS: Brief interventions for alcohol problems: A review. *Addiction* 88:315, 1993.

done, they all work about equally well for almost any kind of patient. Project MATCH (Matching Alcoholism Treatment to Client Heterogeneity) randomized several hundred patients into three therapies: (1) motivational enhancement therapy, which seeks to mobilize the person's own resources to change; (2) cognitive behavioral therapy, which trains patients in skills to cope with situations with risk for drinking; or (3) 12-step facilitation, designed to promote involvement in Alcoholics Anonymous. Outcomes were equivalent across all patient groups and for almost all patient characteristics examined, with a slight advantage for the 12-step facilitation group on some comparisons. In other studies with comparisons with no-treatment control groups; behavioral self-control training; behavioral, marital, and family therapy; the "community reinforcement" approach; and other approaches have all been effective. Given this information, it is reasonable to encourage an alcohol-dependent patient to enter treatment, any treatment, as long as the program appears to fit the patient's needs from both the clinician's and the patient's perspectives. Insurance coverage may be a deciding factor for some patients.

PHARMACOTHERAPY

Pharmacotherapy can be an important part of the primary care management of tobacco and alcohol problems. Nicotine replacement and bupropion have been shown to be efficacious as first-line treatment and clonidine and nortriptyline as second-line treatments to help smokers quit. Naltrexone and disulfiram have proven value in helping alcohol-dependent patients.

NICOTINE REPLACEMENT The efficacy of nicotine replacement therapy (NRT) for smoking cessation has been proven in many randomized clinical trials. NRT appears to blunt the withdrawal symptoms and reduce cravings. The DHHS guideline recommends NRT for all smokers except those with serious medical contraindications. For patients with severe cardiovascular disease, particularly those with severe or worsening angina pectoris, serious dysrrythmias, and recent (less than 4 weeks) myocardial infarction, NRT should be used only after carefully considering the risks and benefits profile. Benowitz and Gourlay report that clinical trials of NRT in patients with stable coronary artery disease suggest that nicotine does not increase cardiovascular risk. Therefore, there is no support for the lay notion that wearing a nicotine patch causes myocardial infarction; smoking, not nicotine, causes myocardial infarction.

Nicotine replacement therapy is proven effective for smoking cessation. Use of the nicotine transdermal patch doubles the 6- to 12-month abstinence rates over those produced by placebo interventions, a conclusion is supported by a meta-analysis including 27 randomized clinical trials. Nicotine gum increases smoking cessation rates by approximately 50 percent compared with control interventions through 12 months of follow-up, a conclusion supported by a meta-analysis including 13 trials. Patients using other forms of NRT (nasal spray and inhaler) appear to have similar quit rates.

Pregnant smokers should first be encouraged to attempt cessation without pharmacologic treatment. Use NRT with pregnant women only after you determine that smoking cessation outweighs the risk of nicotine replacement and potential concomitant smoking. Similar considerations are necessary for lactating mothers.

Nicotine Transdermal Patch. A common form of NRT, the nicotine transdermal patch is applied daily upon awakening in an area that is relatively hairless between the waist and neck. There are no restrictions on activity, but smokers are encouraged not to smoke while on the patch, mainly to avoid relapse. It is important to start with the highest dose. Although it is recommended that patients be treated for 8 weeks, duration of therapy can be individualized.

Nicotine Gum. Nicotine gum is another option for NRT. Proper chewing technique is essential for success using nicotine gum. Chewing nicotine gum in a manner similar to regular chewing gum will produce nicotine toxicity (nausea, hiccups, dyspepsia, etc.). Gum should be chewed slowly until a "peppery" taste emerges, then "parked" between cheek and gum to facilitate nicotine absorption through the oral mucosa. Gum should be slowly and intermittently "chewed and parked" for about 30 min. Acidic beverages such as coffee, juices, and soft drinks interfere with the buccal absorption of nicotine and should be avoided for 15 min before or during gum use. Nicotine gum comes in two doses: 2 mg and 4 mg. The 4-mg dose is most appropriate for highly dependent smokers, those who smoke more than 20 to 25 cigarettes per day, or who smoke within 30 min of awakening. Patients who are particularly concerned about weight gain might benefit from using nicotine gum to prevent weight gain.

Inhalers. Other delivery systems for NRT includes a nicotine inhaler and a nasal spray. Nicotine inhalers deliver 4 mg of nicotine from cartridges with a porous plug containing 10 mg of nicotine. Patients may self-titrate to the level of nicotine they require and should use at least six cartridges per day for the first 3 to 6 weeks of treatment. Frequent continuous puffing is recommended for best effects. Nicotine nasal spray delivers a spray containing 0.5 mg of nicotine. One dose is 1 mg of nicotine (two sprays, one in each nostril). Patients should be started with 1 to 2 doses per hour, which may be increased to a maximum of 40 doses per day (5 doses per hour).

BUPROPION Bupropion (Zyban), in a slow-release (SR) formulation, is the first non-nicotine drug approved by the Food and Drug Administration (FDA) for smoking cessation. For some smokers, it appears to blunt the pleasure pathway related to nicotine intake. One smoker described bupropion's effects as making smoking feel like "sucking hot air." A large randomized clinical trial by Hurt and colleagues found quit rates at 1 year at 23 percent compared to 12 percent with placebo, and demonstrated a reduction in weight gain among those who remained abstinent. This trial excluded smokers who had clinical depression.

Clinicians should start patients on bupropion SR at 150 mg every day for 3 days and then increase to 150 mg twice a day. The smokers should start bupropion SR 1 week prior to their quit day because the drug takes 5 days to achieve steady-state plasma levels. To prevent insomnia, a common side effect, separate doses by 8 h. Giving the second dose 3 to 4 h before bedtime could ameliorate this side effect. Contraindications include seizure disorder, current or prior history of bulimia or anorexia nervosa, concomitant use of monoamine oxidase inhibitors (MAOIs), concomitant use of other forms of bupropion (i.e., Wellbutrin), current other substance abuse, and any other medical conditions that lower the seizure threshold.

In view of the evidence for effectiveness for NRT and bupropion, the patient's preference is the most important consideration. Some patients prefer to take a "pill" and are likely to prefer bupropion, whereas others prefer to use over-the-counter medications and will opt for NRT. If a patient shows evidence of depression, bupropion has the added advantage of being an antidepressant. A smoker who has unsuccessfully tried multiple approaches to quitting may benefit from combined therapy.

CLONIDINE AND NORTRIPTYLINE There is evidence of the efficacy of these two medications for treating tobacco dependence. They are considered second-line medications because the FDA has not approved them for a tobacco dependence treatment indication and there are more concerns about potential side effects than exist with first-line medications. Second-line treatments should be considered for use on a case-by-case basis after first-line treatments have been tried or considered.

NALTREXONE Naltrexone (Revia) is a narcotic receptor blocker used to treat alcohol dependence. Patients are usually given 50 mg daily. How it works is still largely a matter of speculation, but it does work. In two independent randomized clinical trials, both lasting 12 weeks, naltrexone reduced the risk of relapse, defined as drinking more than five drinks on one occasion for men or four for women, from 54 percent to 23 percent in one study and from almost 90 percent to less than 50 percent in the other. In both trials, naltrexone was provided as part of standard alcoholism treatment programs; studies of its use in primary care settings are in progress. Pending the results of these studies, it is reasonable to consider naltrexone along with supportive counseling and frequent follow-up for a patient who is unwilling to accept a referral for specialty care. It is also becoming a regular part of alcohol treatment programs, and we are likely to encounter patients remaining on it in our primary care practices.

About 5 percent of patients enrolled in clinical trials of naltrexone discontinued it because of nausea. Liver toxicity is possible, although more likely with heavy drinking. It is fairly expensive, about $4 per day, but quite cost effective considering the costs of alcoholic beverages, themselves, and the costs of alcohol-related consequences.

DISULFIRAM Disulfiram (Antabuse) prevents drinking not by a pharmacologic action, but by the psychological threat of one. Disulfiram blocks a key step in the metabolism of alcohol, leading to accumulation of toxic amounts of acetaldehyde. Accumulation of acetaldehyde causes an unpleasant and potentially serious reaction characterized by vomiting, headache, hypotension, sweating, and, if enough alcohol is consumed, syncope, arrhythmia, and cardiac arrest. The usual dose is 250 mg daily.

One study by Fuller and co-workers showed little advantage of disulfiram over placebo, but another study by Azrin and associates showed that when given as part of a broader intervention with the family or community, disulfiram was significantly more effective. Particularly notable in the latter study was a suggestive subgroup analysis showing that married male alcoholics whose wives observed their disulfiram dosing each day had outcomes almost as good as a comparison group who received multidimensional community reinforcement therapy, and much better than a third group who received standard outpatient counseling (weekly for 5 weeks, then monthly) and a prescription for disulfiram. Although this approach has not been tested in a primary care practice with the clinician providing (probably briefer) counseling, it may be worth trying in a patient who declines referral for specialized treatment and whose spouse is willing to participate. Disulfiram can affect the liver, but the risk of hepatic damage is greater with continued heavy drinking than with disulfiram.

Step 5: Arrange Follow-Up

The final step in managing patients with problem drinking or who use tobacco is to arrange follow-up. For both problems, follow-up visits improve success. On average, most ex-smokers had three or more serious attempts at quitting before achieving success. The follow-up visits provide opportunities to prevent relapse and to support maintenance of cessation.

For smoking cessation, the first follow-up contact, either in person or by phone, should be scheduled within the first week after the quit date, when the risk of relapse is highest. The second follow-up should be scheduled within the first month after the quit date, if possible. Additional contacts need to be scheduled as necessary. Table 9-8 provides details of potential action during follow-up.

At-risk drinkers who attend booster sessions following a brief clinician intervention have better outcomes, but that may be due to self-selection bias; patients who are more committed to changing their behavior would be likely to attend more follow-up sessions and to be successful in moderating their drinking.

Management of Dual Tobacco and Alcohol Addiction

Tobacco use and problem drinking are both major causes of morbidity and premature mortality in the United States. When a patient has both problems, it is common to focus on just one, but that approach may leave the patient at substantial risk of early death. In one cohort study, patients who had been treated in an inpatient program for alcohol abuse or dependence had a 2.6-fold increase in overall mortality over the subsequent 10 to 20 years. One-third of those deaths were alcohol related, but even more—one-half of them—were tobacco related, according to Hurt and colleagues. The evidence suggests that simultaneously treating both problems improves outcomes. Specifically, Bobo and colleagues found that treating tobacco and alcohol addiction at the same time helps patients quit smoking and does not diminish success regarding alcohol use.

ARNOLD RALPH (CONTINUED) *Mr. Ralph agrees to enroll in the quit smoking program you offer in your practice. He sets a quit date, quits, and uses nicotine gum to help him deal with his craving for cigarettes. He says he will think about cutting back on his beer drinking. Three months later, he*

Table 9-8

Arrange—Schedule Follow-Up Contact

Action	Strategies for Implementation
Schedule follow-up contact either in person or via telephone.	*Timing*—Follow-up contact should occur soon after the quit date, preferably during the first week. A second follow-up contact is recommended within the first month. Schedule further follow-up contacts as indicated. *Actions during follow-up visit*—Congratulate success. If smoking occurred, review circumstances and elicit recommitment to total abstinence. Remind patient that a lapse can be used as a learning experience. Identify problems already encountered and anticipate challenges in the immediate future. Assess nicotine replacement therapy use and problems. Consider referral to a more intense or specialized program.

Source: Adapted from DHHS Smoking Cessation Guideline.

has not smoked a cigarette, and says he has reduced his alcohol intake to two beers a night.

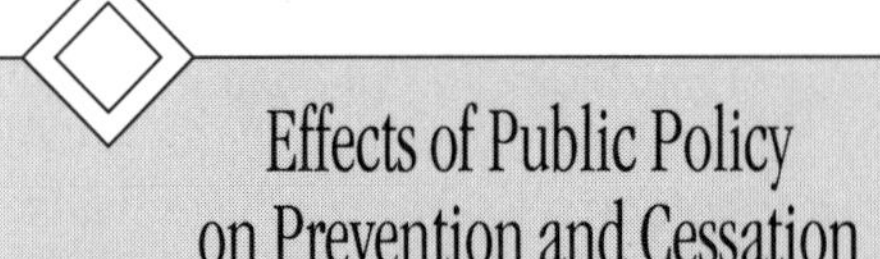

Effects of Public Policy on Prevention and Cessation

For both tobacco use and problem drinking, the benefits of governmental policies are modest, but because the problems are so widespread, the cumulative effects of policies may be substantial. This potential effect has, as yet, only been tested in natural experiments. For example, increasing the price of cigarettes (by taxes) may reduce smoking more among younger persons and members of minority groups than among others. Some research has taken advantage of natural experiments in drinking and driving laws to compare, for example, states with lower thresholds for defining drunk driving to other states. Such analyses have consistently shown benefits. The National Institute on Alcohol Abuse and Alcoholism reports that traffic crash fatalities are reduced by increasing taxes on alcoholic beverages, raising the minimum drinking age, and "zero-tolerance laws" that set the maximum blood alcohol concentration for drivers under age 21 at 0.02 percent or less.

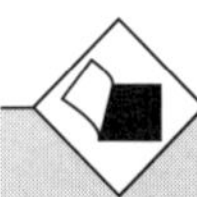

Summary

Alcohol and tobacco are two of the most commonly abused substances in the world. Both are responsible for enormous health problems. Primary care clinicians do not need to feel pessimistic about their ability to help patients reduce or stop their use of these substances—brief office-based interventions are known to be effective, and can be incorporated into almost any primary care setting.

Suggested Reading

The Physicians' Guide to Helping Patients with Alcohol Problems. NIAAA. 1995. Online at http://www.niaaa.nih.gov. Click "publications".

See also "How to cut down on your drinking," a handout for patients, also from NIAAA and on their web site at http://www.niaaa.nih.gov. Click "publications."

Practical advice for the clinician counseling patients about their alcohol use.

Wilk AI, Jensen NM, Havighurst TC: Meta-analysis of randomized control trials addressing brief interventions in heavy alcohol drinkers. *J Gen Intern Med* 12:274, 1997.

Evidence for the effectiveness of brief interventions against alcohol use.

Mayo-Smith MF: Pharmacological management of alcohol withdrawal: A meta-analysis and evidence-based practice guideline. *JAMA* 278:144, 1997.

Evidence for the clinician about managing alcohol withdrawal symptoms.

Surgeon General: Tobacco cessation guideline: New findings about the latest drugs and counseling techniques for treating tobacco use and dependence. Available at http://www.surgeongeneral.gov/tobacco/

The website with the most recent U.S. Public Health Service's guidelines for smoking cessation.

The Tobacco Use and Dependence Clinical Practice Guideline Panel, Staff and Consortium Representatives: A Clinical Practice Guideline for Treating Tobacco Use and Dependence: A U.S. Public Health Service Report. *JAMA* 283:3244, 2000.

Consensus document by the leading experts in tobacco abuse about how to manage this problem in the clinical setting.

Bibliography

Adams A, Ockene JK, Wheeler EV, et al: Alcohol counseling: Physicians will do it. *J Gen Intern Med* 13:692, 1998.

American Psychiatric Association: *Diagnostic and Statistical Manual of Mental Disorders: DSM-IV*, 4th ed. Washington, DC: American Psychiatric Association; 1994.

Azrin NH, Sisson RW, Meyers R, et al: Alcoholism treatment by disulfiram and community reinforcement therapy. *J Behav Ther Exp Psychiat* 13:105, 1982.

Baum-Baicker C: The psychological benefits of moderate alcohol consumption: A review of the literature. *Drug Alcohol Depend* 15:305, 1985.

Benowitz NL, Gourlay SG: Cardiovascular toxicity of nicotine: Implications for nicotine replacement therapy. *J Am Coll Cardiol* 29:1422, 1997.

Bien TH, Miller WR, Tonigan JS: Brief interventions for alcohol problems: A review. *Addiction* 88:315, 1993.

Bobo JK, McIlvain HE, Lando HA, et al: Effect of smoking cessation counseling on recovery from alcoholism: Findings from a randomized community intervention trial. *Addiction* 93:877, 1998.

Buchsbaum DG, Buchanan RG, Centor RM, et al: Screening for alcohol abuse using CAGE scores and likelihood ratios. *Ann Intern Med* 115:774, 1991.

Butler CC, Pill R, Stott NCH: Qualitative study of patients' perceptions of doctors' advice to quit smoking: Implications for opportunistic health promotion. *BMJ* 316:1878, 1998.

Centers for Disease Control and Prevention: Smoking-attributable mortality and years of potential life lost—United States, 1990. *MMWR* 42:645, 1993.

Centers for Disease Control and Prevention: Cigarette smoking among adults—United States, 1994. *MMWR* 45:588, 1996.

Centers for Disease Control and Prevention: State-specific prevalence of cigarette smoking—United States, 1995. *MMWR* 45:962, 1996.

Dawson DA, Grant BF, Chou SP, et al: Subgroup variation in the U.S. drinking patterns: Results of the 1992 national longitudinal alcohol epidemiologic study. *J Subst Abuse* 7:331, 1995.

Department of Health and Human Services: *Reducing the Consequences of Smoking: 25 Years of Progress. A Report of the Surgeon General.* Rockville, MD: Department of Health and Human Services, 1989. Publication no. DHHS (CDC) 89-8411.

Department of Health and Human Services: *The Health Benefits of Smoking Cessation: A Report of the Surgeon General.* Rockville, MD: Department of Health and Human Services, 1990. Publication no. DHHS (CDC) 90-8418.

Dijkstra A, Roijackers J, De Vries H: Smokers in four stages of readiness to change. *Addict Behav* 23: 339, 1998.

Dufour MC, Archer L, Gordis E: Alcohol and the elderly. *Clin Geriatr Med* 8:127, 1992.

Duncan C, Stein MJ, Cummings SR: Staff involvement and special follow-up time increases physicians' counseling about smoking cessation: A controlled trial. *Am J Public Health* 81:899, 1991.

Emont SC, Cummings KM: Weight gain following smoking cessation: A possible role for nicotine replacement in weight management. *Addict Behav* 12:151, 1987.

Fiore MC, Bailey WC, Cohen SJ, et al: *Treating Tobacco Use and Dependence. Clinical Practice Guideline.* Rockville, MD: U.S. Department of Health and Human Services, Public Health Service; June 2000.

Fleming MF, Barry KL, Manwell LB, et al: Brief physician advice for problem alcohol drinkers. *JAMA* 277:1039, 1997.

Flint AJ, Novotny TE: Poverty status and cigarette smoking prevalence and cessation in the United States, 1983–1993: The independent risk of being poor. *Tob Control* 6:14, 1997.

Frazier EL, Okoro CA, Smith C, et al: State-and sex-specific prevalence of selected characteristics: Behavioral Risk Factor Surveillance System, 1994 and 1995. *MMWR CDC Surveill Summ* 46(SS-3):1, 1997.

Fuller R, Branchey L, Brightswell D, et al: Disulfiram treatment of alcoholism—A Veterans Administration Cooperative Study. *JAMA* 256:1449, 1986.

Giovino GA, Henningfield JE, Tomar SL, et al: Epidemiology of tobacco use and dependence. *Epidemiol Rev* 17:48, 1995.

Grady D, Ernster V: Does cigarette smoking make you look ugly and old? *Am J Epidemiol* 135:839, 1992.

Grant BF: Prevalence and correlates of alcohol use and DSM-IV alcohol dependence in the United States: Results of the National Longitudinal Alcohol Epidemiologic Survey. *J Stud Alcohol* 58:464, 1997.

Grant BF, Harford TC, Dawson DA, et al: Prevalence of DSM-IV alcohol abuse and dependence: United States, 1992. *Alcohol Health Res World* 18:243, 1994.

Hart SP, Frier BM: Causes, management and morbidity of acute hypoglycaemia in adults requiring hospital admission. *QJM* 91:505, 1998.

Helzer JE, Pryzbeck TR: The co-occurrence of alcoholism with other psychiatric disorders in the general population and its impact on treatment. *J Stud Alcohol* 49:219, 1988.

Herdman R, Hewitt M, Laschober M: *Smoking-Related Deaths and Financial Costs: Office of Technology Assessment Estimates for 1990.* Congress of the United States, Office of Technology Assessment, 1993.

Hester R, Nirenberg T, Begin A: Behavioral treatment of alcohol and drug abuse: What do we know and where shall we go? In: Galanter M (ed): *Recent Developments in Alcoholism.* New York: Plenum Press; 1990, 305.

Hollis JF, Lichtenstein E, Mount K, et al: Nurse-assisted smoking counseling in medical setting: Minimizing demands on physicians. *Prev Med* 20:497, 1991.

Hopper JL, Seeman E: The bone density of female twins discordant for tobacco use. *N Engl J Med* 330: 387, 1994.

Hughes JR: Clinical implications of the association between smoking and alcoholism. In: Fertig JB, Allen JP (eds): *Alcohol and Tobacco: From Basic Science to Clinical Practice.* Washington, DC: Superintendent of Documents, U.S. Government Printing Office; 1995, pp 171-185. NIAAA Research Monograph No. 30, NIH publication no. 95-3931.

Hurt RD, Offord KP, Croghan IT, et al: Mortality following inpatient addictions treatment. Role of tobacco use in a community-based cohort. *JAMA* 275:1097, 1996.

Hurt RD, Sachs DPL, Glover ED, et al: A comparison of sustained-released bupropion and placebo for smoking cessation. *N Engl J Med* 337:1195, 1997.

Jaén CR: Protecting nonsmokers from environmental tobacco smoke. *J Fam Pract* 43:530, 1996.

Jaén CR, Crabtree BF, Zyzanski SJ, et al: Making time for tobacco cessation counseling. *J Fam Pract* 46:425, 1998.

Jaén CR, Stange KC, Nutting PA: Competing demands of primary care: A model for the delivery of clinical preventive services. *J Fam Pract* 38:166, 1994.

Jaén CR, Stange KC, Tumiel LM, et al: Missed opportunities for prevention: Smoking cessation advice and the competing demands of practice. *J Fam Pract* 45:348, 1997.

Lichtenstein E, Hollis J: Patient referral to a smoking cessation program: Who follows through? *J Fam Pract* 34:739, 1992.

Maclure M: Demonstration of deductive meta-analysis: Ethanol intake and risk of myocardial infarction. *Epidemiol Rev* 15:328, 1993.

Manwell LB, Fleming MF, Johnson K, et al: Tobacco, alcohol, and drug use in a primary care sample: 90-day prevalence and associated factors. *J Addict Dis* 17:67, 1998.

McGinnis JM, Foege WH: Actual causes of death in the United States. *JAMA* 270:2207, 1993.

Miller NS, Gold MS: Comorbid cigarette and alcohol addiction: Epidemiology and treatment. *J Addict Dis* 17:55, 1998.

National Cancer Institute: *Smokeless Tobacco or Health.* Bethesda, Maryland: U.S. Department of Health and Human Services, National Institutes of Health; 1992. NIH publication no. 92-3461 (Smoking and tobacco control monograph no. 2).

National Cancer Institute: *Cigars: Health Effects and Trends.* Bethesda, Maryland: U.S. Department of Health and Human Services, National Institutes of Health; 1998. NIH publication no. 98-4302 (Smoking and tobacco control monograph no. 9).

National Heart Lung, and Blood Institute: *The Sixth Report of the Joint National Committee on Prevention, Detection, Evaluation, and Treatment of High Blood Pressure.* Bethesda, MD: National Institutes of Health, National Heart Lung, and Blood Institute; 1997. NIH publication no. 98-4080.

National Institute of Alcohol Abuse and Alcoholism: *The Physicians' Guide to Helping Patients With Alcohol Problems.* Washington, DC: U.S. Government Printing Office; 1995. NIH publication no. 95-3769.

National Institute on Alcohol Abuse and Alcoholism: *Preventing Alcohol Abuse and Related Problems.* Alcohol Alert: October, 1996; no. 34.

O'Connor PJ, Spann SJ, Woolf SH: Care of adults with type 2 diabetes mellitus: A review of the evidence. *J Fam Pract* 47(suppl):S13, 1998.

O'Malley SS, Jaffe AJ, Chang G, et al: Naltrexone and coping skills therapy for alcohol dependence: A controlled study. *Arch Gen Psychiatry* 49:881, 1992.

Pirkle JL, Flegal KM, Bernett JT, et al: Exposure of the US population to environmental tobacco smoke: The Third National Health and Nutrition Examination Survey, 1988 to 1991. *JAMA* 275:1233, 1996.

Pomerleau OF: Neurobiological interactions of alcohol and nicotine. In: Fertig JB, Allen JP (eds): *Alcohol and Tobacco: From Basic Science to Clinical Practice.* Washington, DC: Superintendent of Documents, U.S. Government Printing Office; 1995, 145. NIAAA Research Monograph No. 30. NIH publication no. 95-3931.

Project MATCH Research Group: Matching alcoholism treatments to client heterogeneity: Project MATCH three-year drinking outcomes. *Alcohol Clin Exp Res* 22:1300, 1998.

Ratcliffe JM, Gladen BC, Wilcox AJ, et al: Does early exposure to maternal smoking affect future fertility in adult males? *Reprod Toxicol* 6:297, 1992.

Response to increases in cigarette prices by race/ethnicity, income, and age groups: United States, 1976–1993. *MMWR* 47:605, 1998.

Rice DP: The economic cost of alcohol abuse and alcohol dependence: 1990. *Alcohol Health Res World* 17:10, 1993.

Rollnick S: Behaviour change in practice: Targeting individuals. *Int J Obesity* 20:S22, 1996.

Shabsigh R, Fishma IJ, Schum C, et al: Cigarette smoking and other vascular risk factors in vasculogenic impotence. *Urology* 38:227, 1991.

Shiffman S, Balabanis M: Associations between alcohol and tobacco. In: Fertig JB, Allen JP (eds): *Alcohol and Tobacco: From Basic Science to Clinical Practice.* Washington, DC: Superintendent of Documents, U.S. Government Printing Office; 1995, p 17–36. NIAAA Research Monograph No. 30, NIH publication no. 95-3931.

Taj N, Devera-Sales A, Vinson DC: Screening for problem drinking: Does a single question work? *J Fam Pract* 46:328, 1998.

Thakker KD: An overview of health risks and benefits of alcohol consumption. *Alcohol Clin Exp Res* 22:285S, 1998.

Thorndike AT, Rigotti NA, Stafford RS, et al: National patterns in the treatment of smokers by physicians. *JAMA* 279:604, 1998.

U.S. Department of Health and Human Services: *Tobacco Use Among U.S. Racial/Ethnic Minority Groups, African Americans, American Indians and Pacific Islanders, Hispanics: A Report of the Surgeon General.* Atlanta: U.S. Department of Health and Human Services, Centers for Disease Control and Prevention, Office on Smoking and Health; 1998.

United States Environmental Protection Agency: *Respiratory Health Effects of Passive Smoking: Lung Cancers and Other Disorders.* Washington, DC: Indoor Air Division, Office of Air and Radiation, U.S. Environmental Protection Agency; 1993. NIH publication no. 93-3605, Smoking and tobacco control monograph no. 4.

Velicer WF, Fava JL, Prochaska JO, et al: Distribution of smokers by stage in three representative samples. *Prev Med* 24:401, 1995.

Volpicelli JR, Alterman AI, Hayashida M, et al: Naltrexone in the treatment of alcohol dependence. *Arch Gen Psychiatry* 49:876, 1992.

Wilk AI, Jensen NM, Havighurst TC: Meta-analysis of randomized control trials addressing brief interventions in heavy alcohol drinkers. *J Gen Intern Med* 12:274, 1997.

Williamson DF, Madans J, Anda RF, et al: Smoking cessation and severity of weight gain in a national cohort. *N Engl J Med* 324:739, 1991.

World Health Organization: *Tobacco or Health: A Global Status Report.* Geneva: World Health Organization; 1997.

Tillman Farley

Grief and Loss

Introduction

Other than being born and eventually dying, grief may be the most universal experience of the human race. Grief occurs throughout all age groups and in all cultures. The burden of suffering caused by grief is impossible to completely quantify, but it is certainly enormous. Grief affects all aspects of a person's functioning and is associated with an increased incidence of illness and disease. Grievers use the health care system more than their numbers predict they should. They are also more likely to miss days at work. Grief has been associated with a decrease in immune function, more clinician visits, poorer physical health and mental health, higher suicide rates, and overall increased mortality. Grief often stresses families to the breaking point and beyond.

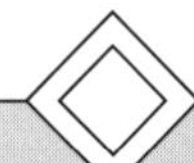

What Is Grief?

Grief is a complex, multifaceted response to loss that is associated with physical, emotional, behavioral, and cognitive symptoms that change over time. The process of grieving involves coming to terms and gradually detaching from the lost person or object, and ultimately reinvesting energy in new relationships. George Engel suggested that grief is actually a disease; it has predictable symptoms, a predictable course, and causes an increase in morbidity and mortality.[1] The central feature of grief is a feeling of sadness.

Grief can be thought of as the response to a loss of meaning. Its resolution "requires individuals to engage in the reconstitution of purpose and meaning in their lives."[2] As we live our lives, we develop our own life stories. With a major loss—through death, divorce, injury, loss of job—our story suddenly no longer makes sense. Grief work is the process of rewriting our story so that it again has meaning and purpose. Sometimes the process is slow; sometimes it moves along quickly; sometimes it stops completely. Some people are never able to weave the threads of their story back into a meaningful tapestry.

Grief Work

Grief work is the process an individual who experienced a loss works through to move on with life. To accomplish grief work successfully, one must achieve four tasks:

1. Accept the loss as real.
2. Experience the pain of the grief.
3. Adjust to a new future without the person or object that has been lost.
4. Redirect energy invested in the lost relationship towards new relationships.

Most grievers are able to accomplish these tasks and move on to a new stage of their lives. Some people, for various reasons, seem to get "stuck" on these tasks, resulting in pathologic grief states.

Grief and Culture

Grief affects people of all cultures. Unlike mourning, which is how the traditions, mores, and customs of a given society dictate that grief should be expressed, grief is a highly individualized response to loss which seems to be independent of culture. Culture can have an important effect on the ability to grieve, however. The Anglo culture of the United States, for example, teaches that grief and other strong emotions are best kept to oneself. Italians, however, often are very expressive about their pain.

Why Do We Grieve?

Grief resulting from a major loss may be the most painful emotion there is; one that cannot be imag-

[1]Engel G: Is grief a disease? A challenge for medical research. *Psychosom Med* 23:18, 1961.

[2]Fulton G, Madden C, Minichiello V: The social construction of anticipatory grief. *Soc Sci Med* 43:1349, 1996.

ined by those who have not gone through it. Yet grieving is probably an adaptive process. Humans are social animals, and derive a large part of their vigor as a species from social cohesion. Grief may be an evolutionary tool that serves the function of helping to maintain social cohesion. It may be adaptive for the species, although it is sometimes maladaptive for certain individuals.

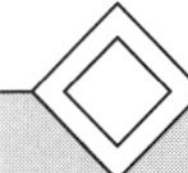

What Are the Effects of Grief?

Grief affects people in many ways, including their health and their interactions with their family. In this section, we discuss the effects of grief, paying special attention to the effects of grief on health, children, and families.

Grief Affects Health

> *"We can hardly doubt that that mental depression is a weighty additive to the other influences favoring the development of the cancerous constitution."*
>
> Sir James Paget, 1870[3]

Severe grief, particularly that associated with death of a spouse or child, increases the likelihood of premature illness and death in survivors. In 1996, Schaefer and colleagues conducted a cohort study of over 12,000 spouse pairs followed for 14 to 23 years. They found a significantly increased mortality rate in bereaved men and women after controlling for race, age, and educational, socioeconomic, and health status. In a study of a widows and widowers, Parkes and Brown found that the bereaved group experienced more sick days and used more alcohol and tobacco than did a matched control group. Biondi and associates have suggested that the stress of the grief response increases the likelihood of activating latent carcinoma. Several studies point to a connection between grief and immune function; they have shown suppression of lymphocyte stimulation as well as diminished activity of natural killer cells in those who are recently bereaved. Although the changes in the immune system are not enough to account for the increased morbidity and mortality in the recently bereaved, there is an identifiable connection between grief and physical health.

There are few published studies on the long-term health effects of grief. In a 1997 study of pathologic grief, Prigerson and co-workers reported that it is not bereavement itself that leads to poor outcomes, but rather the psychiatric sequelae of pathologic grief and depressive symptoms.

MR. FAIR: "I'M NOT DEPRESSED, I'M JUST DONE LIVING." *Mr. Fair had been married for 55 years when his wife suffered a major, debilitating stroke at the age of 82. Mr. Fair himself had been relatively healthy. He was the patriarch of his family. An elder sister lived with him and his wife. He also had a younger brother and a sister who lived about 60 miles away. All his siblings looked up to Mr. Fair as the head of the extended family.*

Mrs. Fair's stroke was right sided, and resulted in a major personality change. Mr. Fair was devastated. He went through the grieving process, trying to cope with the loss of his "normal" wife while at the same time trying to adapt to the seeming stranger who now inhabited his wife's crippled body. He refused to put her in a nursing home, and instead arranged 24-h care at home. He went back and forth through the phases of grief, but maintained a high level of functioning. His major concern became that he would die before his wife, worried that no one could care for her as well as he. Finally, 4 years after the initial stroke, his wife died at home.

Four weeks later, Mr. Fair presented to the emergency room with a massive myocardial infarction. During the week that he was in the hospital, he was able to meet with all his children and grandchildren. His affect was subdued, but he assured everyone that he was not depressed. He reminisced about his wonderful wife, and his large family now gathered

[3]Paget J: *Surgical Pathology*. London: Longman's Green; 1870.

around him. "I have had a great life," he told everyone, "but now it's your turn. I am done living." He lived for 1 week in the hospital, long enough to say goodbye to everyone in the family, and then died.

Eleven days after Mr. Fair's death, his brother died, and 11 days after that, his sister. His last remaining sister suffered a debilitating stroke, and was put in a nursing home. An entire generation passed over the course of a summer.

Bereavement also greatly increases the risk and severity of mental illness. Clayton and colleagues report that as many as 45 percent of widows will experience a major depression at some point within the first year of their loss. Parkes found that the severity of mental illness in the recently bereaved who were admitted for psychiatric hospitalization was more severe than would be expected based on age and social group. Grievers, particularly if the grief response has been blocked or is dysfunctional in some other way, are more apt to present to the clinician's office with somatic complaints, according to Clayton and colleagues.

KIM: "THERE IS ONE THING . . ." *Kim was 19 years old when I first saw her for abdominal pain. She was a high school dropout working at the local convenience store as a cashier. Over the next year, I saw her on multiple occasions for abdominal pain, but could never find any organic cause for her symptoms. Her genogram seemed not to contain any clues, and she continued to reassure me that she was not unduly stressed. Kim was obviously quite intelligent, and I wondered why she had not gone further in her education. After 10 visits over the course of 14 months, she turned to me at the end of a visit and said, "You know how you are always asking me about stress? Well, there is one thing . . ." She then proceeded to relate the following story:*

When Kim was 16 years old, she was a straight-A student at the local high school. Her plan was to go to college, major in business, and "get the heck out of this town." One day she was driving on a side street when a small child darted out from behind a parked car directly into the path of her vehicle. Although she was not speeding, she could not stop in time, and the child was killed. The accident occurred directly in front of the little boy's house, and his parents witnessed the accident. The child's father immediately came running over to Kim's stopped car. He yelled for his wife to call an ambulance, then turned to Kim and said, "It's not your fault."

It turned out that the father of the dead boy was a teacher at Kim's school. He was worried that Kim might feel guilty about this death, so he took it upon himself to look after her at school. Every day when Kim went to school, this teacher would check in on her and make sure that things were going well for her. He even told her at one point that he and his wife considered her like a child of their own. Ultimately, Kim could not deal with this constant reminder of an accident that she felt she should have avoided, and ended up dropping out of school. "He should have yelled at me! I killed his child!" Kim told me.

Shortly after Kim left school, she became pregnant. Her mother was very much against continuing the pregnancy. Reluctantly, Kim agreed to have an abortion. Kim now felt like she had killed two children with no negative consequences. Within a year of the abortion, her chronic abdominal pain started.

After Kim related this story to me, we talked about therapy. She agreed, and began seeing a therapist in my office on a regular basis. Over the next year, I saw her only one time for abdominal pain. When I last saw her, she was planning to get a GED and then go to college.

Grief Affects Families

Grief takes a major toll on families. In a stable family, each member has a role to play. The illness or death of a family member upsets the balance in the family, leaving each member to redefine his or her role. Severe loss can destroy family cohesion, making it difficult for family members to support each other in their grief, which can result in long-term family dysfunction.

It may be that severe grief accentuates both the good and the bad in family functioning. A dysfunctional family is likely to have an increase in dysfunction when dealing with grief, whereas a high functioning family is likely to not only survive the ordeal, but to be strengthened by it. This may explain why, contrary to common belief, the death of a child does not appear to cause an increase in divorce rates. Unfortunately, however, as social and geographic mobility has increased in society, families and family members become more isolated and often have less ability to deal with grief.

Grief Affects Children

Grief in childhood varies depending on the age of the child. Before 5 years of age, children have no real understanding of the permanence of death. They react to separation from their parents and can even grieve, although their grief may take more bodily forms, such as constipation, bedwetting, night terrors, and feeding difficulties. Past the age of 5, most children begin to understand that death is permanent. They are able to understand that the loss of parent due to divorce is different from loss of a parent due to death. The main difference between grieving in children and adults is that children are unable to sustain strong feelings for long periods. The grief reaction thus is more episodic. The florid symptoms of grief in children rarely last longer than a few weeks, and most reach resolution within the first year.

The loss of a parent is likely to result in behavioral problems in children, according to Black. A parent's death may so disturb children's confidence in the world that they may become very worried about the remaining parent. It is common for children to mask their feelings of grief in an attempt to protect the remaining parent. If a sibling has died, the surviving children are likely to feel guilt, thinking they may have some blame in the child's death because of past thoughts or actions.

Adolescents grieve in much the way adults do, except that they tend to have less maturity and fewer resources to help them deal with the problem, DiMinco found. This lack of resources is particularly true if they feel isolated from their families. Behavioral problems are common, and the grieving teen may be more likely to turn to drugs, alcohol, and sexual promiscuity.

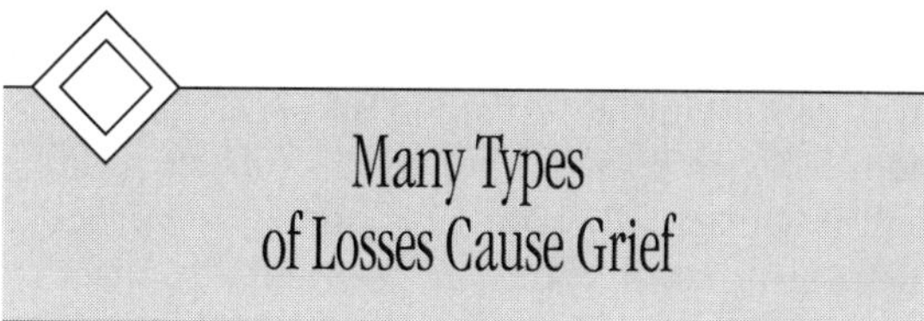

Many Types of Losses Cause Grief

Grief is caused by loss. Death is only one type of loss that each of us must face. At its best, life is a process of continual change. The downside of change is that loss accompanies every change, even a desired change. Coping with loss successfully is one of our main tasks. Losses can be divided into two main categories: loss of others and loss of self.

Loss of Others

Perhaps the most difficult losses are those of family and other supports. This occurs naturally as children grow up and leave home. The child, in exchange for independence, gives up much of the security of the home. The parent, watching a child leave home, is faced with a loss of role, and is made more directly aware of his or her own aging.

Loss of family and supports also occurs through illness and death. Rosenzweig and associates report that fifty percent of women over the age of 65 have lost a spouse to death; at age 85, 81 percent of women have lost their spouse. Alzheimer's disease and stroke can rob us of the people we love without causing death. Accidents and various illnesses can cause the death of loved ones sometimes well before their "time." This is particularly difficult when the death is out of sequence; that is, when the child dies before the parent. Divorce is also a common cause of loss of family and supports, for both children and parents.

Loss of Self

As we move through life, we face changes that cause us to change the way we see ourselves. Some of these changes occur so gradually that we do not notice them, and others happen catastrophically. Humans are granted the dubious honor of being able to contemplate their own demise, a process that for most of us starts long before we actually die. Part of the aging process means moving from the wonderful sense of immortality of youth to the sense that mortality is quite real and perhaps not so far away. Loss of self can be further divided into the categories shown in Table 10-1.

Table 10-1
Categories of Loss of Self

TYPE OF LOSS	EXAMPLES
Loss of function and ability	• Normal aging processes • Disease processes
Loss of role	Changes due to • Normal and desirable events (a child going off to college, or getting married and moving out of the house) • Death of a child or spouse, loss of a job, divorce Losing several roles at once compounds grief, especially when the role changes involve a loss of self-esteem.
Loss of dreams, goals, and hopes	Dreams are lost or modified by • Choice • External rules • Internal limitations Letting go of any dream, no matter how unrealistic, involves some loss
Loss of future	• Due to normal aspects of aging • Prematurely, as the result of illness or injury

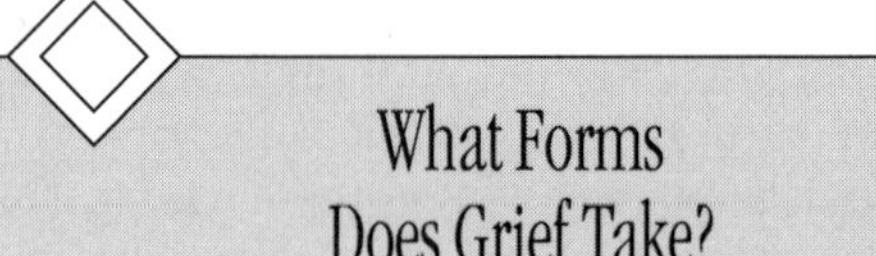

What Forms Does Grief Take?

Grief can be uncomplicated, absent or delayed, acute, distorted, anticipated, or pathologic. Each type presents unique challenges for primary care clinicians.

Grief Can Be Uncomplicated

Uncomplicated grief occurs in phases. Because dying patients also go through a grieving process, it is not surprising that the phases of grief are similar to the psychological phases of dying that Kubler-Ross identified. However, most experts describe the phases of grief with some variation of Brown and Stoudemire's model described in Table 10-2.

CAVEATS

There are several important caveats to this model of the grieving process. First, grieving is individual, and therefore will be different for everyone. Grieving patients should not all be expected to meet the same timeline in processing their grief, nor should they all be expected to fit all the phases of grief exactly. Many grievers will go through phases more closely resembling those of Kubler-Ross (see Chap. 11). Others may not seem to fit any particular model.

Second, grievers will move back and forth between phases. It is unrealistic and incorrect to expect that patients will "complete" a phase and then move on. Patients often move back to an earlier stage, particularly on important "anniversary" dates. In uncomplicated grief, the percentage of time spent in phases 1 and 2 decreases over time, but may never reach zero.

Finally, it is important to note that one does not "get over" a significant loss. Resolution means that one has learned to live with the loss and is able to move on with a somewhat different life. As a

Table 10-2
Phases of Grief

Grief Phase	Description	Common Symptoms
1: Shock	• Begins immediately after the loss and typically lasts up to 2 weeks • Characterized by feelings of numbness and disbelief • An adaptive phase that serves to protect the individual from feeling the intense pain of the loss too quickly • Shock is particularly severe if the loss occurred suddenly or unexpectedly • Patients may continue with normal activities, but commonly deny the death	Throat and chest tightness, dysphagia, nausea, and gastrointestinal disturbances; sense of disorientation and confusion; feelings of relief (after a prolonged illness), anger and guilt, shock
2: Preoccupation with the deceased	• Patients begin to experience the full pain and sadness of the loss • Griever becomes preoccupied with thoughts of the deceased • Feelings of anger and guilt may be quite strong • Phase can last up to 6 months and recurs intermittently for years, particularly on holidays, anniversaries, and other important dates	Insomnia, fatigue, anhedonia, anorexia, and other symptoms of major depression; social withdrawal and increased isolation
3: Resolution	• Griever can recall the deceased with pleasurable feelings, rather than intense sadness • Griever makes social contacts again, begins to reinvest energy into new relationships, activities, and interests • Liberation and relief are also common feelings in uncomplicated grief, which can contribute to guilt feelings in the griever • Griever starts to look at ways of moving on with life without the person or object that has been lost	Diminished intensity of crying spells, feelings of emptiness, and somatic complaints, although they commonly recur intermittently; anger is common, can seem at conflict with grief, and can lead to severe guilt feelings in the survivor

recently widowed patient once told me, "There is life before, and there is life after, but they are not the same life." And in the words of Harold Kushner,[4] author of *When Bad Things Happen to Good People*:

> I am a more sensitive person, a more effective pastor, a more sympathetic counselor because of Aaron's life and death than I ever would have been without it. And I would give up all of those gains in a second if I could have my son back. If I could choose, I would forego all the spiritual growth and depth which has come my way because of our experiences, and be what I was fifteen years ago, an average rabbi, an indifferent counselor, helping some people and unable to help others, and the father of a bright happy boy.

[4]Kushner HS: *When Bad Things Happen to Good People*. New York: Schocken Books; 1981, p 133.

Grief Can Be Absent or Delayed

In delayed grief, patients deny that they feel sad at all. These patients are likely to resume their usual functioning very quickly, and their family, friends, and associates think the patient has managed the loss well. Delayed grief may be a manifestation of prolonged denial and is particularly common in cases where a person is missing, or the body is not recoverable. Delayed grief can also occur when the survivor's subconscious fear of emotions considered unacceptable, such as anger and guilt, causes those emotions to be blocked.

Patients with an absent or delayed grief reaction will commonly have somatic symptoms, and may end up with many symptoms of major depression. The full force of the loss may occur many years after the actual loss itself.

THE JONES FAMILY: "SO TELL ME DOC, HOW DO I QUIT SMOKING?" *I had been taking care of the three young Jones children for about a year when Mrs. Jones began to suffer from severe depression. She underwent several weeks of psychiatric hospitalization, saw a psychiatrist regularly, and was put on appropriate doses of antidepressants. Sadly, nothing seemed to lift her spirits, and 4 months after the initial diagnosis, she committed suicide at home. About 6 months later, her husband presented to my office complaining of fatigue. He voluntarily commented to me that he could not understand why he was fatigued, because "nothing has changed in my life in the past 10 years." I then reminded him gently that in fact everything had changed: his wife was dead, and he was now the sole caretaker of three small children while continuing to work long hours at his job. I went on to suggest that his grief may be compounded and complicated by feelings of anger and guilt. "Well, yeah, there's that," he responded. "So tell me doc, how do I quit smoking?"*

Grief Can Be Distorted

In distorted grief, patients may demonstrate a chronic or prolonged grief reaction that includes somatization that the patient does not associate with the loss. At times, these patients may develop physical symptoms similar to those experienced by the deceased. They may show a behavior pattern of compulsive overactivity without a sense of loss. Deterioration of health is common, and medical illness may develop. Marked social withdrawal and isolation are common, as is severe depression. Unresolved anger is often at the root of a distorted grief reaction.

CAROL VITTI: "THIS HAS NOTHING TO DO WITH HIM!" *When I first saw Carol, I immediately noticed that she had been crying. Her eyes were red and puffy, and her affect was depressed and angry. She handed me a detailed three-page chronology of somatic complaints that she had noticed over the past year. She had seen many clinicians during that time, but had become frustrated with each because they could not cure her. Several had suggested that she see a psychiatrist.*

Judging from her list of complaints, and the vigor with which she denied to me that she had been crying, it was obvious that this would be far more than a simple biomedical problem. As part of each interview, I routinely draw a genogram. Carol was the first patient I had had who became somewhat hostile when I asked questions about her family.

After several visits for various vague somatic complaints, I obtained the following history. About 2 years previously, Carol had been doing the dishes in the kitchen while watching her 5-year-old son play with an aluminum pole in the front yard. While she watched, he suddenly raised the pole up into the air, where it contacted the electric line going into the house. He was electrocuted and died instantly.

About 6 months after his death, Carol began experiencing her somatic symptoms. She had never sought counseling to help with the grief over her son's death, and she became angry with me when I suggested counseling might be helpful. "I am over that!" she snapped at me, "This has nothing to do with him!" I continued as her doctor for about 1 year, never making any headway against her somatic complaints or her refusal to enter counseling. Finally, she asked that her records be transferred elsewhere.

Although distorted grief, particularly in the initial phases, may have many similarities with depression, it is important to recognize them as different entities. In a grief reaction, the patient has a strong feeling of sadness and loneliness. The world feels like an empty place, but there is an effort to find meaning in the loss. Conversely, in depression, there is a feeling of the self being empty. Discouragement degrades into despair, and hopelessness and helplessness predominate as the patient withdraws from social supports and situations.

Unresolved grief can lead to depression, and depression can make the grieving process more difficult. Beutel and colleagues found that when grief is related to spontaneous abortion, risk factors for depressive symptoms include a prior history of depression, lack of social supports, and ambivalent feelings about the pregnancy. In general, initial depressive reaction is predictive of a long-term depressive reaction.

Patients May Anticipate Grief

When a loss can be anticipated, as when a spouse has terminal cancer, grieving generally starts before the actual loss. The survivors experience all the symptoms of grief and generally move back and forth between the phases as if the patient has already died. When the actual death occurs, the ensuing grief process is often fairly short, because much of the grief work has already been done. However, if the illness is prolonged, the survivor can be left in limbo, unable to resolve their grief. In the case described earlier, Mr. Fair began the grieving process shortly after his wife's massive stroke. For 5 years, he processed his grief. He continued to have a very important relationship with his wife, although his role changed from one of equal partner in a loving marriage to caretaker of someone whom he no longer felt he knew. Ultimately, he was not able to put together a new story of his life that made sense to him that did not have his wife in it. After 4 years of a gargantuan caretaking effort, he outlived his wife by only 5 weeks.

Anticipatory grief changes in nature and intensity depending on the certainty in the survivors' minds of the impending death. Family members of a patient who has been told she has breast cancer, for example, may experience anticipatory grief, which will change in intensity with the prognosis of the disease.

Anticipatory grief also varies depending on the nature of the illness and the attitudes of the patient and the survivors. Mr. Fair's wife was a dynamic, well-read, intellectual woman whose greatest fear as she aged was that she would have a debilitating stroke. The fact that she did have a stroke was in many ways more grievous to her husband than if she had died more quickly from some other process. For many people, loss of function, ability, and control are far more frightening than death.

Grief Can Be Acute

People do not often see grief as something that requires a clinician's intervention. After a significant loss, people expect that they will feel badly. However, when acute grief causes physical symptoms, such as chest pain, throat tightness, gastrointestinal disturbances, or shortness of breath, the symptoms often prompt a visit to the clinician. Acute grief also causes psychological symptoms, such as confusion and a sense of disorientation. Clinicians should be aware of the context of every visit. What other factors may contribute to the patient's visit today? Review the patient's family history at each visit.

VICKI: "I MIGHT HAVE CANCER, TOO" *Vicki was a 27-year-old woman who came to the office for evaluation of a breast mass. She was a pleasant woman with a normal affect as we began the medical interview. She first noticed the mass about 2 years previously, but thought that maybe over the past 2 months it had gotten bigger. She was concerned about cancer. This was a natural time to elicit family history, so I started to draw a genogram. There was no family history of breast cancer in Vicki's family, but when I asked about* *her children, she started to cry. One of her children, a 3-year-old daughter, had died of cancer of the blood (leukemia) almost exactly 1 year previously. Although still grieving, she had been managing fairly well, and was starting to look toward the future again. However, as the anniversary of her daughter's death approached (which happened to coincide with Easter), she began to feel more out of control and anxious. She had developed a strong idea that this lump on her breast was cancer, and that she would die and leave her other children without a mother.*

Physical exam immediately showed the mass to be a benign sebaceous cyst in the skin. I offered Vicki the choice of leaving it alone or having it removed. She chose to have it removed, and the procedure was scheduled within a week. More importantly, we talked about whether counseling was something that Vicki had considered to help her to cope with her grief. She was very agreeable to seeing a therapist, so we made an appointment for her to see the psychologist working in my office. She was seen several times over the next 2 months, enough to get her through the anniversary of the death. She continues to check in intermittently, but is on the road to the resolution phase of grief.

Grief Can Be Pathologic

The line between uncomplicated grief and pathologic grief can be difficult to define, but its definition is nonetheless important. Uncomplicated grief is self-limited and does not require therapeutic intervention, whereas pathologic grief is associated with significant morbidity that can sometimes be ameliorated with intensive intervention. The essential component of pathologic grief is enduring dysfunction; the symptoms of pathologic grief persist over time.

Grief is pathologic when it leads to pathologic outcomes. These outcomes may include increased mortality, illness, worsening of immune function, somatization, overuse of the medical system, increased alcohol and drug use, and psychiatric problems. As noted, one study by Prigerson and colleagues has suggested that grief, itself, does not cause pathologic outcomes. Rather, the depressive symptoms and psychiatric sequelae of pathologic grief cause the negative outcomes.

Pathologic grief occurs when the process of grief work stalls. The phases may become abnormally prolonged, or patients may show no manifestations of grief at all. Instead of resolution, patients may fall into a lasting depression. Why do some people move through the grief process in a timely fashion and others do not? What are the implications of pathologic grief? Can we identify patients at higher risk of pathologic grief early enough to initiate preventive interventions?

Risk Factors for Pathologic Grief

Brown and Stoudemire have identified risk factors that may help in the prediction of pathologic grief, which are described below.

CHARACTERISTICS OF THE SURVIVOR Individuals who have suffered a significant loss in childhood, have difficulty expressing their emotions, or have a history of depression or other mental illness are more likely to suffer from a pathologic grief reaction when faced with a loss. Pathologic grief is also more common in patients who suffer multiple losses over a short period of time.

CIRCUMSTANCES SURROUNDING THE DEATH Sudden deaths, deaths following a particularly prolonged or difficult course, and stigmatized deaths (e.g., suicide, AIDS, drug overdoses) are more likely to result in pathologic grief in survivors. If the survivor feels responsible for the death in some way, then pathologic grief is even more likely.

QUALITY OF RELATIONSHIPS BEFORE THE DEATH Pathologic grief is more likely when relationships are characterized by excessive dependence, hostility, ambivalence, or other features that may make it difficult to express grief.

THE SURVIVOR'S SOCIAL AND/OR FAMILY SUPPORT SYSTEM Grievers lacking family and other support people that encourage the expression of grief have been shown to have a higher incidence of pathologic grieving.

Pathologic grief includes any grief process that does not follow a path to resolution within a reasonable period. It follows that pathologic grief can present in several different ways.

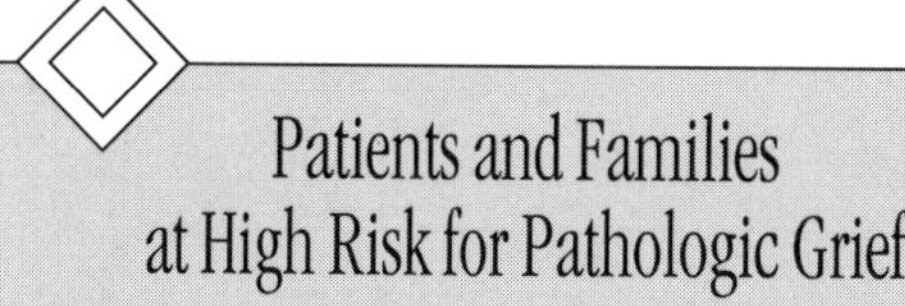

Patients and Families at High Risk for Pathologic Grief

When grief work is unsuccessful, pathologic grief results. Because pathologic grief is associated with a variety of chronic medical and mental health problems, its identification and treatment are important. Certain red flags should trigger a search for underlying pathologic grief, as well as other mental disorders. These red flags include unexplained symptoms, frequent visits, and certain illnesses such as fibromyalgia and chronic fatigue syndrome. Patients with these findings often have a higher incidence of severe life trauma ranging from sexual and physical abuse to severe losses in childhood. It may be worthwhile to use a grief screening tool, such as the Inventory of Complicated Grief, that has been shown to be helpful in identifying dysfunctional grieving (Fig. 10-1).

High-Risk Families

The most important relationships in most peoples' lives are with their family members and significant others. Grief affects families, and the character of each family can predict to some extent whether grieving in that family will be uncomplicated or pathologic. Every clinician should have an understanding of the family structure and relationships of every family under his or her care. Genograms provide an excellent mechanism for obtaining this information, providing a visual illustration of both biomedical history and relationship information. Using genograms, the clinician is able to move easily between "safe" questions, such as, "Does anyone in your family have heart disease?" to less "safe" questions, such as, "Are your parents still married?" to highly "unsafe" questions, such as, "Has your husband ever hit you?" or "Tell me about any significant deaths in your family."

MRS. KIRBY: "WHO AM I TO JUDGE?" *Mrs. Kirby is a 63-year-old woman with chronic back pain secondary to a fall at a department store. I could never find anything on physical exam to support her claims of significant pain, and I felt she was malingering. Nothing I tried seemed to help her. She did not respond to anti-inflammatories or physical therapy. I grew to dread her visits, and we settled into a mutually frustrating patient–clinician relationship.*

When she initiated legal proceedings against the store, it only increased my dislike of her. One day, after I had been seeing her for about a year, I was standing outside her exam room trying to figure out what I could possibly do to get her out of my office, when I noticed with surprise that I had never drawn a genogram of her family. This is something I normally do on every patient within the first several visits. I decided to make that the sole intervention for the day's visit.

Mrs. Kirby was surprised that I was showing interest in other parts of her life besides her back pain and proceeded to relate an amazing life story of loss and grief. She was born in France, where she lived during World War II. Her parents and siblings did not survive the war. She managed to escape to England after the war, where as teenager she married a viciously abusive alcoholic. She had several children with him, one of whom later died in a car accident. Finally, fearing for her life, she managed to leave her husband and flee to the United States, where she again married an abusive alcoholic. She abandoned this marriage after 10 years and had been single ever since. She had few support people in her life and mostly saw herself as a survivor who could take care of herself.

Figure 10-1

Inventory of Complicated Grief

Please fill in the circle next to the answer which best describes how you feel right now.

1. I think about this person so much that it's hard for me to do the things I normally do . . .
   ○ never ○ rarely ○ sometimes ○ often ○ always

2. Memories of the person who died upset me . . .
   ○ never ○ rarely ○ sometimes ○ often ○ always

3. I feel I cannot accept the death of the person who died . . .
   ○ never ○ rarely ○ sometimes ○ often ○ always

4. I feel myself longing for the person who died . . .
   ○ never ○ rarely ○ sometimes ○ often ○ always

5. I feel drawn to places and things associated with the person who died . . .
   ○ never ○ rarely ○ sometimes ○ often ○ always

6. I can't help feeling angry about his/her death . . .
   ○ never ○ rarely ○ sometimes ○ often ○ always

7. I feel disbelief over what happened . . .
   ○ never ○ rarely ○ sometimes ○ often ○ always

8. I feel stunned or dazed over what happened . . .
   ○ never ○ rarely ○ sometimes ○ often ○ always

9. Even since s/he died it is hard for me to trust people . . .
   ○ never ○ rarely ○ sometimes ○ often ○ always

10. Ever since s/he died I feel like I have lost the ability to care about other people or I feel distant from people I care about . . .
    ○ never ○ rarely ○ sometimes ○ often ○ always

11. I have pain in the same area of my body or have some of the same symptoms as the person who died . . .
    ○ never ○ rarely ○ sometimes ○ often ○ always

12. I go out of my way to avoid reminders of the person who died . . .
    ○ never ○ rarely ○ sometimes ○ often ○ always

13. I feel that life is empty without the person who died . . .
    ○ never ○ rarely ○ sometimes ○ often ○ always

Figure 10-1 (continued)

14. I hear the voice of the person who died speak to me . . .
○ never ○ rarely ○ sometimes ○ often ○ always

15. I see the person who died stand before me . . .
○ never ○ rarely ○ sometimes ○ often ○ always

16. I feel that it is unfair that I should live when this person died . . .
○ never ○ rarely ○ sometimes ○ often ○ always

17. I feel bitter over this person's death . . .
○ never ○ rarely ○ sometimes ○ often ○ always

18. I feel envious of others who have not lost someone close . . .
○ never ○ rarely ○ sometimes ○ often ○ always

19. I feel lonely a great deal of the time ever since s/he died . . .
○ never ○ rarely ○ sometimes ○ often ○ always

A grief screening tool, such as the Inventory of Complicated Grief shown here, is helpful in identifying dysfunctional grief. *(Reprinted with permission from Prigerson et al: Inventory of Complicated Grief: A scale to measure maladaptive symptoms of loss.* Psychiatry Res *59: 65, 1995. © Elsevier Science, Inc.)*

This single visit completely changed my relationship with Mrs. Kirby; it created a therapeutic relationship where none had previously existed. I had disliked her, and she had disliked me. By obtaining the information contained in the genogram, however, I showed Mrs. Kirby that I was interested in her as a complete human being. For my part, I began to learn about the arrested grieving that contributed in large measure to Mrs. Kirby's behavior. More importantly, I developed respect for her. Who was I to judge the behavior of someone who had come through such experiences?

Factors that Influence Family Adaptation after Death

According to a scheme developed by Walsh and McGoldrick, four basic factors influence family adaptation to loss due to a death. Primary care clinicians must consider these factors when working with grieving families.

The Nature of the Loss Sudden death or a death after a protracted and difficult illness are most stressful for families. Sudden death prevents the family from preparing for the absence of a loved one and prevents the completion of any "unfinished business." A prolonged illness, on the other hand, is likely to cause significant financial hardship and may overwhelm other family coping resources. For example, families attempting to care for a terminally ill member at home may find that they are unable to do so over the long term. This conflict can lead to feelings of guilt, particularly if the patient is ultimately placed in a nursing home, or if there is strong feeling of relief when the patient finally dies. When difficult questions arise, such as when to turn off life support, or whether to start life supports in the first place, family members may find themselves in conflict. The primary care clinician can help to resolve these issues.

THE FAMILY AND SOCIAL NETWORK The general level of family functioning and the state of family relationships before a loss are important indicators of how well a family will deal with the loss. Family cohesiveness, with family members respectful of the different responses each may have to the loss, is a good prognostic indicator. High degrees of enmeshment or disengagement, on the other hand, are poor prognostic indicators.

Because many losses involve a restructuring of roles, flexibility of family structure to accommodate new role formation is important. Overly chaotic families, in which the roles were never well defined to begin with, or overly rigid families, in which new roles cannot be adopted, do poorly. Families with adequate economic resources and strong outside social support tend to do well.

In the case of a death, it is important for the clinician to understand the prior role of the deceased in the functioning of the family. The loss of an elderly grandparent will generally cause fewer long-term problems than the death of a child or a parent of small children.

Finally, it is important for the clinician to understand the nature of the prior relationships between the deceased and other family members. Conflicted relationships and unresolved hostilities make dysfunction after the death more likely. In cases in which the death can be predicted, it is important for the clinician to help family members resolve these issues before the death. The clinician can refer these families to family therapists, but only if the initial identification of a potential problem has been made.

THE LIFE CYCLE TIMING OF THE LOSS Deaths that occur out of cycle are clearly difficult for the survivors. The death of a child may be the most devastating loss there is. When a loss occurs at the same time as other life stresses, the grief can be compounded. For example, if a husband dies of a heart attack just after the last child has left home and he and his wife were adjusting to a new phase of their lives together, the wife's grief may be more difficult to resolve.

THE SOCIOCULTURAL CONTEXT OF THE LOSS Ethnic, religious, and philosophical beliefs about loss, particularly death, are important in predicting how the family will deal with it. The clinician should have some sense of the family's beliefs about death in general and this death in particular. At times, societal pressures may prevent proper grieving, as with the death of a partner of a gay man who has not told family and friends of his sexual orientation, for example. Parkes refers to this situation as "disenfranchised grief." Finally, there are important cultural gender issues in grieving. Men tend to repress their feelings of grief, while women are more encouraged to grieve openly. Repressing grief is more likely to lead to morbidity than is demonstrating grief.

Identifying Families at Risk for Dysfunctional Grieving

The Family Relationship Index by Moos and Moos has been used to identify families at higher risk for dysfunctional grieving. Kissane and associates divide families into four types based on the results of the Family Relationship Index. *Supportive* and *conflict resolving* families manage grief well, whereas *sullen* and *hostile* families tend to be more dysfunctional when faced with a loss. Families with *intermediate* typology are also prone to dysfunction. Kissane found that by improving communication and problem-solving skills among family members, family cohesion improved and families were able to deal with grief more effectively.

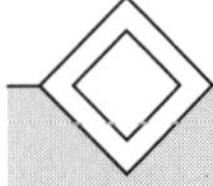

Managing Grief

How does all this translate into action on the part of the primary care clinician? Most grief reactions are self-limited. The griever engages in grief work, processes his or her grief through the various stages, and eventually reaches resolution. It is important to again emphasize that with a major loss, "resolution" in no way indicates that the grieving is over, or that the griever has "accepted" the loss. Rather, it indicates that the griever has learned how to cope with the grief well enough to continue with his life in a productive manner. In working with grieving patients, the clinician's goal should be to support those who are most likely to move on to resolution of their grief in an uncomplicated manner and to identify and intervene with those who are more likely to progress to pathologic grief. The clinician's role is determined largely by the quality of family and other supports available to the patient. The clinician may have a limited role with patients who have strong supports.

The primary care clinician can take several steps to identify individuals and families at greatest risk for dysfunctional grieving and to help promote a more functional grieving process.

Attend to Family Systems

In dealing with loss, the unit of care should be the family. Any significant loss, whether it be a death, the loss of a job, an injury, or illness, will have repercussions throughout the family unit. The loss will affect different people in the family in different ways. To help the family through the loss, it is important for the clinician to be aware of family dynamics. As noted, significant losses such as the death of a child can have a tremendously adverse impact on family cohesion. Genograms should be used to better understand family relationships and roles, and to see how roles may change after the loss.

Hold Family Meetings

Family meetings are possible even in a busy primary care office. Encourage open communication among family members. Elicit each family member's experience of the loss, including the children's. Remember that each family member will cope with the loss differently and proceed along the path to grief resolution at a different pace. Family strengths as well as weaknesses should be identified.

Family meetings do not need to last an hour, and every last cousin does not need to attend. They can be put into the regular office schedule, or can be conducted at the hospital. Invite those family members that can come. Pay attention to who is missing and why; it may reflect important family dynamics. In a sense, these meetings are triage sessions; families that seem at particular risk for dysfunctional grieving can be referred to family therapists.

Communicate

Particularly in the case of terminal illness, it is imperative that the clinician give clear and accurate information to the patient and family members. Terminally ill individuals have a right to know their condition. If handled properly, accurate information will not make them "give up" or in any way hasten death (see Chap. 11). Open and honest communication is imperative in helping a family through the grieving process. Important considerations in breaking bad news are listed in Table 10-3.

Every once in a while, a patient will indicate a preference to not know his or her condition. This preference must be respected, of course, but the need to withhold information may be temporary, and should be revisited periodically. There may be cultural reasons for this preference, which will affect the clinician's communication with family and friends as well.

Listen

A large part of the clinician's role in dealing with grieving patients is simply to listen empathically. Ask questions and listen to the answers. How does this patient feel about her hysterectomy or mastectomy? What was the patient's relationship

Table 10-3
Breaking Bad News

Decide who should be present.
Decide where to meet.
Establish relationship of respect and trust.
Find out what patient and family already know.
Elicit questions.
Use clear, concise, and understandable language.
Don't overwhelm the patient and family with more information than they can handle at one time.
Allow emotions to surface.
Normalize feelings.
Provide as much time as family thinks they need.
Make sure that everyone is safe before ending meeting.
Arrange follow-up.

SOURCE: Reproduced from Parkes CM: Coping with loss: Bereavement in adult life. *BMJ* 316:856; 1998.

with the deceased? Allow patients to cry. Encourage them to express their full range of feelings. Validate and depathologize feelings of relief, anger, and guilt that are so common in grief reactions. It can be helpful to name the feelings associated with the loss, particularly the more conflicted feelings like anger and relief. Do not try to come up with the perfect thing to say. As a patient of mine, whose 15-year-old son was killed in a car accident told me, "Because nobody can understand what this feels like, its okay to say, 'I don't know what to say.'"

Provide Anticipatory Guidance

The grieving process generally has a predictable course. Grievers often relate a feeling of being "crazy," feeling that they are losing control. They may also feel isolated. Primary care clinicians must be able to anticipate these feelings in grievers and help to normalize them. Clinicians should educate the griever as to what to expect in the grieving process. This may be particularly important in helping patients get ready for an inevitable death, or when another significant loss is imminent. It can also be helpful for parents facing the "empty nest syndrome," or patients going through divorces.

Encourage the Use of Rituals

Many people faced with a significant loss find that a ritual can help them to reach some sense of closure. The classic example of this is the scattering of ashes of the deceased. However, there are many other circumstances in which rituals can help with the grieving process. For example, when a perinatal death occurs, the parents should be encouraged to give the baby a name, take photographs, and say goodbye. Help the family decide which rituals, if any, would be helpful.

Maintain Presence

According to Parkes, we must offer grieving people a "secure base," a relationship of respect—with a person who has the time, knowledge, and willingness to remain involved—that will last them through the bad times. When dealing with a patient with serious illness, there is a tendency for primary care clinicians to let specialists take over the patient's care. It is important, however, that primary care clinicians maintain a presence, particularly when they have built a relationship with the patient.

SARA RYAN: "DON'T ABANDON US" *Sara Ryan was a 19-year-old college freshman when I first met her. She had come to the office at the urging of her mother, who told me that Sara had been acting "spacey" and having personality changes. She had already seen a neurologist for this problem, and an MRI had been read as normal. My strong opinion was that the symptoms were psychosocial in nature. Sara's mother had started college at the same time as Sara, and there seemed to be quite a lot of com-*

petition between them. When I talked with Sara alone, told me that she was just "stressed out" by school and her mother.

After finding no abnormalities on physical exam, I raised the idea of family therapy. Sara and her mother were agreeable, although her mother clearly did not believe that family stress was the source of the problem. After several months in therapy, Sara's mother insisted that we obtain another MRI scan of the brain, because Sara's problems were not improving. The scan was done, and again was read as normal. Eight months after the second scan, and again at the insistence of her mother, I sent Sara to another neurologist for a second opinion. This neurologist went back, looked at the MRI scan from 8 months ago, and immediately diagnosed multiple sclerosis.

Thereafter, Sara's disease became rapidly progressive. I felt tremendously guilty about this missed diagnosis, and was content to have the neurologist take over Sara's care. I had not seen Sara or her mother for about a year when her mother scheduled a visit with me. Sara had become very ill since her diagnosis, and it looked like she would die from her disease. The entire purpose of her mother's visit with me, through her anger and grief, was to educate me about the importance of not abandoning my role as Sara's primary care clinician. She explained to me that I was their doctor, and that I needed to maintain a presence as they negotiated the difficult world of subspecialists, hospitalizations, experimental treatments, and end-of-life care. She understood that I felt guilty about Sara's diagnosis, and that it might be easier for me to distance myself from Sara, but she said that I had no right to do so. This is a visit I will never forget—humbling lessons taught by a grieving mother.

Loss can be difficult for the clinician as well as for the patient. We learn in medical school that our role is to heal. We are taught little about how to cope with failure; we often see our inability to eliminate death and disease as the ultimate failure. We work with serious illness and death on an almost daily basis, yet we often are uncomfortable dealing with the affects those conditions bring. To be fully effective in working with grieving patients, we must change our definition of failure. In a sense, this too involves loss, as we modify our expectations of ourselves and our field.

Look for Opportunities for Preventive Intervention

When a significant loss has occurred, the clinician should discuss the grief process with the grievers each time they visit the office for other reasons. It is particularly important to pay close attention to the medical condition of the recently bereaved. It may be necessary to schedule frequent visits in the weeks to months following the loss. Be alert to the need for marriage counseling, particularly after the death of a child. Pay attention to flare-ups of grief around anniversary dates: birthday, wedding, death day, and holidays. Even in uncomplicated grieving, there may be a regression in phases during these periods for several years after the loss. For some patients, early referral to a therapist may be warranted, depending on the counseling skills and interest of the primary care clinician.

Do Not Disturb Normal Grief Processes

Grief is an important and, for the most part, adaptive process. Clinicians should encourage patients to express grief. When a significant loss occurs, it causes pain, and the pain needs to be felt. Our role is to help our patients through to resolution of the pain. Our role is *not* to cover up the pain.

Use Medication as Appropriate

Sometimes medications are appropriate. Selective serotonin reuptake inhibitors (SSRIs) have been shown helpful in depressive symptoms caused by grief, particularly if grief is prolonged. Tricyclic antidepressants (TCAs), on the other hand, have not been shown helpful in correcting the depressive symptoms of grief. When sleep disorder is a major symptom, however, low-dose TCAs can be quite helpful. It is best to avoid benzodiazepines or other medications that are likely to delay the grief response.

Pay Attention to Microculture and Macroculture

Although grief is universal, mourning is culturally determined. A clinician from a stoic mourning culture should not mistakenly believe people from more demonstrative mourning cultures are abnormal grievers. Similarly, clinicians should not protect themselves from their own discomfort with demonstrative mourning by trying to minimize it in their patients.

Refer as Necessary

Counseling has been shown effective for a variety of losses. If possible, counseling can be provided before a loss as well as after; a family expecting a death from chronic disease may be helped by predeath counseling as well as post-death counseling. A diabetic faced with limb amputation likewise can benefit from counseling before the surgery. This counseling may be done by the clinician, although most clinicians will likely want to refer the patient to a mental health specialist. The best solution, if possible, is to provide co-located, collaborative counseling, with the clinician and the mental health provider working together. For clinicians not fortunate enough to have mental health services available in their office, I would encourage the establishment of a referral connection with a good therapist in the area. Let patients know that their providers are working together, and that information obtained by one may be shared with the other. Maintain frequent contact with the therapist so that treatment plans can be agreed upon. The mind–body split is imaginary, and the more we work together with our mental health colleagues, the better care we can provide to our patients.

Besides mental health providers, support groups are also excellent resources for patients. There are support groups in most medium to large cities for almost all chronic diseases, as well as for people suffering from divorce, unemployment, or the death of a child.

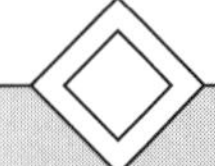

Is Grief a Disease?

George Engel first posed this provocative question in 1961, and the answer remains controversial today. Grief is caused by an identifiable etiologic agent, has a predictable course, causes painful symptoms and functional impairment, and is associated with increased morbidity and mortality. How then can we not consider it "pathologic?" Yet, the DSM-IV gives scant recognition to the problem of grief, listing only "Bereavement," and that under "Other Conditions that may be a Focus of Clinical Attention." Pathologic grief is not listed separately; it is instead lumped into the category of post-traumatic stress disorder (PTSD). Horowitz and co-workers make a convincing argument that neither major depression nor PTSD adequately capture the phenomenon of pathologic grief. They argue for a separate DSM category of "complicated grief," as determined by the Inventory of Complicated Grief. Criteria would include (more than a year after the loss) intense intrusive thoughts, pangs of severe emotion, distressing yearnings, feeling excessively alone and empty, excessive avoidance of tasks reminiscent of the deceased, unusual sleep disturbances, and significant and continuing lack of interest in personal activities. Certainly, this constellation of symptoms describes a population of patients with whom we should intervene, whether or not they are listed in their own category in the DSM-IV.

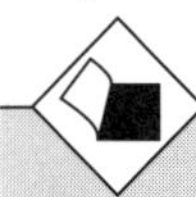

Summary

We tend to find what we are looking for. Grief reactions, both uncomplicated and pathologic, account for a sizable number of visits to primary care clinicians yearly. If we do not look for these reactions, we will be unlikely to find them. There is good evidence, on the other hand, that if we take the effort to identify and intervene as appropriate with grief reactions, we can decrease the associated morbidity among our patients. Primary care clinicians are responsible for identifying acute and pathologic grief because they are the ones to whom these patients will present. The duty of the primary care clinician is to identify grief when it occurs, screen for those patients at higher risk of pathologic grieving, work with patients to try to prevent pathologic grieving, and refer to mental health professionals as necessary.

Suggested Reading

Burnell GM, Burnell AL: *Clinical Management of Bereavement: A Handbook for Healthcare Professionals.* New York: Human Sciences Press; 1989.

This is an excellent book for any healthcare professional who deals with bereaved patients. It is currently out of print, but is available in libraries.

Kushner HS: *When Bad Things Happen to Good People.* New York: Schocken Books; 1981.

This book has been the standard for helping answer its difficult title question since its publication in 1981. The author writes from a first person perspective, having lost his own son to a fatal illness.

McCracken A, Semel M: *A Broken Heart Still Beats: After Your Child Dies.* Center City, MN: Hazelden; 1988.

A collection of stories, essays, and poems by a wide variety of people, including many famous ones, all of whom have lost a child.

Parkes CM, Markus A (eds): *Coping with Loss.* Login Brothers; 1998.

Originally published as a 10-part series in the British Medical Journal in 1998, this excellent book deals with the types of losses often encountered by primary care clinicians, and includes chapters on bereavement, aging, loss of body parts, children and loss, and loss of relationships. The book emphasizes communication skills and the importance of the clinician-patient relationship. There is a comprehensive listing of support organizations in both the UK and USA.

Walsh F, McGoldrick M (eds): *Living Beyond Loss.* New York: Norton; 1991.

Froma Walsh and Monica McGoldrick look at the subject of grief and loss from a family systems perspective. This thorough and well written book should be considered required reading for family clinicians.

Bibliography

Almeida C: Grief among parent of children with diabetes. *The Diabetes Educator* 21:530, 1995.

American Psychiatric Association: Diagnostic and Statistical Manual of Mental Disorders, 4th ed. Washington, DC: American Psychiatric Association, 1994.

Averill JR: Grief: its nature and significance. *Psychol Bull* 70:721, 1968.

Bennet G: Coping with loss: The doctor's losses: Ideals versus realities. *BMJ* 316:1238, 1998.

Beutel M, Deckardt R, von Rad M, et al: Grief and depression after miscarriage: Their separation, antecedents, and course. *Psychosom Med* 57:517, 1995.

Beutel M, Zisook S, Shuchter SR: Depression through the first year after death of a spouse. *Am J Psychiatry* 148:1346, 1991.

Biondi M, Costantini A, Parisi A: Can loss and grief activate latent neoplasia? A clinical case of possible interaction between genetic risk and stress in breast cancer. *Psychother Psychosom* 65:102, 1996.

Black D: Bereavement in childhood. *BMJ* 316:931, 1998.

Brown JT, Stoudemire GA: Normal and pathologic grief. *JAMA* 250:378, 1983.

Burnell GM, Burnell AL: *Clinical Management of Bereavement: A Handbook for Healthcare Professionals.* New York: Human Sciences Press; 1989.

Carmen MB: The psychology of aging. *Psychiatr Clin North Am* 20:15, 1997.

Cavenar JO, Butts NT, Spaulding JG: Grief: Normal or abnormal. *N C Med J* 39:31, 1978.

Clayton PJ, Hirjanic M, Murphy GE: Mourning and depression: Their similarities and differences. *Can J Psych* 19:309, 1974.

Cowles KV: Cultural perspectives of grief: An expanded concept analysis. *J Adv Nurs* 23:287, 1996.

DeMinco S: Young adult reactions to death in literature and life. *Adolescence* 30:179, 1995.

Engel G: Is grief a disease? A challenge for medical research. *Psychosom Med* 23:18, 1961.

Fulton G, Madden C, Minichiello V: The social construction of anticipatory grief. *Soc Sci Med* 43:1349, 1996.

Gamino LA, Sewell KW, Easterling LW: Scott and White Grief Study: An empirical test of predictors of intensified mourning. *Death Studies* 22:333, 1998.

Horowitz MJ, Siegel B, Holen A, et al: Diagnostic criteria for complicated grief disorder. *Am J Psychiatry* 154:904, 1997.

Hunfeld JAM, Wladimiroff JW, Passchier J: The grief of late pregnancy loss. *Patient Education and Counseling* 31:57, 1997.

Irwin M, Weiner H: Depressive symptoms and immune functions during bereavement. In: Zisook S (ed): *Biopsychosocial Aspects of Bereavement.* Washington, DC: American Psychiatric Press; 1987, p 157.

Kissane DW, Block S, McKenzie M, et al: Family grief therapy: A preliminary account of a new model to promote healthy family functioning during palliative care and bereavement. *Psychooncology* 7:14, 1998.

Kubler-Ross E: *Death and Dying.* New York: MacMillan; 1969.

Kushner HS: *When Bad Things Happen to Good People.* New York: Schocken; 1981, p 133.

Maddison D, Walker WL: Factors affecting the outcome of conjugal bereavement. *Br J Psychiatry* 113:1057, 1967.

Maguire P, Parkes CM: Surgery and loss of body parts. *BMJ* 316:1086, 1998.

Moos RH, Moos BS: *Family Environment Scale Manual.* Palo Alto, CA: Consulting Psychologists Press; 1981.

Paget J: *Surgical Pathology.* London, UK: Longman's Green; 1870.

Parkes CM: Recent bereavement as a cause of mental illness. *Br J Psychiatry* 110:198, 1984.

Parkes CM: Bereavement in adult life. *BMJ* 316:856, 1998.

Parkes CM: Facing loss. *BMJ* 316:1521, 1998.

Parkes CM, Brown JT: Health after bereavement. *Psychosom Med* 34:449, 1972.

Prigerson HG, Bierhals AJ, Kasl SV, et al: Traumatic grief as a risk factor for mental and physical morbidity. *Am J Psychiatry* 154:616, 1997.

Prigerson HG, Maciejewski PK, Reynolds CF, et al: The inventory of complicated grief: A scale to measure certain maladaptive symptoms of loss. *Psychiatry Res* 59:65, 1995.

Raphael B, Middleton W: What is pathological grief? *Psychiatr Ann* 20:304, 1990.

Riches G, Dawson P: Lost children, living memories: The role of photographs in processes of grief and adjustment among bereaved parents. *Death Studies* 22:121, 1998.

Rolland J: Helping families with anticipatory loss. In: Walsh F, McGoldrick M (eds): *Living Beyond Loss.* New York: Norton; 1991, p 144.

Rosenzweig A, Prigerson H, Miller M, et al: Bereavement and late life depression: Grief and its complications in the elderly. *Annu Rev Med* 48:421, 1997.

Rynearson EK: Pathologic grief: The Queen's croquet ground. *Psychiatr Ann* 20:295, 1990.

Schaefer C, Quesenbery CP, Dui S: Mortality following conjugal bereavement and the effects of a shared environment. *Am J Epidemiol* 141:1142, 1996.

Schwab R: A child's death and divorce: Dispelling the myth. *Death Studies* 22:445, 1998.

Steeves RH: Loss, grief, and the search for meaning. *Oncol Nurs Forum* 23:897, 1996.

Walsh F, McGoldrick M: Loss and the family: A systemic perspective. In: Walsh F, McGoldrick M (eds): *Living Beyond Loss.* New York: Norton; 1991, p 1.

Zborowski M: *People in Pain.* San Francisco, CA: Jossey-Bass; 1969.

Tillman Farley

End of Life

Man is like a breath
his days are as a fleeting shadow.
In the morning he flourishes and grows up
like grass,
in the evening he is cut down and withers.
So teach us to number our days
that we may get a heart of wisdom.

—Jewish psalm[1]

As medical knowledge progresses and more techniques are found for combating disease, we sometimes lose sight of the fact that death is inevitable. The average life span in the United States is increasing. Over one-third of the population is over the age of 65. The fastest growing part of the population is the "old old," defined as those over the age of 85. However, even as we improve our ability to keep people alive longer, we have not done a good job helping people through that final transition. As a medical culture we have "raged at the dying of the light," often at the expense of helping people die in comfort and with dignity. End-of-life issues confront all clinicians in their professional and personal lives.

In this chapter, we look at issues at the end of life, when the medical focus changes from cure to care. First, we discuss the history of dying in the United States, which helps illuminate why we view dying the way we do. Next, we deal with several ethical issues related to death and dying. We provide guiding principles that will help clinicians better cope with their dying patients and families. Then we focus on stages of death, so that clinicians will understand what dying patients face. Next, we discuss the concept of a good death and the tasks required for a good death. Finally, we discuss end-of-life care with a focus on special circumstances that clinicians will likely encounter.

Death in the United States

History

The concept of death and the manner in which death occurs have changed greatly over the past 100 years. At the beginning of this century, most people died at home, in the presence of family. There were few interventions available to medical science. The clinician's primary roles were to keep the patient comfortable and to comfort the living. Death was regarded as the unavoidable course of things. It was natural, private, and sacred.

With the explosion of modern medical technology following World War II, our concept of death began to change. Individuals began to lose faith in their abilities to administer care to the dying, and instead turned that function over to the medical community. The medical community was making huge strides in combating disease, and began to see death as simply another disease to conquer. Suddenly, there were new options open to patients and families. Medical technologies to forestall death could be brought to bear on the disease process. Deaths began to take place in the hospital under the control of the medical profession. Death was shifting from a private and natural phenomenon to an institutional and artificial one.

In the late 1970s, there was a movement toward empowerment of dying patients and their families, even as medical technology continued to increase exponentially. This was part of a larger consumer movement evident in the United States at the time. Patients became more active in questions regarding their own health and health care. The idea of managed death, "free, conscious, without accident, without ambush"[2] became the standard. Self-determination and patient autonomy became the overriding tenets of end-of-life care.

[1]Myerhoff B: *Number Our Days.* New York: Simon & Schuster; 1978.

[2]Basile CM: Advance directives and advocacy in end of life decisions. *Nurse Practitioner* 23:44, 1998.

Where We Are Today

Both patient autonomy and the idea of accepting death are often in direct conflict with the culture of medicine in the United States. The focus of Western medicine is on curing disease. Organ systems and the pathophysiology of disease often take precedence over the care of the patient, as a whole. Death is often treated as just another disease to be cured, and when death occurs it is seen as failure. We pay little attention to how to deal with patients who are terminally ill. Although the vast majority of medical schools offer some type of death education, most schools do not require a formal course in end-of-life care. In 1975, there were 14 medical schools with a full course on dying, but by 1995, only 9 offered such a course. Clinicians often feel uncomfortable discussing death, both with patients and colleagues. Most clinicians have no forum in which to discuss their own reactions to death. Clinicians' own discomfort with death is often hidden behind a facade of "objective" detachment.

The resulting tension, complicated by fears of malpractice litigation, has largely brought us to where we are today. Lynn and colleagues found that most deaths in the United States occur in hospitals after considerable expense to forestall them. Fewer than half of patients die without being placed on a ventilator, having a feeding tube placed, or undergoing resuscitative efforts. Twenty-seven percent of all Medicare dollars are spent on 5 percent of Medicare patients in their last year of life, and 40 percent of that is spent on patients in the last month of life. Most patients die in pain; 40 percent die in severe pain. Eighty percent complain of severe fatigue in the days and weeks before their deaths. Many others complain of severe dyspnea, anxiety, dysphoria, and other avoidable symptoms that complicate the dying process. Thirty percent of patients express the wish that they would die sooner to avoid such discomfort. Medical care during the dying process occurs contrary to the preferences of 10 percent of patients.

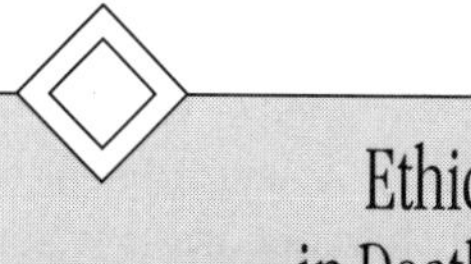

Ethical Issues in Death and Dying

Definition of Death

Most of us probably believe we know how to recognize death, but on closer inspection, the definition of death is not always so clear. What is death? How do we tell when someone has died? These questions form the basis of heated ethical and philosophical debates.

Clinical Death

There are two definitions of death used by clinicians. The first is clinical death, which occurs when the heart stops beating and the patient stops breathing. Before the advent of cardiopulmonary resuscitation (CPR), this was the only definition of death. By the early 1960s, CPR had been developed, along with artificial ventilators. Patients' hearts could be restarted and a machine could do their breathing for them. It appeared that sometimes "dead" patients could be brought back to life. Because death cannot be reversible, a new definition of death was needed. In 1968, a recommendation was put forth that death be redefined to mean brain death. Without immediate intervention, clinical death will always proceed to brain death.

Brain Death

The hallmark of brain death is irreversibility, and it is this definition of death that causes the most debate. What is brain death? How much of the brain has to die for death to be irreversible and brain death to exist? What functions have to be lost? Historically, ethicists and philosophers have used the concept of "whole brain death" to define death. That is, the entire brain has to cease functioning for death to have occurred. Because brain stem function is required for spontaneous breathing, the presence of spontaneous breathing means the patient has not died. A second school of thought posits that death has occurred when there is irreversible loss of all higher mental functions. According to this definition, a patient might still be breathing but be dead. In 1975, Karen Ann Quinlan suffered a respiratory arrest. By the time she was resuscitated, she had incurred significant brain damage and was kept alive by her ventilator. After a lengthy legal battle, her parents were finally given permission to remove her ventilator. At that point, Karen began breathing on her own. She lived another 10 years or so in a persistent vegetative state. According to the "higher brain function" definition of brain death, Karen was dead, although still breathing. According to the "whole brain" definition, she was still alive. Currently, the whole brain definition of death is generally accepted, whereas the higher brain definition is not (although it is gaining credibility).

Guiding Principles

In governing our actions regarding end-of-life care, there are several principles that must be kept in mind:

- Life is good.
- Suffering is bad.
- Death is inevitable.
- Sometimes death is preferable to continued life.

The responsibility of the ethical clinician is to honor the above principles, but overriding consideration must be given to another ethical principal: autonomy.

AUTONOMY

The dominant principle in American medical ethics is that of autonomy. Patient autonomy is defined as "the right to be a fully informed participant in all aspects of medical decision making and the right to refuse unwanted, even recommended and life-saving, medical care."[3] A patient's choice may seem irrational, but the principle of autonomy dictates that we grant that choice as long as a patient is competent to decide and the choice does not cause harm to anyone else. Under the principle of autonomy, it is up to the patient to decide whether and when death is preferable to continued life.

CLOSED AWARENESS VERSUS OPEN AWARENESS

CLOSED AWARENESS In the past, clinicians believed that one could ethically withhold important information from a patient if that information would be likely to hasten death. "Bad news" was routinely kept from patients in the belief that they might "give up" if they knew the true prognosis. Unfortunately, closed awareness prevents patients from making important decisions, not only about their medical care, but also about other end-of-life issues, such as putting personal and relationship affairs in order before dying.

OPEN AWARENESS True autonomy is not possible unless patients are adequately informed of the nature of their illnesses. It is now generally accepted that breaking bad news to patients does not hasten death. When patients know the true extent of their illnesses and the true prognosis, it allows them to attend to important end-of-life tasks. One such task is the formulation of an advanced directive.

Accurate prognostic information is also important in arriving at a meaningful advanced directive. The fact that awareness of prognosis is important to patients' end-of-life decision making is evidenced by the fact that elderly patients will more often choose to forego CPR once they understand the low probability of surviving it.

Advanced Directives

The Patient Self Determination Act, passed by Congress in 1991, requires that every patient admitted to a hospital, long-term care facility, or home health agency be offered an advanced directive. By allowing patients to choose the degree of

[3]Schneiderman LJ, Jecker NS, Jonsen AR: Medical futility: Its meaning and ethical implications. *Ann Intern Med* 112:949, 1990.

medical intervention allowed, it was hoped that advanced directives would prevent painful, futile interventions, support the concept of patient autonomy, and save money. Conflicts can arise when the patient and family disagree with the clinician over treatment options. For example, the patient and their family may overestimate the patient's chance for survival and therefore want "everything" done. Clinicians, in turn, may limit discussion of options that they consider futile, thus effectively removing those options from consideration. Labeling a treatment futile in those cases may be a technique clinicians use to avoid difficult end-of-life discussions. When conflicts between patient and clinician regarding end-of-life care arise, it may help to have an institutional process to mediate such disagreements.

Arguments have arisen over what constitutes futile care, and the definition is often subjective, arrived at after intensive discussion with patient and family. Patients and families may want treatments that the clinician considers futile, or they may reject treatments that the clinician considers worthwhile. Most people agree that any intervention with a less than 1 percent chance of sustaining life for 2 months is futile. Some suggest that any intervention offering less than 13 percent survival for 2 months is futile, and still others argue that any chance at all, however remote, makes the intervention not futile. It is important to note here that the intervention must be aimed at improvement in the patient's overall well-being, and not just at improved functioning of an organ system. For example, giving dopamine for blood pressure support to a brain-dead patient is futile, even though it may have the intended effect on the blood pressure.

Unfortunately, advanced directives may not substantially change how we manage terminally ill patients or how much we spend on end-of-life care. Most people, including those in the hospital, do not have advanced directives. Clinicians remain reluctant to discuss end-of-life issues with patients who are not terminally ill. Studies suggest, moreover, that families and clinicians often ignore the wishes spelled out in the advanced directive. If the family and clinician disagree with the patient's decision, the patient may be unjustly labeled "incompetent."

The Patient Self Determination Act is itself somewhat misguided, because not all patients entering a hospital are ready to discuss their end-of-life wishes. For example, it makes little sense to obtain an advanced directive on a healthy term gravid woman presenting to the hospital in labor. Clinicians should, however, understand the values of their patients on issues concerning end of life, whether or not the patient is at the end of life. Discussion about advanced directives and other end-of-life issues should be ongoing. Family should be involved, even if the patient is able to make his or her own decisions. Although the competent patient has the final say, it is helpful if the family agrees with the decision.

Whether or not advanced directives are achieving their stated goals of saving money by forgoing futile interventions, they offer an opportunity to direct therapeutic end-of-life discussions among clinicians, patients, and family members. These discussions cover difficult and emotionally charged topics that we all too frequently avoid. We need to be careful, however, that in concentrating on the specific treatment decisions of the advanced directive we do not avoid the deeper discussion around values at the end of life.

Euthanasia and Physician-Assisted Suicide

Euthanasia and physician-assisted suicide (PAS) have been topics of heated debate for centuries. After discovery of the atrocities committed by Nazi physicians under the guise of eugenics and medical science, euthanasia and PAS lapsed from public discussion for several decades. Over the past two decades, however, they have moved back into the forefront of public consciousness. A large proportion of physicians report having received a request from a patient for either assistance with suicide or for a lethal injection. Singer and colleagues report that seven percent of physicians report having carried out such a request at least once.

Euthanasia is defined by the New College Edition of the *American Heritage Dictionary* as "the action of inducing the painless death of a person for reasons assumed to be merciful." In the United States, a distinction has been made between "active" and "passive" euthanasia. In active euthanasia, there is an act of commission with a *primary intent* of directly causing the patient to die sooner than the patient otherwise would have. Passive euthanasia occurs when treatment is either withdrawn or not begun, hastening the patient's death. Giving a patient an intravenous injection of morphine with the specific intention of causing respiratory arrest is an example of active euthanasia. Deciding to not put someone on a ventilator in an example of passive euthanasia. Passive euthanasia is now generally considered ethical, moral, legal, and acceptable. Active euthanasia is much more controversial and is currently not legal in any of the 50 United States.

In PAS, the physician is an enabler of the death, unlike in active or passive euthanasia, where the physician is the direct agent. Giving a terminal patient a prescription for enough pain medicine to constitute a lethal dose, knowing full well that the patient is likely to take the lethal dose, is an example of PAS. Currently, Oregon is the only state that explicitly allows PAS. During the first year of the Oregon Death with Dignity Act, 23 people received lethal prescriptions from their physicians, and 15 of those 23 committed suicide with those medications.

Arguments in favor of euthanasia and PAS generally emphasize the principles of patient autonomy, self-determination, and alleviation of suffering. The counterarguments are somewhat more complex, mostly emphasizing the sanctity of human life, the importance of not violating societal taboos against killing people, and the "slippery slope" of deciding whose life is productive and worth living and whose is not. Some have raised concerns that Oregon's Death with Dignity Act would be used disproportionately on poorer, undereducated, and uninsured patients. A study by Chin and colleagues done after the first year that the act was in place showed that socioeconomic factors did not play a role in the decision of the 15 patients who chose to end their lives under the terms of the act. Rather, the most important reason for choosing PAS was the fear of losing autonomy. A complete discussion of euthanasia and PAS is beyond the scope of this chapter. Refer to Fins and Bacchetta's article, "The clinician-assisted suicide and euthanasia debate: An annotated bibliography of representative articles" in the *Journal of Clinical Ethics* for an in-depth discussion of the subject.

PRINCIPLE OF DOUBLE EFFECT

Clinicians caring for patients at the end of life commonly find themselves in a position in which administering enough of a narcotic to adequately control pain or other symptoms is likely to cause respiratory depression to a degree that may hasten death. The principle of double effect states that it is ethical in all circumstances to give a medicine that may hasten death if the primary reason for giving the medication is to control pain, and the medication is used for that purpose. In other words, if a patient's severe pain requires a dose of morphine that renders the patient unconscious and depresses respiration to the point of respiratory arrest, it is still ethical to give that dose of morphine as long as the intended primary direct effect is pain control. However, it would not be considered ethical to give the same patient a lethal dose of potassium chloride, for example, because the direct effect would be death; the indirect effect would be pain control. For a detailed discussion of the principle of double effect and its role at the end of life, see Quill and colleagues.[4]

The preceding section discussed some general ethical issues of dying, including several definitions of death, guiding principles, advanced directives, euthanasia, and PAS. The ethical issues that arise near the end of life are complex and important to consider. Primary care clinicians will need to address these issues repeatedly; each

---

[4]Quill TE, Dresser R, Brock DW: The rule of double effect: A critique of its role in end-of-life decision making. *N Engl J Med* 337:1768, 1997.

case is unique. Remembering the general ethical principles described here may help clinicians effectively deal with end-of-life issues and help patients and their families. Of further assistance in this task is an understanding of the psychological states that patients pass through during the process of dying. The next section discusses these steps in detail.

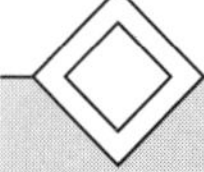

Stages of Dying

The most famous analysis of the process of dying was done by Elizabeth Kubler-Ross[5] in the 1960s. Based on interviews of many dying patients, she concluded that patients go through certain stages of dying. The stages are not necessarily sequential, and patients will move back and forth among the various stages.

Stage I: Denial

I'm not ready to just pack it up and die. I'm a fighter. I don't buy that nothing can be done.
—Terminal metastatic kidney cancer patient[6]

A patient's first reaction to news that he or she has a terminal illness is often denial. Denial has a protective function that prevents patients from being completely overwhelmed by bad news. Denial is therefore adaptive, at least initially. Clinicians should not force a patient to abandon this defense. Even as patients begin to accept their diagnoses, they will from time to time seek refuge in denial.

KEN STRINGER *Ken Stringer was a 54-year-old man who presented to my office with back pain. A chest x-ray revealed a lung mass. CT scan showed numerous masses throughout his abdomen consistent with metastatic lung cancer. He turned out to have brain and bone metastases as well. He was immediately admitted to the oncology service of the University Hospital. When I visited him there 3 days after admission, he explained to me that he was receiving chemotherapy and radiation therapy so that he could go home and "get back to work." We talked about his work and his family, and started the process of life review. I did not try to convince him of his terminal prognosis, or otherwise dissuade him from his idea that he would eventually return to work.*

Stage II: Anger

Do not go gentle into that good night,
Rage, rage against the dying of the light.
—Dylan Thomas

At this stage, the thought process of the dying patient changes from "It can't be me" to "Why me?" The reality of impending death sinks in, and the seeming injustice of death provokes anger. The anger is often unfocused, landing on family, friends, and health care personnel alike. Patients in this stage can be difficult to deal with and require extra patience and understanding.

Stage III: Bargaining

I don't ask for heaven. I'd take hell. Just to be.
—Terminal metastatic kidney cancer patient[7]

This stage is an attempt to gain some control over a largely uncontrollable process. The patient has faced the reality of death, but is placing restrictions on it. "If I can just stay alive until my daughter graduates from college." There is a sense during

[5]Kubler-Ross E: *On Death and Dying.* New York: Simon & Schuster; 1969.

[6]Groopman J: The last deal. *The New Yorker* Sept 8:61, 1997.

[7]Groopman J: The last deal. *The New Yorker* Sept 8:61, 1997.

this stage that good behavior—following clinicians' orders, being nice to people, praying to God—will allow certain conditions to be met. Most of the bargaining is done with God and may be kept secret. Patients in this phase will generally be compliant and easy to get along with. They even may seem to have an optimistic outlook.

Stage IV: Depression

> *Out, out, brief candle!*
> *Life's but a walking shadow, a poor player*
> *that struts and frets his hour upon the stage*
> *and then is heard no more.*
> *It is a tale told by an idiot, full of sound and fury,*
> *signifying nothing.*
>
> —Macbeth

At this stage, the patient may be overwhelmed by a complex array of feelings of powerlessness, hopelessness, guilt, and sadness over past and future losses. It is important to differentiate between anticipatory grief, which is a natural response to impending loss (see Chap. 10) and pathologic depression. Pathologic grief is an understandable but potentially treatable condition, even if the terminal illness and impending death that have triggered the depression are untreatable. Perhaps the most valuable treatment the clinician can offer at this stage is sometimes viewed as no treatment at all—simply listening to the patient, getting the patient to consider his or her death, and finding spiritual meaning in his or her life.

Stage V: Acceptance/Resolution

> *To every thing there is a season, and a time to*
> *every purpose under the sun:*
> *A time to be born, and a time to die . . .*
>
> —Ecclesiastes 3:1, 2

Kubler-Ross called this the stage of acceptance, but I prefer the term *resolution*. The patient has come to terms with his or her death, even though feelings of anger may still be present. The patient has moved along the path toward separation from this life. Hopefully, he or she has found meaning in his or her life and is at peace. Acceptance or resolution does not mean the patient is happy or even content, but is neither overly depressed nor angry. Feelings are blunted during this stage.

RUSSELL KELLY *I first met Russell Kelly when I was an intern covering the medicine floor where Mr. Kelly was a patient. He was 85 years old, and suffering from a blood disorder that caused him to need blood transfusions every few months. Unfortunately, he had quite a rare blood type, and there were only a few donors in the United States from whom he could receive blood. At the time of this hospitalization, none of the donors would be available to donate blood again for several months. Mr. Kelly's hemoglobin during this hospitalization was 5 mg/dL and dropping. It was clear to everyone that he would die and that this would be his last hospitalization. I got to know Mr. Kelly somewhat during my nightly rounds, and I enjoyed my conversations with him very much. He was a quiet, soft-spoken person with an air of wisdom appropriate to his years. He understood completely that he would be dead within a few days, and he accepted this calmly. He had enjoyed his life, but was ready for whatever lay ahead. One night I apologized to him about our inability to find blood. He smiled and told me that he appreciated my concern, but that "Doctors entertain, nature heals." Mr. Kelly died several days later, an example to everyone who knew him of a man at peace with his place in the world.*

It is important to stress that a dying patient does not necessarily progress neatly through these five stages. Expect that a patient will move among the stages during the entire course of his or her illness. The stages simply help us organize our thinking about the various tasks and thought processes that dying patients experience. In the following section, we discuss the these tasks and processes in more detail.

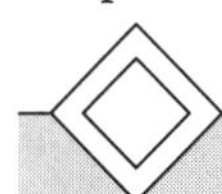

When the Prognosis Is Terminal, What Is the Goal?

Clinicians in our society usually are seen as healers of biomedical disease. When a disease becomes terminal, with no hope for a cure, the clinician's focus should change from curing to caring. The definition of success must change so that death is not seen as a failure. Dylan Thomas aside, our obligation at some point is to help our patients go gently into that good night. This in no way suggests that medical care is any less important. In many ways, terminal care is just as demanding on the clinician's time, energy, and skill as is curative care in the ICU. The goal of terminal care is to achieve a good death, which, in itself, should be considered an important, positive outcome. What is a good death? What factors make the difference between a good death and a "bad" death?

What Defines a Good Death?

According to Singer and colleagues, from the perspective of the dying patient, there are five important requirements in achieving a good death:

1. Adequate pain and symptom management
2. Avoiding inappropriate prolongation of the dying process
3. Achieving and maintaining a sense of control
4. Avoiding or relieving burdens on family and friends
5. The chance to heal and strengthen family relationships

A good death, then, is achieved when one dies without pain, in the presence of friends and family, and with a clear mind. Before death, one has had a chance to heal important relationships, settle unresolved issues, and gain an understanding of one's purpose and meaning in life. One can view death as inevitable and accept it without any sense of depression. The clinician includes the patient in as many decisions as possible and follows the clearly spelled out advanced directive when the patient is no longer able to participate in the decision making.

What Prevents a Good Death?

It is unfortunate that death as described above is not more common. In fact, many people die alone, in pain, with little chance to say goodbye. There is often inadequate documentation of the patient's wishes. Most patients who die in the hospital do not have an advanced directive in place. Family distress and dysfunction may prevent the carrying out of the patient's wishes, even when they are known. Clinicians often focus on cure and not on care, and may be unwilling to change that focus at the end of life.

Both patients and clinicians feel that clinicians often prolong death inappropriately through the use of technology. Patients with terminal illness dying in hospitals continue to receive nonpalliative care even in the last days of life. Because of poor training in palliative care, there may be inadequate control of spiritual, mental, and physical pain. Bereaved family members report dissatisfaction with end-of-life care in general, but particularly because of clinicians' poor communication skills and unwillingness or inability to spend time with dying patients. Paradoxically, clinicians report dissatisfaction with the degree of involvement of patients in end-of-life decisions. Health care providers' own discomfort with end-of-life issues may add to the patient's inability to engage in the spiritual work necessary for a good death. Because of the structure of our health care system, patients may die under the care of clinicians that they have never seen before, clinicians who do not understand these patients' personal histories.

Helping a patient through the transition to death is one of the most important and meaningful tasks in which a clinician can engage. A good death can be a healing experience for both the patient and the family. In contrast, a bad death is painful to watch, and its echoes reverberate throughout the family system for many years. The rest of this chapter will consider the question of a good death, and specifically what primary care clinicians can do to help their patients achieve it.

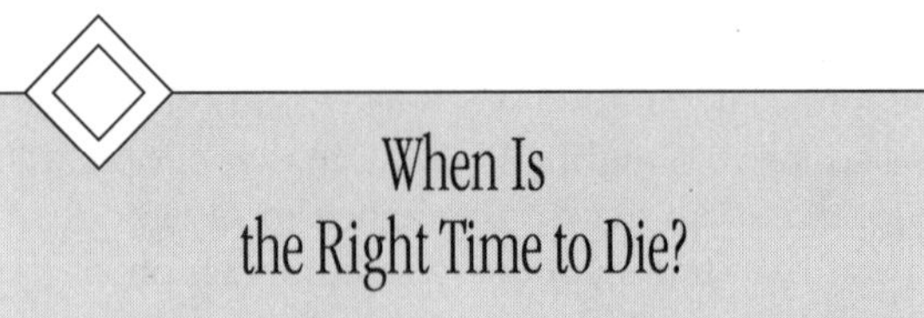

When Is the Right Time to Die?

When should death occur? What is the right length of life? The popular media promotes the sense that life has no natural endpoint; that with medical advances we can live forever. Certainly, the average life span in the United States is increasing. However, with increasing age comes a greater likelihood of widowhood, being a burden on family, losing independence, and suffering prolonged social death. Eighty-one percent of women over the age of 85 are widows. We should note that elderly patients are less likely to suggest that they have lived too long than are their family members. This is particularly true when the surviving family members are not the patients' spouses.

Accepting death is made easier by the accumulation of losses that come with being very old. Before physical death, social death may occur, particularly for elderly patients with prolonged illnesses. Social death involves marginalization from society, with loss of rights and responsibilities accorded the rest of us. There may be a loss of quality of life to such a degree that further living is not reasonable or desirable. Patients often fear social death more than physical death.

LON ROSS *Lon Ross was a 61-year-old man with advanced complications of diabetes when he presented to the hospital emergency room. He had end-stage renal disease that required dialysis, and severe peripheral vascular disease that had caused him to lose several fingers. I had not seen him in the office for several months. He had recently been put into a nursing home because his family was unable to care for him at home. He hated the nursing home and signed himself out against medical advice after several weeks. He returned home where he was essentially bedbound. On my exam, he had numerous gangrenous fingers and toes and a moderate sized sacral decubitus ulcer. He had been dialyzed the day before. His affect was good as I talked with him, but he told me that "I never want to go back to those doctors again." We talked at some length about what kind of interventions he would like to have done. His wife brought me a copy of his living will. That night he developed severe pulmonary edema, became quite lethargic, and ultimately slipped into a coma. A family meeting was held in his room at 2 AM. Ten family members were present. The decision was made that he should have no further interventions of any kind. By the morning, he had 30 family members at his bedside. He died peacefully, with morphine to control dyspnea, about 10 h later.*

Deaths can be categorized as "in phase" or "out of phase." An example of an in-phase death is an 85-year-old woman who dies of cancer. An out-of-phase death is a child who dies before his or her parent, or an adult who dies at an early age. Each type of death can be further categorized as occurring suddenly or gradually. Out-of-phase deaths and sudden deaths are generally considered more difficult to deal with than in-phase deaths and gradual deaths. However, overly prolonged deaths are also difficult for both the patient and family.

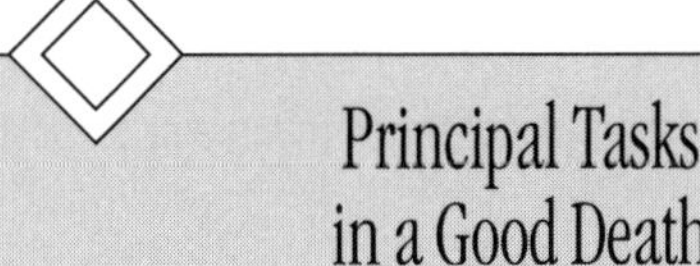

Principal Tasks in a Good Death

To achieve a good death, there are important tasks for the patient, the clinician, and the family. The clinician must be the manager of the various tasks, and, as much as possible, help provide a setting in which the tasks can be accomplished. The tasks are discussed in detail below.

Tasks for the Clinician

As noted, the fact that a patient has a terminal illness does not diminish the role of the clinician. Good end-of-life care is even more intensive than many types of curative care, requiring continual vigilance by a dedicated clinician. One of the most important functions of the clinician is to act as coordinator of a health care team composed of professionals from several different fields. The primary tasks of the clinician are outlined below.

ADDRESS FEARS

Helping patients deal with their fears is an important part of care at the end of life. Fear of death is natural. It is a large component of the survival instinct that keeps any species viable. For humans, who can actually contemplate our own deaths, part of the fear is that of the unknown, and part of the fear comes from being unable to imagine a world without ourselves in it. Dying patients are fearful that they will die in pain, without control, and without dignity. One of the most significant fears of dying patients is the fear of loss of personal identity, which occurs at the end stage of many terminal illnesses.

The most important task in alleviating fears is to discuss them with the patient. The patient may have fears of something the clinician does not expect at all. It is important to ask patients what concerns they have and what they are afraid of. Let the patient direct the conversation. One goal of the conversation is to come up with a concrete list of actions that will help allay the patient's fears; another goal is simply to listen.

COMMUNICATE

Clinicians have a difficult task when facing a patient with a newly diagnosed terminal illness. We are trained to heal; letting patients know that we cannot heal them may be one of the most difficult things we do. However, patients have a right to know, and we have a responsibility to tell. We should discuss the deeper issues as well, and not protect ourselves in the sterile language of medical terminology. The process of discussing the meanings of life and death, and getting some idea of the spiritual and religious inclinations of the patient, should begin as soon as possible. The advanced directive will come out of the deeper discussion. Discussion of advanced directives is necessary but not sufficient.

CONTROL PHYSICAL SYMPTOMS

PAIN Fear of pain is one of the strongest and most prevalent fears of dying patients. Pain control is thus one of the most important tasks of the clinician. Pain may be physical, spiritual, or mental. Mental pain is that which gives rise to psychiatric symptoms and commonly warrants a DSM-IV diagnosis; however, mental pain also includes emotional pain, which presents as emotional distress.

The ability to withstand pain varies. Patients often have a higher tolerance for pain that has a "purpose," such as pain caused by physical therapy, than they do for the physical pain associated with terminal illness or the emotional and mental pain associated with the process of dying.

Physical pain includes nociceptive and neuropathic pain. *Nociceptive pain* is the normal response of healthy nerve endings to the trauma and inflammation of tissue that is common in terminal disease. The pain may be visceral or somatic. An example of nociceptive pain in a terminal patient would be the pain caused by boney metastases. Although this pain is often quite severe, it usually responds well to appropriate doses of narcotics and anti-inflammatory medications. *Neuropathic pain* is caused by damaged or entrapped nerves. It is often difficult to treat, requiring adjuvant drugs such as anticonvulsants and antidepressants. Anti-inflammatory drugs are less useful against neuropathic pain.

When treating physical pain, it is important to use whatever quantity of pain medication necessary. Terminal care is no place for rationing pain medication. The correct dose of medication is the dose that relieves the pain, even if it causes unconsciousness. When adequate control of pain may hasten death, the clinician's ethical duty is to control the pain. It should be considered unethical to let a patient die in pain. The single exception to this principle would be if the patient prefers to tolerate the pain so that his or her sensorium can be clear. For patients with constant pain, adequate doses of pain medicine should be given around the clock rather than only on request.

DYSPNEA Dyspnea is a common and distressing symptom at the end of life. It has many causes, including airway obstruction, excessive secretions, congestive heart failure, chronic obstructive pulmonary disease, restrictive pulmonary disease, central nervous system processes, and anxiety. Dyspnea in a dying patient can cause distress for the family members, even when the patient is unconscious. Dyspnea is present if the patient complains of difficulty breathing, regardless of whether hypoxia is present. Providers should not rely on a pulse oximeter reading to diagnose dyspnea, because dyspnea it is a symptom, not a sign. Adequate doses of morphine should be used to control dyspnea, even if respiratory depression results. If the sensation of dyspnea is being caused by secretions, anticholinergics such as atropine or scopolamine may be helpful.

NAUSEA AND VOMITING Nausea and vomiting are extremely distressing for patients. Not only are they uncomfortable sensations, they also contribute to loss of dignity and control. Friends and family members may not be comfortable in the presence of a patient with uncontrolled nausea and vomiting. This can lead to social isolation at a time when the patient needs as much support at possible.

Nausea and vomiting can be caused by visceral or central nervous system lesions, or they may be iatrogenic. Severe vomiting can lead to metabolic problems that interfere with mental status. There are excellent medications available for nausea and vomiting, and they should be used.

CONTROL PSYCHOLOGICAL SYMPTOMS

The psychological symptoms and needs of a dying patient change with progression of illness and with the patient's degree of acceptance of his or her impending death. A multidisciplinary approach using clergy, social workers, and counselors is probably best. The clinician is directly responsible for controlling anxiety and relieving fear of abandonment.

ANXIETY Anxiety can be caused by brain lesions, physical pain or fear of physical pain, and fear of the unknown. Generalized anxiety is common in patients with a terminal illness. Anxiety is an unpleasant sensation that can interfere with much of the psychologically important work that a dying patient needs to accomplish. With terminally ill patients, there is no concern about addiction, so anxiolytics can be used freely. Use the smallest effective dose, so that cognitive capacities are not diminished more than necessary. Ondansetron, a powerful antiemetic, is also a highly effective medication against anxiety.

FEAR OF ABANDONMENT Fear of abandonment is common among patients facing death. They fear abandonment by friends and family, as well as by the medical community. Clinicians can help allay this fear by providing an environment conducive to visits by friends and family and by encouraging visitation. Visiting hours should not be limited either in time or numbers of visitors allowed, but should be at the discretion of the patient. Close attention should be paid to the personal hygiene of the patient and to the control of symptoms and signs that visitors may find offensive and that may embarrass the patient. Additionally, the clinician needs to be available to the patient to the end. One of the principal ethical obligations of clinicians is to not abandon their patients who are at the end of life.

HELP WITH THE SPIRITUAL WORK OF DYING

The most important spiritual work of dying patients is to gain an understanding of their meaning and purpose in life. The role of the clinician is to initiate and facilitate discussion of spiritual concerns in the context of the patient's particular religious beliefs and to promote discussion between the patient and appropriate family members, friends, or clergy. Respect for the patient's own beliefs is crucial to the success of this process. All patients engage in spiritual work to some degree. Although it is helpful to have some understanding of a patient's religious beliefs, spirituality and religion are not the same. Spirituality can be defined as that which gives life meaning and purpose.

Expressing feelings is important to meaningful spiritual work. Clinicians can help by eliciting feelings. One way to do this is to listen to patients' stories. Anecdotal evidence suggests that by telling their life stories, patients are better able to define their lives and come to an understanding of the meaning and purpose of having lived. Clinicians should help patients review their lives, recalling pleasures, pains, accomplishments, and regrets. Clinicians should not back away from difficult topics. Patients have expressed a need to speak of more serious issues than are usually discussed in conversations with clinicians, family, or even the clergy.

Much of the meaning and purpose in life seems to come from family relationships. For this reason, it is critical for dying patients to have the opportunities to heal rifts with family members. Clinicians should facilitate family meetings. Genograms are helpful in uncovering important relationship information that might otherwise be missed.

Provide Dignity

When caring for a patient near the end of life, it is sometimes easy to forget that the patient was not always ill. This person is a complete human being, who has loved and been loved, who has had hopes and dreams, and who deserves our complete respect. A large part of showing that respect is doing whatever we can to maintain the patient's dignity.

All possible steps should be taken to protect the patient's loss of self-image and self-control. The patient should be bathed as often as necessary, particularly if incontinence is a problem. Patients need to be fully involved, to the extent possible, in decisions regarding their medical care. All options should be explained and the patient's will followed whenever possible. Feelings of isolation should be countered by providing current reading materials, having unlimited visiting hours, and otherwise trying to actively avoid the social death that is so common near the end of life. Listen to the patient's stories, and validate the patient's life by showing interest in it.

Attend to the Family

Death affects the entire family. At times, we are so caught up with the patient that we neglect the family. However, the family plays a huge role in how a patient dies; by ignoring the family we make it more difficult for the patient to achieve a good death. It is generally a family member who assumes the responsibility of making medical decisions once the patient loses capacity to make decisions him- or herself. The family is often burdened with sadness, guilt, relief, anger, and other conflicting emotions that can make decisions difficult.

Family meetings are important on several levels: They help to communicate medical news and answer questions. They can make sure everyone understands and voices opinions on such questions as advanced directives and end-of-life religious rituals. They are also an important opportunity to heal rifts in relationships and to help the patient say goodbye. An excellent video by N. Michael Murphy, entitled *When All is Said and Done: An Introduction to the Family Meeting,*[8] demonstrates one approach to the end-of-life family meeting. Murphy divides the family meeting into five segments (Table 11-1).

Whatever structure one gives to the family meeting, it is an opportunity for the patient to reach closure with important people in his or her life. The five topics that should be covered include the following.

[8]Murphy N: *When All Is Said and Done: An Introduction to the Family Meeting.* [video] Watertown, MA: Vox Populi Productions; 1996.

Table 11-1

Components of a Family End-of-Life Meeting

Story of the wound	At the beginning of the meeting, the dying member describes his or her experience with illness while the family listens.
Worries and fears	The family members have an opportunity to voice their concerns regarding the patient's illness, his or her medical care, and his or her experience at the end of life.
Roots	Recognize and remember other family members who have died. Reminiscing is an important part of the dying process, and goodbyes often follow a pattern.
The family speaks	Near the end of the meeting, ask family members about anything else they would like to say or any other questions or concerns they may have.
Blessings	Blessings are given and goodbyes are said. This part of the meeting stresses ritual as a way of achieving deeper meaning.

1. Forgive me
2. I forgive you
3. Thank you
4. I love you
5. Goodbye

Finally, it is important for the clinician to attend to family needs when the family is caring for the dying patient at home. The family roles need to be supported, even as they are changing in response to the impending death. The clinician needs to be available for urgent end-of-life problems, which are every bit as important emergencies as other types of acute medical problems. As death nears, it is common for the anxiety level in family members to increase. The family needs to be supported during this time. The family will take its cues in large part from the patient. If the patient appears comfortable, the anxiety level will be lower. Although care plans at the end of life must be flexible, they should not change dramatically simply based on the common and expected increase in family anxiety when death is near. As death occurs, the focus of care will shift from the patient to the family.

Tasks for the Patient

> *When Weiran was first diagnosed with cancer, he had a strong will to fight against the disease. He tried many different things, any reasonable treatment to try to overcome his cancer. When his illness got more serious, and he realized that the illness was really terminal, he started to prepare for the end of his life.*
>
> —Yuhua Li, widow of Weiran Lin

Although the clinician can help create conditions that facilitate it, the bulk of the work of dying must be done by the patient. Most of the work of dying is the spiritual work involved in finally coming to the Kubler-Ross stage of acceptance/resolution.

Weiran Lin was a 47-year-old Chinese national working on his doctoral degree at the University of Wisconsin when he developed a rare form of lung cancer. His disease did not respond to treatment by clinicians in the United States or China, and his prognosis was terminal. Over the next 18 months, Weiran and his family went through the stages of grief (see Chap. 10). Weiran himself ultimately reached the stage of resolution regarding his death. He spent a lot of time during his last few months deciding on an epitaph. He originally wrote it in Chinese, but his wife translated it into English for his headstone:

> *Here lies a Red Guard of the Chinese Cultural Revolution. A good man with a good heart, wishing to contribute more. The world is my home.*

The spiritual tasks for the dying patient can be divided into four categories: remembering, reassessing, reconciliation, and reunion. Weiran Lin's epitaph exemplifies these tasks.

REMEMBERING

Here lies a Red Guard of the Chinese Cultural Revolution. . . .

This is the life review, the stereotype of "my life flashing before my eyes." The task during this stage is to make peace with the past and put one's participation in life into a good light. Regrets must be dealt with. The difficulty of this stage is directly related to one's ability to put events into a positive light and understand, accept, and forgive oneself for past regrets.

REASSESSING

. . . A good man with a good heart . . .

Terminal illness destroys accepted notions of self-worth and worth to the world at large. It dramatically changes one's role in the functioning of that world. There are four basic ways that we define ourselves, all of which are affected by terminal illness: our ability to work, our ability to care for others, our intelligence, and our body image. With terminal illness, one can no longer work or care for others. The ability to reason and think logically is eventually lost, as is body image. Successful spiritual work involves reassessing our self-worth such that it is not as dependent on these fairly external qualities.

RECONCILIATION

. . . wishing to contribute more . . .

Reconciliation—the healing of important relationships and coming to terms with regrets—is vital in successful work of dying. This is essentially the task of "cleaning up" and saying goodbye. Reconciliation will vary from patient to patient, but will most often deal with family, God, and the past. Patients will likely want to talk about past hurts. Many times, the only chance for reconciliation lies with a health care provider who is a good and willing listener.

REUNION

. . . The world is my home.

I think of this as the process of coming to terms with death, of reaching the state of acceptance/resolution. As the spiritual work of dying progresses, patients start to detach from this world and ready themselves for whatever lies ahead. Some patients talk of reuniting with loved ones who have died before them. It is important to support patients' religious beliefs during this time. It is just as important not to ascribe our own religious beliefs to the patient or try to "convert" them in any way. Clinicians should support patients where they are.

Completing the tasks required for a good death can be difficult but rewarding. Tasks for clinicians, patients, and families, although all somewhat different, have the ultimate goal of easing the transition from life to death. In the following section, we discuss cultural influences on end-of-life care. These influences will affect the tasks required for a good death in many ways.

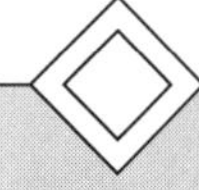

Influence of Culture on End-of-Life Care

With the dramatically changing demographics of the United States, it is important to realize that many attitudes towards end-of-life care are culturally based. For most Americans, autonomy is paramount, and anything other than open awareness and full disclosure is considered unethical. But the clinician must keep in mind that patients ascribing to certain cultural beliefs may not appreciate full disclosure of medical information and may have a much more fatalistic view of life and death. For example, in Japanese society, full disclosure of medical information is not the accepted norm; the belief is that the patient may lose hope and simply give up. In the Navajo culture, it is generally considered inappropriate to discuss all possible bad outcomes of an illness or a medical intervention, because good health is related to thinking positive thoughts.

Furthermore, people of the same ethnicity may think about death very differently. Any approach to dying patients must take into account potential cultural differences while avoiding cultural stereotypes. Patients must be approached as individuals, neither necessarily ascribing to the belief system of any particular cultural group nor to the belief system of the health care provider. The clinician should assess the degree of openness to discussion of diagnosis, prognosis, death, and the relevance of religious beliefs and spirituality. When family is involved, the clinician needs to understand the various roles in the family and the levels at which family decisions are made. Specific issues should be addressed as well, such as what should happen with the body after death. In the Jewish and Muslim cultures, for example, burial generally takes place as soon as possible after death, ideally within 24 h, and autopsy is forbidden.

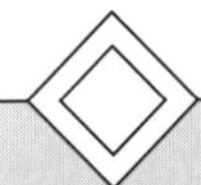

Where Should Death Occur?

As noted, most deaths in the United States currently occur in the hospital. Is this the best place? What are the alternatives?

Hospice

The hospice movement was founded in its current form in England in 1967. The first American hospice opened in Connecticut in 1974. Medicare began offering hospice options only as recently as 1983. The founding principles of hospice care are:

- Effective symptom control
- Care of the patient and the family
- An interdisciplinary approach to care
- Continuity of care
- Bereavement follow-up care of family

Hospice care is available in the patient's home, nursing home, hospital, and sometimes in a dedicated hospice setting. Hospice care is geared entirely toward end-of-life issues, rather than cure. In fact, to qualify for medical hospice benefits, a patient's anticipated life span must be 6 months or less. Hospice care has been shown to be effective in helping patients die well. However, most patients do not die in hospice care. Barriers to hospice care include the following.

- Lack of hospice facilities
- Lack of provider knowledge of hospice resources
- Reluctance of clinicians to change from curative focus to hospice focus
- Lack of payor sources
- Difficulty in estimating 6-month prognosis

Particularly problematic is the ability of clinicians to predict time of death. Hospice care is only open to those with a prognosis of less than 6 months, but clinicians are reluctant to predict time of death that far in advance. Thus, it is not surprising that the most common cause for failure to admit a patient to hospice is the death of the patient before hospice placement.

Home

Dying at home is the choice of many, but not most, people. The advantages are the familiar environment, lack of institutional rules and regulations, and lack of undesired interruptions by staff. The disadvantages are that medical personnel are not on site, there may be a greater delay in responding to end-of-life emergencies, and the family may develop greater anxiety as death approaches. Requirements for managing a dying patient at home are:

- Close contact and frequent meetings with patient and family

- System by which clinician can be reached at any hour of day or night
- Home nursing care (or home hospice, if available)
- Education of family about all available resources, and whom to call if there are any questions

Even with the best preparation and organization, it is common for patients to be transported to the hospital at the last minute to die. This is largely due to the increased family anxiety when the patient nears death, but may also be due to poor communication. For example, if a home nurse or an important family member is not adequately informed of the plan, the resulting confusion may lead to the patient being brought to the hospital. Again, close communication with all parties is critical.

WESLEY WILSON *Wesley Wilson was a 95-year-old man with severe aortic stenosis and congestive heart failure. He had been hospitalized several times for these problems in his last year of life and finally decided, with his family, that he wanted no further interventions. He decided that he preferred to die at home. I made several visits to his house, and he seemed comfortable and in good spirits, surrounded by a supportive family. He had a home nurse who saw him daily. The care plan had been developed during a family meeting.*

One morning I received a call from his daughter saying that Mr. Wilson had developed a worsening cough. We discussed treatment options, and the daughter reiterated that Mr. Wilson wanted to die at home. I called in a prescription for some narcotic cough syrup. However, several hours later the emergency room called me saying that Mr. Wilson had come in by ambulance. Apparently, he and his family developed some last minute anxiety and he decided to come to the hospital. Another family meeting was called in the hospital, and the care plan was adjusted to allow for his death in the hospital. We reassured him that he would remain comfortable. Morphine was used to control cough and dyspnea, and Mr. Wilson died peacefully the next morning. In this case, better control of symptoms may have allowed the patient to die at home, as he wished.

Nursing Home

The advantage of nursing homes is that skilled nursing care is available 24 h a day, but the level of care (and therefore the likelihood of inappropriate medical intervention) is less than in an acute care hospital. Nursing homes require advanced directives, which should spell out in detail the patient's wishes regarding tube feedings, intravenous hydration, blood draws, treatment for symptoms such as cough and dyspnea, and whether the patient should be treated for such potentially reversible conditions as pneumonia. The main drawbacks of nursing homes are that they may have a negative connotation in many patients' minds, and they are difficult to pay for. Medicare does not reimburse for nursing home care. To qualify for Medicaid nursing home benefit, patients must spend down their own resources until they are destitute. This loss of financial resources constitutes a tremendous emotional loss for patients; resources that may have been designated for survivors will instead be spent on end-of-life care.

Hospital

The vast majority of deaths in this country occur in the hospital. As noted, many patients who have stated a preference for dying at home end up dying in a hospital. The primary advantage of hospital care at the end of life is the ready availability of medical personnel to deal with end-of-life problems such as increased pain, anxiety, and dyspnea. However, this may also be a disadvantage. Because medical personnel tend to want to "do something," the patient is at much greater risk of invasive and unwanted interventions, particularly if the personnel at the hospital are not familiar with the patient's condition or wishes. Moreover, Health Care Financing Administration (HCFA) regulations prevent admitting a patient to a hospital unless hospital-based treatments are required. This almost mandates such futile and invasive measures as the placement of an IV, drawing of blood, and other unwanted procedures.

When a terminally ill patient comes to the hospital to die, it is important that the primary clinician be available and closely involved. The patient should be admitted to a private room. The intensive care unit is absolutely the wrong place for a terminally ill patient to die. Plenty of chairs should be available in the room. Interruptions by hospital staff should be kept to a minimum; blood pressures and other vital sign measurements are not needed. Orders should be left for no blood draws or other invasive procedures of any kind. However, the patient should not be ignored, because palliative care for pain and other uncomfortable symptoms is critically important. Because nurses provide most of the care in the hospital, all nursing staff should be apprised of the patient's condition and the plan of care. Regulations regarding visitation should be waived for the terminally ill patient, so that family can be present continually in whatever numbers the patient and family choose. Doses of narcotics should be as high as necessary to control symptoms, even if such doses hasten death. Again, the nursing staff needs to be completely aware of and in agreement with this plan. If a nurse is uncomfortable with the plan, he or she should be able to remove him- or herself from the case without fear of disapproval from other staff or the clinician.

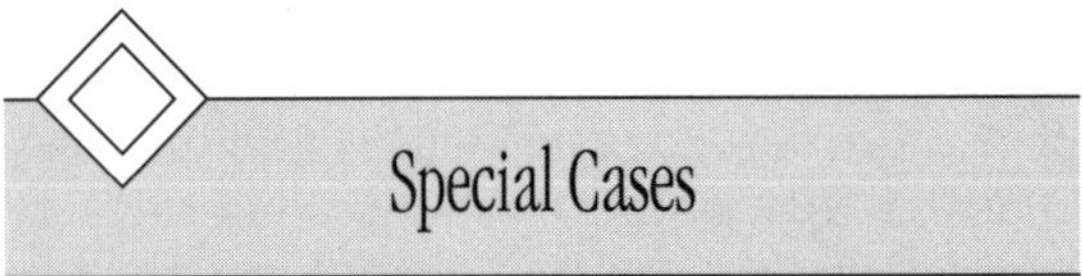

Special Cases

Clinicians will find wide variety in the death experiences of their patients. All cases have unique elements that require special attention, but certain groups of patients require extensive consideration. We discuss several of these types of patients below.

The Dying Adolescent

Working with a dying adolescent is one of the most difficult and emotional tasks in medicine. Dying adolescents are "out of phase," and therefore have a different set of tasks and problems than do the dying elderly. The adolescent with a terminal illness will not be able to accomplish the tasks of adolescence, but is forced instead to deal with end-of-life tasks. Because they are facing death, dying adolescents often have a degree of insight and maturity about death and dying far beyond their years. On the other hand, the dependence caused by the disease process itself, together with the inability to accomplish the task of separating from parents and achieving adult status, can lead to a delay in psychological development in other areas. Social isolation is often a significant concern. Dying adolescents are removed from their peer groups and thus cannot acquire new social skills or try out new roles and values. The social isolation is caused by hospitalizations, missed school from illness, and active avoidance by peers who may be uncomfortable around a dying friend. Clinical depression among dying adolescents is estimated to be as high as 17 percent. Such depression should not be overlooked and should be treated when present.

Working with Dying Adolescents

ALLOW THE ADOLESCENT TO BE "NORMAL" In working with dying adolescents, it is important to help them continue living in as normal a fashion as possible. The tasks of adolescence are important, and the dying adolescent should continue to try to tackle those tasks for as long as possible. School attendance should continue for as long as possible. The importance of school goes far beyond mere academics, and this is no less true for the adolescent with a terminal illness. Independence should be emphasized and promoted.

ENCOURAGE ASKING QUESTIONS AND VOICING FEARS The clinician working with a dying adolescent should have an open, nonjudgmental attitude that encourages the voicing of fears, frustrations, anger, and other strong feelings. Adolescents will commonly choose one person outside the family in whom to confide, and sometimes it is the clinician. This is a position of the highest honor, and should be considered as such. Keep lines of communication open. Always listen to what the teen has to say. Do not be so preoccupied with the disease process that the "person" is neglected. Remember that the teen has not always been ill, and that the illness is probably incompatible with the adolescent's ego. Acknowledge feelings of anger, hopelessness, injustice, frustration, and fear. Do not try to offer solutions where there are none, and do not underestimate the intelligence of the adolescent or the power of the adolescent mind. Avoid any kind of condescending attitude.

MAINTAIN PATIENT CONFIDENTIALITY Parents do not need to know everything. Make sure the teen knows that you treat information as confidential, and only release information that the patient gives permission to be released. Explain this policy early on to both the adolescent and their parents. Make sure that part of each visit with the adolescent is private, with no family in the room.

ENCOURAGE THE TEEN TO KEEP A DIARY OR JOURNAL Teens are often quite worried by the idea that they will not be remembered. Keeping a diary or a journal, making artwork or even a video is something that can help reassure the patient that they will indeed be remembered after they die. This process also helps the teen progress in the spiritual work of dying.

ATTEND TO SYMPTOMS AND FEARS Teens often have very concrete fears: Will I be in pain? Will someone be there when I die? As with adults, symptom control is critical, particularly control of pain. The clinician should be able to assure the patient that pain will always be controlled. Arrangements should be made to make sure family can be in attendance 24 h a day as the time of death draws near. Make sure the adolescent is involved intimately in the care plan. This is an opportunity to promote as much independence as possible.

ATTEND TO THE FAMILY The death of a child is probably the most horrendous experience there is, and those of us who have not been through it cannot even begin to imagine. The family will need support. Do not neglect siblings, who will have their own set of issues (see Chap. 10).

Death and Dying of Young Children

Young children also have a special set of needs and tasks when they are dying. Depending on their age, they may or may not understand that they are dying. The true understanding of death does not occur until after age 10, but the exact timing of this understanding is probably different in every child. Clinicians should treat any cognizant children (age 2 or beyond) as able to know they are dying. If children do not know they are dying, nothing will be lost by treating them as if they do.

In general, clinicians should probably assume that children know that they are dying. Information should be communicated at a level the child can understand, with no attempt to conceal bad news, while allowing the child to determine the pace at which he or she accepts the idea of death. Children under age 10 generally are unable to comprehend their own mortality and may see death as temporary.

As the focus of care shifts from curative to palliative, a family meeting is critically important. The clinician should make sure that everyone in the family understands that the new goal is comfort, not cure. This is likely to take some time for the family to accept. The process of family adjustment should not be forced or hurried, but the clinician should not reinforce false hope in the family.

Dying at home is probably more important for children than for adults. Children need the comfort of home and the attention of family. It is important that medical procedures and medical personnel not interfere with the age-appropriate tasks of childhood. For example, parents need to be allowed to nurture and care for their child. Parental attachment needs to be supported. Finally, as in other cases, the entire family needs to be cared for. Loss of a young child is devastating for parents and siblings. Each will have a different response to the death, and a different set of issues (see Chap. 10).

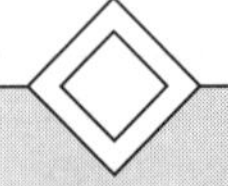

Problems in End-of-Life Care

In delivering end-of-life care, clinicians will face certain barriers or perceived barriers. Some particular situations have the potential to create barriers to the type of care needed when patients are at the ends of their lives. These situations are discussed further in this section.

Corporate Medicine

Caring adequately for patients at the end of life is time intensive. It requires a multidisciplinary effort, a flexible and rapidly responsive care plan, and continuity of care. Unfortunately, these are not words generally used to describe the new medical environment in which many of us practice. The goals of corporate, for-profit medicine often seem to conflict with the type of care required at the end of life. When the treatment of patients is viewed as a cost, it may be more difficult to justify spending money on the devalued life of a terminally ill elderly person. When the goals of corporate medicine are to turn a profit for shareholders, how does one justify the high cost of palliative care, either in the hospital, a hospice, or at home? How can the clinician be allowed to take time away from seeing patients in the office to be with a patient as he or she dies? What happens to continuity of care, so important at the end of life, given the fluidity of provider panels and managed care contracts? The answers to these questions are beyond the scope of this chapter. Suffice it to say that the problems are real and significant, and that current solutions are inadequate, but that commitment to quality care by individual clinicians is essential to success.

Reimbursement

The system of payment for health care services in the United States reflects the values of our medical culture. Curative interventions, no matter how pointless or futile, reimburse well, whereas the kind of intensive, interpersonal care required to usher a patient gently into death is reimbursed poorly—and sometimes not at all. As hospitals try to cut costs by moving patients out of the hospital quickly, terminally ill patients requiring palliative care are left with few options. Sometimes neither hospice nor nursing home care is reimbursable, and hospice beds may be in short supply.

Hospitalist Movement

The trend toward use of hospitalists conflicts with continuity of care at the end of life. The admission of a dying patient to the hospital represents a critical juncture where life transitions to death. To lose one's primary provider during such a time is certain to make the dying process more difficult.

Cost of Care: Can Money Be Saved at the End of Life?

As noted, a large portion of total Medicare dollars are spent on patients in their last year of life. This has led to the suggestion that there are substantial cost savings to be realized by changing the way we manage patients at the end of life. Advanced directives, hospice care, and termination of futile treatment have all been presented as ways to decrease the amount of money that we spend on patients in their last year of life. What are the true economics of dying? Is it possible to save money at the end of life?

In fact, the potential cost savings at the end of life may be less substantial than thought. Several studies suggest that those cost savings are modest at best. Proper end-of-life care is time intensive and therefore can be costly. Timing of death is difficult to predict, and the longer a patient lives in hospice care, the more closely total cost approaches that of patients hospitalized in acute care facilities. Finally, it appears that advanced directives may have a much smaller effect on the cost of care at the end of life than previously thought.

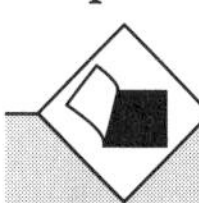

Summary

Good end-of-life care is no less intensive than good curative care, and in fact may be more so. Individual and societal culture must be considered as we deal with patients at the end of life. As much as possible, the autonomy of the patient should be given priority. Clinicians should discuss detailed advanced directives with all patients to fully understand their desires about care at the end of life. At the same time, societal values and the values of the clinician must be balanced with the autonomy of the patient. With few exceptions, honest and open communication with the patient about diagnosis, management, and prognosis is required. Aggressive symptom control to keep the patient comfortable is mandatory, even if it hastens the patient's death. Clinicians should continually monitor and reassess the desires of the patient and then adjust the care plan as necessary. Flexibility of care is important. The dignity of the patient should be maintained, and every effort should be made to help the patient with the spiritual work of dying.

There is no more honorable work than to help patients achieve a good death. The work is difficult and emotional. Most of us will eventually have to deal with our own end-of-life issues. The alternative is to suffer sudden death, which prevents us from completing the important work required to achieve a good death. We should provide for our patients that which we will someday want for ourselves: a caring, empathic clinician who is committed to seeing us gently through the end of life, trusting that our wishes will be honored, our symptoms controlled, that we will be treated with dignity, and that we will never be abandoned.

Suggested Reading

Babbitt N: *Tuck Everlasting*. Toronto: Collins Publishers; 1975.

A remarkable and haunting story written for young adults (of all ages) about the Tuck family, doomed to eternal life after drinking from a magical spring.

Callahan D: *The Troubled Dream of Life: In Search of a Peaceful Death*. New York: Simon & Schuster; 1993.

Written by a medical ethicist, this provocative book examines the way in which death is viewed in the United States, and the manner in which we care for the dying and the critically ill. This book adds greatly to the legal and moral debates surrounding end-of-life issues.

Caring for Patients at the End of Life [special issue]. *West J Med* 1995; vol. 163.

An entire issue of the Western Journal of Medicine *dedicated to end-of-life care.*

End of life care [theme issue]. *JAMA* 284:2411, 2000.

An entire issue devoted to research and commentary on end-of-life issues.

Fins JJ, Bacchetta MD: The clinician-assisted suicide and euthanasia debate: An annotated bibliography of representative articles. *J Clin Ethics* 5:329, 1994.

A comprehensive annotated bibliography of articles about clinician-assisted suicide and euthanasia.

Groopman J: The last deal. *The New Yorker* Sept 8:61, 1997.

This nonfictional piece, written by an oncologist, is the story of one patient's attempt to come to grips with his own terminal illness. Its tragedy, as well as its lessons, lie in the inability of this man to reach the stage of resolution.

Myerhoff B: *Number Our Days*. New York: Simon & Schuster; 1978.

Written by an anthropologist, this book developed out of a study of aging. Although not specifically about death, the lessons about the end of life, taught by the elderly subjects of the book, are profound.

Quill TE, Meier DE, Block SD, et al: The debate over clinician assisted suicide: Empirical data and convergent views. *Ann Intern Med* 128:552, 1998.

An excellent synopsis and analysis of the debate over clinician assisted suicide by well-known experts on end-of-life issues.

Bibliography

Ahronheim JC, Morrison RS, Baskin SA, et al: Treatment of the dying in the acute care hospital: Advanced dementia and metastatic cancer. *Arch Intern Med* 156:2094, 1996.

Barakat LP, Sills R, LaBagnara S: Management of fatal illness and death in children or their parents. *Pediatr Rev* 16:419, 1995.

Bartlett ET: Differences between death and dying. *J Med Ethics* 21:270, 1995.

Bascom PB, Tolle SW: Care of the family when the patient is dying. *West J Med* 163:292, 1995.

Basile CM: Advance directives and advocacy in end of life decisions. *Nurse Practitioner* 23:44, 1998.

Battin MP: Euthanasia: The way we do it, the way they do it. *J Pain Symptom Manage* 6:298, 1991.

Benrubi GI: Euthanasia—The need for procedural safeguards. *N Engl J Med* 326:197, 1992.

Brown JT, Stoudemire GA: Normal and pathologic grief. *JAMA* 250:378, 1983.

Callahan D: Frustrated mastery: The cultural context of death in America. *West J Med* 163:226, 1995.

Carr-Gregg MRC, Sawyer SM, Clarke CF, et al: Caring for the terminally ill adolescent. *Med J Australia* 166:255, 1997.

Carrese JA, Rhodes LA: Western bioethics on the Navajo reservation: Benefit or harm? *JAMA* 274: 826, 1985.

Chin AE, Hedberg K, Higginson GK, et al: Legalized clinician assisted suicide in Oregon: The first year's experience. *N Engl J Med* 340:577, 1999.

Council on Ethical and Judicial Affairs: Medical futility in end of life care: Report of the Council on Ethical and Judicial Affairs. *JAMA* 281:937, 1999.

Derrickson BS: The spiritual work of the dying: A framework and case studies. *Hosp J* 11:11, 1996.

Dickinson GE, Mermann AC: Death education in US medical schools, 1975–1995. *Acad Med* 71:1348, 1996.

Emanuel EJ, Emanuel LL: The economics of dying: The illusion of cost savings at the end of life. *N Engl J Med* 330:540, 1994.

Feldman E: Medical ethics the Japanese way. *Hastings Cent Rep* 15:21, 1985.

Fins JJ, Bacchetta MD: The clinician-assisted suicide and euthanasia debate: An annotated bibliography of representative articles. *J Clin Ethics* 5:329, 1994.

Finucane TE, Harper M: Ethical decision-making near the end of life. *Clin Geriatr Med* 12:369, 1996.

Gavrin J, Chapman CR: Clinical management of dying patients. *West J Med* 163:268, 1995.

Groopman J: The last deal. *The New Yorker* Sept 8:61, 1997.

Hallenbeck J, Goldstein MK, Mebane EW: Cultural considerations of death and dying in the United States. *Clin Geriatr Med* 12:393, 1996.

Hanson LC, Danis M, Garrett J: What is wrong with end-of-life care? Opinions of bereaved family members. *J Am Geriatr Soc* 45:1339, 1997.

Holstein M: Reflections on death and dying. *Acad Med* 72:848, 1997.

Jecker NS: Medical futility and care of dying patients. *West J Med* 163:287, 1995.

Kaye JM, Loscalzo G: Learning to care for dying patients: A controlled longitudinal study of a death education course. *J Cancer Educ* 13:52, 1998.

Kazanjian MA: The spiritual and psychological explanations for loss experience. *Hosp J* 12:17, 1997.

Koenig BA, Gates-Williams J: Understanding cultural difference in caring for dying patients. *West J Med* 163:244, 1995.

Kubler-Ross E: *On Death and Dying.* New York: Simon & Schuster; 1969.

Long MC: Death and dying and recognizing approaching death. *Clin Geriatr Med* 12:359, 1996.

Lubitz JD, Riley GF: Trends in Medicare payments in the last year of life. *N Engl J Med* 328:1092, 1993.

Lynn J, Teno JM, Phillips RS, et al: Perceptions by family members of the dying experience of older and seriously ill patients. *Ann Intern Med* 126:97, 1997.

Lynn J, Teno JM, Harrell FE: Accurate prognostications of death: Opportunities and challenges for clinicians. *West J Med* 163:250, 1995.

Martinson IM: Improving care of dying children. *West J Med* 163:258, 1995.

Meier DE, Emmons CA, Wallenstein S, et al: A national survey of clinician-assisted suicide and euthanasia in the United States. *N Engl J Med* 338:1193, 1998.

Meier DE, Morrison S, Cassel CK: Improving palliative care. *Ann Intern Med* 127:225, 1997.

Miles SH, Koepp R, Weber E: Advance end of life treatment planning: A research review. *Arch Intern Med* 156:1062, 1998.

Miles SH, Weber EP, Koepp R: End of life treatment in managed care: The potential and the peril. *West J Med* 163:302, 1995.

Miller KE, Miller MM, Single N: Barriers to hospice care: Family clinicians' perceptions. *Hosp J* 12:29, 1997.

Murphy DJ, Burrows D, Santilli S, et al: The influence of the probability of survival on patients' preferences regarding cardiopulmonary resuscitation. *N Engl J Med* 330:545, 1994.

Murphy N: *When All Is Said and Done: An Introduction to the Family Meeting.* [video] Watertown, MA: Vox Populi Productions; 1996.

Myerhoff B: *Number Our Days.* New York: Simon & Schuster; 1978.

Nyman DJ, Eidelman LA, Sprung CL: Euthanasia. *Crit Care Clin* 12:85, 1996.

O'Connell LJ: Religious dimensions of dying and death. *West J Med* 163:231, 1995.

Quill TE, Brody RV: "You promised me I wouldn't die like this!" A bad death as a medical emergency. *Arch Intern Med* 155:1250, 1995.

Quill TE, Cassell CK: Nonabandonment: A central obligation for clinicians. *Ann Intern Med* 122:368, 1995.

Quill TE, Dresser R, Brock DW: The rule of double effect: A critique of its role in end-of-life decision making. *N Engl J Med* 337:1768, 1997.

Rhymes J: Hospice care in America. *JAMA* 264:369, 1990.

Rosenzweig A, Prigerson H, Miller M, et al: Bereavement and late life depression: Grief and its complications in the elderly. *Annu Rev Med* 48:421, 1997.

Ross LA: Elderly patients' perceptions of their spiritual needs and care: A pilot study. *J Adv Nurs* 26:710, 1997.

Scitovsky AA: The high cost of dying revisited. *Milbank Q* 72:561, 1994.

Schneiderman LJ, Jecker NS, Jonsen AR: Medical futility: Its meaning and ethical implications. *Ann Intern Med* 112:949, 1990.

Seale C, Addington-Hall J: Dying at the best time. *Soc Sci Med* 40:589, 1995.

Seale C, Addington-Hall J, McCarthy M: Awareness of dying: Prevalence, causes and consequences. *Soc Sci Med* 45:477, 1997.

Sheikh A: Death and dying: A Muslim perspective. *J R Soc Med* 91:138, 1998.

Singer PA, Martin DK, Kelner M: Quality end of life care: Patients' perspectives. *JAMA* 281:163, 1999.

Solomon MZ, O'Donnell L, Jennings B, et al: Decisions near the end-of-life: Professional views on life sustaining treatments. *Am J Public Health* 83:14, 1993.

Sonnenblick M, Friedlander Y, Steinberg A: Dissociation between the wishes of terminally ill parents and decisions by their offspring. *J Am Geriatr Soc* 41:599, 1993.

Stevens ML: The Quinlan case revisited: A history of the cultural politics of medicine and the law. *J Health Polit Policy Law* 21:347, 1996.

Teno JM, Lynn J, Phillips RS, et al: Do formal advance directives affect resuscitation decisions and the use of resources for seriously ill patients? A study from the SUPPORT Investigators. *J Clin Ethics* 5:23, 1994.

Teno JM, Murphy D, Lynn J, et al: Prognosis based futility guidelines: Does anyone win? *J Am Geriatr Soc* 42:1202, 1994.

Tindall G: Decision making at the end of life. *J R Soc Med* 91:166, 1998.

Veatch RM: Brain death and slippery slopes. *J Clin Ethics* 3:181, 1992.

Walling HW: Life's brief candle: A Shakespearean guide to death and dying for compassionate clinicians. *West J Med* 166:280, 1997.

Wanzer SH, Federman DD, Adelstein JJ, et al: The clinician's responsibility toward hopelessly ill patients. *N Engl J Med* 320:844, 1989.

Part 2

Difficult Encounters

Steven R. Hahn

Caring for Patients Experienced as Difficult

Introduction

Today, did you see a patient that you are secretly hoping will not return? About half of primary care clinicians harbor that hope for every sixth patient they see. Were you frustrated, particularly by the patient's vague complaints? Was the patient manipulative, time consuming, self-destructive, or difficult to communicate with? Did the patient make you feel ill at ease and rob you of your enthusiasm to provide care? Ninety percent of your primary care colleagues would share your frustration with this patient, 68 percent because of the patient's vague complaints in particular.

All clinician–patient relationships are vulnerable to problems in communication and to dysfunction in the therapeutic alliance. All clinicians also care for some patients who create a level of distress that transcends ordinary difficulty in the clinician–patient relationship. These patients, who are experienced as difficult, are variously called "hateful," "problem," or "heartsink" patients, or by more overtly hostile names. Although such patients may constitute less than one fifth of a clinician's panel of patients, they exact a disproportionate cost in emotional distress, time, and health care services. Patients experienced as difficult are also of special concern because they are often as dissatisfied with the care they receive as their providers are in giving it, and they have poor health-related outcomes.

The purpose of this chapter is to address difficulties in the clinician–patient relationship using a perspective that can help clinicians to better cope with and care for difficult patients. The most appropriate term for this focus is "patients experienced as difficult." However, the term "difficult patient" will be used interchangeably with "patients experienced as difficult," both to acknowledge that what the clinician experiences is a "difficult patient," and for the convenience of using a less cumbersome phrase.

Although we will not be seeking to fix blame for difficulty, it will be necessary for us to understand why both clinicians and patients have an urge to do just that. If characteristics of difficult patients can be managed or treated medically, then clinicians should do so. If these characteristics are not treatable or manageable problems, then the difficulty is beyond the reach of even the best clinician. However, the question of treatability and manageability is not necessarily clear cut.

Some characteristics of difficult patients, especially somatization and personality pathology, can be managed to some extent, but never completely treated. Furthermore, problems like personality pathology, somatization, and mental disorders are not the kind of problems that general medical clinicians have chosen as the principal focus of their expertise. All clinicians are intuitively aware that it may be possible to manage these difficult characteristics, but many believe that they cannot, and many do not want to try. This awareness contributes to the feelings of inadequacy and guilt that often accompany the experience of caring for difficult patients.

There are two barriers to a proper understanding of difficult patients. The first is that clinicians resist experiencing, acknowledging, and understanding the negative feelings that difficult patients produce. The second is that the difficulty is almost always multifactorial. In proposing a model to assist in caring for difficult patients, both of these barriers must be addressed. This chapter will attempt to provide guidance in identifying and managing clinician's negative emotional responses to difficult patients. Additionally, this chapter will provide a framework for analyzing and understanding the characteristics of difficult patients that contribute to difficulty so that the treatable components can be treated and the remaining components can be managed better.

This chapter will first describe the social roles expected of and by patients and clinicians. Difficulty arises when these roles are violated. However, difficult clinician–patient relationships are not a simple matter of role expectations, and the "difficulty" in the difficult clinician–patient relationship does not reside exclusively in the patient. Characteristics of clinicians themselves also contribute to ordinary difficulties in the clinician–patient relationship. Clinicians' characteristics may affect the threshold for experiencing patients with difficult characteristics as truly difficult. Therefore, this chapter next describes clinicians' emotional responses to patients they experience as difficult.

Similarly, it is clear that patients who produce negative reactions in the clinicians who care for them share certain specific characteristics. In comparison to patients who are not experienced as difficult, difficult patients have twice as many mental disorders, two to three times as many physical symptoms, and three times the prevalence of abrasive personality styles or frank personality pathology. Therefore, this chapter closes with a description of three common characteristics of difficult patients.

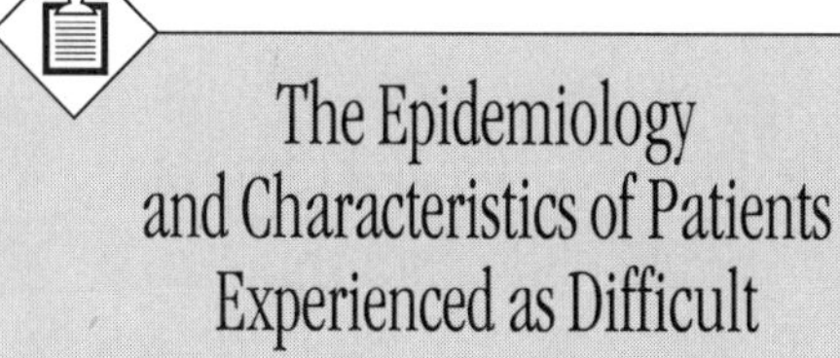

The Epidemiology and Characteristics of Patients Experienced as Difficult

Until recently, our understanding of patients experienced as difficult was based on thoughtful descriptive studies of difficult patients and a few semiquantitative studies. The Difficult Doctor–Patient Relationship Questionnaire or DDPRQ, a self-report questionnaire completed by clinicians after patient visits, was developed for quantitative study of clinician-experienced difficulty. It has proven to be a valid and reliable instrument and has been used in a number of studies, including the PRIME-MD 1000 Study, in which 627 adult patients receiving care in four primary care clinics were assessed by Hahn and colleagues.

Demographics

In the PRIME-MD 1000 study, the mean prevalence of patients experienced as difficult was 15 percent, ranging from 11 to 20 percent in the four clinics. Results demonstrated that clinician-experienced difficulty is not associated with patients' age, gender, race, marital status, or level of education. Rather, clinician-experienced difficulty, as measured by the DDPRQ, is strongly associated with the same characteristics of patients identified in earlier qualitative work, namely major (DSM Axis I) psychopathology, multiple physical (especially somatoform) complaints, and abrasive personality styles.

Major (Axis I) Psychopathology

Patients experienced as difficult are nearly twice as likely as their unaffected counterparts to have a mental disorder (67 vs. 35 percent, $P < .0001$). The odds that a patient with major depressive disorder will be experienced as difficult are three times greater than in patients without major depressive disorder. Multisomatoform disorder, panic disorder, dysthymic disorder, generalized anxiety disorder, and probable alcohol abuse or dependence are also associated with increased risk of clinician-experienced difficulty. Clinician-experienced difficulty increases proportionately with severity of pathology and number of mental disorders.

Abrasive Personality Style

Early descriptive work on clinician-experienced difficulty emphasized abrasive personality styles as a central characteristic of difficult patients. Groves' classic article, "Taking care of the hateful patient," described four "hateful" behavioral styles: (1) the dependent clinger, (2) the help-rejecting complainer, (3) the entitled demander, and (4) the self-destructive denier.[1] These patient behaviors, described in more detail later, all provoke strong negative reactions in clinicians. The dependent clinger is a bot-

[1]Groves JE: Taking care of the hateful patient. *N Engl J Med* 298:883, 1978.

tomless pit of neediness who overwhelms the clinician with multiple, insoluble problems. The help-rejecting complainer demands relief for problems, but finds all the offered treatments to be inadequate or harmful. The entitled demander angrily insists on special treatment and uses intimidation to ensure the clinician's attention. Self-destructive deniers generate feelings of helplessness and guilt by eliciting and then frustrating the clinician's efforts to change the patient's self-destructive health-related behaviors. Most difficult patients display one or more of these behavioral traits.

Other categorizations of personality style have been studied in relation to clinician-experienced difficulty. For example, Schwenk and colleagues studied a group of patients who were identified by their clinicians as "the most difficult patient [seen] today" and observed that many of these patients had abrasive personality styles.[2] In the first study using the DDPRQ, the presence of an abrasive personality was virtually a prerequisite for being experienced as difficult: 90 percent of the patients perceived as difficult met criteria for a personality type compared to 39 percent of not-difficult patients.

Physical Symptoms or Somatization

One of the most important characteristics of difficult patients is an abundance of physical symptoms, especially somatoform symptoms. In the PRIME-MD 1000 Study, a strongly positive correlation was observed between the total number of physical symptoms and those judged to be somatoform by the clinician with DDPRQ difficulty scores (0.39 and 0.37 respectively, $P < .001$ for both). One reason that physical symptoms are associated with difficulty may be their equally strong association with mental disorders, which, as previously discussed, are themselves associated with difficulty. However, even after controlling for the presence of comorbid mental disorders, physical and somatoform symptoms make an independent contribution to difficulty.

Multifactorial Causation of Difficulty in the Clinician–Patient Relationship

Recent studies of the difficult clinician–patient relationship have confirmed that patients who are experienced as difficult confront the clinician with multiple difficult characteristics. Although psychopathology, abrasive personality styles, and physical symptoms may correlate with one another, combinations of variables measuring these three characteristics have explained from one quarter to one third of the variance in difficulty scores.

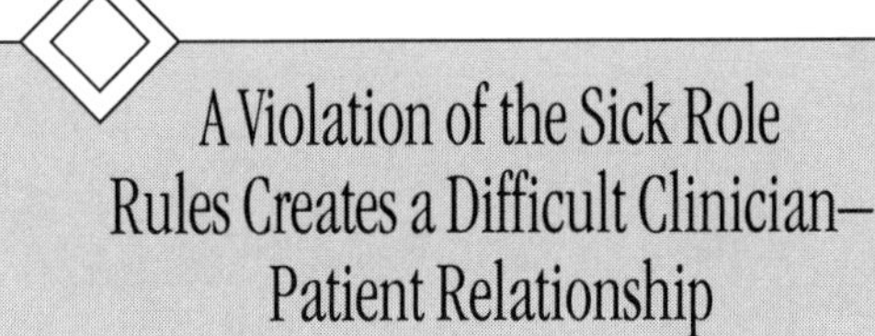

A Violation of the Sick Role Rules Creates a Difficult Clinician–Patient Relationship

Any clinician–patient relationship is vulnerable to problems in communication and in the therapeutic alliance. Therefore, to understand the unique difficulties encountered in caring for patients experienced as difficult, one must understand the structure of the clinician–patient relationship and the social context of each participant's role.

Roles, according to the sociologist Talcott Parsons, are sets of shared expectations, rules, and beliefs that govern action in defined situations.[3] The "sick role" is a temporary role that is conditionally granted to individuals if they have a medical condition, the presence of which is acknowledged to be beyond their control. Individuals remain entitled to the dispensations of the sick role, which include exemption from responsibilities and duties, extra attention and care, financial entitlements, and

[2]Schwenk TL, Marquez JT, Lefever D, et al: Clinician and patient determinants of difficult clinician–patient relationships. *J Fam Pract* 28:59, 1989.

[3]Parsons, T: Definitions of health and illness in the light of American values and social structure. In: Jaco EG (ed): *Patients, Clinicians, and Illness.* Glencoe, IL: The Free Press; 1958, p 165

medical services, as long as they continue to have the medical condition and meet the obligations of the sick role. These obligations include seeking professional help, adhering to the medical regimen, demonstrating a desire to get well, and accepting the stigmatization associated with the sick role. The sick role also requires the patient to have financial access to care. It is assumed that the patient will accept the clinician's definition of the medical problem and will learn enough about the problem to adhere to the medical regimen.

Individuals in the sick role are also entitled to receive medical care from clinicians regardless of the clinician's personal feelings about the patient, as long as the patient does not grossly violate any of the basic rules governing the sick role. Therefore, clinicians are obliged to participate in a relationship that may be personally unpleasant or difficult. The patient, in turn, is obliged to seek care from a clinician, because only a clinician has the power to legitimize the sick role. This social control function is made very explicit by the clinician's role in determinations of disability and eligibility for medical entitlements and is equally important in legitimating the sick role in the eyes of other members of the patient's social system.

Difficulties are created in the clinician–patient relationship whenever the rules governing the sick role are violated. Most violations of the sick role fall into four broad categories: disagreement about the explanatory model of the illness, differing perspectives for evaluating health status, problems with the balance of power between clinician and patient, and subversion of the health care process by "nonmedical" problems. Each of these sick role violations is described below.

Disagreement About the Explanatory Model of the Illness

Patients' ability and motivation to seek help and adhere to treatment depends on understanding their medical problems. Patients often have incomplete and erroneous understandings of their illness, and these errors are often unknown to the clinician. Arthur Kleinman has described a model for understanding and assessing patients' "explanatory model" of the illness that identifies component parts of a functional understanding of the illness (Table 12-1). Concerns about etiology, precipitant, and pathophysiology (items 1 through 5) represent a classical biomedical model of the illness. However, patients develop their understanding from sources that may contradict the clinician's model. Patients' models may be based on folklore or traditional cultural notions; they may espouse "alternative" explanatory models, or most commonly, they may just have an inaccurate understanding of the traditional biomedical model. For example, a patient with hypertension may stop his medication after a normal blood pressure reading because, to him, the normal reading means he is "cured."

Clinicians rarely assess patients' explanatory models and are often unaware of conflicts between their understanding and the patients'. Although patients do not necessarily need a detailed understanding of their illness, inadequate understanding or beliefs that contradict those of the clinician will inevitably create problems. The first five general questions proposed by Kleinman (see Table 12-1) are a good place to begin when the clinician–patient relationship is troubled by problems with cooperation with regimen and should be routinely assessed to prevent confusion.

Differing Perspectives for Evaluating Health Status: The Clinician's "Disease" Versus the Patient's "Illness"

An even more important source of conflict in the clinician–patient relationship is the different emphasis placed by each party on pathophysiologic effects of the "disease" versus the impact of the "illness" on quality of life. Clinicians learn to define health status in terms of control of pathology. Patients, on the other hand, are usually more concerned with their "illness"—how they feel and function.

Table 12-1

Clinician and Patient's Explanatory Models of Illness

Clinician's Model	Patient's Model
Disease concerns	
1. Etiology	1. What do you think caused your problem?
2. Precipitant (onset of symptoms)	2. Why do you think it started when it did?
3. Pathophysiology	3. What do you think your sickness does to you? How does it work?
4. Natural history of the illness: severity, chronicity, impairment, prognosis	4. How severe and impairing is your illness? What do you think will happen?
5. Treatment	5. What is your understanding of treatment options and effects?
Illness concerns	
6. What are the patient's hopes and desires?	6. What are the most important results you hope to receive from this treatment?
7. How is the illness affecting the patient's life?	7. What are the chief problems your sickness has caused for you?
8. What are the patient's fears and anxieties?	8. What do you fear most about your illness?

Source: Adapted from Kleinman A, Eisenberg L, Good B: Culture, illness, and care: Clinical lessons from anthropologic and cross-cultural research. *Ann Intern Med* 88:251, 1978.

Patients' and clinicians' concerns are often diametrically opposed. In patients with hypertension, clinicians worry about blood pressure, an asymptomatic parameter not directly experienced by the patient. By contrast, patients are usually more concerned about the cost, the inconvenience of having to take medicine, or the side effects that make them feel bad or interfere with critical functions. Patients may also be distressed by the stigma and anxiety of thinking of themselves as someone with a medical problem. Patients often find that the adverse effects of treatment are worse than any concern they can muster about the risk of future complications. Even in symptomatic conditions, clinicians will understandably focus on what they can treat and give less attention to the illness concerns that seem beyond their direct influence.

CARL LARSON *Carl Larson has end-stage kidney disease and just finished a treatment in a hemodialysis center.*

Nephrologist: "Hello, how are you doing?"

Carl gives a slightly sad-faced, silent shrug.

Nephrologist (with enthusiasm): "You're doing so well! Your blood pressure was pretty good when you came in today, and so were your blood tests. Now your weight and BP are just fine. I'm really pleased with how it's going."

Carl: "Doc, I feel so washed out all the time, and I hate having to do this."

Nephrologist: Appearing slightly disappointed. "Oh, I know, but you are doing very well with the treatments. I'll see you at your next session."

Although clinicians often cannot help patients with some of their illness concerns directly, patients expect their clinicians to inquire and understand how the illness is affecting them. Clinicians may underestimate the benefit of empathetically witnessing patients' feelings about themselves and the therapeutic alliance. Furthermore, this may be an opportunity to address illness concerns that *are* amenable to medical intervention.

Problems with the Balance of Power Between Patient and Clinician

In medical settings, clinicians generally control the content and form of the interactions. Most of this power and control is produced by socially defined roles, generated without any specific action by the clinician and usually wielded as a matter of course. Although this power gradient has utility and is consistent with the assumption that clinicians know what to say, ask, and do by virtue of their knowledge and training, the power gradient can be a barrier to effective communication when it is uncritically accepted. In general, the power gradient places the patient in a passive, dependent position vis-á-vis the clinician. This passivity may interfere with every step of care, from negotiating an agenda and gathering information, to developing a therapeutic alliance and educating the patient about treatment.

When patients feel powerless to negotiate an agenda and participate in decision making, they may refuse treatment and not participate in their own care. Patients may be afraid to share their explanatory model of the illness for fear of appearing ignorant, foolish, or challenging to the clinician's authority. They may simply not take their medications rather than complain about side effects, or they may refuse treatments altogether because they lack confidence in their ability to influence the particulars of a treatment plan. Rather than feel powerless in the clinician's presence, they may exercise their greatest power by not showing up for their next visit.

Both patients' and clinicians' personalities influence the management of the clinician–patient relationship power gradient. Patients' personalities range from passive and dependent to active and autonomous, and clinicians' styles from collaborative to autocratic. Responses to a dysfunctional balance of power in the clinician–patient relationship will be frustrating and disruptive whether the patient's response is passive withdrawal or more active or aggressive attempts to control.

MERLITA MOUNTOLIVE *Mrs. Merlita Mountolive is a quiet, 68-year-old woman with hypertension that has been gradually coming under control with increasing doses of a diuretic and ACE inhibitor that was added at the last visit.*

Dr. Marks: "How are you today Mrs. Mountolive? Are you having any problems?" Without pausing for an answer, she continues, "How are you doing with your blood pressure medications?"

Mrs. Mountolive: "OK, I guess."

Dr. Marks: "Good, let's see how your blood pressure is." The clinician checks the patient's blood pressure and finds it to be good. "Your blood pressure is excellent today. Congratulations." The clinician completes a brief exam, discusses the need for a mammogram and a Pap test at the next visit, reviews the instructions for and gives the patient cards for stool guaiac, prepares prescriptions, and hands them to the patient. The clinician stands up, extends her hand. "OK, then, I'll see you in 3 months."

Mrs. Mountolive: Still sitting, hands in lap, looking embarrassed. "Please, I need my home care certification form filled out today." Looks in purse and holds out a four-page form.

Dr. Marks: Looking annoyed, then catching herself and readjusting her expression with a sigh. "OK. Let me see it." The clinician takes the form and begins to fill it out.

Mrs. Mountolive: Continuing to look embarrassed, and now a little worried and anxious as well. "By the way, I had some pain last week in the middle of my chest, kind of like squeezing, after I climbed three flights to my daughter's apartment."

Dr. Marks: Looks up from the form, pen frozen in the air.

Mrs. Mountolive: "Do you think it could have anything to do with this dry cough I've been having since the last visit?"

Dr. Marks: Puts pen down and sits back in her chair in silence. "Mrs. Mountolive, tell me about the chest pain."

One of the most common consequences of a passive patient response to the power gradient is an inability to communicate important information or concerns. For example, patients who reveal important concerns at the last minute often do so because desperation finally overcomes the lack of empowerment that prevented them from offering their concern earlier. The initial stages of patient-centered interviewing—welcoming patients, putting them at ease, eliciting concerns, and negotiating an agenda—are specific steps that reset the default assumptions about the balance of power in the clinician–patient relationship so that patients feel empowered to participate actively in the health care process. Passivity severe enough to cause dysfunction in the relationship is more common when it is the result of depression, personality disorder, or physical illness. However, passive communication can also produce serious dysfunction when it is well within the range of normal responses to the default status of the power gradient.

Clinicians can be equally frustrated by patients who employ more active and aggressive strategies in dealing with this power gradient. Patients who perseverate on specific physical symptoms, who are generally demanding or intimidating, who ask detailed questions about seemingly unimportant aspects of care, or who go on and on with extraneous detail are engaged in patterns of communication that wrest control of the content and agenda from the clinician. These communication styles may be employed by abrasive patients with a "normal" personality and behavior. They may also may be the result of personality pathology, organic brain disease, or an Axis I psychopathology.

Subversion of the "Health Care Process" by "Nonmedical" Problems

Establishing the sick role has such a powerful effect on all dimensions of patients' lives that it becomes an interface between the health care process and the patient's entire social system. As a result, aspects of the patient's life not normally related to medical problems may sometimes play a disturbing and hidden role in the patient's health-related behavior. The behavior of patients with factitious illness, using the sick role for financial gain or dispensation from work, is a dramatic example of subversion of the health care process by illegitimate, nonmedical agendas. A more subtle but still disturbing distortion of the health care process is more frequently produced by the use of the sick role to cope with dysfunction in the patient's family system.

ARIANA MARTINEZ *Ms. Ariana Martinez is a bilingual 35-year-old woman who has made an average of 15 visits to the clinic per year for the last several years, not including the 40 visits she made during the past year. She has complained of chronic diarrhea, dyspepsia, severe joint pain, and asthma, but her physical exam and extensive medical work-ups failed to reveal any organic cause for her symptoms. Ariana is frequently called upon to act as a translator for her non-English speaking parents in their dealings with the English-speaking world. Among the many challenges facing the family is medical care for Estelle, the patient's 32-year-old sister, who is blind, deaf, and mildly retarded, has poorly controlled diabetes, and lives with and is cared for by her mother. Ariana's mother relates to all five of her children primarily in terms of their medical and other problems, Estelle's being the most prominent and the one with which other family members must compete if they want their mother's attention. Ariana, who feels oppressed and obligated by the burden of helping her mother care for Estelle, is single and without children. She therefore cannot employ her two other sisters' defense against her mother's pleas for help (their need to attend to "their own" family), an excuse that is automatically honored by their mother. Ariana's only escape from her mother's expectations of assistance, and one that elicits caring and concern from her mother to boot, is to be sick. The frequency of Ariana's visits and the emergence or intensification of her symptoms are closely correlated with variations in Estelle's medical and social functioning.*

The process whereby patients pursue the sick role in an effort to cope with family problems has been called a "compensatory alliance," because patients engage their clinicians in an "alliance" that seeks to compensate for dysfunction or deficit in the family system. The behavior of somatizing patients pursuing a compensatory alliance is disturbing because the patients' hidden objective violates the basic principle that a desire to not be sick is a prerequisite of the sick role. Clinicians' negative reactions to patients who form a compensatory alliance can be particularly intense, because it appears that the patients are pursuing the sick role for secondary gain. An alternative understanding is that patients and their families create compensatory alliances because it is the best that they can do to cope with the overwhelming difficulties and problems that they face, despite limited psychological and concrete resources. The four types of sick role violations (different explanatory model of the illness, different health status perspectives, balance of power problems, and nonmedical problems) cause difficulties in the clinician–patient relationship. Throughout the rest of the chapter, specific characteristics of patients experienced as difficult will be discussed. It is important to remember the role issues that were discussed in this section; however, it is not just the patients' actions that strain the relationship. Clinicians' emotional responses, which are mostly unconscious, greatly affect their interactions with patients. The next section of this chapter addresses clinicians' emotional response.

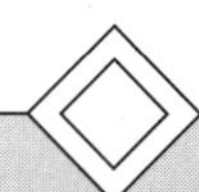

Clinicians' Emotional Responses to Patients Experienced as Difficult

Interacting with difficult patients requires clinicians to do something they have never been taught to do—manage their own emotional response to patients and patient care. Success in coping with all difficult personality styles depends on clinicians' ability to manage their own negative emotional responses.

TOM CONAN *It is 2:15 PM and Dr. Smith is running about 15 minutes behind schedule. She greets her next patient at the door of the waiting room. Another person in the waiting room, a middle-aged man in a business suit, approaches her. Ignoring the fact that Dr. Smith is greeting her patient, he speaks.*

Tom: "Excuse me, I'm Mr. Conan. Tom Conan." With a big smile, and no eye contact with the patient Dr. Smith has just greeted, he reaches out his hand just as she has let go of the other patient's, and in a voice that is at once a little too intimate, too confident, and falsely conspiratorial speaks again. "I have a 2:30 appointment and I just wanted to know if you were going to see me on time today. I have some very complicated and important problems to call to your attention, but my schedule this afternoon is very tight." Voice growing just a bit more conspiratorial, he suppresses a downward glance at the patient Dr. Smith just greeted, who is standing next with a meekly baffled expression and says, "I'm sure you understand."

The Clinician's Primitive Physical Reaction, Primitive Emotional Response, and Primitive Impulse to Act

Encounters such as this provoke an immediate "primitive physical reaction." Most clinicians report sensations of muscular tension, accelerated breathing, flushing of the face, and edginess upon merely reading the vignette. The physiologic reaction is rapid and virtually impossible to prevent. The physical reaction is generated by a preconscious understanding of what is happening and is full blown well before the clinician can put his or her internal experience into words.

The primitive physical reaction soon generates an equally "primitive emotional response." In this case, clinicians almost universally report feelings of anger. Some clinicians can also identify feelings of fear or anxiety when they sense that this patient's bullying may extend to them. In particular, they are afraid of Mr. Conan's response when he is told he will have to wait.

The primitive emotional response in turn immediately generates a "primitive impulse to act."

When questioned, one clinician's response to this vignette was "I just want to smack him!" At once a key feature of the problem emerges: both the primitive emotional response and especially the primitive impulse to act are emotionally unacceptable to clinicians. Feelings of anger or rage and a wish to lash out at a patient are deeply antithetical to clinicians' concept of how they should behave and who they are. The contradictions between clinicians' primitive emotional responses and impulses and their self-concept are so profound that awareness of the primitive emotional response and impulse to act is suppressed or repressed. In effect, unless given permission to do so, clinicians may be largely unaware of their negative reactions to patients with abrasive personality styles.

Clinicians learn to suppress awareness of a variety of emotional experiences that might interfere with effective functioning, including unpleasant odors, horrible wounds, expressions of pain, and their own fear and anxiety. Clinicians are particularly likely to suppress a special class of negative emotional responses: those that are associated with guilt or shame. Although there is nothing shameful in having a negative emotional response to a positive HIV test or seeing a horrible wound, realizing that you are so angry with a patient that you want to "smack him" so goes against our notion of patients as objects of care and concern that we almost inevitably feel guilt and shame.

Hateful or negative thoughts and feelings toward patients produce guilt, even though under some circumstances such thoughts and feelings are common, understandable, and essentially normal. Nevertheless, the internal guilt response to initial primitive emotional reactions and impulses generates an immediate and largely unconscious disavowal and suppression of those thoughts and feelings. This suppression prevents those thoughts and feelings from becoming conscious enough to be examined. In fact the whole sequence—initial primitive emotional response and impulse to act, followed by guilty self-censoring and suppression of the awareness of the primitive impulses—is largely automatic and unconscious.

This sequence has two important consequences. First, because clinicians cannot allow their true feelings to guide their behavior, they must rely on the more superficial and less flexible guide of "proper professional behavior" (i.e., be polite, courteous, patient, and thorough). However, with truly difficult patients, the formalities of proper professional behavior are no match for the suppressed negative emotional responses and impulses that the clinician harbors. In fact, the suppression of these feelings makes their ultimate communication to the patient through tone of voice, facial expression, and a cold, aloof, professional distance all the more likely, because clinicians cannot monitor the effect of feelings that they cannot acknowledge having.

The second consequence of suppressing awareness of negative feelings is that clinicians are denied the opportunity to examine the initial emotional response and recognize that such feelings are common, understandable, and essentially normal. As a result, the important distinction between *having* a feeling, thought, or impulse, and *acting* on it cannot be appreciated. Acknowledging the acceptability of negative feelings, and developing confidence that those feelings will not be acted on, is critical to self-acceptance, diminishing feelings of guilt and shame, and developing consistently effective professional behavior. Otherwise, a vicious cycle ensues: negative feelings lead to guilt and shame, which prevent examination of the feelings; inability to examine the feelings prevents internal acceptance of the feelings and confidence that they will not be acted on; failure to develop self-acceptance and confidence leads to the persistence of the guilt, which in turn maintains the inability to examine the guilt-inspiring feelings.

Abrasive Patients Behave Stereotypically, and Clinicians Typically Respond in the Worst Possible Way

Patients with personality pathology have a limited repertoire of behaviors; that is what gives them a specific "style" or personality. The consistency of the abrasive behavior is the cause of the universal negative reaction that patients with personality pathology produce in everyone around them. Unfortunately, and not surprisingly, the clinician behavior that results from suppressed primitive emotional responses and impulses, even when tempered by adhering to appropriate professional behavior, is usually a counterproductive response to the patient's behavior.

TOM CONAN (CONTINUED) *Dr. Smith: Acting a little flustered in response to suppressed primitive emotions and impulses. "Excuse me, I don't believe we've met, I'm . . ."*

Tom: "Yes I know, Dr. Smith, . . . look, I . . ."

Dr. Smith: "Excuse me, you are?"

Tom: "I told you, Tom Conan, call me Tom, O.K?"

Dr. Smith: "Well, Mr. Conan, as you can see I was just introducing myself to Ms. Jones, who happens to be next on my schedule, and I will see you as soon as I can."

Tom: (back to the conspiratorial, "of course you understand," tone of voice and facial expression): "I hope it won't be too long because I have some very important issues to address with you and a busy afternoon. I'm closing an important deal at lunch with some big backers and..."

Dr. Smith: "Mr. Conan, I understand your concern about waiting, I'll do the best I can, but you'll just have to wait your turn." She then abruptly turns around and marches through the door with her patient.

With her boundaries threatened, feeling attacked, and desperately wishing to reestablish limits, Dr. Smith fights the impulse to put the patient in his place, ("Just who do you think you are? I can't believe how rude you're being to Ms. Jones, and how disrespectfully you are behaving! You're no more important than *any* of my patients, and I don't like your behavior [or you]"). Instead, she struggles to be polite while firmly setting limits. However, unable to either express her true feelings or make a different response to the patient's abrasive behavior, Dr. Smith's underlying anger shows through. Afterward, Dr. Smith's response to the situation is more polarized and she anticipates the visit itself with dread. Already she is experiencing shame and guilt without really understanding why. She reflexively suppresses these feelings, along with any further attempts to analyze the emotional transaction.

The escalation observed in this encounter is inevitable with the truly abrasive patient unless the underlying dynamic is understood, because the final compromise between the primitive emotions and impulses to act and "professionally acceptable behavior" does not succeed in preventing the communication of the clinician's concealed emotions. Neither does it change the patient's behavior. So far, as we have traced the evolution of the clinician's response to abrasive behavior. What is missing is a consideration of the emotional needs and conflicts that underlie the patient's abrasive behavior.

The powerful negative emotions and impulses generated by the patient's behavior tend to usurp a more compassionate consideration of the patient's inner struggles and needs. For example, in the case of Mr. Conan, who acts in a demanding and entitled manner, the last thing in the world that you will feel like doing is to tell him that he *is* entitled, and yet that is exactly what you must do. Any attempt to set limits with an "entitled demander" that precedes acknowledgment of his true entitlement will be met with renewed demands and entitled attacks.

Furthermore, those attacks will be expertly executed, because patients with personality pathology expect and anticipate the response they receive and are ready to handle it. Patients with personality pathology have accumulated a lifetime of expertise in staying a step ahead of the sequence of behaviors they generate. The patient with an abrasive personality disorder is like a tennis player with a difficult and effective "first serve," who knows that if the opponent can return the serve at all, it is likely to come to the same place over the net. Thus, he or she can calmly wait for that return, racquet in hand, to put the ball away.

Understanding how clinicians react to patients they experience as difficult is an important first step in understanding the complex dynamic of clinician–patient relationships. The next step is to learn more about specific characteristics of difficult patients and how to manage the patients (and the clinicians' responses) to improve the relationship and interaction.

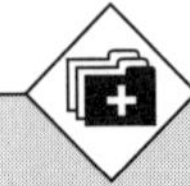

Common Characteristics of Difficult Patients

Effective management of patients experienced as difficult requires attention to each of the characteristics that contribute to the difficulty.

Major (Axis I) Psychopathology

Perhaps the most straightforward task required in managing difficult patients is to detect and treat mental disorders. Two decades of studies have demonstrated that approximately one quarter of all patients seen in general medical settings suffer from a mental disorder meeting DSM criteria. Another 10 to 15 percent have subthreshold mental disorders that also affect health-related quality of life and may contribute to clinician-experienced difficulty. Although the percentage of mental disorders detected by primary providers does not differ between difficult and not difficult patients, mental disorders are suspected in only half of these patients, and a much smaller proportion receive a correct specific diagnosis.

New tools, such as the PRIME-MD and the SDDS-PC, have been developed to aid the primary care provider in diagnosing mental disorders. Awareness of subjective distress in caring for a patient should immediately prompt clinicians to reassess the presence of Axis I psychopathology using one of these reliable instruments or an equivalent. Assessment for less common disorders not covered by these instruments such as obsessive-compulsive disorder, should also be considered. Detection, evaluation, and management of many mental disorders are addressed in detail in other chapters of this book.

Abrasive Personality Styles and Personality Pathologies

The second common characteristic of patients experienced as difficult is that they have abrasive personality styles or personality pathologies. Groves, in his classic description of the "hateful" patient, described four personality styles in a model that has great value for understanding and guiding behavior with difficult patients:

1. The dependent clinger,
2. The help-rejecting complainer,
3. The entitled demander, and
4. The self-destructive denier.

These four types can be identified by their *overt behavior*, the *primitive emotional responses and impulses to act* that they provoke in the clinician, and the typical and usually countertherapeutic *behavioral response* they evoke in the clinician. Identifying the patient's basic emotional needs and psychological issues will lead to a better understanding of the patient's behavior. There is a contradiction between the message conveyed by patient's unspoken clinical behavior and the patient's overt verbal communications. Knowing this helps the clinician to understand why he or she finds the patient's behavior difficult. Clinicians can develop alternative responses to the patient when they understand the patient's emotional needs, the contradictions between the patient's spoken and behavioral messages, and the quality of the clinician's own primitive emotional reaction to the patient's behavior.

There are three internal conflicts or contradictions that are structurally the same for all four personality types. First, in each case the patient's overt verbal behavior contradicts the implicit behavioral message. For example, dependent clingers ask you to make all their symptoms better, despite the fact that their endless new symptoms make it clear that you never will be successful. Second, the patient's emotional needs are thwarted by the clinician's typical behavior. For example, help-rejecting complainers need to retain the sick role, but the clinician persists in efforts to eliminate the patient's symptoms and make the sick role unnecessary. Third, the patient's behavior provokes an emotional state in the clinician that makes the therapeutic clinical response the last thing the clinician wants to do. For example, an entitled demander infuriates with his or her demanding and self-centered behavior, and the last thing the clinician feels like doing is validating the entitlement, but that is exactly what must be done.

PORTRAIT OF THE DEPENDENT CLINGER

The prototypical dependent clinger is a patient with multiple physical complaints who requests treatment for all of them and is grateful for any intervention offered (Table 12-2). The symptoms often respond to treatment, but dependent clingers either return or new symptoms emerge. A variation is patients with a symptom that just will not go away, and reassurance is only partially and transiently effective. They usually bring the same problem to many different clinicians. These patients present their complaints with the expectation that the clinician will make them all go away and seem to imply by their hopeful attitude that the clinician should succeed. Dependent clingers can bring a long written list of items, too numerous to remember without writing down, and go through the list without any concern about its possibly being too long. These patients' lack of self-restraint in making a large number of requests seems to communicate the belief that the clinician can and should give them as much attention as is necessary to satisfy them completely.

Dependent clingers are grateful for all their clinician's efforts and do not blame their clinician if a treatment does not work or produces an adverse secondary effect. Their expectation of unlimited attention seems naive and passive. They do not insist, but act as though they can assume that the clinician will continue until the list of complaints is exhausted. They are the patient waiting outside the exam room with "just one more" question or concern. When clinicians attempt to end the visit, the patients' emotional response is one of surprise, disbelief, or, at worst, feeling hurt. They will not be indignant, angry, bitter, or relieved.

Underlying dependent clingers' behavior is a childlike need to be taken care of and a fear of being abandoned. Childish behaviors include the patients' wish that all their problems be attended to right away, their naive surprise or disappointment when these expectations are not met, and their inability to discern and respond to normal social cues indicating that the visit should end. Their symptoms are a surrogate—an effort to obtain reassurance that they themselves are deserving of love and attention—and are overtures to the clinician to demonstrate a commitment to caring for them.

Treating the dependent clingers' specific symptoms is not as important as the act of caring. Acknowledging that the *symptom* is serious, important, and worthy of attention reassures the patients that *they* are important and worthy of attention as well. Structurally, dependent clingers' desire to receive the clinician's attention is indistinguishable from the legitimate desires of any patient. It is the intensity of childlike expectation that transforms the clinician–patient relationship from a vehicle for addressing the patients' medical problems into a source of emotional fulfillment from the relationship with the clinician itself.

Dependent clingers are exhausting. They make clinicians feel depleted, overwhelmed, and defeated, because the patients' requests make it seem as though only complete relief will count as success. These patients' behavior generates a desire to escape the burden and frustration of struggling with their endless problems. The last thing in the world that a clinician will spontaneously feel like doing with dependent clingers is to give them what they really want: a promise to always take care of them and give them the attention they need. In short, the patients' behavior produces an emotional state in the clinician that makes the clinician want to do exactly the opposite of what the patient hopes for.

Typically, clinicians initially set out to meet all the dependent clinger's requests. However, the number, vagueness, and refractoriness of the

Table 12-2

Characteristics of Difficult Personality Types and Clinician Responses: The "Dependent Clinger"—Multiple Complaints and Requests, Gratitude for All Attention

Patient's			Clinician's		
Overt Behavior	Implicit Behavioral Message	Emotional Need[a]	Primitive Emotional Response/Impulse[b]	Typical Behavioral Response[a]	Alternative Therapeutic Behavioral Response[b]
I have many needs and problems. Please take care of me, give me all the attention and treatment that I need.	Neverending complaints communicate the message: *You will never be able to give me enough attention, care, or treatment*. But I think you are a great clinician anyway.	1. *A need to be cared for (loved), and a fear of being abandoned.* Unconsious fear they are unworthy of love. Each complaint is a request to be cared for. 2. *A need to alter interpersonal relations by occupying the sick role* and therefore to remain symptomatic (see section on somatization).	*Emotion:* drained, defeated, and depleted. The unchallenged implicit request to make *everything* better creates feeling of failure. Patient's gratitude defuses anger. *Impulse:* End the visit, walk away, get rid of, abandon. *Do anything but promise never to abandon, always be there, and respond to the patient's needs.*	*Initially try to treat all problems and symptoms.* Inevitably, limits must be set: some symptoms are minimized or ignored, and underlying impatience and frustration cannot be concealed. Long visit intervals.	1. *State your intention to never abandon the patient, but admit to not being able to treat all of their problems.* 2. *Conditionally but explicitly give permission to occupy the sick role*. Set short visit intervals independent of symptoms. 3. Reframe attention to underlying psychosocial issues, empathically witness the patient's efforts to cope, and refer for appropriate family or individual counseling (see section on somatization).

[a]The key feature of the patient's emotional need (italicized), is the exact opposite of the clinician's typical response (italicized).
[b]The clinician's primitive impulse (italicized), is the exact opposite of what the alternative therapeutic response requires (italicized).

requests soon become overwhelming. Unable to acknowledge the primitive emotional response and impulse to abandon the patient, the clinician struggles to adhere to principles of proper professional behavior and attempts to remain attentive, courteous, and thorough. Clinicians may select some symptoms to focus on and minimize others. However, setting limits with the dependent clinger will almost certainly be experienced as rejection and abandonment unless preceded by proper attention to the patient's underlying emotional needs. Unfortunately, the clinician's emotional state makes paying attention to the patients' emotional needs almost impossible. Despite the clinician's best efforts, impatience and frustration will show through in tone of voice, facial expression, moments of abruptness, and long intervals between visits. The patient will perceive any effort to set limits as further proof that the clinician is ready to abandon him.

An alternative therapeutic response to the dependent clinger is to address the patient's underlying emotional need by separating the patient from the symptom. This requires reframing the therapeutic alliance in two fundamental ways. First, the clinician should realize that although patients express needs in the language of symptoms, what they really need to hear is that they will be cared for. Second, the clinician must explicitly redefine success as caring for the patient whether or not a symptom can be diagnosed and treated. The three most important statements the clinician can make to a dependent clinger are:

1. "I understand that you are suffering from the many serious problems that you have."
2. "I may not be able to make all of your *symptoms* and problems go away, but I will always take care of *you*."
3. "I will always do the best that can be done to understand what your problems are, help you get the most relief possible, and help you learn to live as best you can with what cannot be relieved."

The most important "don't" in working with dependent clingers is do not minimize the importance of the patient's symptoms. For example, when reassuring the patient, never say that a problem is not serious. Instead, say that the symptom is not a sign of some more serious problem that will create additional difficulties. When setting limits, first declare commitment to caring for the patient and couch the limits in terms of that caring. For example, in addressing a patient who waits outside your door with "just one other problem," you could reply: "I really want to do a good job of *taking care of you*. For me to do that, I need to have enough time to *care for you* properly. So, rather than trying to address your additional problem when I don't have enough time to care for you, let's either schedule another visit soon or discuss this problem at our next visit." Involve the patient in setting the next date, which should be sooner rather than later so that the patient will not be driven to have a new symptom to justify a visit earlier than scheduled.

Portrait of the Help-Rejecting Complainer

Like dependent clingers, help-rejecting complainers have multiple physical complaints. Unlike dependent clingers, help-rejecting complainers complain about the care they receive and will often blame the treatments as the cause of their problems. These patients insist that their problems be relieved and seem to believe that any technically competent clinician who is not withholding could do so. Unlike the grateful and appreciative dependent clinger, the help-rejecting complainer generally seems angry and dissatisfied with clinicians (Table 12-3).

As with other abrasive personality styles, help-rejecting complainers' behavior contradicts their verbal requests. Although these patients ask for and expect treatment and relief, all treatments seem to repeatedly fail, and the patients develop adverse secondary effects with a regularity that defies both logic and probability. These indications convey a message contrary to the patient's request for relief: "I don't really want treatment, I don't want to be better." And although the patients seem to assume that clinicians can be efficacious,

Table 12-3

Characteristics of Difficult Personality Types and Clinician Responses: The "Help-Rejecting Complainer"—Multiple Complaints, All Treatments Fail or Make the Patient Worse

Patient's			Clinician's		
Overt Behavior	Implicit Behavioral Message	Emotional Need[a]	Primitive Emotional Response/Impulse[b]	Typical Behavioral Response[a]	Alternative Therapeutic Behavioral Response[b]
I have serious problems and I want treatment. I know you can make me better (if you are smart and caring).	Inevitable treatment failure and side effects communicate the message: *You are a bad clinician, you cannot make any of my problems better. In fact, you make them worse.* Persistent request despite past failure communicates: *Relief may be possible; therefore, your failure means you are withholding or incompetent.*	1. Feelings of powerlessness and anger, in a world of withholding and inadequate caretakers. 2. *A need to alter interpersonal relations by occupying the sick role* (see section on somatization). Unresolved symptoms are needed to preserve the sick-role therefore all treatments will fail.	*Emotions:* Frustration, failure, and anger. Anger feelings produce guilt. Guilt increases vulnerability to accusations of being uncaring. *Impulses:* Abandon, strike back, or passive sadistic thoughts ("Complain of atypical chest pain one more time and I'll cath you even though I know you don't need it!"). Because failure to provide relief equals personal failure, *do anything* but *admit not being able to eliminate symptoms.*	Initially try to make the patient better. In response to treatment failure or side effects, treatment is changed and/or intensified. Persistent failure leads to minimizing symptoms, referral to specialists, appeasement treatment and testing, long visit intervals. Nonverbal signs of anger cannot be concealed.	1. Acknowledge suffering, reassure as appropriate, then *acknowledge that symptoms cannot be completely eliminated:* a) I'm sorry that I can't make your problem completely better. b) I'll do everything to make it better. c) I will do what I can to help you cope. 2. These interventions *conditionally give explicit permission to occupy the sick role.* 3. Reframe attention to underlying psychosocial issues, empathically witness the patient's efforts to cope, and refer for appropriate family or individual counseling (see section on somatization).

[a]The key feature of the patient's emotional need (italicized), is the exact opposite of the clinician's typical response (italicized).
[b]The clinician's primitive impulse (italicized), is the exact opposite of what the alternative therapeutic response requires (italicized).

the same help-rejecting behaviors communicate the message that clinicians do more harm than good, and their clinician, in particular, is either incompetent, withholding efficacious treatment, or both.

Help-rejecting complainers' behavior is an unconscious response to their basic emotional experience: an angry sense that others will not give them what they need unless they are made to do so. Both help-rejecting complainers and dependent clingers are concerned with getting their dependency needs met, but with very different emotional tones. The dependent clinger is passive and accepting, whereas the help-rejecting complainer is passive and aggressive. At a spiritual level, the help-rejecting complainer seems to say, "I suffer and ask God, *why me?*" while the dependent clinger will say, "I suffer, as God wills it." Help-rejecting complainers' illnesses are a solution to both their sense of powerlessness and their need to vent their anger. Help-rejecting complainers use the power of the sick role to get others to address their needs. At the same time, the sick role permits withdrawal from usual responsibilities without loss of self-esteem.

In applying this understanding of the motivation and utility of help-rejecting behavior and legitimization of the sick role, it is important to avoid thinking that all these powerful effects are simply "secondary gain" for the patient. As will be discussed in the section on somatization, the sick role cannot be sustained through somatization unless it serves some purpose for the entire family system. Careful analysis of the family system will usually reveal the ways in which the entire family "needs" the patient to be ill, albeit at significant cost to both the family and the patient.

Help-rejecting behavior creates a profound sense of frustration, anger, and guilt in the clinician. The patients' words imply, but never state outright, a belief that clinicians could make them better if only they were any good. Clinicians pick up on this implication and experience their inability to provide relief as a personal failure. Therefore, in addition to feeling the frustration of repetitive failure, the covert personal attack contained in the patient's ingratitude and complaints generates tremendous anger.

All these negative feelings make clinicians want to abandon their help-rejecting patients. Unconscious guilt about a wish to get rid of patients is one reason that clinicians spend an inordinate amount of time with help-rejecting complainers. Clinicians also want to avoid confirming their patients' implicit accusation that they are uncaring and withholding. They feel driven to do more and try harder, because the unspoken dynamic established by the patients' abrasive behavior makes failure to eliminate symptoms a sign of the clinicians' inadequacy. Under these circumstances, the last thing clinicians want to do is admit to being unable to completely relieve symptoms, because such an admission is experienced as a confession of personal failure.

Unable to abandon the patient, retaliate, or admit to the truth (that the symptoms cannot be completely eliminated), clinicians' typical response to help-rejecting complainers is to try even harder to make the patients better. However, unless they offer treatments designed to alleviate symptoms with the proper conditions, the treatment will fail, because they threaten to deprive the patients of entitlement to the sick role. The patient's requests for relief fulfill the sick role requirement that the patient try to become healthy and the "complaints" localize the blame for staying in the sick role with the clinician, while the persistence of the symptom perpetuates the sick role.

In the face of persistent failure and complaints, even the most determined clinicians will not be able to avoid "acting out" their feelings of anger and frustration. The patient feels rejected by referrals to specialists, the clinician's inevitable comments that minimize some symptoms, and long visit intervals. Although clinicians try not to take the patient's complaints personally, angry defensive statements are almost inevitable ("I gave you Tylenol precisely because it doesn't upset most patients' stomachs; it's not like the Motrin we tried before!")

What then can clinicians do? Unable to give up trying to satisfy the patients' demands for symptom relief; determined to suppress their own angry feelings, but doomed to act them out anyway; hoping to minimize contact with the patient, but discovering that long visit intervals just intensify somatization; how can clinicians alter the pattern of interaction and offer a truly therapeutic response? *The key to defusing the struggle with help-rejecting complainers is to conditionally accept the patients' need to be in the sick role by stating that it will probably not be possible to completely eliminate their symptoms.* The emotional challenge for clinicians is to defuse their own anger, not by suppressing, gritting their teeth, or "white knuckling" through it, but rather by being able to explicitly define the inability to relieve the patients' suffering as a shortcoming of medicine rather than as their personal inadequacy. At the same time, understanding the true nature of the patients' emotional needs and conditionally accepting their need to be in the sick role opens the door to some truly therapeutic, even symptom-reducing interventions.

Help-rejecting complainers are caught in a terrible bind. They do not want to suffer, but they may be forced to suffer if that is what it takes to maintain the sick role. Paradoxically it is only after being promised that they will not "get better," defined as improvement to the point of no longer needing to be in the sick role, that they will allow their symptoms to improve at all. After acknowledging that the patients' symptoms probably cannot be completely or even satisfactorily reduced, the clinician can do several therapeutic things:

1. Prescribe treatment but make it clear that symptoms will probably not be completely resolved (something to "take the edge off the symptom.")
2. Reassure the patients that the symptom does not point to any other condition that will make their health any worse. When the symptom is part of a problem that might indeed become worse, appropriate prognostic reality testing is in order.
3. Empathetically witness the patients' suffering and compliment and support their efforts to cope: "I am so impressed with how well you are doing despite all that is troubling you." This "empathic witnessing" is an essential part of an approach to understanding the patients' symptoms in the context of their interpersonal relationships and will be discussed in greater depth later.

Portrait of the Entitled Demander

Tom Conan from the earlier case scenario is the prototype of the entitled demander. Patients like Mr. Conan demand time and attention and state or imply that they and their problems are more important than those of others. These patients regard their requests as obvious and ordinary, and do not think of them as demanding, but to clinicians the requests are clearly entitled demands. Although the importance of their needs should be obvious, their need to *demand* attention communicates a belief that the clinician will not otherwise respond to their obvious needs. To enforce their demands, they may drop the names of important individuals or threaten to call superiors, speak with patient relations, or call regulatory agencies. The reason that these patients feel such a need to demand remains unstated, but the threatening or angry tone of the entitled demanding creates the impression that it must be because clinicians are incompetent, uncaring, and/or withholding. This can be particularly surprising when the entitled demanding begins even before the patient has any experience with the clinician upon which to base a judgment (Table 12-4).

Entitled demanders typically offer another threatening contradiction between words and action. They demand the clinician's attention, but simultaneously question the clinician's qualifications and competence, leaving the impression that they would like someone better qualified. In training environments they are likely to refuse evaluation by medical students, and residents are particularly vulnerable to these challenges. However, even the patients' own attending clinicians will not be immune to challenges to their competence.

In addition to fear and anxiety about any illness that they may have, entitled demanders are distinguished by an unconscious belief that they are

Table 12-4

Characteristics of Difficult Personality Types and Clinician Responses: The "Entitled Demander"—Entitled Angry Threatening Demands for Care on the Patient's Terms. Implicit or Explicit Undermining of Clinician's Competence or Authority

Patient's			Clinician's		
Overt Behavior	**Implicit Behavioral Message**	**Emotional Need**[a]	**Primitive Emotional Response/Impulse**[b]	**Typical Behavioral Response**[a]	**Alternative Therapeutic Behavioral Response**[b]
It should be obvious that I have serious, important problems, I deserve your attention and you should take care of me now.	Entitled demands communicate the message: *I don't believe you will acknowledge that my problems and I are worthy of your attention*. Accusations of inadequate care communicate: *I want someone better than you to take care of me.*	*Feeling undeserving and fearing that needs will not be met* because others perceive them as unworthy or undeserving. Setting limits is experienced as denial of care, and confirmation that their entitlement to care is not respected.	*Feelings:* Anger and fear in response to the usurpation of control of the health care process and the challenge to competence. Anger at the patient's assault on the rights of other patients, staff, and society. Fear increases in proportion to limit setting, anger increases in proportion to compromise and capitulation. *Impulse:* Counterattack and "put the patient in his place." *Do anything* but *endorse the patient's entitlement.*	Initially, attempt to control anger, limit setting alternating with capitulation. Limits usually articulated as "rules" to be followed. Anger, communicated despite efforts to be "professional," combined with rule-based limit setting *confirms patient's fear that needs will not be met*. Intermittent capitulation to demands reinforces the patient's belief that demands are necessary.	First *tell the patients that they* are *entitled* to the very best quality medical care and that you are determined to give it to them. Then, *describe limits as the conditions necessary in order for them to receive the care to which they are entitled*. Say, "*You deserve* the very best quality care and I am determined to provide it. In order for me to give you the care to which *you are entitled* we will have to . . ." Do not say, "if you want to get your care here, you will have to follow the (our) rules."

[a]The key feature of the patient's emotional need (italicized), is the exact opposite of the clinician's typical response (italicized).
[b]The clinician's primitive impulse (italicized), is the exact opposite of what the alternative therapeutic response requires (italicized).

actually undeserving and unworthy. Were this not so, they would be able to relax with confidence that their obvious needs and right to be cared for would be responded to without their own insistence. Coupled with this underlying problem with self-esteem is the conviction that other people, including those who are supposed to be committed to caring and helping, are untrustworthy, uncaring, and withholding. The patients' demands are extreme because they constantly need to test their clinicians' willingness to provide care. As with other disordered personality styles, the strategy employed to achieve the objective not only fails to achieve its goal, it makes matters worse. In fact, the emotional state evoked in clinicians by entitled demanders' abrasive behavior virtually guarantees that clinicians will confirm the patients' worst fears.

Clinicians typically respond with anger and fear to the entitled demanders' assault on their professional self-esteem and commandeering of the health care process. The more clinicians "take the easy way out" and capitulate to the patients' demands, the angrier the clinicians will feel. On the other hand, the clinicians' fear is likely to increase if they try to set limits and the patients intensify their assault. The patients' behavior creates an impulse to counterattack by setting limits on the patients' demands and to "put the patient in his place." What clinicians truly feel like saying, (but hopefully do not), is something like: "Just who do you think your are? You are no more important than any of my patients. You are not entitled to special treatment, and you cannot expect me to do whatever you say and give you whatever you want whenever you want it." *The very last thing that clinicians are inclined to do is tell these patients that they are entitled to care.*

Because clinicians cannot act out their impulse to "put the patient in his place," they will adopt "appropriate professional behavior" and try to remain calm, polite, and "professional." At the same time, clinicians cannot avoid setting limits on patients' entitled demands. Despite clinicians' best efforts to constrain and conceal their anger and fear, their true feelings will be transparent to the practiced eyes of entitled demanders. The patients will experience the cool if not cold tone, the "white knuckled" and clenched jawed self-restraint, as sure signs of their worst fear: a disposition to withhold the care they are entitled to. The most devastating consequence of clinicians' suppressed anger and fear will be the transformation of every attempt to set limits into an act that, in the end, tells patients that they are *not entitled* to the treatment they demand. "You will *have to wait* until it is your turn." "You *cannot have* an MRI just because it is safe and you think it might show something—it is a very expensive test."

In fact, limits must be set. Entitled demanders leave clinicians no choice. By their very nature, limits are a deprivation, so how can clinicians set limits without depriving patients of something that they feel entitled to? The format of the solution is the same as with other difficult personality styles: address patients' underlying emotional needs. In this case, clinicians will have to do the one thing that they are least likely to do given the emotional state produced by the difficult patients' behavior: tell entitled demanders that they are entitled! Clinicians will be able to do this only by understanding that the patients truly *are* entitled to the very best quality medical care. *Limit setting must be reframed as the conditions under which the very best quality of medical care can be provided*:

> "*You are entitled to the very best quality medical care*, and that is what I am determined to provide to you. For me to give you the care that you deserve, I need to have enough time to address your problems properly and to be free from distractions. So I will need to see you at the scheduled time rather than before, so that I can care for you in the way that you deserve."
>
> "*You are entitled to the very best quality medical care*, and that includes the prevention of the risks associated with unnecessary medical tests and medicines."
>
> "*You are entitled to the very best quality medical care*, and that includes avoiding unnecessary medications that might cause side effects. You deserve to be free of avoidable medication side effects."

> "*You are entitled to the very best quality medical care*, and that can best be provided when decisions about care are made by a clinician whose knowledge of your case is as complete as possible. Therefore, the use of too many specialist consultations may fragment your care and increase the risk that treatments are started with incomplete knowledge of your medical history and conditions."

One device that may be helpful when feelings of anger or fear threaten to get the upper hand during limit setting is to develop the habit of beginning *every* response with the phrase, "You are entitled to the very best quality medical care, and for me to provide that to you. . . ."

A final and critical caveat in the management of entitled demanders is that although clinicians need to have considerable control over the health care process and also need to feel confident in their clinical judgment, these needs are not absolute. Excessive need for control and overconfidence from clinicians will deny patients their proper voice and participation in the health care decision making process. Autocratic and arrogant clinician behavior can transform an otherwise collaborative and cooperative patient into a defensively insistent one who appears to be an entitled demander. If a clinician finds a disproportionate number of patients are entitled demanders, the clinician should seek to confirm this impression through consultation with colleagues and be prepared to examine his or her own style for signs of excessive autocracy.

Portrait of the Self-Destructive Denier

Some patients appear to be doing everything in their power to hasten their own demise at the same time as they seek medical care (see Chap. 8, 9, and 13). Examples include patients with chronic obstructive pulmonary disease who smoke, patients with type I diabetes who will not maintain a reasonably regular meal and activity pattern, and patients with substance abuse problems. Self-destructive patients often visit their clinicians voluntarily and request medical care (Table 12-5). In some cases, the consequences of their self-destructive behavior bring them to emergency rooms, clinics, and hospitals involuntarily. Initially, clinicians usually respond "normally," as though the patients were asking for medical care and would accept the expectations of the sick role. It later becomes clear that this is not so. The patients do not act as though they want to get better, they do not cooperate with the treatment regimen, and they do not acknowledge and agree to stop adverse health-related behaviors. Clinicians are frustrated by the contradiction between the stated, implied, or assumed agreement to adhere to the obligations of the sick role and the patients' rejection of those obligations as demonstrated by self-destructive behavior. Clinicians need to understand or accept patients' underlying emotional needs and problems, which include:

1. Addiction or dependency on substances or behavior,
2. Denial about their addiction/dependency, and
3. Feelings of hopelessness and helplessness.

Self-destructive deniers are addicted to their substances of abuse or to habitual behaviors that are not compatible with proper management of their disease. These patients *need* their alcohol, or the food they are not supposed to eat, or freedom from a regimented life style. Further, they do not want to experience the anxiety and stress of changing their behavior. Self-destructive deniers accomplish this by avoiding situations that will confront them with the need to change, suppressing awareness of the need to change, and, as the name implies, denying the self-destructive behavior.

Denial is a powerful and baffling psychological defense mechanism that causes great confusion and frustration for clinicians. Denial alters self-awareness at the level of *perception*, and allows individuals to remain unaware of aspects of their behavior that may be obvious to others. It can be extremely difficult to believe that patients in denial are not more self-aware. However, patients who are in denial about their alcohol abuse, for example, are not lying; they report the truth

Table 12-5

Characteristics of Difficult Personality Types and Clinician Responses: The "Self-Destructive Denier"—Substance Abuse or Dysfunctional Health-Related Behaviors

Patient's			Clinician's		
Overt Behavior	Implicit Behavioral Message	Emotional Need[a]	Primitive Emotional Response/Impulse[b]	Typical Behavioral Response[a]	Alternative Therapeutic Behavioral Response[b]
I am here, take care of me. I will be your patient and will accept the responsibilities of the sick role. *Please save me from my self-destructive behavior.*	I am not responsible for my own medical problems. My substance abuse or dysfunctional health-related behavior does not exist or is not significant. I will continue with my substance abuse or dysfunctional behavior. *You cannot save me from my self-destructive behavior.*	*Dependence* on the substance of abuse, or the gratification of dysfunctional health-related behaviors. *Need to be in denial,* i.e., experience the cause of problems as something other than the substance abuse or inability to follow self-care regimen.	*Emotions:* Failure, resentment, and anger. Bad outcomes are experienced as personal failure. This causes anger and resentment. *Impulse:* A wish that the self-destructive patient would go away or, in extreme cases, "get it over with and die already." *Do anything but empathetically accept the dependency and denial as the problem to be addressed.*	Initially, tell the patient to *give up their dependency,* i.e., stop their substance abuse or dysfunctional health-related behavior, and *abandon their denial.* Clinician's reflexive assumption of responsiblity for outcomes combines with the patient's denial to blur awareness of who is in charge of deciding what changes will occur.	*Empathically accept the patient's dependency and denial as the problem that needs to be addressed.* Determine the patient's "stage of readiness for change" and redefine the objective of care and success as progression through stages rather than an immediate change in the self-destructive behavior. Accept the limitations of power to change patient's habitual behavior without abandoning efforts. Return responsibility for change to the patient.

[a]The key feature of the patient's emotional need (italicized), is the exact opposite of the clinician's typical response (italicized).
[b]The clinician's primitive impulse (italicized), is the exact opposite of what the alternative therapeutic response requires (italicized).

as they experience it. Because denial does not depend on the patient's conscious efforts or skills, it can be hypervigilant, indefatigable, and smart, even in individuals who display none of those characteristics in other aspects of their behavior. Even though denial may have survival value in acute situations where full awareness of risks and odds would be counterproductively paralyzing, it can be just as powerful a barrier to change when a full appraisal of a situation would be beneficial.

Clinicians may be tempted to collude with their patients' denial because it allows them to avoid addressing self-destructive behavior. For example, clinicians may focus on the medical sequelae of alcohol abuse without addressing the alcohol abuse or lecture diabetics about monitoring and medication regimens when habitual behavior is the barrier to control.

Clinicians' emotional response to self-destructive denial is driven by two factors: first, the frustration of feeling forced to continue providing care despite the apparent impossibility of "success"; and second, the sense that failure is caused by the patients' unwillingness to live up to their end of the bargain by meeting the obligations of the sick role. Both of these factors generate anger, and, because clinicians are not supposed to feel anger toward their patients, guilt.

Ordinarily, clinicians focus first on what is wrong with patients' current behavior and the advantages of changing those behaviors. However, the source of patients' ambivalence lies elsewhere; that is, in the reasons that patients *do not* want to change and in the attractions and gratifications of their self-destructive behavior. Typically clinicians would rather dismiss than explore the "pros" of staying the same and the "cons" of changing, despite the fact that these issues are the source of the patients' ambivalence. In effect, when clinicians avoid patients' reasons for not changing and proceed as though changing behavior is simply a matter of rational choice, they are exhibiting a form of *clinician denial* that complements the patients' denial.

In addition to perpetuating an implicitly judgmental environment, telling patients that they must stop their self-destructive behavior or that they must follow a well-understood regimen that they are not following reinforces the patients' passivity and low self-efficacy. When a patient whose diabetes has been poorly controlled for many years says, "I don't know, what do you think?" in response to being asked what they want to do about her illness, the clinician should not answer the question. Rather the clinician should kindly but firmly insist that the patient answer the question in terms of the patient's own concerns and perceptions of the barriers to change.

The alternative therapeutic response to the self-destructive denier requires clinicians to do the one thing they are most unprepared to do: accept the self-destructive behavior and denial itself as the real problem. First and most important, clinicians must create an environment where patients are truly comfortable expressing all their feelings about their self-destructive behavior, including reasons that they *want to persist* in the self-destructive behavior. The keys to working with self-destructive deniers are to:

1. Accept the health-related behavior itself as existing for good reasons that will require the clinician's compassionate understanding and attention.
2. Assess the patient's readiness for change, as outlined by Prochaska and DiClemente,[4] and use interventions that are appropriate for the patient's stage (discussed in Chap. 8). Define success as progression from one stage to the next. Patients' ability to change habitual behavior is limited, and clinicians' ability to produce that change even more limited.
3. Resist the temptation to tell the patient what to do and maintain a focus on returning the responsibility for making change to the patient.

This section described four types of personality pathologies. These abrasive personality types make

[4]Prochaska JO, DiClemente CC, Norcross JC: In search of how people change. Applications to addictive behaviors. *American Psychologist* 47:1102, 1992.

up the second common characteristic of patients experienced as difficult. In the following section, we discuss the third common characteristic: somatization.

Somatization

Somatization and subversion of the health care process by "nonmedical problems" (the cause of one fourth of the general problems in the clinician–patient relationship) have a common feature: the need of patients and their families to cope with life stress by attributing the sick role to the patients. Somatization is discussed in detail in Chap. 15. The present chapter will only deal with two aspects of somatization that render patients particularly difficult. The first is somatization in the context of the patient's family system. The second is somatization as an adaptive strategy—achieved at great cost to somatizing patients and representing the best the patients and their families can do to cope with circumstances whose demands exceed their ability to cope in other ways.

When somatization is associated with particularly high levels of clinician frustration or difficulty, the clinician should initially proceed as outlined in the chapter devoted to that subject. Additionally, four further steps should be taken:

1. *Analyze* the family system and bring the pain into the room.
2. *Reframe* attention to underlying psychosocial issues as worthy of attention in their own right.
3. *Empathetically witness* the patient's and family's efforts to cope with their difficulties.
4. *Refer* for further treatment: family or individual therapy, self-help group, or other treatment program.

These steps are discussed in detail below.

Step 1: Analyze the Family System and Bring the Pain into the Room

Because somatization is embedded in family dynamics, clinicians need to discover how the physical symptoms and the sick role they create are needed and sustained by the patterns of interaction in the patient's family system. One technique for analyzing a family system is to conduct a "genogram-based interview." In this instance, the clinician draws a family tree with the patient and discusses the role of illness in the family, particularly the responses of other members of the family to the patient's symptoms and sick role status. Once the genogram is constructed it is usually possible to anticipate the areas of psychosocial stress by examining the family's life cycle stage and considering the tasks that are inevitably challenging during that stage.

MARIA COSTELLO *Maria Costello is a 32-year-old single mother with hypertension and classic tension headaches. Her mother lives alone nearby. Maria lives with her three daughters, ages 16, 4, and 2, who have two different fathers. She has seen many clinicians for her chronic headaches, and she has had extensive work-ups, including several MRIs. Her headaches respond intermittently to nonsteroidal anti-inflammatory medication or Tylenol. She is a one-recurring-symptom dependent clinger: always grateful for the clinician's attention, never angry or dissatisfied, resigned to the inevitable recurrence of her headaches, and always needing to talk for what feels like a very long time about how bad they are. Her genogram is shown in Figure 12-1.*

Maria's family can be characterized by two family life cycle stages: Maria is a single mother with young children and a teenager. Primary tasks for these life cycle stages include providing childcare for the young children and guiding the teenager in developing independence outside the immediate boundaries of the family.

A few screening questions can rapidly test the hypotheses that are generated by examining the genogram. These questions have to do with the life cycle tasks, the effect that the somatic symptoms have on accomplishing these tasks, and the responses of other family members to the symptoms. For example, the clinician could ask the following questions:

- How are you doing with taking care of the young ones?

Figure 12-1

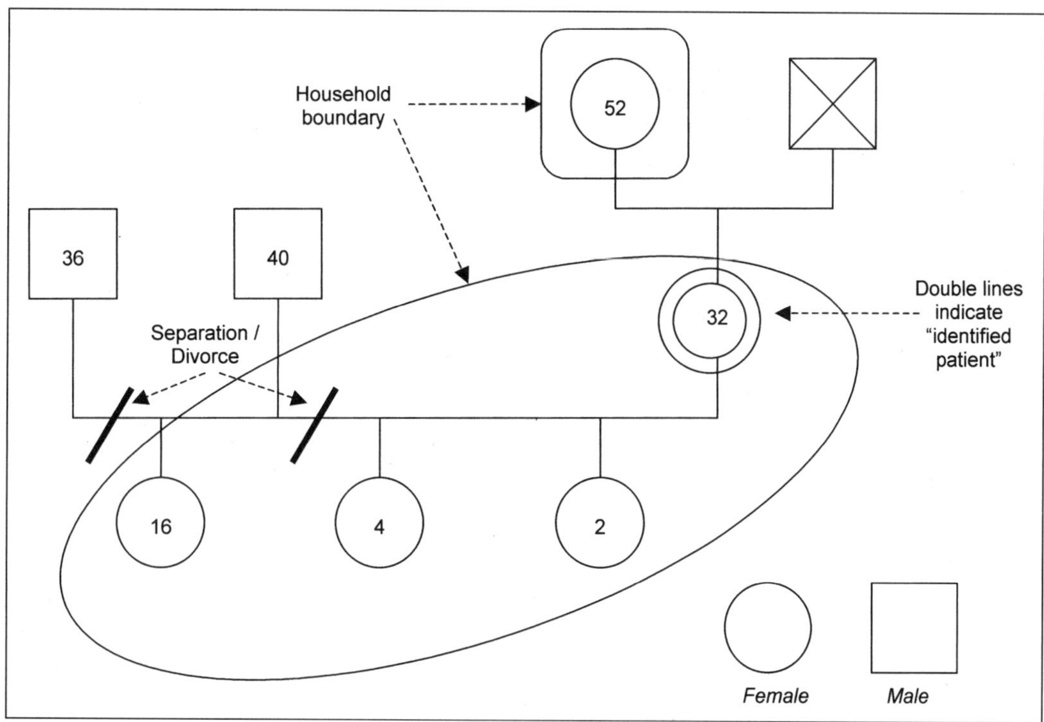

Genogram of a single mother with headaches.

- When you have a headache, how does it affect your ability to take care of your 2- and 4-year-olds?
- When you are having difficulty with your headache, what does your mother say or do?
- When you have the headaches, who helps you out with the young children?

In Maria's case it is not surprising to learn that she is willing to ask her mother for help with the children when she has a headache but not otherwise, and that her mother will help when asked but never volunteers. Maria's 16-year-old engages in the usual arguments with her mother about freedom of action, but will back off if she sees that her mother has a headache. She is also more willing to care for her younger half sisters when her mom is not feeling well.

As the patient tells her story, it is critical to support expression of the feelings associated with the story. It is necessary to "bring the pain into the room" (the clinician's office), because the pain and distress caused by the family dysfunction will be the motivation and rationale for the second and third steps of the intervention. This step is complete when the clinician (1) understands the basic nature of the family dysfunction, (2) understands how the symptom and associated sick role function in the family system, and (3) has helped the patient to express the emotional distress associated with the family dysfunction.

Step 2: Reframing Attention to the Underlying Psychosocial Issues

The task of reframing is simply to establish that the psychosocial issues are important in their own right, in addition to the physical symptoms. The clinician could say, "It seems to me that the difficulties you are having caring for your three daughters are at least as painful as your headaches and are worth paying attention to." In reframing, it is helpful to distinguish between the somatizing patient's goal and the patient's strategy. For example, one of Maria's goals is to obtain assistance in caring for her young children, and her strategy is to adopt the sick role so that others will be willing to help her. The appropriate reframe would include a statement such as, "You know, even if you are the picture of perfect health and never have a headache, you will still need some assistance in caring for your children so that you can take care of some of the other important needs you have in your life."

Step 3: Empathic Witnessing

Empathic witnessing is a powerful intervention that takes the generic form, "I am truly impressed with how well you are doing (or how hard you are trying), despite all the difficulties you have to deal with." This statement can be tremendously empowering if it is based on the kind of authentic understanding achieved by analyzing the patient's family system and bringing the pain into the room. For example, "Maria, I am tremendously impressed by how well you are able to manage with your children despite having so little assistance." It is useful to validate and praise the patient's motivation, and this can be done even if the patient is failing. If, in fact, you are not impressed with how well Maria is doing, and both of you know it, then the proper form of the empathic witnessing would be, "I can see that you very much want to be good mother." Empathic witnessing also helps clinicians address problems that they believe are beyond their expertise. Primary care clinicians need to be relieved of the burden of feeling that it is their role to fix the psychosocial problems that they encounter in their patients, but need to have some alternative response to do so.

Step 4: Referral for Further Treatment

Once clinicians decide that a patient should be referred for further treatment, they must decide how to approach the topic with the patient. Referrals to mental health resources that are presented in terms of the psychosomatic hypothesis (i.e., that the patient's physical symptoms are due to psychological distress) are often resisted and rejected. Reframing can go a long way in destigmatizing a mental health referral, because it bases the referral on an understanding of the patient's problems shared during the family assessment interview rather than on a stigmatizing diagnostic label. Empathically witnessing the patient's efforts to cope can also destigmatize the intervention by supporting the patient's "healthy" efforts at dealing with an overwhelming problem. The advantage of reframing is that the patients do not have to accept that their symptoms have anything to do with their family problems; they only have to accept that the family problems themselves are worthy of attention.

Very often patients will reject a referral for mental health intervention no matter how skillfully and empathically executed. However, once the clinician has engaged in all four steps of the family intervention, the clinician–patient relationship is irrevocably changed. On subsequent visits the encounter can begin with an inquiry about the family situation. Another full family assessment is not needed because the initial assessment will be remembered if the pain was brought into the room. Therefore, the clinician can quickly move on to restate the reframe, empathically witness the patient's efforts, and inquire about the patient's pursuit of therapy.

MARIA COSTELLO (CONTINUED) *Dr. West: "Maria, how are things going with the childcare situation?"*

Maria: "I'm still only getting help from Mom when she knows I have a headache."

Dr. West: "It must be so difficult for you having to take care of your children with so little help. I'm impressed with how much you respect your mother's time and with how hard you have to work to take care of your family. Have you followed up with that referral for therapy?"

Maria: "Not yet, I've been so busy."

Dr. West: "I understand, you're really in a jam. You have difficulty asking your Mom for help, so you don't have the time to follow up on therapy, and that's where you might be able to learn how to ask for help a little better."

Maria: "I know, kind of stupid, huh?"

Dr. West: "Not at all stupid, very understandable and difficult, but maybe you could work it out to get some help at the community mental health center like we talked about."

Maria: "I'll try, thanks."

Dr. West: "OK then, let's check your blood pressure."

Eventually Maria will go for therapy. In the meantime the clinician's encounters with her have radically changed. What used to be a prolonged discussion of physical symptoms has now become a brief but sympathetic update on her family problems. The discussion does not need to be long because both patient and clinician have the shared experience of the initial family assessment interview. Treatment of depression has also lessened the intensity of Maria's distress, and the clinician is no longer experiencing as much difficulty in caring for Maria, even though her symptoms are unresolved.

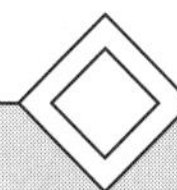

Developing Expertise in Managing Patients Experienced as Difficult

Patients experienced as difficult bring an intense burden of psychiatric and behavioral pathology into the primary care encounter. The prevalence of these problems in primary care patients is high enough to make basic expertise in the management of common psychiatric and behavioral disorders a necessary part of the primary care armamentarium. Nevertheless, the severity and complexity of the psychosocial problems encountered in patients experienced as difficult can easily exceed the skills and knowledge of a well-trained primary care clinician. Therefore, it is useful to develop a multidisciplinary team or consultation and referral resources to help manage patients experienced as difficult. Members of such a team will vary according to the setting, but could include psychiatrists, psychologists, social workers, substance abuse counselors, and treatment programs. Although mental health professionals may have expertise in the diagnosis and management of psychopathology, family systems dysfunction, or substance abuse, they may not be attuned to the needs of a primary care provider trying to untangle the effects that this pathology has on the clinician–patient relationship. The primary care provider may need to help consultants develop an interest in providing clinician–patient relationship-centered assistance rather than just patient-centered consultative assistance.

Encounters with difficult patients offer clinicians an opportunity to discover a great deal about themselves and about the struggles of life in general. Caring for patients experienced as difficult requires sensitivity to internal emotional experience and understanding of the connection between feelings and actions. Caring for difficult patients can heighten admiration for the creative determination of the human spirit struggling to cope with adversity despite limited resources. Taking care of patients experienced as difficult offers an opportunity to contemplate healing where the pursuit of cure and the power of treatment begin to falter. The challenge of caring for difficult patients may prove to be a gift, a high road for personal growth and development, and a nudge toward self-exploration that has benefit far beyond the particular situations described in this chapter.

Suggested Reading

Carter EA, McGoldrick M: *The Changing Family Life Cycle: A Framework for Family Therapy,* 2nd ed. New York: Gardner Press; 1988.

The conceptual model of a family life cycle is a powerful guide to understanding sources of stress and dysfunction in family systems.

Groves JE: Taking care of the hateful patient. *N Engl J Med* 298:883, 1978.

A classic description of difficult personality types in medical care.

Hahn SR: The difficult doctor-patient relationship questionnaire: DDPRQ. In: Maruish M (ed): *Handbook of Psychological Testing in Primary Care Settings.* Mahwah, NJ: Lawrence Erlbaum; 2000.

A detailed summary of the research literature on clinician-experienced difficulty, including a description of the Difficult Doctor Patient Relationship Questionnaire.

Hahn SR: Working with specific populations: Families. In: Feldman MD, Christensen JF (eds): *Behavioral Medicine in Primary Care: A Practical Guide.* Stamford, CT: Appleton & Lange; 1997, p 57.

An overview of a family system approach to patients in primary care.

Hahn SR, Kroenke K, Williams JBW, et al: Primary care evaluation of mental disorders: PRIME-MD. In Maruish M (ed): *Handbook of Psychological Testing in Primary Care Settings.* Mahwah, NJ: Lawrence Erlbaum; 2000.

An overview of the epidemiology, diagnosis, and management of psychopathology in the primary care setting.

McGoldrick M, Gerson R: *Genograms in Family Assessment.* New York: Norton; 1985.

How to explore family systems using genogram based interviewing and the family life cycle.

Prochaska JO, DiClemente CC, Norcross JC: In search of how people change. Applications to addictive behaviors. *Am Psychol* 47:1102, 1992.

An introduction to the concept of stages of behavioral change in helping patients with habitual health related problems.

Bibliography

Groves JE: Taking care of the hateful patient. *N Engl J Med* 298:883, 1978.

Hahn SR: Working with specific populations: Families. In: Feldman MD, Christensen JF (eds): *Behavioral Medicine in Primary Care: A Practical Guide.* Stamford, CT: Appleton & Lange; 1997, p 57.

Hahn SR, Feiner JS, Bellin EH: The doctor-patient-family relationship: A compensatory alliance. *Ann Intern Med* 109:884, 1998.

Hahn SR, Kroenke K, Williams JB, et al: Primary care evaluation of mental disorders (PRIME-MD). In: Maruish ME (ed): *The Use of Psychological Testing for Treatment Planning and Outcomes Assessment,* 2nd ed. Mahwah, NJ: Lawrence Erlbaum; 2000.

Hahn SR, Kroenke K, Spitzer RL, et al: The difficult patient: Prevalence, psychopathology, and functional impairment. *J Gen Intern Med* 11:1, 1996.

Hahn SR, Thompson KS, Stern V, et al: The difficult doctor-patient relationship: Somatization, personality and psychopathology. *J Clin Epidemiol* 47:647, 1994.

Jackson JL, Kroenke K: Difficult patient encounters in the ambulatory clinic: Clinical predictors and outcomes. *Arch Intern Med* 159:1069, 1999.

Kleinman A, Eisenberg L, Good B: Culture, illness, and care: Clinical lessons from anthropologic and cross-cultural research. *Ann Intern Med* 88:251, 1978.

Kroenke K, Jackson JL, Chamberlin J: Depressive and anxiety disorders in patients presenting with physical complaints: Clinical predictors and outcome. *Am J Med* 103:339, 1997.

Kroenke K, Spitzer RL, Williams JBW, et al: Physical symptoms in primary care: Predictors of psychiatric disorders and functional impairment. *Arch Fam Med* 3:774, 1994.

Lin EHB, Katon W, Von Korff M, et al: Frustrating patients: Clinician and patient perspectives among distressed high users of medical services. *J Gen Intern Med* 6:241, 1991.

McGaghie WC, Whitenack DC: A scale for measurement of the problem patient labeling process. *J Nerv Ment Disord* 170:598, 1982.

Merrill JM, Laux L, Thornby JI: Troublesome aspects of the patient-clinician relationship: A study of human factors. *S Med J* 80:1211, 1987.

Schwenk TL, Marquez JT, Lefever D, et al: Clinician and patient determinants of difficult clinician–patient relationships. *J Fam Pract* 28:59, 1989.

Sharpe M, Mayou R, Seagroatt V, et al: Why do doctors find some patients difficult to help? *Q J Med* 87:187, 1994.

Parsons, T: Definitions of health and illness in the light of American values and social structure. In: Jaco EG (ed): *Patients, Clinicians, and Illness.* Glencoe, Il: The Free Press; 1958, p 165.

Prochaska JO, DiClemente CC, Norcross JC: In search of how people change. Applications to addictive behaviors. *Am Psychol* 47:1102, 1992.

Spitzer RL, Williams JBW, Kroenke K, et al: Utility of a new procedure for diagnosing mental disorders in primary care: The PRIME-MD 1000 study. *JAMA* 272:1749, 1994.

Weissman MM. Broadhead WE, Olfson M, et al: A diagnostic aid for detecting (DSM-IV) mental disorders in primary care. *Gen Hosp Psychiatry* 20:1, 1998.

Kelly Derbin
Allen Perkins

Noncooperation

Introduction

Doctor Hibbert: Homer, I'm afraid you'll have to undergo a coronary bypass operation.
Homer: Say it in English, Doc.
Doctor Hibbert: You're going to need open heart surgery.
Homer: Spare me your medical mumbo-jumbo.
Doctor Hibbert: We're going to cut you open and tinker with your ticker.
Homer: Could you dumb it down a shade?

—"Homer's Triple Bypass"
The Simpsons

The teenaged parents in the emergency room with a sick child, the 55-year-old Hispanic female with a strong family history of breast cancer, the homeless patient with active tuberculosis (TB), and the 40-year-old heavy smoker with early emphysema all have one thing in common. Their doctor will ask them to embark on a course of treatment or to change their behavior. They may choose to follow the doctor's instructions, but it is almost as likely that they will not. Failure to follow the prescribed course of action may place them at risk of worsening health, disability, and even death. The clinician may never know if these patients cooperate.

The purpose of this chapter is to give the primary care clinician an appreciation of the scope of patient noncooperation, the factors that contribute to this phenomenon, and a useful management plan to minimize its effect. We will start with a discussion of the importance of noncooperation. This includes the prevalence, cost, morbidity, and mortality associated with clinician–patient noncooperation. In the next section we identify some key concepts, including a quick review of the evolution of the concept of noncooperation, a brief discussion of the concept of "readiness to change," and the different models of the clinician–patient relationship and how this relationship can affect cooperation.

We will then discuss specific types of clinical interventions and how noncooperation might alter outcomes. These include medication use, diagnostic testing, and life-style changes. Within each of these categories we will pay specific attention to clinician, patient, clinician–patient, and system barriers.

The next section is a discussion of special problems including literacy, racial and ethnic issues, and the role of religious beliefs or differing values. Finally, we will suggest specific recommendations that all have a basis in the evidence-based scientific literature, although not all are equally tested. These are arranged in tabular form for easy review and discussed in depth in the text. The chapter concludes with a summary of the important points.

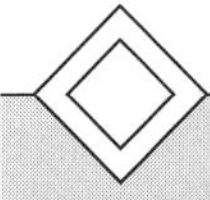

What Is Noncooperation in Primary Care?

Noncooperation affects all aspects of clinical care, and attention to it is of paramount importance in daily interactions with all patients. Like a child's fever, noncooperation is only a symptom that requires further investigation into its cause. Table 13-1 describes the different faces of noncooperation.

Scope of Noncooperation

Between 10 and 20 percent of appointments made by patients are not kept. When the patient is sent for a diagnostic test, nonattendance jumps even higher. When you send a patient home with a prescription, about 30 percent of patients will not get it filled, and for those who do, the chances of them completing a 10-day course of therapy are only about 80 percent. Patients placed on long-term medication for a chronic disease will take the prescribed medication 50 percent of the time. Life-style changes can be even more chal-

Table 13-1
The Different Faces of Noncooperation

Type of Interaction	Example of Potential Problem
Clinician does not ask about medication coverage. Patient does not fill prescription.	The parents of a 2-year-old discharged from ED do not pick up the prescribed antibiotic because they cannot afford it.
Clinician does not write out instructions. Patient doesn't take medication properly.	The patient with hypertension who only takes medication when symptoms occur.
Clinician does not encourage feedback about medication side effects. Patient discontinues medication without consulting clinician.	A 45-year-old man discovers the β-blocker given post-MI has caused impotence.
Patient doesn't refill medication.	A prescription expires and the patient cannot get a follow-up appointment for 3 weeks, so goes without.
Patient does not follow-up as recommended.	A 3-month-old treated for an ear infection misses 2-week follow up appointment because the mother has no transportation.
Patient does not have recommended test done.	A 55-year-old woman on estrogen replacement doesn't show up for scheduled mammogram.
Patient does not go to specialty appointment.	A 45-year-old woman with breast mass does not show for surgical appointment for fear of cancer.
Patient does not make life-style changes recommended.	A 25-year-old smoker with bronchitis refuses to consider quitting.
Clinician does not address the patient's concerns about therapy. Patient seeks unconventional therapy.	A 44-year-old goes to pharmacy inquiring about herbal hormone replacement therapy.

lenging; 30 percent of patients succeed in changing diet, and only 5 percent give up tobacco. If you recommend a mammogram, there is only a 30 percent chance the patient will have it done, according to Nockowitz.

Generally, clinical providers markedly underestimate the prevalence of noncooperation, but the problem is pervasive in clinical medicine. When clinicians formulate a therapeutic plan, they must consider noncooperation as part of every aspect of their patient's care. The differential diagnosis of treatment failure or recurrence of disease must include noncooperation.

To further complicate matters, it is difficult to predict which patients will have trouble following a treatment plan. Unfortunately, patients' attitudes in the office are not an accurate indication of their cooperation once they leave. In fact, it would not be overly pessimistic to determine which patients will follow treatment plans by flipping a coin.

How to Detect Noncooperation

Attempting to objectively quantify noncooperation is not clinically useful. Measurement techniques used in clinical trials, such as medication refill rates, pill counts, and electronic medication monitors, are not practical for the daily practice routine, although computerized tracking systems may change this. A better way to identify medication compliance is to ask, in a nonjudgmental way, "Many people have difficulty taking medications. Has this been a problem for you?" Approximately 55 percent of partially or totally noncompliant patients will identify themselves in response to such a question. However, Steiner found that they will tend to overestimate how often they are capable of cooperating.

The other measure of cooperation is therapeutic response to treatment. When a patient fails to improve, we are trained to reconsider our diagnosis and treatment. We should also remember to consider and explore cooperation issues.

What Is the Cost of Noncooperation?

The total direct dollar cost of noncooperation is difficult to estimate. For the patient, costs include loss of treatment benefit as well as increased morbidity and mortality. Clinician costs include duplicated efforts, diminished job satisfaction, and unnecessary expenses for patients whose care is covered by capitated contracts. The cost to the system is one of decreased efficiency and excess capacity. Direct costs of noncooperation to the entire community include the costs of up to 33 percent of all prescription medications that are filled but not used, the cost of the 5 percent of all hospital admissions that could have been avoided, and the cost of unmeasured long-term disability and premature deaths, according to Nockowitz.

What Are the Effects on Morbidity and Mortality?

Total morbidity and mortality as a consequence of noncooperation is unknown. For each type of disease studied, there is a measurable increase in morbidity when the clinician's treatment plan is not followed. For some infectious diseases, such as tuberculosis and HIV, the consequences of noncooperation not only accrue to the patient but to other members of society. For chronic diseases, such as diabetes mellitus, the consequences of noncooperation may not become apparent for decades, but include significant complications such as limb amputation, dialysis, and premature death. Noncooperation during acute illnesses leads to negative consequences sooner. For example, if pneumonia is only partially treated, it will result in delayed recovery with further loss of work time. Thus, noncooperation in contagious, chronic, and acute illness leads to significant morbidity and mortality.

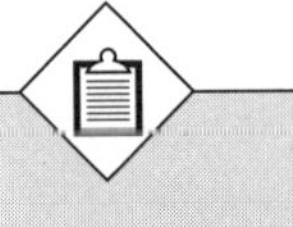

Definitions and Underlying Concepts

As it became possible to significantly alter the course of disease with medication, it became increasingly important for patients to cooperate with a treatment plan. Patients who did not take medications as directed did not achieve the full benefit of therapy. The problem was labeled failure to adhere to the therapeutic regimen; no one stopped to consider whether these patients were influenced by their belief system, life circumstance, or clinical understanding.

Traditionally, noncooperative behavior was thought of as a patient problem. Patients who did not adhere to their treatment regimen were labeled as noncompliant, nonadherent, or "difficult." The term we prefer to use is *noncooperation,* which implies the problem is not the sole responsibility of the patient, but lies with the clinician–patient dyad. As stated by Steiner, "Compliance is a crucial link between the process of medical care (the interaction between clinician and patient) and the outcomes of care (the physiologic and functional consequences of treatment)."[1]

Noncooperation can be simplistically viewed as the patient's defiance of the clinician's order,

[1]Steiner JF: Compliance. In: Fihn SD, DeWitt DE (eds): *Outpatient Medicine,* 2nd ed. Philadelphia, PA: Saunders; 1998, p 773.

or it can be less judgmentally defined as the extent to which a person's behavior fails to coincide with medical advice. In a more complex model, called the Therapeutic Decision Model, there are three responses to therapeutic recommendations: *rejection, acceptance,* or *modification* of the clinician's advice and instructions (Fig. 13-1).

Some patients feel that accepting treatment signifies accepting an illness. They may thus symbolically deny their illness by rejecting treatment. Dowell and Hudson found that for these patients, encouraging "just" a trial period of the treatment regimen could lead to more genuine acceptance of the treatment. For example, a depressed patient who does not feel comfortable acknowledging his mood disorder may agree to test a selective serotonin reuptake inhibitor (SSRI) for 3 months, receive real benefits from the course of medication, and then accept the need for continued treatment.

What truly constitutes noncooperation? Is it simply not taking a medication? Eating "forbidden" foods? Skipping a follow-up appointment? Refusing chemotherapy for cancer? Before we, as clinical practitioners, decide what constitutes noncooperation, we must first ask ourselves if there is evidence that the treatment we are recommending is beneficial. Would refusing this treatment be a reasonable choice for the patient? Clinician and patient may agree that *nontreatment* is a valid option. Refusing chemotherapy, for example, can be a carefully considered decision and not noncooperation at all.

Over the past several decades, medicine has removed its emphasis on the paternalistic clinician and now stresses patient autonomy and empowerment. This means that even when our patients make choices that we do not agree with, we must respect them as people. When their deci-

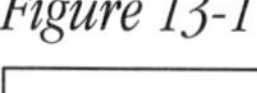

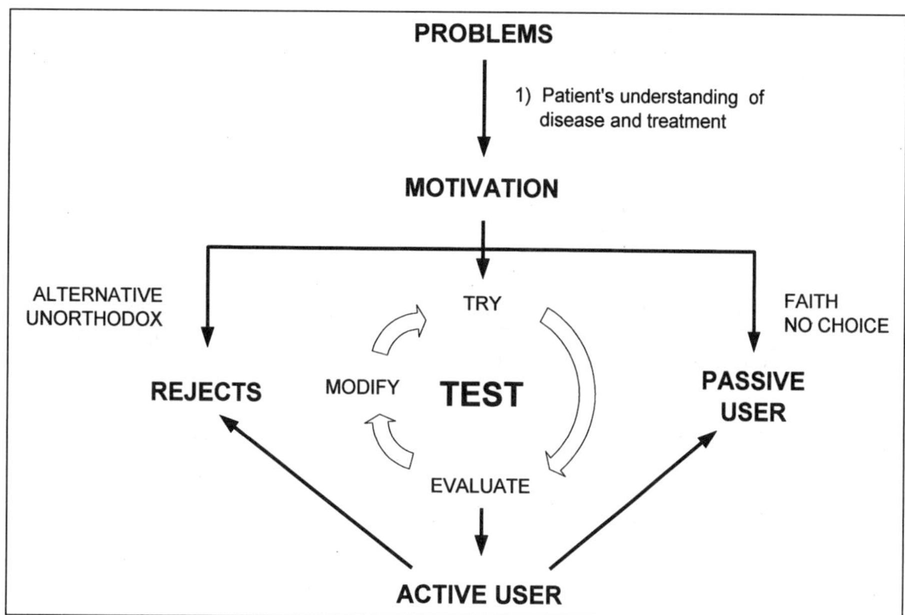

Patients respond to therapeutic recommendations in one of three ways: *rejection, acceptance,* or *modification.* While some patients accept and follow their clinician's recommendations, others symbolically deny their illness by rejecting treatment, and still others modify the clinician's recommendations to a way they find acceptable. *(Adapted from Dowell J, Hudson H: A qualitative study of medication-taking behaviour in primary care. Family Practice 14:369, 1997.)*

sions conflict with our personal belief systems, this can be a daunting task.

What Is "Readiness to Change"?

Some of the most difficult and frustrating "prescriptions" we give our patients are for changes in life style or behavior. DiMatteo reports that more than 70 percent of patients do not actually follow recommended life-style changes such as dietary recommendations. When the recommended changes involve ending addictive behavior such as tobacco use, the rates of noncooperation increase to 90 to 95 percent, according to O'Connell. Counseling such patients can seem nothing short of futile; however, understanding their readiness to change may help both patients and clinicians.

DiClemente and Prochaska proposed that patients move through predictable stages in their paths to change.[2]

These stages are:

- Precontemplation
- Contemplation
- Preparation/determination
- Action
- Maintenance
- Relapse

Familiarity with this model can allow the clinician to determine a patient's progression toward change and assist with predictable pitfalls and relapses.

Patients in the precontemplation stage have a problem, but they minimize or deny it and may get defensive when asked about it. Patients might be so embarrassed or demoralized that it is difficult to identify their stage. The clinician should always express concern and inquire about the patient's feelings. Clinicians may identify extremely defensive patients as precontemplative, but they may actually be at the relapse or contemplation stage.

Patients in the contemplation stage are actively thinking about the problem and its solution. This stage can last for many years. Patients who appear suddenly to throw away their cigarettes or quit drinking have probably been silently in the contemplation stage for quite some time. The clinician's role here is to offer support and encourage action.

Patients really begin to pick up energy and commitment in the preparation stage. They begin to make specific plans of action and should be encouraged to do so. The clinician can play an important role in helping to point out potential pitfalls, especially in regard to the patient's "support network." For example, the patient's spouse who smokes can sabotage the patient's efforts to quit smoking and spouses of alcoholics may not cope well with their recovering alcoholic partner.

In the action stage, patients follow the plan they have created. The patient's strategy may not correspond exactly to the plan you recommended. The 20 minutes of daily exercise you advised may become twice weekly water aerobics. It is important not to criticize or minimize the progress the patient has made. In the action stage, the patient may suffer from second thoughts and will need high levels of support from everyone. A clinician should be watchful if a patient is well into the action stage without a long-term plan to avoid relapse.

Patients in the maintenance stage have managed a period of success. Now they must be prepared for both expected and unexpected obstacles to ultimate success. At this point, patients may grow weary, and their desire to maintain improvement may decline. The clinician and the patient should not become discouraged by the most likely outcome of the initial attempt at behavior change—relapse.

Relapse is a natural part of the model. Life-style changes and addictive behavior often require several unsuccessful attempts before a patient achieves long-term success. The clinician can help keep the patient from becoming too discouraged. Each relapse should be regarded as a learning opportunity for future success.

Effects of the Clinician–Patient Relationship

The clinician–patient interaction is the basis upon which "the accuracy and completeness of patient

[2]DiClemente CC, Prochaska JO. Self-change and therapy change of smoking behavior: A comparison of processes of change in cessation and maintenance. *Addictive Behaviors* 7(2):133, 1982.

data, diagnostic accuracy, efficiency in the encounter, compliance, patient understanding of problems, and patient and clinician satisfaction"[3] are determined. The framework for the clinician–patient relationship is the medical interview, where up to 80 percent of diagnoses are made. The interview sets the tone and content for the problems that will be addressed.

Clinicians may view the interview as uncomplicated, but to many patients, the act of presenting for care is merely one step in a very complex illness event. A defective clinician–patient interaction will sabotage the therapeutic relationship. Patient satisfaction with the clinician–patient relationship has been shown by Lipkin to be one of the most powerful predictors of cooperation. The patient may not feel comfortable with advice the clinician gives and may elect to disregard all the recommendations.

Researchers have studied this relationship for many years and have identified elements and functions of the interview that, when used, improve outcomes. Knowing what works well during patient interviews helps identify what does not work—that is, the barriers to effective clinician–patient interaction.

Lipkin organizes these barriers into three categories: physical, psychological, and social. Physical barriers include disabilities that prevent clear communication and environmental obstacles, such as a noisy emergency room. Psychological barriers are conditions that cloud the relationship, such as depression, anxiety, or lack of trust. Social barriers are those caused by differences in language and culture. Other barriers to cooperation may be discordant expectations for the interaction or poor communication on the part of the clinician or patient.

In the past two decades, the relationship in Western medicine has changed from predominantly clinician paternalism to one with greater emphasis on patient autonomy. Table 13-2 illus-

Table 13-2

Four Models of Clinician–Patient Relationship

Model	Goals, Obligations, Values
Paternalistic	1. Clinician determines interventions based on patient needs and well-being 2. Clinician presents limited information to enlist patient compliance. 3. Shared objective criteria for best therapy is assumed; thus, there is no need for patient input.
Informative	1. Clinician provides all options, patient makes decision, and clinician executes. 2. Clinician must give patient all pertinent information as he or she is sole decision maker; clinician interpretation of patient values not relevant. 3. Assumes clinician acts as purveyor of technical expertise only. 4. Clinician is obligated to provide truthful information, sufficient technical skills, and referral when appropriate.
Interpretive	1. Clinician must elucidate patient values and help patient to understand and use them. 2. Obligation of clinician similar to informative. 3. Clinician acts as a counselor or adviser of the patient.
Deliberative	1. Clinician elucidates patient values and identifies which are most helpful for the particular clinical situation. 2. Clinician and patient engage in a discussion of moral self-development and coercion is avoided. 3. Clinician acts as a friend or teacher.

Source: Modified from Emmanuel EJ, Emmanuel LL: Four models of the physician-patient relationship. *JAMA* 267:2221, 1992.

[3]O'Connell D: Behavior change. In: Christensen JF (ed): *Behavioral Medicine in Primary Care A Practical Guide.* Stamford, CT: Appleton & Lange; 1997, p 345.

trates four models of provider–patient relationships. These theoretical models contain one spectrum of patient "self-governing" and another of clinician involvement. The ideal relationship would be of one of shared decision making with mutual participation and respect. Of course, no single model is ideal, and aspects of each are appropriate in different clinical scenarios.

LESLIE TOLER *Leslie Toler was having problems early in pregnancy. On ultrasound, there is an intrauterine sac but no fetus, and her primary clinician was following labs to determine if she had an ectopic pregnancy. The patient later presented in the middle of the night to the emergency room with a low blood pressure, abdominal pain, and a large volume of fluid in the cul-de-sac. After only the briefest explanation of what was going on, Ms. Toler was hurriedly given a consent form, told to sign at the bottom, and rushed to the operating room where she underwent emergency surgery for a ruptured ectopic pregnancy.*

In this situation, it was not appropriate to engage in a long dialogue about treatment options. The clinician acted in a "paternalistic" manner and the patient received life-saving treatment without delay. However, in most clinician–patient encounters, attention to the entire provider–patient relationship is necessary.

An effective approach to clinical relationships recommended by Lowes is one of accountability. Both patient and clinical provider must work to create a clinician–patient *partnership*, with patient-centered care as the emphasis. Clinicians should encourage patients to be actively involved in planning their health care and to take responsibility for their health. This clinician–patient relationship is very complex, reflecting therapeutic needs, societal changes, and the individual biases of both the clinician and the patient.

Poor communication is commonly at the root of noncooperation, according to Joos and colleagues. Even optimal communication can be negated by a lack of trust by one party toward the other. Should the interaction take place in a setting of limited continuity, such as the emergency room, the clinician who does not initially work to establish trust will commonly find patients not cooperating. Patients seek to identify clinicians who are worthy of their trust and will dismiss advice from clinicians who fail their test. One study by Beardon and associates linked nonredemption of prescriptions with level of training of the clinician. It was suggested that the patient's lack of confidence in an inexperienced clinician might increase the risk of noncooperation.

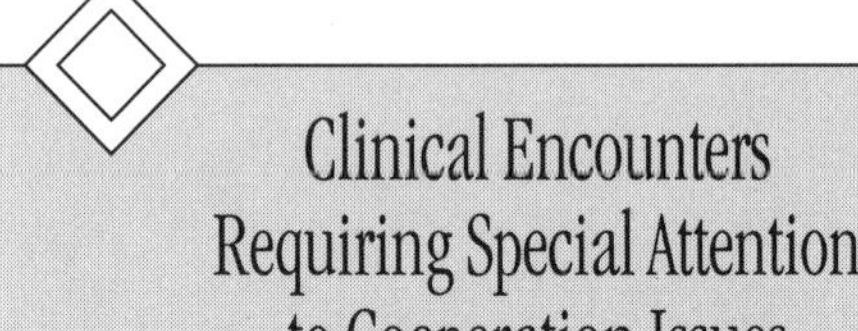

Clinical Encounters Requiring Special Attention to Cooperation Issues

In this section, we describe clinical encounters around three issues: medication use, diagnostic testing, and what we call "special issues." Each of these types of encounters requires attention to the patient–clinician relationship to encourage cooperation.

Medication Use

When you recommend the use of medication, writing a prescription for your patient is only the first step. The prescription may never be filled, or if filled, never taken. The patient may take it improperly, discontinue the medication prematurely, or fail to refill the prescription as directed. Patients are less likely to cooperate if the treatment is long term, requires multiple medications and doses (more than 1 to 2 per day), or has poorly tolerated side effects.

Nonredemption of prescriptions has been reported to range from 18 to 30 percent. It has been hypothesized that reduced cost of medication or free medication would improve these rates; however, there are conflicting data on whether reducing costs increases the rate at which people redeem prescriptions. Several studies reviewed by Haynes failed to show an increase in cooperation when medications (prenatal vitamins and antipsychotic medications) were provided free or at a markedly reduced rate. Thus, the reasons for nonredemption of prescriptions are still not fully understood.

It has been shown that cooperation is generally better with short-term regimens than long-term regimens. DiMatteo reports that approximately 80 percent of patients follow through on short-term medication regimens, while the rate decreases to 50 to 60 percent for patients on long-term medications. Leenen and colleagues report a modest difference in cooperation rates between once daily and twice daily medications, but this rate markedly declines with greater than twice daily dosing.

How do we define medication cooperation? Most studies rely upon the same definition used in clinical trials: taking more than 80 percent of prescribed medication is considered full cooperation, taking 20 to 79 percent is considered partial cooperation, and taking less than 20 percent is noncooperation. The rates of medication cooperation included in the "fully cooperative" category is sufficient to maintain the therapeutic effect for most drugs. Partially cooperative patients take their medications in an erratic manner, with correspondingly variable therapeutic results. Those in the noncooperative group take little or no medication, thus receiving no therapeutic benefit.

When medical conditions pose a public health threat, 80 percent compliance is not acceptable. The treatment of active TB inherently carries multiple risk factors for noncooperation, including multiple medications, unpleasant side effects, and extensive length of treatment. Yet, inadequate treatment of active TB creates a 50 percent risk of death for the patient and the resulting contagion puts the entire community at risk. To ensure adequate cooperation, directly observed therapy must be used in some cases. Although this is obviously an expensive and perhaps extreme solution, it is one option in a spectrum of management modalities for noncooperation.

Another disease process being targeted for cooperation interventions is AIDS. Even small lapses in cooperation can facilitate the emergence of drug resistant viruses and treatment failure. Research reveals that AIDS patients have somewhat different cooperation issues than other patients. The most important issues among AIDS patients are (1) how well the regimen "fits" with the their routine and (2) the patient's understanding that cooperation is directly related to viral resistance. Noncooperation among AIDS patients occurs for reasons different than among the general population. For this specific population, alcoholism and untreated depression are especially linked to noncooperation.

Patients with mental disorders such as schizophrenia require additional attention to facilitate cooperation. Although the affliction is symptomatic when not treated, effects of the disease, medication side effects, complex regimens, denial, and secondary gain from being ill all combine to make noncooperation a major source of treatment failure.

Clinician Barriers to Medication Use

There are many clinician-related barriers to cooperation surrounding medication use. The clinician, faced with competing demands for time, may fail to uncover the patient's unspoken concerns about the disease or treatment. According to Lipkin, patients commonly complain that clinicians do not provide them with enough information, a factor strongly linked to patient satisfaction. If the clinician does not listen to patients or discover their real agenda, the patients will leave dissatisfied with the interaction and may intentionally not cooperate with the therapeutic regimen. The intentional noncooperation may manifest itself as altering how the therapeutic regimen is carried out or not following the treatment plan at all.

PENELOPE LYLE *Penelope Lyle is 35 years old and has headaches. You learn that Penelope has a high school education and is a single mother of two children under the age of 5. She is working two jobs to cover day care costs, rent, and food. The father of the children is minimally involved and is not paying child support. When you initially evaluate her, she describes a pattern of* *headaches that is entirely consistent with tension headaches, and you prescribe your favorite remedy for these. You find out later that Penelope left dissatisfied and never filled her prescription. You were certain of your diagnosis, but Penelope continued to worry about the brain tumor she is sure that you failed to discover.*

How could this have been avoided? The patient may or may not have revealed her true concern. An astute clinician might sense the patient's hesitation and delve deeper to uncover the patient's belief system. One approach is simply to ask, "What are you worried about?" or "What do you think is wrong?"

Of course, the clinician's time is a valuable commodity with many competing demands upon it. It is understandable that he or she would hesitate to become involved in what may be perceived as time-intensive gathering of nonessential information. However, information gathering may not be as time costly as the clinician thinks. Lipkin found that generally, clinicians tend to *overestimate* the amount of time they spend conveying information to their patients and *underestimate* the amount of information their patients desire. We should be mindful of past criticism and make sure to spend enough time explaining diagnoses, prognoses, treatment options, and diagnostic procedures to our patients.

Clinicians are also at risk of providing information that is unintelligible to their patients. Although we have been socialized into a field with its own language and explanatory models, we are required to be the interface between illness, technology, and the patient. It is critical to avoid jargon or unnecessary complexity. However, "dumbing down" information for a knowledgeable patient can also be damaging. The interaction requires that clinicians understand the patient's level of knowledge and understanding.

Patient Barriers to Medication Use

Patient barriers can be divided into several areas: social circumstances, cultural background, and individual patient's attitudes or beliefs about illness. "Social circumstance" is a catchall term that includes factors related the individual (education and literacy), the family (support and/or dependency of other family members), and the community (community support and financial resources).

Finances can create an especially difficult barrier. Many patients do not have the health insurance they need to access the health care system. They therefore avoid health care until they perceive they are sick enough to warrant emergency department visits. Because there are not established clinician–patient relationships in the emergency department, these individuals are at even greater risk for noncooperation. Patients may not be able to pay for an expensive medication or even to afford the copayment for medication covered by insurance. It is our experience that patients will not voice these concerns unless they are comfortable with the clinician and the encounter.

Juan Ortiz *Juan Ortiz is a 45-year-old migrant farm worker who has been suffering from headaches, intermittent blurred vision, and fleeting episodes of chest pain over the past month. He is the sole income earner for his wife and three children. He is also trying to save money to send home to Mexico City so that his brother can come to the United States to make a better living. He was hiding his symptoms from his wife because he knew that they could not afford an expensive medical bill. Mr. Ortiz finally mentioned his symptoms in passing because his chest pain lasted longer than usual. His wife was angry and demanded that he go to the emergency department immediately. On arrival to the emergency department (ED) his blood pressure was 170/110. The ED physician did the usual tests looking for end organ damage from elevated blood pressure, which were unremarkable. Mr. Ortiz was discharged and told to follow-up next week with his primary care clinician. This was Mr. Ortiz' first contact with the U.S. medical system, and although he was not sure what a primary care clinician was, he was too embarrassed to ask. Because the ED discharged him, Mr. Ortiz decided that he must be fine and returned to work the next day. He did not schedule a follow-up clinic appointment to seek treatment for his hypertension.*

Cultural background may affect the patient's willingness to accept treatment out of the realm of familiar, traditional modalities, such as folk remedies. A clinician may inadvertently criticize a traditional treatment that the patient has been using at home. Additionally, some patients may have difficulty trusting a clinician from a different culture. For example, as described by Damrosch, some Vietnamese immigrants believe that Western medicine is too strong for them because they are constitutionally smaller and may decrease the dose any recommended medication by as much as half. Dowell and Hudson report that patients commonly seek health advice from practitioners outside the conventional health care system, in addition to accessing care from medical doctors. Patients who do not feel that the clinician validates their beliefs may not commit to the prescribed regimen.

If the patient's attitudes and beliefs are not addressed, the clinician–patient interaction is doomed from the beginning. Damrosch describes multiple theories regarding patient beliefs, including the Health Belief Model, self-efficacy theory, and the theory of reasoned action. She emphasizes five major factors that affect cooperation. Patients are more likely to cooperate when:

1. They perceive a high severity of illness and consequences.
2. They feel they are highly susceptible to the disease.
3. They are capable of performing a behavior to reduce their risk.
4. They are confident the treatment will reduce their risk.
5. They intend to perform the behavior.

Patients have an inherent desire to control aspects of their illness or treatment. As described earlier in the Therapeutic Decision Model, they may retain some measure of control by testing and modifying a treatment regimen (see Fig. 13-1).

We intuitively feel that educating patients about their diseases will increase cooperation. However, evidence shows that although patients who understand their illness have a higher rate of cooperation than those who do not, even highly knowledgeable patients will fail to follow instructions. While we should always make sure our patients receive adequate education about their disease process, that alone may not be sufficient to ensure cooperation.

Patient literacy may be a hidden barrier for some patients. You should consider literacy issues when offering written patient education materials or instructions. Trombatore reports that more than 40 million Americans are functionally illiterate. Many patients may try to hide the fact that they cannot read. We should be aware of this possibility and keep instructions simple as well as ask patients questions to verify them understanding. These issues are discussed further in the section on literacy.

Patient cooperation tends to decay over time. For patients on a limited course of therapy, this probably does not affect outcome to any large extent. For those who require lifetime therapy, however, cooperation decay can be a problem. We know that many patients tend to be partially cooperative, with better cooperation around certain days and times of day. Patients are often more cooperative in clinical trials than in practice settings. We do not have tools that are sensitive or specific enough to allow us to detect those patients who will not fully cooperate. Fortunately, many patients obtain benefit from partial cooperation. Selection of a medication with fewer side effects may be especially important with long-term regimens.

System Barriers to Medication Use

Our current health care system has many potential obstacles to medication cooperation, including, but not limited to, lack of health insurance (or underinsurance), frequent insurance policy changes (especially for employees whose employers are mandating changes), and lack of understanding about how to access care. One glaringly obvious barrier to cooperation in health care is the lack of access to health care for over 40 million uninsured Americans. These patients rarely have the opportunity to develop a longitudinal relationship with any clinical provider. How can a person that begins with this disadvantage navigate through the health care system and cooperate with treatment and follow-up? The health care system can present a confusing picture to patients or families who have limited experience with the system.

The increasing presence of managed care organizations and competition for company contracts can lead employers to jump from one health insurance plan to another, each of which offers different clinician panels. These changes lead to forced discontinuity for covered employees and the attendant negative influences on the clinician's knowledge of the patient, communication, and coordination of care. Both the clinician and the patient must work to overcome this obstacle. All of us have experienced the initially hostile patient who is frustrated by the health care system red tape. We, ourselves, may find the bureaucracy extremely irritating. It is important that both parties get past the frustration so it does not interfere with the care offered or the patient's willingness to accept it.

Diagnostic Testing

Much of what we do as clinicians is focused on data gathering. The history and physical exam provide the initial data for diagnosis and treatment. Diagnostic testing will further confirm or refute a clinical diagnosis, or identify disease in the asymptomatic individual through routine screening. To acquire this additional information, the clinician must first understand the various testing modalities and use them appropriately. The patient must then accept the necessity for the test and take the steps necessary to complete it. System barriers between the clinician, the patient, and the test can trigger noncooperation with diagnostic testing.

Clinician Barriers to Diagnostic Testing

The clinician's attitude affects the patient's decision to follow through with diagnostic and preventive services. If the clinician does not emphasize the need for the study or shows skepticism about its effectiveness, the patient is less likely to follow through. When the test is for screening purposes, patients who identify with a clinician are more likely to participate. If you personally recommend an annual Pap smear during a patient's visit, she will be more likely to present for one than if you merely send a postcard or rely on public health advertisements.

Patients being screened are often asymptomatic and clinicians must remind patients to take advantage of screening technology. The clinician who successfully offers screening is knowledgeable about screening protocols, takes advantage of all opportunities, selectively orders tests based on priorities, and has the medical record arranged to facilitate compliance with screening recommendations. The recommendations a clinician offers should be based on evidence and should link cooperation with acceptable outcomes.

Patient Barriers to Diagnostic Testing

Clinicians expect patients to complete the diagnostic work-up. If patients are concerned about the disease process, they are more likely to follow through with recommended tests. But if patients become convinced that their symptoms are not serious, or that the clinician is being overly cautious, they will be less likely to cooperate. The astute clinician is aware of potential barriers to finishing the testing, including transportation, logistics, child care, and other issues, and is willing to work with patients to overcome any roadblocks. The clinician may also consider a compromise with patients, perhaps postponing or canceling tests that present major obstacles.

Asymptomatic patients are most likely to fail to complete a diagnostic or screening work-up. They must independently complete a number of complex steps when complying with recommended guidelines for preventive services, such as scheduling an appointment time, arranging transportation and child care, and so on. If they are not sure their health insurance will pay for a recommended test on someone who "is not really sick," it only makes matters worse.

A system built around motivating patients should take the Health Belief Model into account. The patient should be allowed to modify recommendations within reason to take into account personal preferences, health beliefs, and shared decision-making. The clinician should take advantage of every opportunity to educate patients, recognizing that it may take several visits before the patient becomes an active partner.

Successful screening programs must rely heavily on external pressure. The patient obtaining annual cervical cancer screening is likely to be motivated by the desire to continue on oral contraception as much as she is motivated by her fear of cervical cancer. Postmenopausal women do not present as regularly for such screening, possibly because they no longer need contraception. If a system does not rely on pressure to encourage cooperation, the perceived risk must be high enough to encourage patients to work to overcome barriers such as transportation and childcare. For example, Ore and colleagues report that a system offering free mammography screenings for breast cancer only approached a 45 percent participation rate, even when written invitations were sent.

System Barriers to Diagnostic Testing

An obvious system barrier to the delivery of diagnostic services is the cost. Most diagnostic tests cost money, and many patients are unable or unwilling to pay large out-of-pocket costs for what they perceive to be a small benefit. The clinician is often asked to make a judgment for the patient regarding the relative value of a recommended test. The use of shared decision making in this setting will often help to release the clinician from dogmatic adherence to conventional recommendations.

More difficult to navigate are the structural barriers imposed by our changing health care system. Insurance companies continue to increase the barriers between the clinician and the desired test. Some of these are relatively minor, such as preauthorization based on standard protocols, or the need for approval by the primary care clinician for tests ordered by consultants. These barriers necessitate additional staff time and often result in minor delays in receiving care, but are easily surmountable if both the clinician and patient are motivated.

More worrisome is the tactic of reducing services by limiting the clinicians who can provide the service. This results in more lengthy delays of service and often creates insurmountable obstacles for patients. The clinician must work with the insurer to elucidate the consequences of delayed or absent care.

Finally, changes in monetary incentives that reward clinicians who severely limit diagnostic testing are a subtle but important potential obstacle. Patients should be able to trust the clinician to act in their best interest. Clinicians should not be rewarded for increasing barriers to care.

Life-Style Changes

A chapter on noncooperation would be incomplete without a discussion of life-style issues. Over 50 percent of excess morbidity and mortality in the United States can be attributed to unhealthy life-style choices, according to McGinnis. Whether consciously or unconsciously, many Americans choose to smoke, drink, drive recklessly, eat unhealthy foods, live violently, and otherwise risk premature death or long-term disability. For many diseases, life-style modification can be used therapeutically to prevent progression or cause regression. As clinicians, our most difficult task is to foster cooperation among our patients who must make life-style changes to prevent or alter the course of their disease. Some of these problems are discussed in Chap. 8.

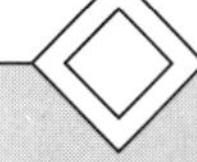

Special Issues in Noncooperation

Literacy and cultural issues play an important role in patients' ability to cooperate with clinicians' care recommendations.

Patients with Poor Literacy Skills May Fail to Cooperate

A large portion of the patient population is assumed to be literate but is not. Poor literacy skills affect one in five adults in the United States. There are multiple risk factors for low literacy, including low socioeconomic status, ethnic minority classification, immigrant status, unemployment, less than a high school education, and being over 60 years of age. A common misconception is that the number of years of education completed is a reliable predictor of reading ability. Lasater and Mehler report that estimating literacy based on the highest level of education obtained may overestimate reading level by four to five grade levels. People can become very skilled at hiding their illiteracy. Many gainfully employed members of high socioeconomic status are unable to read.

Limited literacy skills is a problem that can affect more than a patient's ability to read; it has been independently associated with poor health. Limited literacy interferes with the fundamentals of patient cooperation, treatment and access to care, and indeed affects the most basic communication. The social stigma that is associated with low literacy often prevents the low literacy patients from identifying themselves, even when asked directly. Patients who are labeled as "poor historians" may have limitations in their vocabulary, making it impossible for them to verbalize their symptoms. All too often, this common obstacle to receiving comprehensive care goes unrecognized.

A heightened awareness by the medical community is critical. Patients may signal to clinicians that you need to consider literacy skills as a barrier to care. For example, Mayeaux and colleagues report that people with impaired literacy skills may easily become overwhelmed and not ask many questions. They may create excuses not to read printed material at the point of care, such as, "I forgot my reading glasses," or "I'll take this home to read more thoroughly later."

To address literacy issues, effective patient education should include both oral and written forms. Patients with reading level below the fifth grade may be completely dependent on verbal communication. In any case, printed material should never be the sole source of patient education, regardless of the level of the patient's apparent reading ability. Oral communication should be presented slowly, in a culturally sensitive manner, in short sentences, and with simple language. The following are more specific guides for presenting patient education.

- Prioritize the information (most important information first).
- Repeat the material.
- Involve the patient in the interaction.
- Request feedback and reiteration by the patient.
- Split the material into several sessions.
- Use visual aids and graphics.
- Include a family member or friend.

In summary, limited literacy skills are a highly prevalent yet often unrecognized barrier to care that interfere with patients' ability to cooperate with many aspects of their medical care. Patients who cannot read the prescription bottle are unable to take medication as directed. If they cannot read printed material to follow instructions, they may not follow clinicians' recommendations about blood work, screening, and diagnostic tests. They may be unable to attend referral appointments or follow-up with their primary care clinician if they are unable to read street signs or a bus schedule. Therefore, literacy should be included in the differential of any cooperation problems in patient care.

Cultural Issues Affect Cooperation

Patient cultural background has an important influence on beliefs about health, illness, treatment, and health care practitioners who offer care. In contrast to ethnicity, which is a racial designation, culture has implications regarding values, beliefs, and traditions that affect how a patient reacts to situations. Reactions to illness are strongly influenced by cultural factors, as are health practices. It is also important to be aware that some cultures have their own health practitioners and traditional remedies. If the clinician overlooks how a patient's cultural values inform her attitude toward health care, both parties may wind up frustrated. Cultural conflict may make the patient uncomfortable with the clinician's health care recommendations. Historical perspectives may give insight into a particular culture; issues such as discrimination, oppression, forced relocation, and immigration all affect interactions between patients and health care providers.

When individuals adapt to customs, behaviors, language, and values of the local culture, they are said to be acculturated. A common misconception is that the length of time an individual has spent in a new country will indicate his or her degree of acculturation. According to Falvo, some of the other factors affecting acculturation are:

- The patient's age at the time of immigration.
- Family influences.
- Education.
- Socioeconomic status.

The younger a person is at the time of immigration, the more likely she or he is to become acculturated. A close knit family that isolates itself or remains within a "local community" from the same culture is less likely to become acculturated than a family that immigrates alone. Opportunities for education and travel, which give a broader exposure to many different cultures, make acculturation easier. The point here is that acculturation is a complex, multifactorial process requiring individual evaluation by the clinician to weigh the likelihood that cultural factors will affect cooperation.

Barriers to effective communication include conflicts between the health practitioner's values and the patient's values—the patient's preconceived notions of culture, such as myths and stereotypes. Clinicians must acknowledge that there is diversity within each particular culture. When practitioners treat patients as cultural stereotypes rather than as individuals, or rush through encounters with no attempt to consider cultural relevance, the result is often alienation of their patients.

It is important not to make the mistake of interpreting limited English language skills as lack of intelligence. A language barrier should remind you that there is a large cultural gulf between you and your patient. An interpreter may translate words into English but probably will not capture the complexity of the clinician–patient interaction. Interpreters may even create problems by adding their personal bias to the translation. If you use an interpreter, remember to direct your nonverbal contact toward the patient. However, nonverbal communication also has cultural variations. Factors such as the practitioner's tone and inflection of voice, amount of eye or body contact, even where you sit in the room can all affect the patient's comfort level.

It is not possible for clinicians to be familiar with every culture and its beliefs, but it is possible to be aware of how cultural factors can influence the outcome of health care interactions. It is vital not to discount or discredit your patients' cultural beliefs. Acknowledge their beliefs and strive to understand them. Try to differentiate between behavior that is culturally based and behavior that is individually based.

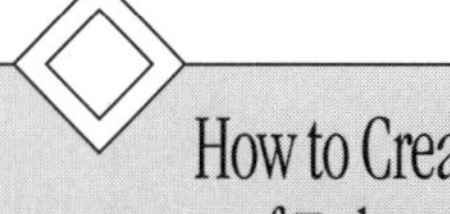

How to Create an Atmosphere of Enhanced Cooperation

Only suggest therapy when clinical judgment or evidence suggests that the intervention will alter the course of disease. As patients often defer to their clinician's judgment, it is the clinician's responsibility to base therapeutic recommendations either on the best available evidence, or on sound and careful clinical reasoning. The patient takes your therapeutic recommendations very seriously. If you successfully enlist or even coerce the patient into cooperation with a regimen that in hindsight was ineffective or even harmful (e.g., thalidomide), then you bear responsibility for the outcome (Table 13-3). Many studies have documented that some clinicians fail to follow established guidelines and prescribe ineffective or even dangerous therapy. Always try to base therapy on available evidence.

Table 13-3

Optimizing Clinician–Patient Cooperation: Some Suggestions from the Literature

- Only suggest therapy when clinical judgment or evidence suggests that intervention will alter course of disease.
- Think noncooperation.
- Offer patient information on disease and treatment.
- Consider therapeutic goals, then elicit feedback on ability to achieve goals.
- Renegotiate goals based on patient feedback and clinician constraints; accept outcome.
- Elicit commitment to therapy.
- Maintain contact: every encounter is an opportunity to identify and expand on behavior that allows achievement of goals.
- Keep care inexpensive and simple.
- Support and empathize with patient.
- Encourage positive life-style modifications.
- Add therapy in a step-wise fashion until goals are achieved.
- Focus on overall quality of life for the patient.
- Be willing to stop unsuccessful therapy and try different approach.
- When prescribing medications
  - Integrate medication into daily routine; encourage keeping a diary to monitor therapy.
  - Anticipate adverse effects and adjust therapy to prevent, minimize or ameliorate.
  - Use written instructions, both for prescriptions and all other therapy.
- Identify barriers; offer assistance with overcoming them.
- Be positive about ability to achieve goals.
- Use ancillary staff; take advantage of every encounter to focus on achieving goals.
- Inquire about accomplishment of goals at every visit in a nonjudgmental way.

Think noncooperation. Whenever the therapeutic goal is not being met, you should consider noncooperation in the differential diagnosis at every encounter. Remember to be nonjudgmental. This allows the patient to discuss problems and barriers without feeling threatened.

Offer patients information about the disease and treatment options. Educating patients is necessary for informed consent and choice, as well as for effective patient negotiation. The encounter should include communication about diagnostic significance of the problem; appropriate diagnostic interventions, treatments; and preventive measures, as well as discovering the social and psychological context of the disease and treatment. Patients can only share in decision making if they understand the implications of diagnosis, diagnostic inquiry, treatment, and prognosis. Those patients who have adequate knowledge and who are able to take an active role should be more satisfied and have better outcomes.

Consider therapeutic goals, then elicit patient feedback on the ability to achieve goals. Determining the therapeutic regimen is only the first step. The patient must next agree with treatment goals and be willing to cooperate with the therapeutic interventions necessary to achieve them. Patients seeking care for acute illness, chronic illness, and prevention all have different goals. If patients seek care for an acute illness, their goal will likely be to resume their previous healthy state after a finite course of therapy. A chronic illness is more complex; the clinician may seek to return the patient to physiologic normalcy, but the patient may be more concerned about eliminating undesired side effects of medication. A patient with a family history of breast cancer may ask for preventive screening. Often a single encounter has components of acute, chronic, and preventive services.

Renegotiate goals based on patient's feedback and clinician's constraints; accept outcome. At every visit, both patient and clinician should renegotiate the relative importance of all the identified goals and how each goal fits into the broad therapeutic picture. This negotiation is a long-term process; the cooperative relationship should unfold over a series of encounters. Remember Damrosch's Health Belief model: patients will cooperate according to their perception of the disease's severity and their own ability to bring about change. The clinician must be flexible and allow the patient to direct which goals are possible.

A clinician may become frustrated if, once goals are identified, the patient fails to give them priority. In such cases, remember the stages of change model. If the desired behavior change is introduced gradually, the clinician can often assist the patient in moving toward the action phase. The uncompromising clinician who insists on addressing behaviors that the patient is not yet willing to change will only succeed in increasing the patient's resistance to change.

Elicit commitment to therapy. Once the clinician and the patient have successfully negotiated their differences and established a course of action, it is important that patients restate the goals and their commitment to achieving these goals. This relatively simple step may identify problem areas that need to be renegotiated. At this time, the clinician can clear up any confusion and permit further compromise when possible.

Maintain contact: every encounter is an opportunity to identify and expand on behavior that allows achievement of goals. Patients who abuse tobacco and alcohol tend to present more frequently for illness care and become involved with complex medical regimens. When a patient is attempting to alter life style, every encounter is an opportunity to reinforce cooperation and reduce barriers to cooperation. "Encounters" can include phone contacts, blood pressure checks, and acute care visits for other problems. Try not to give negative feedback but instead focus on positive reinforcement for desirable behavior. As an example, patients who have lost weight should get positive reinforcement for weight loss at every encounter. If they mention an exercise routine, all of the staff should make every effort to encourage further efforts.

Keep care inexpensive and simple. The literature is very clear on this point: patients will follow inexpensive regimens more frequently than expensive ones and will favor simple regimens over complex ones. If given a choice, remember the principles of parsimony and KISS ("keep it simple, stupid"). Even in nonpharmacologic interventions, these principles should be followed. If giving an exercise prescription, for example, you are much more likely to engender cooperation by incorporating walking into an established gardening routine than by trying to get the patient to purchase a new exercise cycle.

Support and empathize with the patient. The clinician should use the principles of motivational interviewing when attempting to enhance cooperation. These include accurate empathy, reflective listening, and an attitude of accepting but not necessarily approving the patient's choices. The clinician should highlight any discrepancy between current behavior and future goals. Never argue with a patient; instead, shift strategies as resistance occurs. Above all, leave patients with the message "If you choose to change, I will help you to change yourself."

Encourage positive life-style modifications. Whether we think in terms of cooperation or noncooperation, we tend to consider it the role of the patient to present with a problem and the role of the clinician to coordinate a therapeutic plan, which may include life-style modifications and medications. Clinicians often focus on medication—this is the aspect over which they believe they have the most control. However, the importance of encouraging and rewarding positive life-style modifications should not be underestimated. Approximately half of all premature deaths can be directly attributed to life-style choices. Managing the consequences of life-style choices with medication, no matter how cooperative the patient, is the equivalent of putting a Band-Aid on a bedsore. Every positive change in life style should be sought and rewarded, as these changes are incremental in nature and often require many false starts before ultimately being successful.

Add therapy in a step-wise fashion until goals are achieved. Despite the principle of diagnostic parsimony, ambulatory patients commonly carry more than one diagnosis. These diagnoses often have a common life-style component, but may have separate medical management. Clinicians may get caught in the trap of trying to offer therapy for every condition identified and may become frustrated when patients fail to cooperate with every intervention. Managing patients with chronic medical problems is a long-term process, and successfully reducing risk can take decades. Do not attempt to institute therapy for all problems at the first visit. First educate the patient about modifying life-style risks common to all diseases. Then prioritize the diagnoses based on immediate risk and institute therapy incrementally.

Focus on the overall quality of life for the patient. Unfortunately, as clinicians we sometimes focus more on the act of cooperation than on the consequences of noncooperation. We should remember that we want the effect of our therapy not only to lengthen the patient's life but also improve it. This means that we should temper our recommendations with common sense, appreciate our patients' concerns, and work on a plan that our patients will feel comfortable with. Do not pressure patients to cooperate with a therapy that may offer only a marginal benefit, such as uncomfortable cancer screening procedures for a very elderly patient.

Be willing to stop unsuccessful therapies and try different approaches. Even the best treatment plans may fail. Even if you suspect noncooperation, do not assign blame. The patient, the clinician, or the therapy itself may be the cause of failure. If, after an adequate trial, it becomes clear that the therapy is ineffective, it is important to move on to something new. Trying to force an ineffective therapy to work leads to frustration, mistrust, suspicion, and ultimately the breakdown of the therapeutic relationship.

When prescribing medications, integrate medications into daily routine, use a diary, anticipate adverse effects, take efforts to ameliorate adverse effects, and use written instructions. Few clinicians think twice about writing a prescription. Based on our understanding of the disease process, we select a medication that we think will improve our patient's health. The patient, however, must always decide whether or not to cooperate with the therapy. Then, after testing the therapy, they will either reject it outright, accept it with modifications, or accept it without reservations—a complex interaction (see Fig. 13-1).

We must stress the severity of the illness and the consequences of noncooperation. The best way to secure the patient's commitment is to offer positive assertions, such as assurance that cooperation will result in personal benefits to the patient. If patients feel the medication is important to their health, then they are more likely to enter the testing phase. Even motivated patients may have difficulties during the testing stage. When prescribing medication, we should anticipate problems and be proactive.

The initial step, particularly when starting a long-term therapy, is to encourage the patient to incorporate the medication into a daily routine. Offer the simplest regimen possible. Once a day is easier than twice a day, one pill is easier than two pills, and so on. After establishing the regimen, offer suggestions to help the patient include it in daily life. A simple plan might involve mealtimes or a daily task like brushing teeth. Patients on a more complex regimen may want to consider a pill diary. Acknowledge the difficulty of a complicated regimen and be willing to negotiate simplification.

The testing phase will reveal any side effects of the prescribed medication. If these are unanticipated or severe, the patient may discontinue the medication. Always discuss the common side effects of any medication you prescribe and discuss the patient's experiences at follow-up visits. Patients are better able to tolerate side effects and subsequent reduction in the quality of life if the patients have anticipated them.

Offer written instructions. Immediately following the average encounter with a physician, patients retain only about 50 percent of what is said. To make sense of the retained information, they may inappropriately apply those instructions they recall. Often these "creative" instructions may be quite different from yours. Providing written directions may forestall confusion. (Of course, literacy issues may interfere with this approach.)

Identify barriers and offer assistance with overcoming them. Unfortunately, there are many obstacles that prevent even highly motivated patients from successfully following a treatment plan. These can be roughly divided into financial, cultural, and class barriers. Financial barriers are fairly straightforward, but we often fail to consider them. We write a prescription for an expensive fourth-generation cephalosporin instead of a generic drug and wonder why the patient did not improve. We scribble instructions for a costly diagnostic test and wonder why the patient does not keep the appointment. The astute clinician should inquire about financial barriers rather than wait for the patient to volunteer the information.

Be positive about ability to achieve goals. After a treatment plan has been negotiated, the clinician takes on the role of cheerleader. Even if you are not convinced the patient will be able to improve, never reveal your pessimism. Every pound lost, every cigarette not smoked is a victory. Remember that this is a long-term commitment.

Use ancillary staff; take advantage of every encounter to focus on achieving goal. "So you're still not smoking—good for you!" This is what you should say to your former smokers. It is also what staff nurses can say if you give them the chance. The entire office should be involved in eliciting patient cooperation. The temptation to revert to old behaviors or to forget new habits is strong. Think of how powerful it would be for your patients to get positive feedback from everyone they encounter during their visit to your office. Your staff can also help with preventive measures that you may be too busy to consider, such as immunizations or cancer screening. Encourage your staff to see patient health as a common objective.

Inquire about accomplishment of goals at every visit in a nonjudgmental way. Once you and the patient have agreed on the plan, every visit is an opportunity to encourage cooperation. However, you should do this in a way that allows the patient to bring up any problems without forcing them into an uncomfortable situation. For example, almost all patients will list smoking cessation as a therapeutic goal. As the patient passes from precontemplation through contemplation and preparation to action, both patient and clinician will have different concerns. If you do not bring up the issue of smoking at each visit, you will not know what stage of consideration your patient has reached.

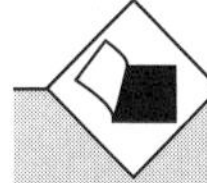

Summary

Prescribing a particular therapy for a specific disease is the focus of 4 years of medical school and the majority of the postgraduate training that physicians receive. Such training, however, has not traditionally focused on ensuring that patients cooperate with the therapy. Patient cooperation takes on more importance for practicing clinicians, when they notice that without cooperation, their patient's health does not improve. We hope that our brief introduction into the field of cooperation will encourage clinicians to avoid cynicism and instead, embrace the spirit and the science of cooperation as a tool to improving their patients' well-being.

Suggested Reading

Sackett DL, Haynes RB, eds. *Compliance with Therapeutic Regimes.* Baltimore, MD: Johns Hopkins University Press, 1976.

The seminal work on the scientific basis of the study of patient compliance written from an epidemiologic perspective.

DiMatteo MR, DiNicola DD. *Achieving Patient Compliance.* New York: Pergamon Press, 1982.

Although almost 20 years old, this book still contains excellent ideas that we would be wise to become aware of and use in our practice.

Family Practice Management (Journal)

This journal is published by the American Academy of Family Physicians. It offers clinicians practical solutions to common practice problems. It is available online at http://aafp.org/fpm/. *Following are two representative articles from the journal that address patient compliance:*

Funnell MM. Helping patients take charge of their chronic illnesses. *Fam Pract Manag* (March, 2000).

Lowes R. Patient-centered care for better patient adherence. *Fam Prac Manag* (March, 1998).

Roter D, Hall J, Merisca R, Nordstrom B, Cretin D, Svarstad B: Effectiveness of interventions to improve patient compliance: A meta-analysis. *Medical Care 36*(8):1138, 1998.

This meta-analysis looks at all of the literature through 1998 in a systematic fashion to evaluate the effectiveness of interventions to improve compliance. Dr. Debra Roter has worked extensively to identify the scientific basis upon which the recommendations regarding enhancing patient cooperation are based.

Falvo D, ed: *Effective Patient Education: A Guide to Increased Compliance,* 2nd ed. Gaithersburg, MD: Aspen Publishers; 1994.

One of the keys to an enhanced cooperative relationship is improving the education of your patients regarding their disease and treatment. This book outlines issues, concerns, and solutions regarding patient education and has an especially useful chapter on literacy.

Bayer Institute for Health Care Communication

A not-for-profit organization whose mission is to improve the quality of health care through education, research, and advocacy for improved provider-patient communication. www.bayerinstitute.com

This web site provides tools and resources for providers and patients as well as recommended books and videos.

Bibliography

Beardon PHG, McGilchrist MM, McKendrick AD, et al: Primary non-compliance with prescribed medication in primary care. *BMJ* 307:846, 1993.

Carr V: The role of the general practitioner in the treatment of schizophrenia: Specific issues. *MJA* 166:143, 1997.

Chaulk CP, Kazandjian VA: Directly observed therapy for treatment completion for pulmonary tuberculosis: Consensus statement of the Public Health Tuberculosis Guidelines Panel. *JAMA* 279:943, 1998.

Clark L: Improving compliance and increasing control of hypertension: Needs of special hypertensive populations. *Am Heart J* 121:664, 1991.

Damrosch S: Facilitating Adherence to preventive and treatment regimens. In: Wedding D (ed): *Behavior and Medicine,* 2nd ed. St. Louis, MO: Mosby; 1995, p 537.

DiMatteo RM: Adherence. In: Feldman MD, Christensen JF (eds): *Behavioral Medicine in Primary Care: A Practical Guide.* Stamford, CT: Appleton & Lange; 1997, p 345.

Dowell J, Hudson H: A qualitative study of medication-taking behaviour in primary care. *Family Practice* 14:369, 1997.

Duncan J: Medication compliance in patients with chronic schizophrenia: Implications for the community management of mentally disordered offenders. *J Forensic Sci* 43:1133, 1998.

Ely JW, Goerdt J, Bergus GR, et al: The effect of physician characteristics on compliance with adult preventive care guidelines. *Family Med* 30:34, 1998.

Emanuel EJ, Emanuel LL: Four models of the physician-patient relationship. *JAMA* 267:2221, 1992.

Falvo D: Illiteracy in patient education and patient compliance. In: Falvo D (ed): *Effective Patient Education: A Guide to Increased Compliance,* 2nd ed. Gaithersburg, MD: Aspen; 1994, p 330.

Falvo D: Multicultural issues in patient education and patient compliance. In: Falvo D (ed): *Effective Patient Education: A Guide to Increased Compliance,* 2nd ed. Gaithersburg, MD: Aspen; 1994.

Fenton W, McGlashan T: Schizophrenia: Individual psychotherapy. In: Kaplan H, BJ S, (eds): *Comprehensive Textbook of Psychiatry.* Baltimore, MD: Williams and Wilkins; 1995, p 2804.

Flocke S, Stange K, Zyzanski S: The impact of insurance type and forced discontinuity on the delivery of primary care. *J Fam Pract* 45:129, 1997.

Friedman I: Promoting adolescents' compliance with therapeutic regimens. *Pediatr Clin North Am* 33:955, 1986.

Greenfield S, Kaplan S, Ware JE, et al: Patients' participation in medical care: Effects on blood sugar control and quality of life in diabetes. *J Gen Intern Med* 3:448, 1988.

Harbarth S, Siegrist C, Schira J, et al: Influenza immunizations: Improving compliance of healthcare workers. *Infect Control Hosp Epidemiol* 19:337, 1998.

Haynes B: Strategies to improve compliance with referral, appointments, and prescribed medical regimens. In: Haynes B, Taylor W, Sackett D (eds): *Compliance in Health Care.* Baltimore, MD: The Johns Hopkins University Press; 1979, p 516.

Hiatt R: Behavioral research contributions and needs in cancer prevention and control: Adherence to cancer screening advice. *Prev Med* 26(suppl):S11, 1997.

Insull W: The problem of compliance to cholesterol altering therapy. *J Intern Med* 241:317, 1997.

Jecker N, Carrese J, Pearlman R: Caring for patients in cross-cultural settings. *Hastings Cent Rep* 25:6, 1995.

Joint National Committee on Prevention, Evaluation, Detection, and Treatment of High Blood Pressure: *Sixth Report of the Joint Committee on Prevention, Detection, Evaluation, and Treatment of High Blood Pressure.* Bethesda, MD; 1997. NIH Publication 98-4080.

Joos S, Hickman D, Gordon G, et al: Effects of a physician communication intervention on patient care outcomes. *J Gen Intern Med* 11:147, 1996.

Kaplan De-Nour A: Foreword. In: Gerber K, Nehemkis A (eds): *Compliance: The Dilemma of the Chronically Ill.* New York, NY: Springer; 1986, p 239.

Kingsbury K: Taking AIM: How to teach primary and secondary prevention effectively. *Can J Cardiol* 14(suppl A):22A, 1998.

Kuttner R: The American health care system. *N Engl J Med* 340:163, 1999.

Lasater L, Mehler P: The illiterate patient: Screening and management. *Hosp Pract (Off Ed)* 33:163, 1998.

Leard L, Savides T, Ganiats T: Patient preferences for colorectal cancer screening. *J Fam Pract* 45:211, 1997.

Leenen FHH, Wilson TW, Larochelle P, et al: Patterns of compliance with once versus twice daily antihypertensive drug therapy in primary care: A randomized clinical trial using electronic monitoring. *Cardiovasc Med* 13:914, 1997.

Lipkin M: Physician-patient interaction in reproductive counseling. *Obstet Gynecol* 88(3):31S, 1996.

Lipkin M: Patient education and counseling in the context of modern patient-physician-family communication. *Patient Educ Couns* 27:5, 1996.

Lowes R: Patient-centered care for better patient adherence. *Fam Pract Manag* 5:46, 1998.

Mayeaux E, Murphy P, Arnold C, et al: Improving patient education for patients with low literacy skills. *Am Fam Physician* 53:205, 1996.

McGinnis MJ: Actual causes of death in the United States. *JAMA* 270:2207, 1993.

Nockowitz R: Enhancing patient compliance with treatment recommendations. *Am J Med* 79(suppl 6A): 34, 1985.

O'Connell D: Behavior change. In: Christensen JF (ed): *Behavioral Medicine in Primary Care A Practical Guide.* Stamford, CT: Appleton & Lange; 1997, p 345.

Ore L, Hagoel L, Shifroni G, et al: Compliance with mammography screening in Israeli women: The impact of a pre-scheduled appointment and of the letter-style. *Isr J Med Sci* 33:103, 1997.

Roter D, Hall J, Merisca R, et al: Effectiveness of interventions to improve patient compliance: A meta-analysis. *Med Care* 36:1138, 1998.

Safran DG, Taira DA, Rogers WH, et al: Linking primary care performance to outcomes of care. *J Fam Pract* 47:213, 1998.

Setter S: Improving compliance with estrogen therapy for osteoporosis. *The Female Patient* 23:29, 1998.

Steiner JF: Compliance. In: Fihn SD, DeWitt DE (eds): *Outpatient Medicine,* 2nd ed. Philadelphia, PA: Saunders; 1998, p 773.

Stephenson J: AIDS researchers target poor adherence. *JAMA* 281:1069, 1999.

Stern TA, Herman JB, Slavin PL (eds): *MGH Guide to Psychiatry in Primary Care.* New York, NY: McGraw-Hill; 1998, p 696.

Street R: Physicians' communication and parents' evaluation of pediatric consultations. *Med Care* 29: 1146, 1991.

Trombatore K: Missed messages. *American Medical News* July 28, 1998.

U.S. Preventive Services Task Force: *Guide to Clinical Preventive Services,* 2nd ed. Baltimore, MD: Williams & Wilkins; 1996.

Vollmer S: Compliance: A physician's problem. *Family Practice Recertification* 20:91, 1998.

Womeodu R, Bailey J: Barriers to cancer screening. *Med Clin North Am* 80:115, 1996.

Part 3

Psychological Problems

Carlos M. Grilo

Eating and Weight Disorders in Adults

Introduction

The goal of this chapter is to present evidence-based recommendations for the assessment and treatment of adults with obesity and eating disorders. Eating disorders—which are classified as psychiatric disorders—are characterized by abnormal eating behaviors and beliefs regarding eating, weight, or shape. This chapter also discusses several other eating disorders including "binge eating," anorexia nervosa, and bulimia nervosa. Obesity, a weight disorder classified as a general medical condition, is an extremely common problem that is associated with significant morbidity and mortality. It will be discussed first.

For each eating and weight problem, the empirical literature will be reviewed with the view of addressing practical issues for assessment and treatment of eating and weight disorders faced by primary care providers. Then, a brief overview of the clinical and associated features, assessment, and treatment will be provided.

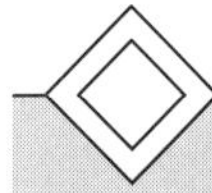

Obesity

MARGARET BELL *Margaret Bell's blood sugar is high. She was at the Health Fair last week, where they checked her glucose and told her that she needed to come in for a checkup—and be sure to bring the glucose lab result. Ms. Bell is 40 years old, and says she's "as healthy as a horse." She gained 50 pounds with each of her two pregnancies, and lost less than half of it each time. So now she thinks she is about 60 pounds overweight, and wants to do something about it. She wonders if her blood sugar is high because of her weight. She does not have any other health problems, and takes no medications. You estimate that she eats about 2500 calories a day. She gets almost no exercise.*

Ms. Bell is 5'5" tall and weighs 190 pounds. You calculate her body mass index (BMI) at 32. Her physical exam is otherwise entirely normal. Her lab work is also normal, except for a HbA1c of 9.0. You reassure yourself that she is motivated to change her weight, give her a questionnaire on eating and weight patterns to complete at home, instruct her to maintain a careful eating diary, and to return to your office in 2 weeks.

Obesity is a physical problem, defined as excess adipose tissue resulting from excess energy intake relative to energy expenditure. Obesity is also a major public health problem. Despite pervasive sociocultural pressures to be thin and high rates of dieting, 97 million Americans (55 percent of adults) are overweight or obese, and this number continues to increase. Obesity is associated with increased risk for morbidity and death, and results in staggering economic health costs.

Overweight is defined as excess deviation of body weight above some standard ("ideal") for height. Excess weight does not always reflect excess fat (e.g., some extremely muscular athletes may be overweight but not obese). Nonetheless, the various indices of weight by height, correlate with direct measurements of body fat. These indices include percent overweight, weight divided by height, and BMI, which is weight in (kg) divided by the square of height in meters.

Obesity experts most frequently uses BMI as the standard measurement. Figure 14-1 shows the widely used Bray nomogram for BMI. In 1998, the National Institutes of Health, in its *Clinical Guidelines on the Identification, Evaluation, and Treatment of Overweight and Obesity,* adopted a threshold BMI of above 25 to define overweight, and defined a BMI of 30 or higher as signifying obesity.

In addition to measures that estimate the body fat, it is also important to consider the distribution of the fat. Upper body fat distribution (abdominal or android type) is associated with greater morbidity and mortality than is lower-body (hip or gynoid-type) obesity. Abdominal fat distribution is more common in men than in women, but its presence in both genders is associated with increased morbidity and mortality. Thus, although in general a

Figure 14-1

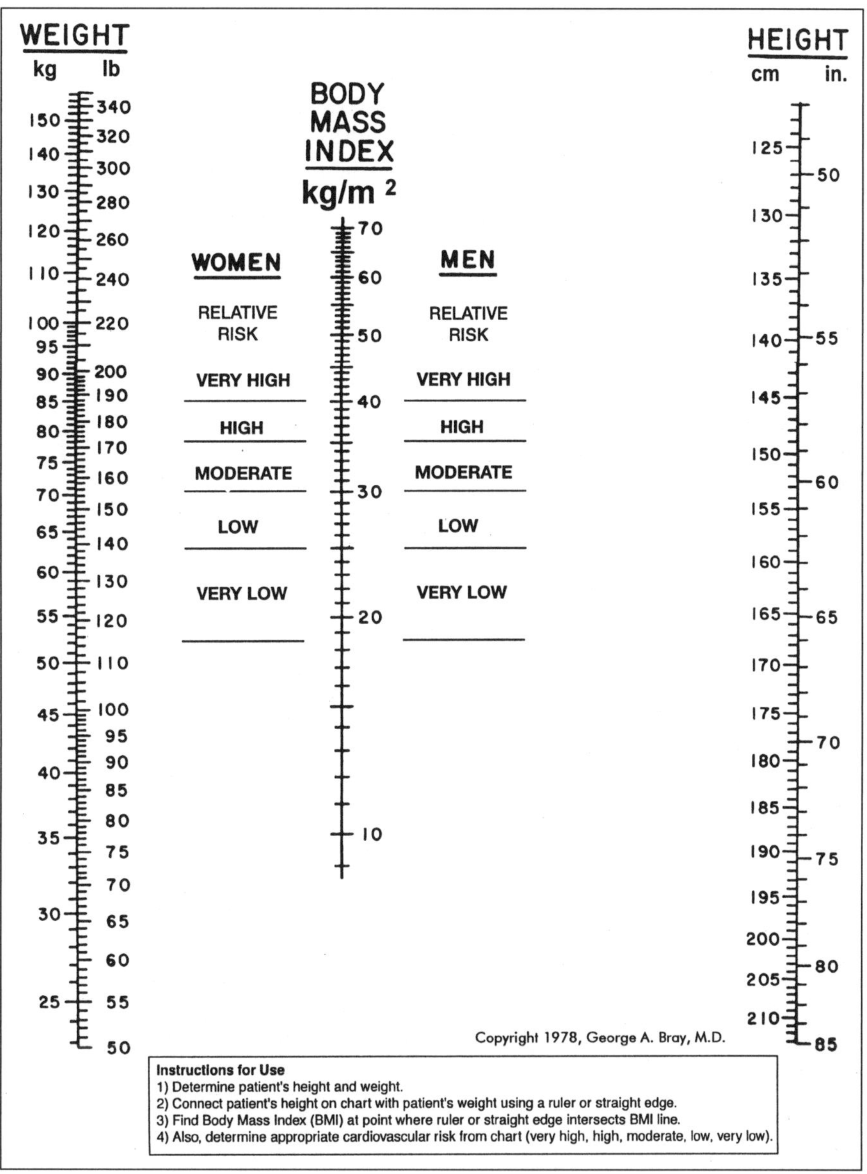

Know your body mass index.

BMI of 30 or higher is associated with an increase in health risks, waist-to-hip ratio (WHR) is actually a stronger predictor of health risk (especially cardiovascular disease) than is body weight, body fat, or BMI. WHR is considered an adequate estimate for intra-abdominal obesity, the measurement of which would otherwise require sophisticated and expensive methods. Figure 14-2 also shows Bray nomogram for WHR and recommendations for intervention. The United States Department of Health and Human Services (USDHHS) guidelines note that a WHR over 40 in men and

Figure 14-2

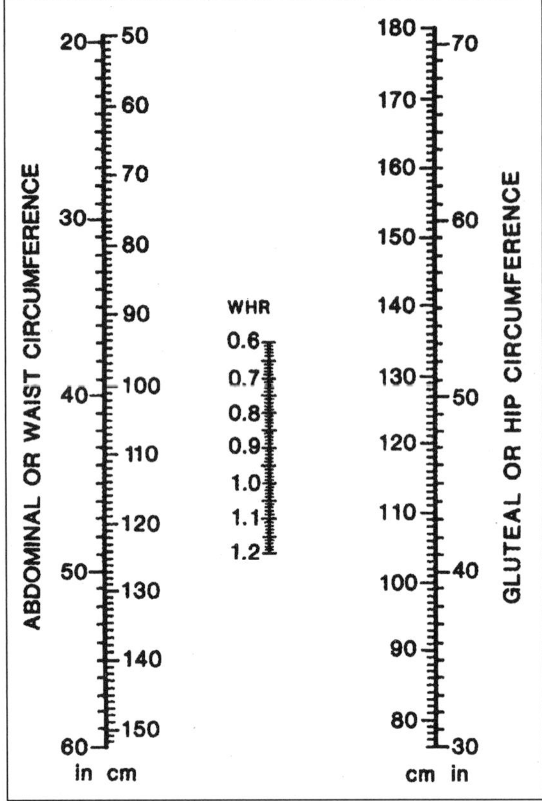

Bray nomogram for waist-to-hip ratio.

over 35 in women indicates increased medical risk in persons with BMI greater than 25.

Medical Assessment

In general, increasing obesity, and especially WHR, are associated with greater risk for morbidity and mortality. In particular, obesity is associated with heart disease, high blood pressure, and diabetes. Table 14-1 summarizes factors recommended by Weisner to consider in the medical assessment of obese patients. Table 14-2 summarizes these recommendations for laboratory assessment of medical conditions associated with obesity.

Psychological Functioning and Assessment

Research by Friedman and Brownell has found that obese and nonobese persons differ little in psychological and psychiatric functioning. If one excludes patients with anorexia nervosa and morbid obesity, obese and nonobese people generally show similar rates of psychological and psychiatric disorders. There are, however, two important caveats to this generalization. First, some studies have found that obese persons may have lower self-esteem and higher rates of dissatisfaction with body image. Second, and of particular relevance, Grilo and colleagues found that obese persons who binge eat represent a subgroup of obese patients characterized by high rates of psychological and psychiatric problems.

Determining which overweight patients may have psychological or psychiatric problems is important. One self-report instrument that is useful for this determination is the Questionnaire on Eating and Weight Patterns-Revised (QEWP-R). The QEWP-R, a psychometrically standardized by Nangle and colleagues, yields information regarding weight and dieting history, weight cycling, body image, and binge eating. In addition to information about obesity and eating habits, the QEWP-R also produces necessary information for generating two specific eating disorder diagnoses-binge eating disorder and bulimia nervosa (both discussed later).

General Treatment Issues and Interventions

MARGARET BELL (CONTINUED) *Ms. Bell returns as requested. Her QEWP-R indicates that she has no concurrent eating disorders, that she has never seriously tried to diet, that most of her weight gain occurred during her pregnancies with minor gains before and after, and that her obesity creates moderate self-esteem problems for her. Her desired weight loss would put her at a BMI of 22, close to ideal body weight. She is eating about 2200 calories a day, with a wide variation from day to day. You prescribe a balanced diet of 1200* *calories, a brisk 2-mile walk each evening with her neighbor, encouragement to continue keeping a compulsive food diary, and ask her to return in 2 weeks to see how she is doing. You advise her that this may be easier if she joins a support group, and you provide her with information about such groups. You also warn her that achieving and maintaining her ideal weight will be a lifelong process—that the biggest challenge is to not regain the weight lost initially.*

A brief overview of some common issues and general guidelines for working with obese patients

Table 14-1

Factors to Be Considered in the Medical History of an Obese Patient

- Factors predisposing to/associated with obesity
  - Family history of obesity (number of first-degree relatives who are obese)
  - Age of onset
  - In children: growth patterns; mental and physical maturation
  - Potential endocrine abnormalities
    - *Hypothyroidism:* symptoms include cold intolerance, menstrual abnormalities, constipation, weakness
    - *Cushing's syndrome:* symptoms include hypertension, glucose intolerance, menstrual dysfunction, weakness, back pain, compression fractures, bruising
    - *Polycystic ovarian syndrome:* symptoms include reduced/absent menses shortly after menarche, hirsutism
  - Life style changes concurrent with onset of weight gain (e.g., job change, marriage/divorce, childbirth, relocation)
  - Dietary pattern (best reviewed with diet records)
  - Pattern of physical activity (best reviewed with exercise records)
- History of medical complications of obesity
  - Cancer (especially of endometrium and breast)
  - Glucose intolerance and diabetes mellitus
  - Hepatobiliary disease (especially gallstones, hepatic steatosis and enlargement)
  - Hypertension, hyperlipidemia, coronary artery disease
  - Osteoarthritis (especially, but not exclusively, of weight-bearing joint)
  - Respiratory disease (especially periodic apnea due to obstruction, or alveolar hypoventilation)
- Previous treatment responses
  - Past successes, failures; weight-cycling pattern
  - Past medical and surgical therapies for obesity
- Factors warranting precaution/precluding weight reduction
  - <20 or >65 years of age
  - History of anorexia nervosa
  - Pregnancy or lactation

SOURCE: Reprinted with permission from Weinsier RL: Clinical assessment of obese patients. In: Brownwell KD, Fairburn CG (eds): *Eating Disorders and Obesity.* New York: Guildford Press; 1995.

Table 14-2

Laboratory Assessment of Medical Conditions Associated with Obesity

IF SUSPICION OF . . .	CONSIDER . . .
Cushing's syndrome	24-h urine collection to be tested for free cortisol (>150 μg/24 h; abnormal) plus low-dose dexamethasone suppression test of milligrams every 6 h for 2 days, with collection of 24-h urine to test for 17-hydroxy-corticosteroid levels on second day (>3.5 mg/24 h; abnormal)
Hypothyroidism	Serum TSH level (normal, general <5 μU/mL)
Diabetes	Fasting serum glucose level
Hyperlipidemia	Fasting total levels of cholesterol, triglycerides, HDL cholesterol
Gallstones	Ultrasonography
Periodic/sleep apnea	Sleep studies for oxygen desaturation; ENT exam for upper airway obstruction

NOTE: ENT, ear, nose, and throat; HDL, high-density lipoprotien; TSH, thyroid-stimulating hormone.
SOURCE: Table reprinted with permission from Weinsier RL: Clinical assessment of obese patients. In: Bromwell KD, Fairburn CG (eds): *Eating Disorders and Obesity.* New York: Guildford Press; 1995.

follows. Above all, it is important to remember the strong social stigma faced by obese persons. In addition, it is important to be sensitive to patients' frustrations regarding previous unsuccessful "diets."

CALORIE GOALS AND NUTRITION

Substantial variation exists in how behavioral weight loss programs make nutritional and caloric recommendations. Most university-affiliated programs recommend roughly a 1200 to 1500 kcal/day goal for producing weight loss. Given gender and individual differences in metabolic processes and energy expenditure, Grilo and Brownell recommend the following general approach to estimate calorie goals for a patient. First, begin with a 1500 kcal/day goal for men and a 1200 kcal/day goal for women and carefully monitor all food intake in a food diary. This information will allow for the calculation and readjustment of caloric intake necessary to accomplish weekly weight loss goals. This approach assumes intra-person variability over time due to changes in water loss, metabolic shifts, lean tissue loss, and changes in activity levels, and will produce a more individualized caloric estimate.

Research has documented limitations in the reliability of dietary self-report and has challenged claims that certain "diet-resistant" obese persons do not eat substantially more than lean persons. Both lean and obese persons underestimate caloric intake, but the underestimation by obese persons is generally greater than by lean persons. For example, Lichtman and colleagues found that a sample of diet-resistant obese patients underestimated the amount of food they ate during a 2-week period by 47 percent and overestimated their level of physical activity by 51 percent. Such findings suggest that the failure to lose weight or sustain weight loss may be due mostly to overeating and underactivity (i.e., noncompliance). The implication is that professionals should devote time to detailed descriptions of caloric measurement and repeatedly focus on the value of careful ongoing self-monitoring and record keeping.

In addition to total caloric expenditure, any weight control program must consider balanced nutrition practices. The U.S. Department of Agriculture published the Food Guide Pyramid, which is now widely disseminated on many food packages. The Food Guide Pyramid schematically shows recommended dietary guidelines with clearly specified daily servings for all five food groups.

Exercise

Increased physical activity is a critical component of any for weight loss program. Exercise alone, however, without dietary changes, is insufficient to produce significant weight loss in many obese persons. The combination of exercise and diet, on the other hand, although not consistently associated with short-term weight loss, is usually associated with successful longer-term weight loss and maintenance of weight loss. Moreover, exercise predicts weight maintenance across different forms of dietary interventions.

Physical activity and fitness are themselves associated with decreased morbidity and mortality through a number of possible mechanisms. Exercise can result in health improvement even with only minimal weight loss. The benefits of exercise may be especially salient in obese patients with poor health risk factor profiles. Moreover, studies from the Cooper Institute have provided impressive evidence that fitness protects against health risks even in overweight persons.

Recent findings from well-controlled studies suggest that even modest levels of physical activity may be sufficient to produce improvements in health. Two randomized controlled clinical trials suggest that life style physical activity (physical activity in the course of one's daily routine) interventions may be as effective as structured exercise programs. Dunn and colleagues reported that in previously sedentary healthy adults, life style exercise was similar in efficacy to a structured exercise program in improving physical activity, cardiorespiratory fitness, and blood pressure. Anderson and colleagues reported that the addition of life style exercise or structured exercise to a behavior therapy program produced similar improvements in obese women.

Weight Loss Goals

Weight losses of as little as 10 percent may result in significant health benefits. According to Sjostrom. The so-called 10 percent solution has increasingly been promoted by obesity experts, based on emerging but as yet uncertain evidence for the beneficial effects of weight loss of as little as 10 percent. Such weight losses, however, are cosmetically and psychologically disappointing to the majority of obese patients entering treatment. Greater attention needs to be paid to the multiple benefits (e.g., health profile, fitness, psychological benefits) of behavioral and life style change—instead of solely on the traditional focus on weight loss for health.

Overview of Obesity Treatment Options

Numerous treatments exist for obesity, including self-help programs, self-help groups, commercial programs, dietary programs, behavioral treatments, very-low-calorie diet programs, pharmacotherapy, and surgery. This brief review focuses selectively on those interventions that have received the most study (behavioral treatments, very-low-calorie diets, exercise, and pharmacotherapy). Overall, the treatment literature is characterized by two general findings: First, significant short-term weight loss can be achieved via a number of treatment approaches. Second, for many patients, weight loss is difficult to maintain over time.

Behavioral Treatment

Early applications of behavior therapy focused primarily on modifying specific eating behaviors and occurred separately or in parallel to nutritional and exercise interventions. Over the years, the different approaches have been integrated and today the application of behavioral therapies generally occurs as an integrated approach in combination with dietary/exercise interventions.

The efficacy of behavioral treatments for obesity has been studied and reviewed extensively. Overall, most behavioral treatments produce significant short-term weight losses, but are characterized by substantial weight regain after treatment. Studies generally found that during the first year after treatment, patients regain, on average, one-third to one-half of the weight they lost, and most patients regain their entire weight loss by 5 years.

The inability to produce lasting weight loss led to investigations of relapse and ways to improve weight maintenance. Treatments have become longer and relapse prevention techniques have become standard components. Treatments have shown slight trends toward greater weight losses, but the observed increases in weight losses appear to be primarily a function of the longer rather than more effective treatment.

Very-Low-Calorie-Diets

Very-low-calorie-diets (VLCD) were widely used and studied during the mid 1980s and early 1990s. VLCDs involve fasting (calorie levels generally between 400 and 800 kcal/day) with protein supplements. Wadden and Bartlett's critical review of randomized clinical trials of VLCDs concluded that they produce rapid and substantial weight losses, but are characterized by poor maintenance of lost weight. Although combining behavior therapy with VLCD regimens decreases weight regain during the year following treatment, studies with 3- to 5-year follow-up periods found that for most patients, all of the weight lost was regained. Wadden and colleagues found that the combination of a VLCD and behavior therapy had no long-term advantage over the combination of a conventional balanced moderate deficit diet plus behavior therapy.

Pharmacotherapy

There is currently no accepted role for pharmacotherapy alone as the treatment of obesity. The National Heart Lung and Blood Institute, together with the National Institute of Diabetes and Digestive and Kidney Diseases, in the first federal obesity clinical guidelines, stated that the most effective approach to weight loss includes caloric reduction, increased physical activity, and behavior therapy to enhance eating and activity changes. These guidelines, reviewed by 115 health experts and endorsed by representatives from 54 organizations, recommended that professionals prescribe a life style behavioral approach for at least 6 months prior to attempting an obesity medication trial. In general, pharmacologic agents should be reserved for use as additional tools (i.e., as part of a comprehensive weight management program) to help selected patients achieve successful long-term weight management.

Obesity medications are recommended for use only in individuals who have a BMI of at least 30 or have a BMI of at least 27 with at least two obesity-related morbidities. The following patients should not be treated with obesity medications: pregnant or lactating women, those under age 18 or over 65, those with severe systemic illness or cardiac-related conditions, those on other medication regimens that might adversely interact with (e.g., monoamine oxidase inhibitor, antidepressants), and those with uncontrolled high blood pressure. Additional (less absolute) contraindications to consider include a history of certain severe mental illnesses (most notably psychosis, bipolar disorder, anorexia nervosa) and any current severe mental disorders (in addition to the ones noted, significant depression, anxiety, or substance use problems) that dictate more immediate intervention than treatment of obesity.

Currently, there are approximately 12 medications approved by the Food and Drug Administration (FDA) for weight control in the United States. Ten medications are centrally active adrenergic drugs, one medication (sibutramine) is a centrally active combined adrenergic and serotenergic drug, and one (orlistat) is the first locally active medication approved that works by altering absorption of dietary fat calories. These medication types are discussed below.

ADRENERGIC MEDICATIONS Of the centrally active adrenergic drugs, three (amphetamine, methamphetamine, phenmetrazine) are classified as Drug Enforcement Agency (DEA) Schedule II, four (benzphetamine, chlorphentermine, chlortermine, phendimetrazine) as DEA Schedule III, and three (diethylpropion, mazindol, phentermine) as DEA Schedule IV. DEA schedule II and III drugs (reflecting high potential and some potential for abuse, respectively) are generally not recommended and are no longer used. If prescribed, adrenergic drugs are recommended and approved for only very short use. Reviews of over 200 studies with adrenergic drugs have noted that in approximately 40 percent of controlled studies, the active drug produced significantly more weight loss than placebo, which across studies averaged 0.5 lb/week more weight loss.

The most carefully studied adrenergic drug is phentermine, which is approved by the FDA only for short-term treatment (i.e., 3 months or less). Currently, seven pharmaceutical companies distribute phentermine, and it is available in either resin (Ionamine) or hydrochloride (Adipex-P, Banobese, Fastin, Obenix, Oby-Cap, Oby-Trim, Zantryl) form. The two forms are roughly similar in safety and efficacy. Current manufacturers' recommended doses are 15 to 30 mg/day for the resin form and 18.75 to 37.5 mg/day for the hydrochloride. Phentermine is associated with the following common side effects (observed more frequently than placebo): rapid heart beat, increased blood pressure, restlessness, constipation, and diminished sexual arousal.

SEROTONERGIC DRUGS Particular attention has been paid to three serotonergic medications: sibutramine, fenfluramines, and fluoxetine. Sibutramine is an inhibitor of both serotonin and noradrenaline reuptake. The fenfluramines were approved by the FDA and subsequently withdrawn from the market; fluoxetine has not been approved for weight loss (and thus will not be reviewed here).

The fenflurances (fenfluramine and dexfenfluramine) are no longer available because their use was associated with primary pulmonary hypertension and heart value abnormalities. The problems were of particular concern because many cases occurred in average weight persons using the medications for cosmetic reasons. Serious questions confronted the field, including what are adequate length drug trials to determine safety; who should or should not be prescribed obesity medications; and how to consider potential benefit-cost ratios.

Subsequently, sibutramine (Meridia), an inhibitor of serotonin and noradrenaline reuptake, was approved by the FDA for the treatment of obesity. Sibutramine has demonstrated efficacy for acute weight loss in several randomized placebo-controlled trials. Doses of 10 mg and 15 mg once daily have similar efficacy and tolerability and are superior to placebo. Compared to weight losses of less than 1 kg among subjects using placebo pills, 10 mg- and 15 mg-dosing of sibutramine produce roughly 6 kg of weight loss, with most of the weight loss occurring within the first 12 weeks.

The manufacturer of sibutramine (Knoll Pharmaceuticals) notes that the most common side effects include mild degrees of dry mouth, constipation, and insomnia. Some reports indicate sibutramine increases the heart rate and the 10- and 15-mg doses of sibutramine increase systolic and diastolic blood pressure roughly 2 mm Hg in patients with normal blood pressure. Roughly 12 percent of patients experience clinically significant rises in blood pressure. Interestingly, in patients with hypertension, Lean reports that sibutramine seems to produce slight decreases in blood pressure. Valvular heart disease has been observed in 2.3 percent of patients treated with sibutramine versus 2.6 percent of patients treated with placebo.

Noncentrally Acting Drugs That Influence Nutrition Partitioning (Orlistat)

The FDA approved orlistat (Xenical) for the treatment of obesity in April 1999. Orilstat is a lipase inhibitor; that is, it inhibits the activity of pancreatic and gastric lipases and thereby inhibits digestion and absorption of dietary fat. Orlistat has demonstrated efficacy for acute weight loss in several randomized placebo-controlled trials and for longer-term weight control (over a 2-year period). Studies have observed up to 30 percent reduction in the absorption of fat with a 120 mg three times per day dosing schedule.

Orlistat is associated with gastrointestinal side effects. Because considerable fat passes through the intestines, stool softening, oily stools and soiling, and increased stool size are common. It is also possible that some percentage of important nutrients such as fat-soluble vitamins are lost. Therefore, patients taking orlistat should also take vitamin supplements.

Medication Summary

Obesity treatment is complex; obesity is a heterogeneous disorder and patients' needs vary greatly. In general, risk-benefit ratios should be considered in matching patients and available treatments. A moderately obese patient with significant medical comorbidities would warrant consideration of more aggressive and comprehensive treatment (including possibly medication) than would a slightly overweight person with no comorbid conditions or other risk factors.

MARGARET BELL (CONTINUED) *Ms. Bell returns in 2 weeks, having lost 5 pounds, and at 2 months having lost 10 pounds. She is discouraged that she has begun "slipping" off her diet. You reinforce her success and refer her to a weight loss group, consisting of patients from your practice, that meets once a week. She asks about medication, but agrees to withhold this option unless she fails to continue her weight loss. She agrees to return in 3 months, sooner if she falls off her regimen.*

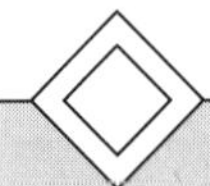

Binge Eating Disorder

Binge eating was originally recognized as a problem in obese persons by Stunkard, and has recently been identified as an important clinical problem with significant implication for treatment. Binge eating disorder, defined as recurrent binge eating in the absence of compensatory purgative practices, coupled with distress around the binges, was added as a "research diagnostic category" to the DSM-IV.

Spitzer and colleagues found that binge eating disorder may be present in as many as one-fourth to one-third of obese patients who present to university-based weight control programs and roughly 3 percent of persons of the community. Binge eating disorder is associated with increased BMI and obesity and may represent a risk factor for subsequent weight gain. Obese binge eating disorder patients have higher levels of psychopathology, greater body image dissatisfaction, and poorer psychological functioning than do obese patients without binge eating problems. Binge eating disorder patients also have cognitive symptoms (i.e., dysfunctional attitudes regarding eating and overvalued ideas regarding weight and shape) comparable to those of patients with bulimia nervosa.

Patients with binge eating disorder are characterized by problems in three domains: (1) binge eating, associated dysfunctional attitudes about eating, and overvalued ideas regarding weight and shape; (2) elevated levels of psychological and psychiatric symptoms; and (3) obesity and associated physical morbidities.

In the first comprehensive literature review of binge eating and obesity treatment, Yanovski evaluated the treatment responses of obese binge eaters versus non-binge eaters to different types of weight control programs. Although not definitive, some studies found that obese binge eaters benefited less than nonbingers from a variety of weight control programs.

Pharmacotherapy

Pharmacotherapy has been compared to placebo for binge eating disorder in five studies, and pharmacotherapy in combination with either cognitive behavioral therapy or behavioral weight loss has been tested in three studies. Overall, these pharmacotherapy trials have been of short duration, with short follow ups, and have used relatively narrow outcome measures. Few pharmacotherapy studies, however, have reported data across domains.

One study by McCann and Agras found that desipramine (Norpramin) was significantly superior to placebo for reducing binge eating disorder. Unfortunately, the study subjects relapsed to baseline levels within 4 weeks of discontinuing the medication. Another study by Alger and colleagues found that two different medications, the tricyclic antidepressant imipramine (Tofranil) and the opioid antagonist naltrexone (Revia) produced substantial reductions in binge eating (but not weight), but the reductions were not greater than those observed with placebo. All three conditions produced roughly 70 percent reductions in binge eating. Hudson and colleagues found that 45 percent of patients receiving fluoxamine and who completed a 9-week treatment program stopped binge eating compared to 24 percent of patients on placebo. Patients receiving fluoxamine lost an average of 2.7 pounds and those receiving placebo lost 0.3 pounds. McElroy and colleagues found that sertraline produced significantly greater reductions in binge eating and BMI than placebo. More study is needed to determine the role of medications for binge eating disorder.

Cognitive Behavioral Therapy and Behavioral Weight Loss

Cognitive behavioral therapy (CBT), well-established as a treatment for bulimia nervosa, has been tested in a number of controlled trials of treatment for binge eating disorder. CBT has been compared to wait-list controls in four studies, behavioral weight control in three studies, and interpersonal psychotherapy in one study.

In all of the controlled trials reported to date, CBT for binge eating disorder has resulted in significantly superior reductions and abstinence rates in binge eating and greater improvements in psychological measures than wait-list controls. Available follow-up data suggest that the improvements were maintained for at least 6 months after treatment.

Marcus and colleagues reported that individual behavioral weight loss therapy (moderate calorie reduction plus nutrition and exercise components) was comparable to CBT in reducing binge eating. However, whereas the CBT produced no weight loss, the behavioral weight loss treatment resulted in an average weight loss of 21.6 pounds, the majority of which was maintained during the year after treatment. A second, smaller study by Porzelius and associates, however, reported that obese patients with binge eating disorder lost more weight in CBT than behavioral weight loss, whereas obese patients who did not binge benefited equally from the two approaches.

Combined or Sequenced Treatments

Weight loss represents an important clinical need for obese patients with binge eating disorder. Many experts have recommended addressing the binge eating first rather than making weight loss the focus. Their recommendations are based on the first generation of binge eating disorder treatment findings and the initial promise of CBT and pharmacologic interventions adapted from bulimia nervosa. Recent findings, however, have raised questions about the ideal use and sequence and treatments for binge eating disorder.

Only one controlled trial with DSM-IV-defined binge eating disorder has reported significant weight loss with CBT. Marcus and colleagues, in an unpublished study, reported that binge eating disorder patients receiving 6-month behavioral weight loss treatment lost an average of 21.6 pounds, whereas the subjects receiving CBT showed no weight change (the two treatments produced comparable and impressive reductions in binge eating).

Controlled trials directly comparing pharmacologic and psychological treatments in combination are ongoing. Although comparison across studies warrants caution, overall CBT trials tend to have lower attrition, more robust short-term outcomes, and are superior in terms of maintenance. To date, three studies have tested whether adding antidepressants to either cognitive behavioral therapy or to behavioral weight loss treatments produced any added benefit. Fluvoxamine, fluoxetine, and desipramine did not seem to contribute much long-term benefit to either cognitive behavioral or weight control treatments for reducing binge eating, although a slight advantage for producing short-term weight loss was observed. Further research is needed to determine the optimal combination and/or sequence of treatments for obese binge eaters to reduce binge eating, improve psychological functioning, and to produce lasting weight loss.

Exercise for weight control may also be critical for obese binge eating disorder patients. One study by Levine and co-workers reported that the addition of programmed exercise to behavioral weight loss treatment significantly enhanced the effect on binge eating and weight loss.

Self-Help and Guided Self-Help

Empirical research has provided impressive support for the use of self-help materials and guided-self-help for binge eating disorder. For example, in a particularly impressive study, Carter and Fairburn evaluated the effectiveness of two methods of administering a self-help CBT program to binge eating disorder patients. This controlled study was designed to examine effectiveness in "real-world" practice of self-help CBT in community and primary care settings. Seventy-two women with binge eating disorder were randomly assigned to one of three treatment groups for 12 weeks: (1) pure self-help, (2) guided self-help, or (3) a wait-list control. Participants in the pure-self help group were mailed the CBT manual and instructed to read the book and "do their best" to follow it for 12 weeks; no other advice was given and no other contact occurred. In the guided self-help group, female facilitators without any clinical training met with each patient between six and eight times for 25 min during the 12-week period to provide support in the use of the CBT program. The overall attrition rate was quite low (12 percent). The pure self-help and the guided self-help groups produced significant reductions in binge eating that were significantly greater than seen in the wait-list group. Specifically, 50 percent of the guided self-help group and 43 percent of the pure self-help group stopped binge eating versus 8 percent of those on the waiting list. The improvements in binge eating were accompanied by improvements in associated eating psychopathology, overvalued ideas regarding weight and shape, and general psychiatric functioning. The improvements were well maintained at 6-month follow-up.

Table 14-3 summarizes empirically supported self-help programs for binge eating disorder. Also shown are self-help programs relevant for weight control and body image. Patients may benefit from using such programs alone or with some guidance, even if non-specialists provide the guidance. The reported outcomes compare favorably with those reported in pharmacotherapy trials.

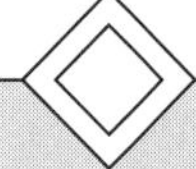

Anorexia Nervosa

Anorexia nervosa is characterized by a refusal to maintain a minimal normal body weight (defined as 15 percent below average weight for height), an intense fear of becoming fat, and (in females) amenorrhea for at least 3 months. Additionally, persons with anorexia nervosa have a disturbance in body image (the way in which body weight or shape is experienced), their weight and shape concerns unduly influence self-image, or they deny the seriousness of their low body weight.

The current Diagnostic and Statistical Manual (the DSM-IV) specifies two subtypes of anorexia nervosa: "restricting type" and "binge-eating/purging type." The majority of cases of anorexia nervosa are classified as "restricting type"; these individuals achieve their abnormally low weight by severe diet-

Table 14-3

Evidence-Based Self-Help Programs for Bulimia Nervosa and Binge Eating Disorders

- Agras WS, Apple RF: *Therapist Guide: Overcoming Eating Disorders: A Cognitive-Behavioral Treatment for Bulimia Nervosa and Binge Eating Disorders*. San Antonio: Graywind Publications; 1997.
- Apple RF, Agras WS: *Client Workbook: Overcoming Binge Eating: A Cognitive-Behavioral Treatment for Bulimia Nervosa and Binge Eating Disorder*. San Antonio: The Psychological Corporation and Graywind Publications; 1997.
- Cooper PJ: *Bulimia Nervosa and Binge Eating: A Guide to Recovery*. London: Robinson; 1995.
- Fairburn C: *Overcoming Binge Eating*. New York: Guilford Press; 1995.
  (A self-help version of the cognitive behavioral therapy for bulimia nervosa and binge eating disorder that has been most widely studied. This manual has received empirical support in efficacy and effectiveness studies via both self-help and guided self-help).
- Schmidt UH, Treasure JL: *Getting Better Bit(e) by Bit(e)*. London: Erlbaum; 1993.

Obesity and Weight Control

- Brownell KD: *The LEARN Program for Weight Control*. Dallas: American Health Publishing; 1996.
  (The most widely used behavioral weight loss treatment at major research facilities. This comprehensive manual focuses on moderate caloric restriction embedded within a model of sustained life style change. Includes attention paid to behavioral, cognitive, and physical activity domain in addition to the nutritional components).
- Blair SN: *Living With Exercise: Improving Your Health Through Moderate Physical Activity*. Dallas: American Health Publishing; 1991.
  (Although not considered a treatment for binge eating disorder, balanced life style exercise may contribute to successful weight loss and enhanced well-being).

Related Problems

- Cash TF: *The Body Image Workbook: An 8-Step Program for Learning to Like Your Looks*. New Harbinger Publications; 1997.
  (Body image dissatisfaction is frequently present in eating disordered patients and in overweight persons. Body dissatisfaction is also experienced by persons without eating disorders and by normal weight individuals. This CBT self-help manual is based on extensive empirical research).

SOURCE: Adapted with permission from Grilo CM: Self-help and guided self-help treatments for bulimia nervosa and binge eating disorder. *J Prac Psych* 6:18, 2000.

ing, fasting, and often by exercising compulsively. In advanced cases, patients will refuse to eat and can starve to death or die from medical complications.

The second subtype of anorexia nervosa, the "binge-eating/purging type," is characterized by low weight and binge eating or purging through vomiting or misusing laxatives, enemas, or diuretics. Classification into one of the two subtypes is based on current symptoms. It is common for patients with anorexia nervosa to alternate between the restricting and the binge-eating/purging subtypes at different points in their illness. Bulik found that about 50 percent of anorexia nervosa patients develop bulimia nervosa (described below).

Epidemiology

Anorexia nervosa is a relatively rare disorder. Epidemiologic research has not yet ascertained conclusive estimates of incidence (number of new cases per year) or prevalence (actual number of cases at a certain time point in a given population). Available data from Hoek suggest that the prevalence of anorexia nervosa is slightly less than 1.0

percent of adolescent and young adult females. Most cases (90 percent) of anorexia nervosa are found in women; the majority are Caucasian and come from middle-class or higher socioeconomic groups. Anorexia nervosa develops most frequently during adolescence. The mean age of onset is 17 years with bimodal peaks at ages 14 and 18 years.

Anorexia nervosa is more prevalent in industrialized countries that share Western views regarding thinness as an ideal. Epidemiologic research indicates that the prevalence of anorexia nervosa has remained constant over the past few decades. One notable change, however, is the higher incidence of the disease in women over age 30, although this population group still represents a minority of cases.

Medical Assessment

Medical assessment of anorexia nervosa is a complex process. Although some patients with anorexia nervosa show no evidence of medical problems, prolonged starvation affects most organ systems and a wide array of significant medical problems tend to be present. Frequent medical findings include leukopenia, anemia, dehydration, hypercholesterolemia, abnormal liver and thyroid function, electrolyte imbalances, low estrogen levels in females, osteoporosis, and cardiovascular problems (sinus bradycardia, severe hypotension, and arrhythmias). Anorexia nervosa patients who purge are at especially high risk for developing serious medical problems. Table 14-4 summarizes the common physical complications of anorexia nervosa and species organ system, symptoms, signs, and relevant laboratory test findings.

Psychological Functioning and Assessment

Anorexia nervosa is associated with high rates of psychiatric morbidity. Persons with anorexia nervosa frequently display symptoms of depression (e.g., depressed mood, loss of interest, social withdrawal, insomnia, difficulty concentrating) and anxiety. Clinicians may have difficulty determining whether these symptoms reflect secondary effects of the starvation or the coexistence of those psychiatric disorders. The restricting type of anorexia nervosa is generally associated with obsessiveness, rigidity, perfectionism, and over-control, whereas the binge-eating/purging subtype is associated with greater mood lability and impulsivity across a wide range of areas, including substance abuse.

Etiology, Maintenance, and Course

The etiology of anorexia nervosa is not yet understood but likely involves a complex combination of genetic, familial, psychological, and sociocultural factors. First-degree relatives of persons with anorexia nervosa have an increased risk of developing anorexia nervosa.

Some individuals may be especially susceptible to Western society's pervasive emphasis on thinness as the ideal. These individuals may have low self-esteem or may be perfectionistic or obsessive. Their families may be rigid or overly involved, or may display poor communication or high achievement demands.

The onset of anorexia nervosa tends to follow a period of dieting and is frequently triggered by stressful life events or transitions. Initially, a person finds that weight loss and dieting provide a sense of control or mastery over the body, which represents an escape from distress and uncertainty regarding other life circumstances. Soon, however, the dieting behaviors, perfectionistic and obsessional styles, and the overvalued ideas regarding weight and shape become intertwined and result in a vicious and self-maintaining spiral of weight loss. With more weight lost, the fear of fatness seems to intensify and perfectionistic standards regarding weight or shape become more difficult to attain, while the importance of perceived control and the influence of weight and shape on self-evaluation magnify.

Anorexia nervosa tends to be a chronic refractory condition associated with considerable morbidity. Even with intensive treatment, most studies

Table 14-4

Physical Complications of Anorexia Nervosa

Organ System	Symptoms	Signs	Laboratory Test Results
Whole body	Weakness, lassitude	Malnutrition	Low weight/BMI, low body fat percentage per anthropometrics or underwater weighing
Central nervous system	Apathy, poor concentration	Cognitive impairment; depressed, irritable mood	CT scan: ventricular enlargement; MRI: decreased gray and white matter
Cardiovascular and peripheral vascular	Palpitations, weakness, dizziness, shortness of breath, chest pain, coldness of extremities	Irregular, weak, slow pulse; marked orthostatic blood pressure changes; peripheral vasoconstriction with acrocyanosis	ECG: bradycardia, arrhythmias, Q-Tc prolongation (dangerous sign)
Skeletal	Bone pain with exercise	Point tenderness; short stature/arrested skeletal growth	X-rays or bone scan for pathologic stress fractures; bone densitometry for bone mineral density assessment for osteopenia or osteoporosis
Muscular	Weakness, muscle aches	Muscle wasting	Muscle enzyme abnormalities in severe malnutrition
Reproductive	Arrested psychosexual maturation or interest; loss of libido	Losses of menses or primary amenorrhea; arrested sexual development or regression of secondary sex characteristics; higher rates of pregnancy and neonatal complications	Hypoestrogenemia; prepubertal patterns of LH, FSH secretion; lack of follicular development/dominant follicle on pelvic ultrasound
Endocrine, metabolic	Fatigue; cold intolerance; diuresis; vomiting	Low body temperature (hypothermia)	Elevated serum cortisol; increase in rT_3 ("reverse" T_3); dehydration; electrolyte abnormalities; hypophasphatemia (especially on refeeding); hypoglycemia (rare)
Hematologic	Fatigue; cold intolerance	Rare bruising/clotting abnormalities	Anemia; neutropenia with relative lymphocytosis; thrombocytopenia; low erythrocyte sedimentation rate; rarely clotting factor abnormalities
Gastrointestinal	Vomiting; abdominal pain; bloating; obstipation; constipation	Abdominal distention with meals; abnormal bowel sounds	Delayed gastric emptying; occasionally abnormal liver function test results
Genitourinary		Pitting edema	Elevated BUN; low glomerular filtration rate; greater formation of renal calculi; hypovolemic nephropathy
Integument	Change in hair	Lanugo	

Source: Reprinted with permission from *Practice Guidelines for the Treatment of Patients with Eating Disorders–Revision* (APAPG 2000).

find that only approximately 50 percent of anorexia nervosa patients recover and that 25 percent show a chronic and disabling course. Sullivan estimates mortality from anorexia nervosa at 5.6 percent per decade. Indeed, Harris and Barraclough report that the excess mortality rate of eating disorders (along with substance use disorders) is the highest of all psychiatric disorders, with most deaths resulting from starvation, starvation-related cardiac events, or suicide.

Treatment

Because the starvation and weight loss can be life threatening, initial treatment efforts need to focus on weight gain and the reestablishment of regular eating patterns. Inpatient hospitalization is frequently necessary to prevent continued weight loss, stabilize the weight and any medical comorbidities, and initiate the nutritional rehabilitation. Recent changes in the mental health care delivery system have greatly modified and shortened inpatient treatments, resulting in the need to create intensive interventions using multidisciplinary treatment teams or partial hospital programs to treat severe eating disorders. Patients usually resist the initial period of weight stabilization and nutritional rehabilitation, and are typically emotionally upset. Clinicians should focus on consistency and structure during this time period. This approach is essential for the patient's success. Family therapy is also helpful to family members during this difficult time.

Patients with anorexia nervosa often have significant psychological issues that may eventually require treatment. The negative effects of starvation on psychological and cognitive functioning, in addition to the obsessive preoccupation with food and weight, preclude any meaningful psychotherapy. Once weight gain is achieved, psychotherapies can begin to be useful, although relatively few controlled systematic studies of well-defined treatments have been conducted with anorexia nervosa. Available evidence supports the use of CBT. Some evidence supports the potential usefulness of family therapy.

Numerous medications (antipsychotics, antidepressants, anxiolytics, appetite-enhancing agents, prokinetic agents) have been tested for the treatment of anorexia nervosa. Overall, although there are hints of potential efficacy, most researchers have found that anorexia nervosa is relatively refractory to medication. It is generally held that medication is potentially useful as one component of therapy, but there is no reason to support this position. A report by Kaye and associates suggests the possible role for fluoxetine for preventing relapse in weight-restored anorexia nervosa patients. Relapse rates are high for patients with anorexia nervosa. Relapse is most common during the year following treatment, although it can occur even years later. Overall, patients who achieve normal weight during treatment and are able to maintain that weight have the best long-term prognosis.

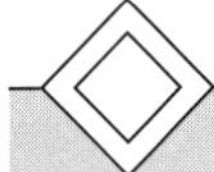

Bulimia Nervosa

Bulimia nervosa is characterized by recurrent episodes of binge eating (eating unusually large amounts of food in a discrete period while experiencing a sense of lack of control over the eating), the regular use of extreme weight compensatory methods (self-induced vomiting; abuse of laxatives, diuretics, or diet pills; severe dieting or fasting; vigorous exercise), and dysfunctional beliefs about weight and shape that unduly influence self-evaluation or self-worth. The binge eating and inappropriate compensatory behaviors both occur, on average, at least two times per week over the previous 3 months. If anorexia nervosa is also present, then the anorexia nervosa diagnosis is given (anorexia nervosa "trumps" bulimia nervosa based on severity).

The DSM-IV specifies two subtypes of bulimia nervosa, "purging type" and "nonpurging type." The "purging type" regularly engages in self-induced vomiting or the misuse of laxatives, diuretics, or enemas, whereas, the "nonpurging type" uses the other forms of inappropriate weight compensatory behaviors such as severe dieting or fasting.

Epidemiology

The DSM-IV specifies that bulimia nervosa occurs in roughly 2 percent of adolescents and adults. It is most common in women (90 percent of cases) and in Caucasian and middle-class or higher socioeconomic groups. The prevalence of bulimia has increased over the past few decades; persons born after 1960 have a higher rate of developing bulimia than those born before 1960.

Medical Assessment

Although less dangerous than anorexia nervosa, medical complications can occur in bulimia nervosa because of the extreme dieting, binge eating, and purging. Frequent exposure of the teeth to vomit causes dental erosion and periodontal problems. Vomiting can also cause electrolyte imbalance and dehydration, resulting in serious medical complications including cardiac arrhythmias. In rare cases, esophageal bleeding and gastric ruptures occur from forceful vomiting. Table 14-5 summarizes the common physical complications of bulimia nervosa and species organ system, symptoms, signs, and relevant laboratory test findings as reported in the *Practice Guidelines for the Treatment of Patients With Eating Disorders* (revised).

Psychological Functioning and Assessment

The majority of persons with bulimia nervosa are of average weight, although frequent weight fluctuations are common. The preoccupation with weight and shape, coupled with considerable shame and guilt regarding their eating practices, contribute to frequent interpersonal and social difficulties and may account for the relatively low rates of treatment seeking. Persons with bulimia nervosa have high rates of depression, anxiety, and substance abuse problems.

Etiology, Maintenance, and Course

The etiology of bulimia nervosa is uncertain, but likely results from a combination of genetic, familial, psychological, and sociocultural factors. Risk factor studies of bulimia nervosa by Fairburn and colleagues have found that family histories of bulimia and obesity and negative experiences such as teasing about weight and shape may precipitate dieting and bulimia nervosa. Strict dieting is thought to represent a major risk factor for the development of bulimia. Although many persons have weight concerns and diet, the development of bulimia nervosa is thought to develop only in vulnerable individuals. Once developed, bulimia nervosa is a self-maintaining vicious cycle of emotional fear of weight gain that results in strict dieting and food deprivation. These behaviors trigger binge eating, which is followed by purging to undo to caloric intake, followed by shame and disgust, followed again by strict dieting.

Treatment

In contrast to anorexia nervosa, the past 20 years have witnessed the development of effective pharmacologic and psychological treatments for bulimia nervosa. Based on qualitative reviews, quantitative analysis, and expert consensus, CBT appears to be the treatment of choice for bulimia nervosa. CBT is superior to other forms of psychological treatment.

Treatment with antidepressant medication is also effective (relative to placebo) for bulimia nervosa, but less so than CBT. A combination of antidepressant treatment and CBT is superior to antidepressant treatment alone, but is generally comparable to CBT alone. Two studies, though, reported a slight advantage for the combination for some symptoms. Moreover, although few

Table 14-5

Physical Complications of Bulimia Nervosa

Organ System	Symptoms	Signs	Laboratory Test Results
Metabolic	Weakness, irritability	Poor skin turgor	Dehydration (urine specific gravity; osmolality); serum electrolytes: hypokalemic, hypochloremic alkalosis in those who vomit; hypomagnesia and hypophosphatemia in laxative abusers
Gastrointestinal	Abdominal pain and discomfort in vomiters; occasionally automatic vomiting; obstipation; constipation; bowel irregularities and bloating in laxative abusers	Occasionally blood-streaked vomitus; vomiters may occasionally have gastritis, esophagitis, gastroesophageal erosions, esophageal dysmotility patterns (including gastrophageal reflux, and, very rarely, Mallory-Weiss [esophageal] or gastric tears); may have increased rates of pancreatitis; chronic laxative abusers may show colonic dysmotility or melanosis coli	
Reproductive	Fertility problems	Spotty/scanty menstrual periods	May be hypoestrogenemic
Oropharyngeal	Dental decay; pain in pharynx; swollen cheeks and neck (painless)	Dental caries with erosion of dental enamel, particularly lingular surface of incisors; erythema of pharynx; enlarged salivary glands	X-rays confirm erosion of dental enamel; elevated serum amylase associated with benign parotid hyperplasia
Integument		Scarring on dorsum of hand (Russell's sign)	
Cardiomuscular (in ipecac abusers)	Weakness: palpitations	Cardiac abnormalities; muscle weakness	Cardiomyopathy and peripheral myopathy

SOURCE: Reprinted with permission from *Practice Guidelines for the Treatment of Patients with Eating Disorders – Revision* (APAPG 2000).

pharmacotherapy studies have reported longer term outcomes, it is generally believed that relapse is frequent upon drug discontinuation.

It is critical to note here that although effective treatments for bulimia nervosa have been established, the majority of patients who present to bulimia specialists for further treatment have not received those efficacious treatments. Crow and colleagues examined the frequency with which patients who had previously been treated for bulimia nervosa had received adequate pharmacotherapy trials or CBT. Of bulimia nervosa patients with prior treatment, 96.5 percent received some form of psychotherapy but only 6.9 percent reported having received CBT. Only two-thirds received pharmacotherapy, with fluoxetine being the most frequently reported medication. Of those respondents who received a trial with fluoxetine, only 36.6 percent reported having been on a minimum of 60 mg/day, which is the dosage that is considered adequate for treatment of bulimia. Thus, the majority of patients with bulimia nervosa appear to receive inadequate pharmacotherapy (insufficient dosing and or inadequate duration) or unspecified psychotherapies lacking empirical support.

These results suggest the need for education of clinicians to enhance knowledge of appropriate treatment. In the case of pharmacotherapy, if the primary care clinician chooses to implement treatment instead of referring to a psychiatrist, the treatment literature suggests the importance of high dose (i.e., 60 mg/day) of fluoxetine compared to the standard 20 mg/day starting dose for depression.

Fairburn also noted that the desire for secrecy among persons with bulimia nervosa and binge eating represents a potential obstacle to their seeking professional help. Consistent with this finding is the report by Masheb and co-workers, documenting higher levels of shame in binge eaters than in those with other medical problems. Indeed, studies have documented that individuals with bulimia nervosa—in spite of its seriousness—demonstrate lower rates of treatment seeking than those with other psychiatric disorders. Despite increased public awareness of the problem, research still shows that the vast majority of those with bulimia nervosa are not in treatment at all.

Self-Help Treatments

Self-help and guided self-help interventions may be particularly useful for bulimia nervosa. In one study, Treasure and associates randomized 110 women with bulimia nervosa to receive either 16 weeks of CBT or a sequential treatment involving 8-week self-help CBT followed by, if necessary, 8 weeks of therapist-administered CBT. Both approaches to treatment produced 30 percent remission rates, and no significant differences were observed immediately after treatment or at the 18-month follow up. Follow up revealed that 40 percent of the self-help/sequential CBT condition and 41 percent of the therapist-led CBT condition were symptom free. These findings suggest that the effects of CBT are well maintained during the follow-up periods and that some patients continue to improve over time.

One controlled study has compared the efficacy of fluoxetine to self-help CBT, and measured their relative efficacy alone and in combination. In that study Mitchell and associates randomized patients with bulimia nervosa to one of four treatments: placebo only, fluoxetine only, placebo plus self-help, or fluoxetine plus self-help. Initial unpublished analyses suggest that self-help and fluoxetine were no more effective than placebo, but that the combination of self-help and medication had the best outcome.

Table 14-3 provides a listing of empirically supported self-help treatments for bulimia nervosa as reviewed by Grilo. These resources can be given to patients themselves (pure self-help) or be used collaboratively with nonspecialist facilitators (guided self-help). If used in a guided self-help format, the health care professional can provide structure and support and attend to motivational issues.

Table 14-6

Common Presentations and Symptoms of Eating and Weight Disorders

Obesity	Anorexia Nervosa	Bulimia Nervosa	Binge Eating Disorder
• Request for weight loss • Patients frequently underestimate overeating and overestimate physical activity • Overweight • Body image concerns • Concerns regarding health problems	• Denial of problem, deny complaints, or concern regarding low body weight • Patients secretive regarding extent of dieting and weight control; frequently hide emaciated state with baggy clothing • Thin • Variety of somatic complaints including fatigue, headaches, abdominal pain, constipation, cold intolerance, sleep disturbance, and amenorrhea • Irritability, depression, perfectionism, obsessionality	• Ambivalence about seeking treatment • Patients may be secretive about disordered eating, bingeing, and purging; high levels of shame and embarrassment • Mostly normal weight • Body image concerns • Fatigue, decreased energy, constipation, swelling of hands, feet and throat, heartburn and GI complaints, and irregular menses • Depression, substance abuse, and impulsivity	• Request for diet advice • Patients may be secretive about binge eating or may not realize its significance • Frequently overweight • Request for weight loss • Weight cycling and recent weight gain • Depression and anxiety

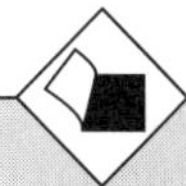

Summary

This chapter has reviewed some of the major issues regarding the assessment and treatment of eating and weight disorders. Anorexia nervosa is a difficult to treat chronic disorder with high levels of morbidity and mortality. Bulimia nervosa is more common than anorexia nervosa and a number of effective treatments have been developed. Overweight and obesity are the most common problems, affecting over 55 percent of adults in the United States. Some of the common ways in which patients with eating and weight disorders present for care are summarized in Table 14-6.

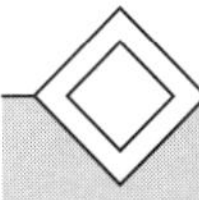

Acknowledgment

Preparation of this chapter was supported by NIH grant DK49587 and Donaghue Medical Research Foundation Investigator Award.

Suggested Reading

Brownell KD, Fairburn CG (eds): *Eating Disorders and Obesity: A Comprehensive Handbook.* New York: Guilford Press, 1995.

This edited volume contains 101 brief but authoritative chapters provided by experts. The chapters provide clear overviews of the nature, assessment, and treatment of eating disorders and obesity. The chapters include annotated reference lists describing the major references.

Official web site of the National Institute of Diabetes and Digestive and Kidney Diseases of the National Institutes of Health. http://www.niddk.nih.gov

This web site contains up-to-date health information for practitioners and patients with questions about obesity and eating problems. Federal guidelines and statements can be found here.

Official web site of the Academy for Eating Disorders. www.acadeatdis.org

The Academy for Eating Disorders is a multidisciplinary professional organization focused on treatment and research of eating disorders. The web site contains links to other web sites including a number of respected networks and organizations. A link to the International Journal of Eating Disorders *is also included.*

Official web site of the North American Association for the Study of Obesity (NAASO). www.naaso.org

NAASO is an interdisciplinary society with the goals of developing and disseminating knowledge in the field of obesity. The web site has frequent updates of developments in the field and information on conferences and meetings. NAASO is also the publisher for the journal Obesity Research *and a link to the journal may be found on the web site.*

Bibliography

Abenhaim L, Moride Y, Brenot F, et al: Appetite-suppressant drugs and the risk of primary pulmonary hypertension. International Primary Pulmonary Hypertension Study Group. *N Engl J Med* 335: 609, 1996.

Agras WS, Rossiter EM, Arnow B, et al: Pharmacologic and cognitive-behavioral treatment for bulimia nervosa: A controlled comparison. *Am J Psychiatry* 149:82, 1992.

Agras WS, Telch CF, Arnow B, et al: One year follow-up of cognitive-behavioral therapy for obese individuals with binge eating disorder. *J Consult Clin Psychology* 65:343, 1997.

Agras WS, Walsh T, Fairburn CG, et al: A multicenter comparison of cognitive-behavioral therapy and interpersonal psychotherapy for bulimia nervosa. *Arch Gen Psychiatry* 57:459, 2000.

Agras WS: Pharmacotherapy of bulimia nervosa and binge eating disorder: Longer-term outcomes. *Psychopharmacol Bul* 33:433, 1997.

Alger SA, Schwalberg MD, Bigaouette JM, et al: Effect of a tricyclic antidepressant and opiate antagonist on binge-eating behavior in normal weight bulimic and obese, binge-eating subjects. *Am J Clin Nutrition* 53:865, 1991.

American Psychiatric Association: *Diagnostic and Statistical Manual of Mental Disorders,* 4th ed. Washington, DC: American Psychiatric Association; 1994.

Ames-Frankel J, Devlin MJ, Walsh BT, et al: Personality disorder diagnoses in patients with bulimia nervosa: Clinical correlates and changes with treatment. *J Clin Psychiatry* 53:90, 1992.

Andersen RE, Wadden TA, Bartlett SJ, et al: Effects of lifestyle activity vs structured aerobic exercise in obese women: A randomized trial. *JAMA* 281:335, 1999.

Andersen RE, Wadden TA, Bartlett SJ, et al: Relation of weight loss to changes in serum lipids and lipoproteins in obese women. *Am J Clin Nutrition* 62:350, 1995.

Atkinson RL: Use of drugs in the treatment of obesity. *Annu Rev Nutrition* 17:383, 1997.

Atkinson RL, Blank RC, Loper JF, et al: Combined drug treatment of obesity. *Obes Res* 3:497S, 1995.

Attia E, Haiman C, Walsh BT, et al: Does fluoxetine augment the inpatient treatment of anorexia nervosa? *Am J Psychiatry* 155:548, 1998.

Barlow CE, Kohl HW III, Gibbons LW, et al: Physical fitness, mortality and obesity. *Int J Obes Relat Metab Disord* 19: S41, 1995.

Beck AT, Ward CH, Mendelson M, et al: An inventory measuring depression. *Arch Gen Psychiatry* 4:561, 1961.

Berman R, Grilo CM, Daniels E, et al: Pindolol augmentation of fluoxetine treatment for bulimia nervosa. Paper presented at the Eighth New York International Conference on Eating Disorders. New York: April 1998.

Beumont PJ, Russell JD, Touyz SW: Treatment of anorexia nervosa. *Lancet* 341:1635, 1993.

Blackburn GL: Effect of degree of weight loss on health benefits. *Obes Res* 3:211S, 1995.

Black CMD, Wilson GT: Assessment of eating disorders: Interview versus questionnaire. *Int J Eat Disord* 20:43, 1996.

Blair SN: Living with exercise: Improving your health through moderate physical activity. Dallas, TX: American Health; 1991.

Bray GA: Definitions, measurement, and classification of the syndrome of obesity. *Int J Obesity* 2:99, 1978.

Bray GA: Evaluation of drugs for treating obesity. *Obes Res* 3:425S, 1995.

Bray GA: Obesity: A time bomb to be defused. *Lancet* 352:160, 1998.

Bray GA, Blackburn GL, Ferguson JM, et al: Sibutramine-dose produces response-related weight loss. *Obes Res* 7:189, 1999.

Bray GA, Gray DS: Obesity: Part I—Pathogenesis. *West J Med* 149:429, 1988.

Bray GA, Ryan DH, Gordon D, et al: A double-blind randomized placebo-controlled trial of sibutramine. *Obes Res* 4:263, 1996.

Brody ML, Walsh BT, Devlin MJ: Binge eating disorder: Reliability and validity of a new diagnostic category. *J Consul Clin Psychol* 62:381, 1994.

Brownell KD, Rodin J: Medical, metabolic, and psychological effects of weight cycling. *Arch Intern Med* 154:1325, 1994.

Brownell KD, Wadden TA: Etiology and treatment of obesity: Understanding a serious, prevalent, and refractory disorder. *J Consult Clin Psychology* 60: 505, 1992.

Brownell KD: LEARN Program for weight control. Dallas, TX: American Health Publishing; 1996.

Brownell KD, Fairburn CG (eds): *Comprehensive Textbook of Eating Disorders and Obesity.* New York: Guilford; 1995.

Brownell KD, Rodin J: The dieting maelstrom: Is it possible and advisable to lose weight? *Am Psychol* 49:781, 1994.

Brownell KD, Stunkard AJ: Couples training, pharmocotherapy, and behavior therapy in the treatment of obesity. *Arch Gen Psychiatry* 38:1224, 1981.

Brownell KD, Wadden TA: The heterogeneity of obesity: Fitting treatments to individual. *Behav Ther* 22:153, 1991.

Bulik CM, Sullivan PF, Fear J, Pickering A: Predictors of the development of bulimia nervosa in women with anorexia nervosa. *J Nerv Ment Dis* 185:704, 1997.

Calfas KJ, Long BJ, Sallis JF, et al: A controlled trial of physician counseling to promote the adoption of physical activity. *Prev Med* 25:225, 1996.

Carter JC, Fairburn CG: Cognitive-behavioral self-help for binge eating disorder: A controlled effectiveness study. *J Consult Clin Psychology* 66:616, 1998.

Carter JC, Fairburn CG: Self-help and guided self-help for binge eating disorder. Paper presented at the 7th International Conference on Eating Disorders: New York, 1996.

Casper RC, Davis JM: On the course of anorexia nervosa. *Am J Psychiatry* 134:974, 1977.

Casper RC, Eckert ED, Halmi KA, et al: Bulimia: Its incidence and clinical importance in patients with anorexia nervosa. *Arch Gen Psychiatry* 37:1030, 1980.

Castonguay LG, Eldredge KL, Agras WS: Binge eating disorder: Current state and future directions. *Clin Psychol* Rev 15:865, 1995.

Cheng TL, DeWitt TG, Savageau JA, et al: Determinants of counseling in primary care pediatric practice: Physician attitudes about time, money, and health issues. *Arch Ped Adolesc Med* 153:629, 1999.

Cohen J, Cohen P: *Applied Multiple Regression for the Behavioral Sciences.* Hillsdale, NJ: Elbraum; 1983.

Cohen J: *Statistical Power Analysis for the Behavioral Sciences.* New York: Academic Press; 1977.

Colditz GA: Economic costs of severe obesity. *Am J Clin Nutrition* 55:503S, 1992.

Comuzzie AG, Allison DB: The search for human obesity genes. *Science* 280:1374, 1998.

Connolly HM, Crary JL, McGoon MD, et al: Valvular heart disease associated with fenfluramine-phentermine. *N Engl J Med* 337:581, 1997.

Cooper PJ, Coker S, Fleming C: An evaluation of the efficacy of supervised cognitive behavioral self-help for bulimia nervosa. *J Psychosom Res* 40:281, 1996.

Cooper PJ, Coker S, Fleming C: Self-help for bulimia nervosa: A preliminary report. *Int J Eat Disord* 16:401, 1994.

Cooper PJ, Taylor MJ, Cooper Z, et al: The development and validation of the Body Shape Questionnaire. *Int J Eat Disord* 6:485, 1987.

Cooper Z, Cooper PJ, Fairburn CG: The validity of the eating disorder examination and its subscales. *Br J Psychiatry* 154:807, 1989.

Craighead LW, Stunkard AJ, O'Brien RM: Behavior therapy and pharmacotherapy for obesity. *Arch Gen Psychiatry* 38:763, 1981.

Crisp AH, Callender JS, Halek C, et al: Long-term mortality in anorexia nervosa. A 20-year follow-up of the St. George's and Aberdeen cohorts. *Br J Psychiatry* 161:104, 1992.

Crow S, Mussell MP, Peterson C, et al: Prior treatment received by patients with bulimia nervosa. *Int J Eat Disord* 25:39, 1999.

Davidson MH, Hauptman J, DiGirolamo M, et al: Weight control and risk factor reduction in obese subjects treated for 2 years with orlistat: A randomized controlled trial. *JAMA* 281:235, 1999.

de Zwaan M, Mitchell JE, Seim HC, et al: Eating related and general psychopathology in obese females with binge eating disorder. *Int J Eat Disord* 15:43, 1994.

de Zwaan M, Mitchell JE: Binge eating in the obese. *Ann Med* 24:303, 1992.

de Zwaan M, Nutzinger DO, Schoenbeck G: Binge eating in overweight women. *Compr Psychiatry* 33:256, 1992.

Devlin MJ, Walsh BT: Pharmacotherapy and psychotherapy for obese patients with binge eating disorder. Annual meeting of the American Psychiatric Association, Miami, FL: May 1995.

Drent ML, Van der Veen EA: Lipase inhibition: A novel concept in the treatment of obesity. *Int J Obes Rel Metab Disord* 17:241, 1993.

Drouin P, Hanotin C, Courcier S, et al: Efficacy and tolerability of sibutramine in weight loss: A dose-ranging study. *Int J Obes Rel Metab Disord* 22(1):32, 1998.

Duncan JJ, Gordon NF, Scott CB: Women walking for health and fitness: How much is enough? *JAMA* 266:3295, 1991.

Dunn AL, Marcus BH, Kampert JB, et al: Comparison of lifestyle and structured interventions to increase physical activity and cardiorespiratory fitness: A randomized trial. *JAMA* 281:327, 1999.

Eckel RH, Krauss RM: American Heart Association call to action: Obesity as a major risk factor of coronary heart disease. *Circulation* 97(21):2099, 1998.

Eckel RH: Obesity in heart disease: A statement for healthcare professionals from the Nutrition Committee, American Heart Association. *Circulation* 96:3248, 1997.

Eckert ED, Halmi KA, Marchi P, et al: Ten-year follow-up of anorexia nervosa: Clinical course and outcome. *Psychol Med* 25:143, 1995.

Eisler I, Dare C, Russell GF, et al: Family and individual therapy in anorexia nervosa: A 5-year follow-up. *Arch Gen Psychiatry* 54:1025, 1997.

Fairburn C, et al: Cognitive behavioral therapy for binge eating and bulimia nervosa: A comprehensive treatment manual. In: Fairburn C, Wilson GT (eds): *Binge Eating: Nature, Assessment, and Treatment.* New York: Guilford Press; 1993.

Fairburn CG: *Overcoming Binge Eating.* New York: Guilford Press; 1995.

Fairburn CG: Self-help and guided self-help for binge eating problems. In: Garner DM, Garfinkel PE (eds): *Handbook of Treatment for Eating Disorders.* New York: Guilford Press; 1997.

Fairburn CG, Beglin SJ: Assessment of eating disorders: Interview or self-report questionnaire? *Int J Eat Disord* 16:363, 1994.

Fairburn CG, Belgin SJ: Studies of the epidemiology of bulimia nervosa. *Am J Psychiatry* 147:401, 1990.

Fairburn CG, Cooper Z, Doll HA, et al: The natural course of bulimia nervosa and binge eating disorder in young women. *Arch Gen Psychiatry* 57:659, 2000.

Fairburn CG, Cooper Z: The schedule of the Eating Disorder Examination. In: Fairburn CG, Wilson GT (eds): *Binge Eating: Nature, Assessment, and Treatment.* New York: Guilford Press; 1993.

Fairburn CG, Cooper Z, Doll HA, et al: Risk factors for anorexia nervosa: Three integrated case-control comparisons. *Arch Gen Psychiatry* 56:468, 1999.

Fairburn CG, Doll HA, Welch SL, et al: Risk factors for binge eating disorder: A community-based, case-control study. *Arch Gen Psychiatry* 55:425, 1998.

Fairburn CG, Jones R, Peveler RC, et al: Three psychological treatments for bulimia nervosa: A comparative trial. *Arch Gen Psychiatry* 48:463, 1991.

Fairburn CG, Welch SL, Doll HA, et al: Risk factors for bulimia nervosa: A community based case-control study. *Arch Gen Psychiatry* 54:509, 1997.

Fairburn CG, Wilson GT (eds): *Binge Eating: Nature, Assessment and Treatment.* New York: Guilford Press; 1993.

First MB, Spitzer RL, Gibbon M, et al: *Structured Clinical Interview for DSM IV Axis I Disorders (SCID-I).* New York: New York Biometrics Research Department, 1995.

Flegal KM, Carroll MD, Kuczmarski RJ, et al: Overweight and obesity in the United States: Prevalence and trends, 1960–1994. *Int J Obes Relat Metab Disord* 22:39, 1998.

Fontaine KR, Faith MS, Allison DB, et al: Body weight and health care among women in the general population. *Arch Fam Med* 7:381, 1998.

Friedman MA, Brownell KD: Psychological correlates of obesity: Moving to the next research generation. *Psychol Bull* 117:3, 1995.

Garfinkle PE, Kaplan AS: Starvation based on perpetuating mechanisms in anorexia nervosa and bulimia. *Int J Eat Disord* 4:651, 1985.

Garner DM, Bemis KM: A cognitive-behavioral approach to the treatment of anorexia nervosa. *Cogn Therapy Res* 6:123, 1982.

Garner DM, Vitousek KM, Pike KM: Cognitive-behavioral therapy for anorexia nervosa. In: Garner DM, Garfinkle PE (eds): *Handbook of Treatment for Eating Disorders.* New York: Guilford Press; 1997.

Garrison RJ, Castelli WP: Weight and thirty-year mortality of men in the Framingham Study. *Ann Intern Med* 103:1006, 1985.

Gibbons RD, Hedeker D, Elkin I, et al: Some conceptual and statistical issues in analysis of longitudinal psychiatric data. Application to the NIMH treatment of Depression Collaborative Research Program Dataset. *Arch Gen Psychiatry* 50:739, 1993.

Gibbons RD, Hedeker D, Waternaux C, et al: Random regression models: A comprehensive approach to the analysis of longitudinal psychiatric data. *Psychopharmacol Bull* 24:438, 1988.

Gladis MM, Wadden TA, Foster GD, et al: A comparison of two approaches to the assessment of binge eating in obesity. *Int J Eat Disord* 23:17, 1998.

Gold PW, Gwirtsman H, Avgerinos PC, et al: Abnormal hypothalmic-pituitary-adrenal function in anorexia nervosa. Pathophysiologic mechanisms in underweight and weight-corrected patients. *N Engl J Med* 314:1335, 1986.

Greeno CG, Marcus MD, Wing RR: Diagnosis of binge eating disorder: Discrepancies between a questionnaire and clinical interview. *Int J Eat Disord* 17:153, 1995.

Grilo CM: Self-help and guided self-help treatments for bulimia nervosa and binge eating disorder. *J Prac Psych* 6:18, 2000.

Grilo CM, Levy KN, Becker DF, et al: Comorbidity of DSM-III-R axis I and II disorders among female inpatients with eating disorders. *Psychiatr Serv* 47:426, 1996.

Grilo CM, Masheb RM: Onset of dieting vs binge eating in outpatients with binge eating disorder. *Int J Obes Relat Metab Disord* 24:404, 2000.

Grilo CM, Pogue-Geile MF: The nature of environmental influences on weight and obesity: A behavior genetic analysis. *Psychol Bull* 110:520, 1991.

Grilo CM: Physical activity and obesity. *Biomed Pharmacother* 48:127, 1994.

Grilo CM, Berman R, Daniels ES, et al: Cognitive behavioral therapy and fluoxetine treatment for binge eating disorder. Paper presented at the Eighth New York International Conference on Eating Disorders. New York: April 1998.

Grilo CM, Brownell KD: Interventions for weight management. In: *ACSM Resource Manual for Guidelines for Exercise Testing and Prescription,* 3rd ed. Philadelphia: Lea & Febiger; 1998.

Grilo CM, Devlin MJ, Cachelin FM, et al: Report of the NIH Workshop on the development of research priorities in eating disorders. *Psychopharmacol Bull* 33:321, 1997.

Grilo CM: The assessment and treatment of binge eating disorder. *J Prac Psychiatry Behav Health* 4:191, 1998.

Gwirtsman HE, Guze BH, Yager J, et al: Fluoxetine treatment of anorexia nervosa: An open clinical trial. *J Clin Psychiatry* 51:378, 1990.

Halmi KA, Eckert E, LaDu TJ, et al: Anorexia nervosa: Treatment efficacy of cyproheptadine and amitriptyline. *Arch Gen Psychiatry* 43:177, 1986.

Halmi KA, Eckert E, Marchi P, et al: Comorbidity of psychiatric diagnoses in anorexia nervosa. *Arch Gen Psychiatry* 48:712, 1991.

Halmi KA, Sunday SR: Temporal patterns of hunger and fullness ratings and related cognitions in anorexia and bulimia. *Appetite* 16:219, 1991.

Hanotin C, Thomas F, Jones, SP, et al: Efficacy and tolerability of sibutramine in obese patients: A dose-ranging study. *Int J Obes Relat Metab Disord* 22:32, 1998.

Harp JB: An assessment of the efficacy and safety of orlistat for the long-term management of obesity. *J Nutr Biochem* 9:516, 1998.

Harris EC, Barraclough B: Excess mortality of mental disorder. *Br J Psychiatry* 173:11, 1998.

Herzog DB, Dorer DJ, Keel PK, et al: Recovery and relapse in anorexia and bulimia nervosa: A 7.5-year follow-up study. *J Am Acad Child Adolesc Psychiatry* 38:829, 1999.

Herzog DB, Keller MB, Lavori PW, et al: The prevalence of personality disorders in 210 women with eating disorders. *J Clin Psychiatry* 53:147, 1992.

Herzog DB, Nussbaum KM, Marmor AK: Comorbidity and outcome in eating disorders. *Psychiatr Clin North Am* 19:843, 1996.

Hoek HW: The incidence and prevalence of anorexia nervosa and bulimia nervosa in primary care. *Psychol Med* 21:455, 1991.

Hoek HW: Review of the epidemiological studies of eating disorders. *Int Rev Psychiatry* 5:61, 1993.

Hoek HW: The distribution of eating disorders. In: Brownwell KD, Fairburn CG (eds): *Eating Disorders and Obesity: A Comprehensive Handbook.* New York: Guilford Press; 1995.

Hoffman-La Roche: *Orlistat monograph.* Basel, Switzerland; 19XX.

Hollander PA, Elbein SC, Hirsch IB, et al: Role of orlistat in the treatment of obese patients with type 2 diabetes. A 1-year randomized double-blind study. *Diabetes Care* 21:1288, 1998.

Hsu LK, Crisp AH, Harding B: Outcome of anorexia nervosa. *Lancet* 1:61, 1979.

Hudson JI, McElroy SL, Raymond NC, et al: Fluvoxamine in the treatment of binge eating disorder: A multicenter placebo-controlled, double-blind trial. *Am J Psychiatry* 155:1756, 1998.

Jakicic JM, Wing RR, Butler BA, et al: Prescribing exercise in multiple short bouts versus one continuous bout: Effects on adherence, cardiorespiratory fitness, and weight loss in overweight women. *Int J Obes Relat Metab Disord* 19:893, 1995.

Jakicic JM, Winters C, Lang W, et al: Effects of intermittent exercise and use of home exercise equipment on adherence, weight loss, and fitness in overweight women: A randomized trial. *JAMA* 282: 1554, 1999.

Jones SP, Newman BM, Romanec FM: Sibutramine hydrochloride: Weight loss in overweight subjects. *Int J Obes* 18:61, 1994.

Jones SP, Smith IG, Kelly F, et al: Long term weight loss with sibutramine. *Int J Obes* 19:41, 1995.

Kaplan AS, Garfinkle PE (eds): *Medical Issues in Eating Disorders.* New York: Brunner/Mazel; 1993.

Kassett JA, Gwirtsman HE, Kaye WH, et al: Pattern of onset of bulimic symptoms of anorexia nervosa. *Am J Psychiatry* 145:1287, 1988.

Kaye WH, Gwirtsman HE, George DT, et al: CSF 5-HIAA concentrations in anorexia nervosa: Reduced values in underweight subjects normalize after weight gain. *Biol Psychiatry* 23:102, 1998.

Kaye WH, Weltzin TE, Hsu G, et al: Relapse prevention with fluoxetine in anorexia nervosa: A double-blind placebo-controlled study. In: *1997 Annual Meeting New Research Program and Abstracts.* Washington, DC: American Psychiatric Association; 1997, p 178.

Kazdin AE: Comparative outcome studies of psychotherapy: Methodological issues and strategies. *J Consult Clin Psychology* 54:95, 1986.

Knoll Pharmaceuticals: *Meridia monograph.* Mt. Olive, NJ; 1997.

Knoll Pharmaceutical Company: *Meridia.* Mount Olive, NJ; 1998.

Kuczmarski RJ, Flegal, KM, Campbell SM, et al: Increasing prevalence of overweight among U.S. adults: The National Health and Nutrition Examination Surveys, 1960 to 1991. *JAMA* 272:205, 1994.

Kuczmarski RJ: Prevalence of overweight and weight gain in the United States. *Am J Clin Nut* 55:495S, 1992.

Kuehnel RH, Wadden TA: Binge eating disorder, weight cycling, and psychopathology. *Int J Eat Disord* 15:321, 1994.

Kurz X, Van Ermen A: Valvular heart disease associated with fenfluramine-phentermine. *N Engl J Med* 337: 1772, 1997.

Lean MEJ: Sibutramine-A review of clinical efficacy. *Int J Obes Relat Metab Disord* 21:S30, 1997.

Lee CD, Jackson AS, Blair SN: US weight guidelines: Is it also important to consider cardiorespiratory fitness? *Int J Obes Relat Metab Disord* 22:S2, 1998.

Levine MD, Marcus MD, Moulton P: Exercise in the treatment of binge eating disorder. *Int J Eat Disord* 19:171, 1996.

Lichtman SW, Pisarska K, Berman ER, et al: Discrepancy between self-reported and actual caloric intake and exercise in obese subjects. *New Eng J Med* 327:1893, 1992.

Loeb KL, Pike KM, Walsh BT, et al: Assessment of diagnostic features of bulimia nervosa: Interview vs self-report format. *Int J Eat Disord* 16:75, 1994.

Long BJ, Calfas KJ, Wooten W, et al: A multisite field test of the acceptability of physical activity counseling in primary care: Project PACE. *Am J Prev Med* 12:73, 1996.

Luscombe GP, Slater NA, Lyons MB, et al: Effect on radio labelled-monoamine uptake in vitro of plasma taken from healthy volunteers administered the antidepressant sibutramine HCl. *Psychopharmacology* 100:345, 1990.

Manson JE, Faich GA: Pharmacotherapy for obesity—Do the benefits outweigh the risks? *N Engl J Med* 335:659, 1996.

Manson JE, Willett WC, Stampfer MJ, et al: Body weight and mortality among women. *N Engl J Med* 333:677, 1995.

Marcus MD: Adapting treatment for patients with binge eating disorder. In: Garner DM, Garfinkel P (eds): *Handbook of Treatment for Binge Eating Disorders*, 2nd ed. New York: Guilford Press; 1997.

Marcus MD, Wing RR, Ewing L, et al: Psychiatric disorders among obese binge eaters. *Int J Eat Disord* 9:69, 1990.

Marcus MD, Wing R, Fairburn C: Cognitive treatment of binge eating versus behavioral weight control in the treatment of binge eating disorder. *Ann Behav Med* 17:S090, 1995.

Marcus MD, Wing RR, Ewing L, et al: A double-blind, placebo-controlled trial of flouxetine plus behavior modification in the treatment of obese binge-eaters and non-binge-eaters. *Am J Psychiatry* 147:876, 1990.

Marks IM, Swinson RP, Basoglu M, et al: Alprazolam and exposure alone and combined in panic disorder with agoraphobia: A controlled study in London and Toronto. *Br J Psychiatry* 162:776, 1993.

Marshall JB, Russell JL: Achalasia mistakenly diagnosed as eating disorder and prompting prolonged psychiatric hospitalization. *South Med J* 86:1405, 1993.

Masheb RM, Grilo CM: Binge eating disorder: The need for additional diagnostic criteria. *Compr Psychiatry* 41:159, 2000.

McCann UD, Agras WS: Successful treatment of non-purging bulimia nervosa with desipramine: A double-blind, placebo-controlled study. *Am J Psychiatry* 147:1509, 1990.

McCann UD, Seiden L, Rubin LJ, et al: Brain serotonin neurotoxicity and primary pulmonary hypertension from fenfluramine and dexfenfluramine. A systemic review of the evidence. *JAMA* 278:666, 1997.

McElroy SL, Casuto LS, Nelson EB, et al: Placebo-controlled trial of sertraline in the treatment of binge eating disorder. *Am J Psych* 157:1004, 2000.

Mitchell JE, Pyle, RL, Eckert ED, et al: A comparison study of antidepressants and structured intensive group therapy in the treatment of bulimia nervosa. *Arch Gen Psychiatry* 47:149, 1990.

Nangle DW, Johnson WG, Carr-Nangle RE, et al: Binge eating disorder and the proposed DSM-IV criteria: Psychometric analysis of the Questionnaire of Eating and Weight Patterns. *Int J Eat* Disord 16:147, 1994.

Ockene IS, Hebert JR, Ockene JK, et al: Effect of physician-delivered nutrition counseling training and an office support program on saturated fat intake, weight, and serum lipid measurements in a hyperlipidemic population: Worchester Area Trial for Counseling in Hyperlipidemia (WATCH). *Arch Intern Med* 159:725, 1999.

Pate RR, Pratt M, Blair SN, et al: Physical activity and public health. A recommendation from the Centers for Disease Control and Prevention and the American College of Sports Medicine. *JAMA* 273:402, 1995.

Patrick K, Sallis JF, Long B, et al: A new tool for encouraging activity: Project PACE. *Physician Sports Med* 22:45, 1994.

Pavlou KN, Krey S, Steffee WP: Exercise as an adjunct to weight loss and maintenance in moderately obese subjects. *Am J Clin Nutr* 49:1115, 1989.

Perri MG, Nezu AM, Viegener BJ: *Improving the Long-Term Management of Obesity: Theory, Research, and Clinical Guidelines*. New York: Wiley; 1992.

Peterson C, Mitchell J, et al: Group cognitive behavioral treatment of binge eating disorder: A comparison of therapist-led vs. self-help formats. Paper presented at 7th International Conference. New York: 1996.

Peterson CB, Mitchell JE, Engbloom S, et al: Group cognitive-behavioral treatment of binge eating disorder: A comparison of therapist-led versus self-help formats. *Int J Eat Disord* 24:125, 1998.

Polivy J, Herman CP: Etiology of binge eating: Psychological mechanisms. In: Fairburn CG, Wilson GT (eds): *Binge Eating: Nature, Assessment, and Treatment.* New York: Guilford Press; 1993, p 173.

Porzelius LK, Houston C, Smith M, et al: Comparison of a standard behavioral weight loss program and a binge eating weight loss treatment. *Behav Ther* 26:119, 1995.

Powers P: Management of patients with comorbid medical conditions. In: Garner DM, Garfinkle PE (eds): *Handbook of Treatment for Eating Disorders.* New York: Guilford Press; 1997.

Pyle RL, Mitchell JE, Eckert ED, et al: Maintenance treatment and 6-month outcome for bulimia patients who respond to initial treatment. *Am J Psychiatry* 147:871, 1990.

Quesenberry CP Jr., Caan B, Jacobson A: Obesity, health services use, and health care costs among members of a health maintenance organization. *Arch Intern Med* 158:466, 1998.

Rabkin SW, Mathewson FA, Hsu PH: Relation of body weight to development of ischemic heart disease in a cohort of young North American men after a 26-year observation period: The Manitoba Study. *Am J Cardiol* 39:452, 1977.

Ratnasuriya RH, Eisler I, Szmukler GI, et al: Anorexia nervosa: Outcome and prognostic factors after 20 years. *Br J Psychiatry* 158:495, 1991.

Rimm EB, Stampfer MJ, Giovannucci E, et al: Body size and fat distribution as predictors of coronary heart disease among middle-aged and older US men. *Am J Epidemiology* 141:1117, 1995.

Rippe JM, Ward A, Porcari JP, et al: Walking for health and fitness. *JAMA* 259:2720, 1988.

Rosen JC, Vara L, Wendt S, Leitenber H: Validity studies of the Eating Disorder Examination. *Int J Eat Disord* 9:519, 1990.

Rosenberg M: *Society and the Adolescent Self Image.* Princeton, NJ: Princeton University Press; 1965.

Russell GF, Szmulker GI, Dare C, et al: An evaluation of family therapy in anorexia nervosa and bulimia nervosa. *Arch Gen Psychiatry* 44:1047, 1987.

Schmidt U, Tiller J, Treasure J: Self treatment of bulimia nervosa: A pilot study. *Int J Eat Disord* 13:273, 1993.

Schwartz MB, Wilfley DE, Spurrell EB, et al: Using the eating disorder examination to identify the specific psychopathology of binge eating disorder. Paper presented at the Eighth New York International Conference on Eating Disorders. New York: April 1998.

Scoville BA: Review of amphetamine-like drugs by the Food and Drug Administration: Clinical data and value judgements. In: GA Bray (ed): *Obesity in Perspective.* Washington DC: US Government Printing Office. (DHEW publication (NIH) No 75-708); 1975.

Seagle HM, Bessesen DH, Hill JO: Effects of sibutramine on resting metabolic rate and weight loss in overweight women. *Obes Res* 6:115, 1998.

Schocken DD, Holloway JD, Powers PS: Weight loss and the heart: Effects of anorexia nervosa and starvation. *Arch Intern Med* 149:877, 1989.

Sharp CW, Freeman CP: The medical complications of anorexia nervosa. *Br J Psychiatry* 162:452, 1993.

Sjostrom LV: Mortality of severely obese subjects. *Am J Clin Nutrition* 55:516S, 1992.

Sjostrom L, Rissanen A, Anderson T, et al: Randomized placebo-controlled trial of orlistat for weight loss and prevention of weight regain in obese patients. European Multicentre Orlistat Study Group. *Lancet* 352:167, 1998.

Spitzer R, Yanovski S, Wadden T: Binge eating disorder: Its further validation in a multisite study. *Int J Eat Disord* 13:137, 1993.

Spitzer RL, Devlin MJ, Walsh BT, et al: Binge eating disorder: A multisite field trial of the diagnostic criteria. *Int J Eat Disord* 11:191, 1992.

Steinhausen HC, Rauss-Mason C, Seidel R: Follow-up studies of anorexia nervosa: A review of four decades of outcome research. *Psychol Med* 21:447, 1991.

Stice E: A review of the evidence for a sociocultural model of bulimia nervosa and an exploration of the mechanisms of action. *Clin Psychol Rev* 14:663, 1994.

Strober M, Freeman R, Morrell W: The long-term course of severe anorexia nervosa in adolescents: Survival analysis of recovery, relapse, and outcome predictors over 10–15 years in a prospective study. *Int J Eat Disord* 22:339, 1997.

Strober M, Morell W, Burroughs J, et al: A controlled family study of anorexia nervosa. *J Psychiatr Res* 19:239, 1985.

Stunkard AJ, Berkowitz, F, Tanrikut C, et al: D-Fenfluramine treatment of binge eating disorder. *Am J Psychiatry* 153:1455, 1996.

Stunkard AJ, Messick S. The three-factor eating questionnaire to measure dietary restraint, disinhibition, and hunger. *J Psychosom Res* 29:71, 1985.

Sullivan PF: Mortality in anorexia nervosa. *Am J Psych* 152:1073, 1995.

Tanofsky MB, Wilfley DE, Spurrell EB, et al: Comparison of men and women with binge eating disorder. *Int J Eat Disord* 21:49, 1997.

Telch CF, Agras WS, Rossiter EM, et al: Group cognitive-behavioral treatment for the non-purging bulimic: An initial evaluation. *J Consult Clin Psychol* 58:629, 1990.

Telch CF, Agras WS: Obesity, binge eating, and psychopathology: Are they related? *Int J Eat Disord* 15:53, 1994.

Telch CF, Christy F, Agras WS, et al: Binge eating increases with increasing adiposity. *Int J Eat Disord* 7:115, 1988.

Thiels C, Schmidt U, Treasure J, et al: Guided self-change for bulimia nervosa incorporating use of a self-care manual. *Am J Psychiatry* 155:947, 1998.

Treasure J, Schmidt U, Troop N, et al: Sequential treatment for bulimia nervosa incorporating a self-care manual. *Br J Psychiatry* 168:94, 1996.

Treasure J, Schmidt U, Troop N, et al: First step in managing bulimia nervosa: Controlled trial of therapeutic manual. *BMJ* 308:686, 1994.

United States Department of Agriculture: Food guide pyramid. In: *Home and Garden Bulletin Number 252.* Washington, DC: Human Nutrition Information Service, 1992.

US Department of Health and Human Services, Center for Disease Control and Prevention, and National Center for Chronic Disease Prevention and Health Promotion: *Physical Activity and Health: A Report of the Surgeon General.* Atlanta, GA: USDHHS; 1996.

US Department of Health and Human Services: National Institutes of Health and the National Heart, Lung and Blood Institute: *Clinical Guidelines on the Identification, Evaluation and Treatment of Overweight and Obesity in Adults-the Evidence Report.* Bethesda, MD: NIH Press, Publication No. 98–4083, 1998.

Vanderecycken W, Kog E, Vanderlinden J: *The Family Approach to Eating Disorder.* New York: PMA; 1989.

Vogler GP, Sorensen TI, Stunkard AJ, et al: Influences of genes and shared family environment on adult body mass index assessed in an adoption study by a comprehensive path model. *Int J Obesity Relat Metab Disord* 19:40, 1995.

Wadden TA, Berkowitz RI, Vogt RA, et al: Lifestyle modification in the pharmacologic treatment of obesity: A pilot investigation of a potential primary care approach. *Obes Res* 5:218, 1997.

Wadden TA, Steen SN, Wingate BJ, et al: Psychosocial consequences of weight reduction: How much weight loss is enough? *Am J Clin Nutrition* 63:461S,1996.

Wadden TA, Van Itallie TB, Balckburn GL: Responsible and irresponsible use of very-low-calorie diets in the treatment of obesity. *JAMA* 263:83-5, 1990.

Walsh BT, Hadigan CM, Devlin MJ, et al: Long-term outcome of antidepressant treatment for bulimia nervosa. *Am J Psychiatry* 148:1206, 1991.

Weintraub M: Long-term weight control: The National Heart, Lung, and Blood Institute funded multimodal intervention study. *Clin Pharmacol Ther* 51:581, 1992.

Weisner RL: Clinical assessment of obese patients. In: Brownwell KD, Fairburn CG (eds): *Eating Disorders and Obesity: A Comprehensive Handbook.* New York: Guilford Press; 1995.

Wilfley DE, Agras WS, Telch CF, et al: Group cognitive-behavioral therapy and group interpersonal psychotherapy for the nonpurging bulimic individual: A controlled comparison. *J Consult Clin Psychol* 61: 296, 1993.

Wilfley D, Grilo C, Rodin J: Group psychotherapy for the treatment of bulimia nervosa and binge eating disorder. In: Spira J (ed): *Group Therapy for the Medically Ill.* New York: Guilford Press; 1997.

Wilfley DE, Cohen LR: Psychological treatment of bulimia nervosa and binge eating disorder. *Psychopharmacol Bull* 33:437, 1997.

Wilfley DE, Schwartz MB, Spurrell EB, et al: Assessing the specific psychopathology of binge eating disorder patients: Interview or self-report? *Behav Res Ther* 12:1151, 1997.

Williamson DF: Pharmacotherapy for obesity. *JAMA* 281:278, 1999.

Williamson DF, Kahn HS, Remington PL, et al: The 10-year incidence of overweight and major weight gain in U.S. adults. *Arch Intern Med* 150:665, 1990.

Wilson GT: Behavioral treatment of obesity: Thirty years and counting. *Advan Behav Res Therapy* 16:31, 1994.

Wilson GT, Fairburn CG, Agras WS: Cognitive-behavioral therapy for bulimia nervosa. In: Garner DM, Garfinkel P (eds): *Handbook of Treatment for Eating Disorders.* New York: Guilford Press; 1995.

Wilson GT, Fairburn CG: Cognitive treatments for eating disorders. *J Consult Clin Psychol* 61:261, 1993.

Wolf AM, Colditz GA: Current estimates of the economic cost of obesity in the United States. *Obes Res* 6:97, 1998.

Wonderlich SA, Swift WJ, Slotnick HB, et al: DSM-III-R personality disorders and eating-disorder subtypes. *Int J Eat Disord* 9:607, 1990.

Wood PD, Stefanick ML, Williams PT, et al: The effects on plasma lipoproteins of a prudent weight-reducing diet, with or without exercise, in overweight men and women. *N Engl J Med* 325:461, 1991.

Yanovski S: Binge eating disorder: Current knowledge and future directions. *Obes Res* 1:306, 1993.

Yanovski SZ, Gormally JF, Leser MS, et al: Binge eating disorder affects outcome of comprehensive very-low-calorie diet treatment. *Obes Res* 3:205, 1994.

Yanovski SZ, Nelson JE, Dubbert BK, et al: Association of binge eating disorder and psychiatric comorbidity in obese subjects. *Am J Psychiatry* 150:1472, 1993.

Zhang Y, Proenca R, Maffei M, et al: Positional cloning of the mouse obese gene and its human homologue. *Nature* 372:425, 1994.

Kurt Kroenke

Unexplained Physical Symptoms and Somatoform Disorders

Introduction

Symptoms are the body's mother tongue; signs are in a foreign language.
—John Brown, *Horae Subsecivae*

Early in their training, clinicians are taught to distinguish subjective data from objective data. The distinction lies between information that patients actively communicate (subjective data) versus information they passively relinquish as clinicians examine their bodies (objective data). Obtaining subjective data requires dialogue; collecting objective data merely requires tacit consent and physical contact. Ironically, however, a hierarchy has evolved in which we respect objective data more; it is regarded as more trustworthy, valid, and unbiased. Physical and laboratory findings are considered "hard" data, and patient-reported information is perceived as "soft." Symptoms that are not confirmed by physical signs or laboratory evidence are labeled as *functional* instead of *organic*. In busy practice settings, this may lead to truncation of the interview.

A Hindu proverb says, "Ask the patient, not the clinician, where the pain is." Yet the patient's symptoms may be difficult to sort through for several reasons. First, symptoms often present *undifferentiated*, with the cause not obvious, even after a medical work up. Second, there is *inadequate research* on symptoms in comparison to research on diseases. The lack of research makes evaluating and managing the patient who complains of dizziness, fatigue, or back pain less straightforward than caring for the patient with diabetes, hypertension, or rheumatoid arthritis. Practice guidelines are unavailable for most symptoms, because guidelines require rigorous evidence. A third reason symptoms are clinically challenging is that to understand them requires inquiry into *psychosocial factors*. Clinicians may not explore these factors because they are concerned about the time it takes to elicit them, and uncertain about what to do with the information. Despite these barriers, recent advances in our understanding of common symptoms may mitigate some of the frustration clinicians experience. A review of some salient findings will set the stage for a clinical approach to the patient with unexplained physical complaints.

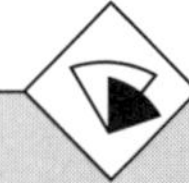

Prevalence of Symptoms in the United States

Symptoms account for over one-half of all reasons for visits to outpatient clinics. In the United States alone, this amounts to nearly 400 million clinic visits annually according to the National Ambulatory Care Survey. The reasons for the rest of the encounters are divided between visits for diagnosed disease, diagnostic or screening tests, preventive interventions, treatment, injuries, adverse effects, and others. Approximately one-half of the visits for symptoms are for pain complaints (e.g., headache, chest pain, abdominal pain, joint pains), one-quarter are for upper respiratory symptoms, and the remaining quarter are nonpain, non-upper respiratory symptoms, such as fatigue, dizziness, dyspnea, and palpitations.

Yet the symptom episodes of patients who present to the clinic represent only a small fraction of symptomatic episodes in the population as a whole. The high prevalence of various common symptoms in both clinical and community populations is well established. Banks and colleagues did a prospective study in which 516 British women kept a 1-month health diary. They found that the women tended to have a symptom episode 1 out of every 3 days, with the average episode lasting 1.6 days. One in 37 symptom episodes resulted in a health care visit. Clearly, most people recognize symptoms as ubiquitous, self-limited events and allow for spontaneous resolution or home remedies.

The subset of people presenting for care is more relevant to the clinician than the prevalence in the community. The frequency of symptoms seen in general medical practice has been examined by chart review, cross-sectional surveys, and prospective cohort studies. Bothersome symptoms appear to be far more prevalent than what providers detect, and what patients volunteer as their chief complaint fails to capture numerous symptoms. On the other hand, checklists may capture an excessive amount of symptoms: using checklists of 15 to 20 common symptoms, individuals will identify a median of 4 symptoms as bothersome. The inflated list may then require the clinician to disentangle the significant from the trivial to eliminate the "background noise."

Prognosis for People Who Have Symptoms

About 75 percent of outpatients presenting with physical complaints will experience improvement within 2 weeks. Kroenke and Jackson examined the 3-month outcomes. Of patients not improved at 2 weeks, 60 percent improve within 3 months. Moreover, relapse in patients initially better at 2 weeks is uncommon (6 percent) in the ensuing several months.

In a prospective study, Kroenke and Jackson determined the symptom improvement for 500 general medical patients presenting with physical complaints. At 2 weeks, improvement was most likely in patients whose symptoms had been present only a few days (91 percent), with recovery rates slightly lower for symptoms present 3 to 14 days (80 percent), and lowest when duration exceeded 2 weeks (55 percent). Interestingly, 2 weeks represented a sort of cutoff level: improvement rates were similar whether a symptom has been present 2 to 4 weeks (56 percent), 1 to 12 months (57 percent), or longer than a year (49 percent). Thus, even among patients whose symptoms were chronic, nearly half reported improvement 2 weeks after their clinic visit. At 2 weeks and 3 months, patients who identified multiple physical symptoms (more than 5 on a 15-symptom checklist) were less likely to improve than patients with fewer symptoms. Although improvement varied somewhat by type of symptom, no specific symptom had a 2-week improvement rate of less than 50 percent.

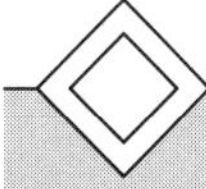

Unexplained Symptoms

Symptoms that are unexplained, for which a specific physical disorder is not easily identified, are most troublesome for the clinician and the patient.

Prevalence

In four separate studies examining a variety of symptoms, Kroenke and colleagues found that at least one-third of the symptoms seen in primary care are medically unexplained. Table 15-1 shows the proportion of specific types of unexplained symptoms in three of the four studies described. Wide differences among the three studies relate to methodological differences, including (1) whether symptoms were volunteered as chief complaints by patients or elicited by a checklist, (2) whether an unexplained status was assigned by investigators interpreting what was documented in the chart rather than directly interviewing clinicians or patients, and (3) how systematically psychiatric disorders (particularly depression and anxiety) were pursued and, if detected, whether such disorders precluded or permitted classification of a symptom as unexplained.

How Does Diagnostic Imprecision Affect Care?

Classifying symptoms into specific categories is often more an approximate than an exact process. A number of established symptom categories are more descriptive than etiologic. Our pathophysiologic understanding of symptoms is often poor, so what we have is a phenomenologic classifica-

Table 15-1

Proportion of Symptoms That Are Unexplained

Symptom	Kroenke and Mangelsdorff[a]	Kroenke et al.[b]	Kroenke and Price[c]
Population	Clinic	Clinic	Community
Number of subjects	1000	1000	13,538
Method	Chart review	Clinician inquiry	Patient inquiry
Symptom	Complaint	Checklist	Checklist
Unexplained Symptoms (%)			
Abdominal pain	90	21	27
Back pain	90	16	18
Chest pain	83	27	35
Constipation	100	22[d]	59
Dizziness	80	27	33
Dyspnea	73	19	32
Fatigue	66	19[e]	59
Headache	75	30	53
Insomnia	47	17[e]	87
Joint or limb pain		17	13
Palpitations		26	56

[a]Kroenke K, Mangelsdorff AD: Common symptoms in ambulator care: Incidence, evaluation, therapy, and outcome. *Am J Med* 86:262, 1989.

[b]Kroenke K, Arrington ME, Mangelsdorff AD: The prevalence of symptoms in medical outpatients and the adequacy of therapy. *Arch Intern Med* 150:1685, 1990.

[c]Kroenke K, Price RK: Symptoms in the community: Prevalence, classification, and psychiatric comorbidity. *Arch Intern Med* 153:2474, 1993.

[d]Included constipation *or* diarrhea.

[e]Not classified as unexplained if due to mood or anxiety disorder.

tion based on symptom characteristics, aggravating and alleviating factors, associated symptoms, and other historical data. Physical examination and laboratory tests are often not helpful. A prime example of this is dizziness.

Although dizziness can be a nebulous symptom to classify, one of the more discrete subtypes is vertigo. *Vertigo* refers to dizziness experienced by the patient as a sensation of motion, often rotary, but sometimes rocking, tilting, or another type of movement. *Vestibulopathy* (vestibular system dysfunction, either peripheral or central) is considered the predominant pathophysiologic lesion producing vertigo, but it too is rather generic: many different disorders can produce a vestibulopathy, and up to one-half of cases remain poorly understood, "nonspecific" vestibulopathies. Moreover, dizziness can be more confidently ascribed to a vestibulopathy when, in addition to a vertiginous sensation, the clinician documents other objective findings like nystagmus on physical examination or an abnormal electronystagmogram. Benign positional vertigo (BPV), *Meniere's disease*, and *labyrinthitis* are the more common specific types of peripheral vestibulopathy, yet these diagnoses still rely substantially on the patient's description and history. BPV may have nystagmus and vertigo reproduced by the head-hanging (Hallpike) maneuver, but in half of the cases, this maneuver is negative. Patients with Meniere's disease ultimately develop characteristic findings on audiography, but are typically absent early in the course of the disease. Thus, the progressive refinement of a particular patient's diagnosis from dizziness to vertigo to peripheral vestibulopathy to BPV or Meniere's disease shows the vital role of history as well as the high potential for diagnostic imprecision in symptom classification. Unlike diseases, there are no clear diagnostic tests for symptoms.

Migraine headaches, mechanical low back pain, nonulcer dyspepsia, myofascial pain syndromes, and costochondritis are only a few examples of other diagnoses with which symptomatic patients are commonly labeled but for which diagnostic criteria are typically vague. In some cases, they exaggerate our pathophysiologic understanding of a symptom, suggesting that we know with confidence a patient's back pain is "mechanical" in origin, or that a person's chest pain is due to inflammation of a costochondral junction, or that a person's myalgias are due to myofascial irritation. The liberal application of these labels to a wide variety of patients also raises questions on how good the agreement would be between two clinicians independently evaluating the same symptomatic patient. In one of the few instances where this has been rigorously studied, Kroenke and associates found that three experts reviewing the same data on the same patients and using explicit diagnostic criteria demonstrated only modest inter-observer agreement on classifying the cause of dizziness in specific patients. Diagnostic heterogeneity is probably quite common in labeling symptomatic patients in practice. This in turn may lead to considerable variability in diagnostic testing and treatment approaches.

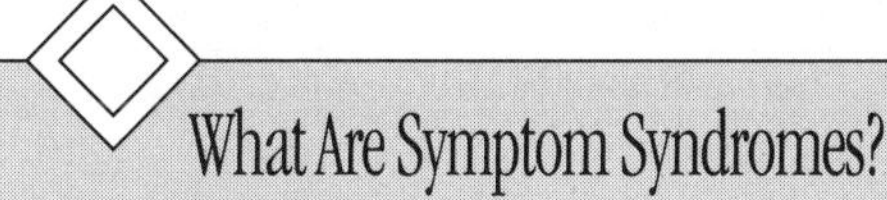

What Are Symptom Syndromes?

The frequency of patients presenting with symptoms in practice, coupled with our limited pathophysiologic understanding, has resulted in efforts to operationalize certain symptom patterns into *symptom syndromes*. Common examples include irritable bowel syndrome, fibromyalgia, chronic fatigue syndrome, temporomandibular joint syndrome, and premenstrual syndrome. Several recent monographs have collectively reviewed some of the more prevalent syndromes. Explicit criteria (still predominantly symptom based) have been published for irritable bowel syndrome, chronic fatigue syndrome, fibromyalgia, and others. Although useful in research, they tend to be loosely applied in clinical practice. Some of these symptom syndromes may turn out to have clear biomedical etiologies that we simply have not yet clarified. Others may represent a form of somatization, and many may actually be a combination of problems. In reality, the presence or absence of a clear biomedical cause for the symptoms may have little effect on the way the symptoms are experienced by the patient or managed by the clinician, unless a treatment tied to the biomedical cause can be developed.

What Happens When Syndromes Become Extinct?

Certain syndromes have emerged to explain constellations of symptoms, yet the syndromes fade and eventually disappear. Chronic brucellosis in the 1950s, hypoglycemia in the 1960s, mitral valve prolapse in the 1970s, and candidiasis hypersensitivity syndrome (the "yeast connection") were all commonly applied to patients with fatigue, episodic weakness, autonomic symptoms, neurocognitive complaints, and other nonspecific symptoms. Two main factors are probably responsible for emergence of these "fad" diagnoses. First, clinicians and patients alike prefer a discrete biomedical explanation of symptoms. Second, the four examples cited resulted from the co-occurrence of laboratory findings and symptoms common in the general population; "fad" diagnoses emerge from misinterpreting this co-occurrence as causation. The demise of these syndromes occurred rather rapidly once controlled studies were conducted.

When Syndromes Change Names

Sometimes a symptom syndrome remains intact, but name changes reflect changing theories regarding etiologic agents or causal mechanisms. In the late nineteenth century, George Beard popularized the diagnosis of "neurasthenia" for patients with chronic fatigue, because he believed the illness resulted from injury to the nervous system. During the first half of the twentieth century, use of the term "neurasthenia" waned; although it remains a psychiatric diagnosis in the ICD-9 classification system but not in DSM-IV. Postinfectious causes of chronic fatigue began to gain prominence in the 1930s and 1940s following outbreaks of illnesses characterized by fatigue and muscle pain, variously labeled neuromyasthenia, myalgic encephalitis, and postviral fatigue. Viral causes for chronic fatigue then became less fashionable until the 1980s, when a wave of "chronic mononucleosis" swept across the United States due to over interpretation of positive serology for Epstein-Barr virus. Subsequently, a series of laboratory studies with asymptomatic controls and negative clinical trials of antiviral therapy diminished the popularity of this hypothesis. New viral theories, however, continue to emerge, as do immunologic, endocrine, and psychiatric disturbances as potential causes of chronic fatigue. Indeed, immunologic advocates now propose that chronic fatigue syndrome be renamed *chronic fatigue and immune dysfunction syndrome* (CFIDS).

Other Controversial Syndromes

In addition to syndromes no longer extant, several contemporary syndromes engender considerable debate. One is the general category of *environmental illness*, the study of which is sometimes referred to as *clinical ecology*. Traditional medical organizations have expressed skepticism about the scientific evidence supporting the proposed syndromes. This controversy includes two of the more familiar environmental illnesses, *multiple chemical sensitivity* (MCS) and *sick building syndrome*. Little evidence to date supports MCS as a valid syndrome. Sick building syndrome should be differentiated from building-related illnesses for which there is a known specific cause, such as Legionaire's disease, Pontiac fever, and hypersensitivity pneumonitis. There is a larger group of patients who have nonspecific symptoms (e.g., fatigue, memory loss, headaches, dry skin, and irritated eyes) that are attributed to "sick buildings." Here, a specific causal relationship between building characteristics and symptoms has not been well established.

War syndromes are another example of a recurring constellation of symptoms given a variety of labels and purported causes. Hyams and colleagues recently reviewed war-related illnesses from the Civil War through the Persian Gulf War, including Da Costa syndrome (irritable heart), neurocirculatory asthenia, battle fatigue, combat exhaustion, Agent Orange syndrome, post-traumatic stress disorder, and Gulf War syndrome. These syndromes share similar symptoms, including fatigue, headache, sleep disturbances, memory and concentration difficulties, and shortness of breath. No specific physical or laboratory abnormality has been documented in any of these syndromes. Recent analyses of symptoms in Gulf War veterans show a high prevalence of common somatic symptoms and symptom syndromes, inadequate evidence for a toxic cause, and prominent psychological factors that are likely contributory.

How Does Overinterpretation of Diagnostic Tests Affect Care?

Historical examples have already been cited in which laboratory tests led to pseudo-epidemics of "chronic brucellosis" in the 1950s and "chronic mononucleosis" in the 1980s. Lyme disease may be the present-day equivalent. No one contests the fact that *Borrelia burgdorferi* causes Lyme disease in a certain number of exposed individuals, characterized by annular skin lesions, arthralgias and, in a small proportion of cases, neurologic and cardiac complications; however, much larger number of persons with fatigue, musculoskeletal pains, and other nonspecific symptoms have been misdiagnosed as having Lyme disease because of abnormal serologic test results. The limitations of laboratory testing in

Lyme disease include the inability of serologic tests to distinguish active from inactive infection and marked interlaboratory and intralaboratory variability in test results.

Proliferation of diagnostic testing has yielded a burgeoning number of false-positive results that may then be mistakenly linked to nonspecific symptoms. This co-occurrence of a common laboratory or radiologic finding with a prevalent symptom may be misinterpreted as causal. One example is the attribution of low back pain to disc abnormalities seen on magnetic resonance imaging (MRI), a diagnosis complicated by the fact that according to Jensen and colleagues, 40 percent of asymptomatic individuals have some degree of disc abnormality on MRI.

When Syndromes Overlap

Patients suffering from one symptom syndrome often meet criteria for other syndromes. For some syndromes, a particular symptom will be present in 100 percent of afflicted patients because it will be the defining symptom: bowel symptoms for irritable bowel syndrome, myalgias for fibromyalgia, fatigue for chronic fatigue syndrome. What is striking, however, is the high prevalence of various symptoms in each of the syndromes. Because patients appear to be "polysyndromic" more often than monosyndromic, clinicians should not be surprised when individuals with one syndrome appear months or years later complaining of symptoms in a different area. This may allow for less diagnostic testing in some cases. For example, a patient with known irritable bowel syndrome who later presents with headache, myalgias, or fatigue is more likely than the average primary care patient manifest another symptom syndrome rather than a new potentially serious medical disorder.

Why has this substantial overlap of syndromes only recently become apparent? One reason may be the migratory nature of physical complaints in somatizing and symptom-prone patients. Such patients may have a predominant complaint or syndrome for a certain period of time and unless we take a longitudinal rather than cross-sectional view (years instead of weeks or months), we may overlook the accumulating evidence. Second, Beckman and Frankel found that the time constraints of outpatient practice may compel clinicians to truncate the open-ended introductory part of the interview. Once the first symptom is elicited, a busy clinician may quickly move to close-ended questioning and clarification to achieve diagnostic closure and management decisions. Third, research on symptom syndromes has largely been conducted by subspecialists who naturally focus on syndromes relevant to their discipline. Future research on a particular symptom syndrome should systematically evaluate patients for other syndromes as well.

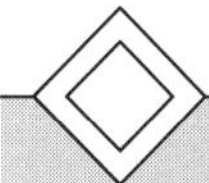

What Is Somatization?

Somatization is the process whereby individuals experience and report physical symptoms that cannot be fully explained by a known general medical condition after appropriate investigation. Earlier definitions of somatization required not only the absence of an explanatory medical condition but also the presence of psychological factors causing or contributing to the symptom. Confirming that psychological factors are the actual cause of physical symptoms rather than a consequence or simply coexisting conditions may not be easy. Also, somatizing patients may strenuously resist efforts to attribute their symptoms to nonphysical causes.

What Are the Health-Related Consequences?

Somatization is associated with increased health care utilization, functional impairment, provider dissatisfaction, and psychiatric comorbidity (Table 15-2). The latter is so consequential it will be discussed in a separate section of this chapter. Indeed,

Table 15-2

Signs Associated with Somatization

	Description	Effects
Health care utilization	Somatizing patients use more health care resources than other patients (high rates of clinic and emergency visits, diagnostic testing, subspecialty referrals, and polypharmacy). Moreover, care of the somatizing patient is frequently fragmented owing to the number and diversity of health care providers involved.	This "balkanization" of care makes it especially difficult to control medication prescribing, test ordering, and other medical costs.
Functional impairment	Symptoms are sometimes dismissed as "minor illness," particularly in the absence of an explanatory organic cause. Diagnoses such as irritable bowel syndrome convey the message that, "Your symptoms are nothing serious. We needn't worry about them any more."	However, symptoms can be quite disabling and cause substantial disability. Patients with multiple unexplained symptoms have particularly high levels of impairment.
Provider dissatisfaction	Patients with multiple or unexplained symptoms are considered especially difficult. In one study of 500 patients who completed a 15-symptom checklist, Jackson and Kroenke found that the proportion of visits that clinicians rated difficult was 6%, 13%, 23%, and 36%, among patients who endorsed 0–1, 2–5, 6–9, and ≥ 10 physical symptoms, respectively. Somatization is considered more difficult to deal with than most other mental disorders. Thus, although the presence of depression or anxiety made it almost three times more likely that an encounter would be rated as difficult, the presence of somatization made it nearly nine times more likely. This may be because effective treatments, particularly pharmacotherapy, are less established for somatoform disorders. Also, somatizing patients are more reluctant to accept a pyschological basis for their symptoms. Difficulty may also be related to overly long clinic visits, patient personality factors, provider feelings of incompetence, and pressures to contain costs. Do somatizing patients express dissatisfaction with their care commensurate with the frustration experienced by their providers? Intuitively, it would seem that the repeated visits for persistent symptoms, demands for further testing, unresponsiveness of symptoms to treatment trials, resistance to reassurance in those with hypochondriacal concerns, and seeking care from multiple providers ("clinician shopping") either reflect or result in dissatisfaction with care. However, several studies of somatoform disorders that have simultaneously examined patient and provider satisfaction have found a link between somatization and provider satisfaction, but not patient satisfaction.	Three separate studies involving over 1500 primary care patients demonstrated that clinicians experience one out of six clinic visits as "difficult." In a study of 627 primary care patients conducted by Hahn and associates, the odds ratios for patients with a specific type of mental disorder being experienced as difficult was 8.9 for somatoform disorders, 2.9 for depressive disorders, and 2.8 for anxiety disorders.

comorbid depressive and anxiety disorders are partly responsible for the excess utilization and impairment seen in somatizing patients. However, not all somatizing patients qualify for a depressive or anxiety diagnosis, and somatizing tendencies amplify the health-related consequences and illness behavior seen in depressed or anxious patients.

How to Diagnose Somatization

There are various clinical clues that heighten the suspicion of somatization, some of which are illustrated in Table 15-3.

JOYCE STILLMAN *Joyce Stillman is a 34-year-old woman who comes to your clinic for an unsched-*

Table 15-3

Clinical Indications of Somatization

Clinical Cue	Description	Example from Joyce Stillman
Chronicity	*Symptoms over time:* either a single persistent symptom, or more "migratory" complaints. Symptoms in a person without previous somatization require vigilance for potential medical causes and treatable depressive and anxiety disorders. Past unexplained symptoms and negative work ups indicate a patient's current symptoms may be somatoform. Somatization is a diagnosis best made longitudinally rather than at a single point in time.	She has a history of chronic headaches and persistent fatigue over the past few years.
Provider suspicion	Follow-up studies confirm that the clinician's initial judgment that a symptom is nonorganic is usually correct. When serious organic causes are considered doubtful after initial evaluation, they rarely emerge later.	Joyce's clinician may think her symptoms have a somatic component, as indicated by asking about mood changes.
Patient defensiveness	Patients may be reluctant to consider that psychological factors may be contributing to (if not causing) their symptoms. When simple questions about depressed mood, anxiety, or stress elicit a defensive response in a patient with unexplained symptoms, the likelihood of somatization increases.	When her clinician asked her about any changes in mood or recent stresses, Joyce defensively replies, "Everything is fine. I'm not depressed."
Medication history	*Several patterns are common in patients with chronic somatization:* polypharmacy, multiple drug intolerance, multiple drug failures, and use of psychotropic and controlled drugs. See Table 15-4 for more details.	Joyce's medications are disproportionately numerous for her age and predominantly target symptoms or symptom syndromes.
Psychosocial evidence	Depressive and anxiety disorders commonly underlie medically unexplained symptoms. Childhood family problems, particularly physical or sexual abuse, but also alcoholic parents and family dysfunction are risk factors for adult somatization. Current stressors at home or work in a patient with vague complaints may imply a connection.	

uled visit complaining of dizzy spells for the past 6 weeks. Her dizziness is not really vertigo but more of a lightheadedness that may last minutes to hours and is unrelated to position or exertion. You see that she has a history of chronic headaches for which she takes ibuprofen and propoxyphene and, sometimes, acetaminophen-oxycodone (Percocet) when pains are severe. When you ask whether she needs medication refills she says, "I need some more Percocet; I have plenty of my other medications."

She has also noted persistent fatigue for the past few years, but trials of several different antidepressants were discontinued because even at low doses she reported that, "They make me feel worse." Your previous work ups for her fatigue and arthralgias have included a normal ANA, TSH, complete blood count, and joint x-rays. Other medications she takes chronically include psyllium and Imodium for irritable bowel syndrome, an H_2- blocker for dyspepsia, multivitamins, and St. John's wort. You recently referred her to gynecology to rule out endometriosis as a cause of her chronic pelvic pain. When you ask about any change in mood or recent stresses, she tersely replies, "Everything is fine. I'm not depressed."

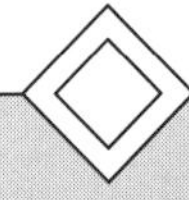

What Are Somatoform Disorders?

A classification of somatoform disorders relevant to the primary care clinician is available in the *Diagnostic and Statistical Manual of Mental Disorders, 4th Edition: Primary Care Version*, known as the DSM-IV-PC. We do not exhaustively review these disorders here, because in practice most clinicians do not use a precise classification system such as DSM-IV-PC, nor has it been proven that criteria-based diagnoses of somatoform disorders improve patient management. Instead, practical issues related to the more common disorders will be discussed. Table 15-4 outlines an algorithm for classifying somatoform disorders.

Table 15-4

Unexplained Physical Symptoms Algorithm

Step 1
Consider the role of a *general medical condition or substance use* and whether the unexplained symptoms are better accounted for by another *mental disorder*.
- A. Symptoms due to a general medical condition
- B. Substance-induced (including medication) symptoms
- C. Other mental disorders

Step 2
If the predominant symptom is an unexplained, *apparently neurologic symptom*, consider *conversion disorder*.

Step 3
If the predominant symptom is *pain*, and if the clinician suspects psychological factors are playing a role in the onset, severity, or exacerbation of the pain, consider *pain disorder*.

Step 4
If there is excessive *preoccupation with the fear of having a disease*, consider *hypochondriasis*.

Step 5
If *multiple unexplained physical symptoms* are present, consider
- A. *Undifferentiated somatoform disorder*
- B. *Somatization disorder*

Step 6
If the clinician suspects that physical symptoms are *intentionally feigned*, consider
- A. Malingering
- B. Factitious disorder

Step 7
If clinically significant symptoms are present but the *criteria are not met for any of the previously described disorders*, consider *somatoform disorder not otherwise specified*.

Step 8
If the clinician has determined that a disorder is not present but wishes to note the presence of *symptoms*, consider *unexplained general medical complaint*.

SOURCE: Adapted from American Psychiatric Association: *Diagnostic and Statistical Manual for Mental Disorders*, 4th ed: Primary Care Version. Washington, DC: American Psychiatric Association; 1995, p 65.

Somatization Disorder

Somatization disorder (SD) is one of the better validated somatoform diagnoses, and the major criterion has always been the presence of a large number of medically unexplained symptoms (Table 15-5). Somatization disorder is associated with high rates of psychiatric comorbidity (particularly depressive and anxiety disorders), functional impairment, and excessive health care costs and utilization. Patients with SD commonly undergo unnecessary diagnostic and surgical procedures. Age of onset is typically less than 30 years of age, and SD is much more common in women than in men. With a prevalence in primary care of around 1 percent, SD accounts for only a minority of the clinically significant somatization seen in the general medical setting.

Subthreshold Somatization

Subthreshold somatization diagnoses of several types have been proposed to classify the substantial number of patients with multiple unexplained symptoms who do not meet the symptom threshold for SD. The DSM-III-R added *undifferentiated somatoform disorder*—a somatoform diagnosis that requires only a single unexplained symptom persisting for 6 or more months. However, this threshold may be too low. The diagnosis appears to be inconsistently applied in clinical practice and not well validated.

In a series of studies, Escobar described and validated an *abridged somatization disorder* (ASD), defined as 6 to 12 lifetime unexplained symptoms in women (4 to 12 in men). ASD is at least 10 times more prevalent than SD (10 to 15 percent of primary care patients) and is associated with psychiatric comorbidity, functional impairment, and utilization less than SD but substantially greater than that occurring in nonsomatizing clinic patients.

Another subthreshold somatization diagnosis has recently been proposed—*multisomatoform disorder* (MSD)—defined as three or more current unexplained symptoms and a somatization history of at least 2 years. Diagnosing MSD requires asking about 15 physical symptoms (derived from the PRIME-MD instrument) that may be currently present, whereas ASD is derived from a 37-symptom checklist and requires inquiry about lifetime prevalence. Thus, MSD may be diagnosed more quickly, and it appears to identify a similar group of patients as ASD.

The distinction between these subthreshold somatization disorders may, in fact, be relatively unimportant for the clinician not enamored with nosological subtleties. Recent data suggest that somatization is a continuous rather than categorical variable and that psychiatric comorbidity, functional impairment, and utilization progressively increase as the number of unexplained symptoms

Table 15-5

Diagnostic Criteria for Somatization Disorders

		Subthreshold Somatization		
Disorder	**Somatoform Disorder (SD)**	**Undifferiated Somatoform Disorder**	**Abridged Somatization Disorder (ASD)**	**Multisomatoform Disorder (MSD)**
Diagnostic criteria	History of eight symptoms (four pain, two gastrointestinal, one sexual or reproductive, and one pseudoneurologic (conversion) (DSM-IV criteria).	One unexplained symptom persisting for 6 or more months.	Six to 12 lifetime unexplained symptoms in women (4–12 in men).	Three or more current unexplained symptoms and a somatization history of at least 2 years.

increase in an almost dose–response fashion. Recognizing that a patient has "multiple unexplained complaints" without taking an exact inventory of those complaints may identify clinically significant somatization just as well as the proposed diagnostic categories, although this remains to be verified.

Hypochondriasis

Although it has a precise meaning in the DSM-IV classification scheme, the term "hypochondriac" has historically accrued such pejorative connotations among the medical profession and lay public alike that a clinician should think twice about placing this label in the patient's medical record. The precise meaning, however, describes a clinically important characteristic in a subgroup of somatizing patients, namely, a preoccupation with the fear of having a serious disease.

Hypochondriasis is not about the number of symptoms but the patient's conviction that his or her symptoms portend an undiagnosed yet grave disease. Patients with other somatoform disorders may frustrate the clinician with their unexplained symptoms, but those with hypochondriasis are the most insistent for further testing or referral. Despite repeated evaluations the hypochondriac is relatively refractory to reassurance.

Compared to other somatoform disorders, hypochondriasis does not occur disproportionately in women and occasionally begins in middle-aged or older persons. Depressed patients can sometimes develop hypochondriacal concerns about their somatic symptoms, and hypochondriasis can also co-occur with acute or chronic medical disorders. These secondary forms of hypochondriasis have a more favorable prognosis for resolution.

Pain Disorder

Psychogenic pain disorder in DSM-III was renamed "somatoform pain disorder" in DSM-III-R and simply "pain disorder" in DSM-IV. This change to a more etiologically neutral name may reflect, in part, how sensitive patients with chronic pain are to having their symptoms labeled as psychogenic. Nonetheless, one DSM-IV criterion for pain disorder is that "psychological factors are judged to have an important role in the onset, severity, exacerbation, or maintenance of pain." Another criterion is that "the pain is not better accounted for by a mood, anxiety, or psychotic disorder."

How accurately and reliably can clinicians judge whether it is psychological factors causing the pain, or vice versa? Although depression and anxiety are common in chronic pain patients, the patients legitimately ask, "Wouldn't you be depressed (or anxious) if you had constant pain?"

Diagnosing pain disorder as a somatoform diagnosis is further complicated by the fact that pain is the most common symptom in primary care: headache, back pain, abdominal pain, chest pain, arthralgia, and myalgia account for many millions of primary care visits in the United States alone each year. Therefore, it can be difficult to decide whether a patient with chronic pain has a somatoform diagnosis or a nonpsychiatric diagnosis of chronic back pain, tension headache, atypical chest pain, or another pain syndrome.

Less Common Symptom Disorders

Conversion disorder is characterized by one or more symptoms affecting voluntary motor or sensory function—that is, *pseudoneurologic* symptoms such as aphonia, paralysis, blindness, and seizures. The lifetime occurrence of at least one conversion symptom is required for somatization disorder, and one-third or more of patients with conversion symptoms may meet criteria for somatization disorder. However, somatization disorder differs from conversion disorder in that it is multisymptomatic and chronic. The prognosis for conversion disorder is variable but appears more favorable than somatization disorder, and patients infrequently develop serious medical disorders at follow up.

Intentional production or feigning of symptoms characterizes *malingering* and *factitious dis-*

order. Both disorders are in fact uncommon; most somatizing patients are not "faking" their symptoms or illness. The DSM-IV-PC distinguishes the two disorders as follows:

> Malingering should be strongly suspected if any combination of the following is noted: 1) medicolegal context of presentation (e.g., the person is referred by his or her attorney to the clinician), 2) marked discrepancy between the person's claimed stress or disability and the objective findings, 3) lack of cooperation during the diagnostic evaluation and in complying with the prescribed treatment regimen, and 4) the presence of antisocial personality disorder. Malingering differs from factitious disorder in that the motivation for the symptom production in malingering is an external incentive, whereas in factitious disorder the motivation is a psychological need to maintain the sick role.
>
> Factitious disorder is often characterized by objective findings such as nonhealing ulcers, hematuria, infected urine, or fevers, all of which the patient creates through various deceptions (for example, self-inflicted wounds; putting blood or fecal matter in one's urine; heating up a thermometer).

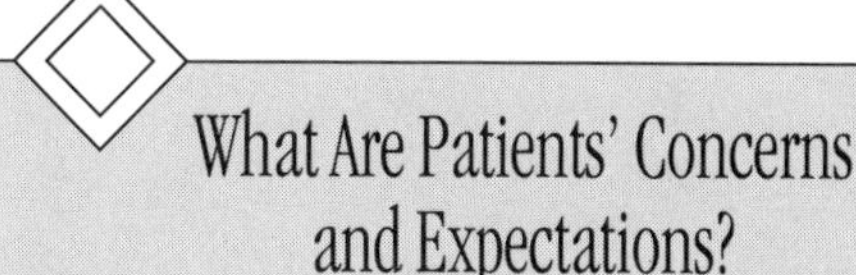

What Are Patients' Concerns and Expectations?

CURTIS MILLER *Curtis Miller is a 42-year-old man who comes to your office because he has had low back pain for 4 weeks. He tells you his symptoms are partially alleviated by ibuprofen purchased at his local pharmacy, and he has not had to miss any work. Although he does not recall any injury, his pain was greatest in the first week and has declined since then to being about a "3 on a scale of 10." When you ask what prompted him to seek care now he replies, "After it didn't go away in the first few weeks, I started to worry." You ask him what, specifically, he is worried about he says, "I don't know—maybe a slipped disc, or arthritis, or my kidneys." When you ask about the latter concern, Curtis reports that his father died of renal cell carcinoma 1 year ago, which began as back pain that had initially been attributed to muscle spasms. After finding nothing abnormal during the exam, you reassure Curtis that his symptoms appear to be musculoskeletal, and prescribe a muscle relaxant along with instructions on back strengthening exercises. Because Curtis does not seem entirely reassured, you ask, "Was there anything else you thought might be helpful?" He replies, "I don't know. Do you think I should have a CT scan or at least see a urologist?"*

Although symptoms are ubiquitous, only a small proportion of individuals seek health care for their complaints. In short, only a minority of symptomatic *persons* become true *patients.* Although this can be prompted by symptom severity or persistence, many individuals come to the clinic because of symptom-related concerns and expectations. Serious illness worry is one of the most common concerns, either disease specific ("Could this headache be a brain tumor?") or generic ("I don't know what this might be, but is it something to worry about?") Patients commonly expect providers to prescribe medication, order diagnostic tests, or refer to subspecialists. Prognosis is another frequent concern: "How long is this likely to last? Will it interfere with my work or recreational activities?"

Patients frequently do not reveal their concerns and expectations unless specifically invited to do so, and clinicians often fail to elicit them. Patients may be reluctant to volunteer their "hidden agenda" because of embarrassment ("Are my concerns foolish or unreasonable?"), intimidation ("Will I be wasting this busy clinician's time? Will I insult him or her by 'playing clinician' myself?"), or the mistaken assumption that if it is important, the clinician will ask. Clinicians may not detect patients' unique concerns or expectations because they use a biomedical rather than biopsychosocial approach, they feel their time is limited, and they are reluctant to open Pandora's box ("What if this patient asks for an antibiotic or CT scan or subspecialty referral that I do not agree with? Will this cause an uncomfortable confrontation?").

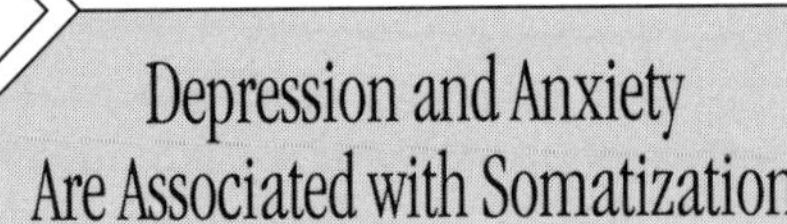

Depression and Anxiety Are Associated with Somatization

Depressive and anxiety disorders are strongly associated with somatization. This association does not pertain only to symptoms that are part of the diagnostic criteria for a psychiatric disorder (e.g., fatigue and insomnia in depressive disorders). Rather, a depressive or anxiety disorder is two to three times more likely in a person with *any* given symptom (compared to persons without that symptom). When the symptom is unexplained, the likelihood of depression or anxiety is even greater. Although the specific type of symptom is not particularly important in terms of predicting depression or anxiety, the number of symptoms is. There is a dose–response relationship between the number of physical symptoms endorsed by patients as currently bothersome and the likelihood of a coexisting depressive or anxiety disorder (Table 15-6). This dose–response relationship is for total symptom count, both medically explained as well as unexplained. Although limiting the count to unexplained symptoms further strengthens the relationship with depression and anxiety, the total symptom count itself is a powerful predictor and does not require the clinician to go through the time-consuming and somewhat subjective process of adjudicating the somatoform nature of each symptom.

The physical symptom count is in some respects a "sed rate" for potential psychopathology: it is nonspecific, but the higher the count the greater the likelihood of a coexisting depressive or anxiety disorder. One common question is: What about the person with multiple medical conditions? Couldn't the person with heart disease, chronic lung disease, esophageal reflux, and osteoarthritis be bothered by multiple physical symptoms? Although this is theoretically true, the reality is that patients with multiple medical problems will typically only endorse a limited number of symptoms as currently bothersome on a symptom checklist; offered a menu, they will focus on a few predominant complaints. In fact, physical symptom count has a much stronger relationship with depressive and anxiety disorders than with the number of medical disorders.

Table 15-6

Number of Physical Symptoms and Association with Anxiety and Depressive Disorders[a]

	Number (%) of Patients		Percent with Disorder					
			Anxiety Disorder		Depressive Disorder		Any Disorder	
Number of Symptoms	**Study 1 (n = 1000)**	**Study 2 (n = 499)**	**Study 1**	**Study 2**	**Study 1**	**Study 2**	**Study 1**	**Study 2**
0–1	215 (22)	106 (21)	1	3	2	3	7	4
2–3	225 (23)	131 (26)	7	8	12	13	22	18
4–5	191 (19)	129 (26)	13	13	23	32	35	31
6–8	230 (23)	96 (19)	30	26	44	42	61	52
≥9	139 (14)	37 (7)	48	51	60	57	81	78

[a]Study 1 is the PRIME-MD 1000 study, a mental survey of 1000 patients seen in 4 primary care clinics (Kroenke et al., 1989). Study 2 evaluated 500 patients presenting to a general medicine walk-in clinic with a physical complaint (Garro et al., 1994). In both studies, all patients completed the PRIME-MD, which included a checklist of 15 physical symptoms as well as clinician-administered modules, which made DSM-IV criteria-based diagnoses of anxiety and depressive disorders.

Impact of Gender on Somatizaton

Gender has an important relationship to symptom reporting. Women report most symptoms at least 50 percent more often than men do. Although depressive and anxiety disorders are also more prevalent in women and account for a substantial amount of the increased somatization, gender affects symptom reporting whether or not there is psychiatric comorbidity. Gender is the demographic factor with the greatest influence on symptom reporting.

Abuse and Somatization

Abuse (sexual or physical), particularly during childhood, has increasingly been shown to have a strong relationship with somatization as an adult. This not only includes complaints like chronic abdominal or pelvic pain but other unexplained symptoms, too. Moreover, there is a dose–response relationship between symptom counts and likelihood of abuse.

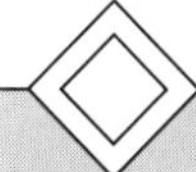

How to Manage Somatic Disorders

A practical approach to the patient with unexplained symptoms is outlined in Fig. 15-1. First, it consists of seven key questions to which an affirmative answer may provide a "skip out" to a specific clinician action or treatment.

Seven Key Questions to Ask

Is the Symptom Medically Explained?

Frequently, the cause or at least etiologic category of the symptom will be apparent with a focused history and physical examination.

Could the Symptom Be Acutely Serious?

Some symptoms are intrinsically more worrisome; for example, chest pain, syncope, dyspnea, and acute abdominal pain. Even when mentioned as incidental, end-of-the-visit complaints, these symptoms require at least a few additional questions to determine whether an expedited or routine evaluation is appropriate. In contrast, symptoms such as arthralgias or myalgias, chronic abdominal pain, most headaches, and fatigue are seldom harbingers of an urgent condition; usually, a subsequent visit can be scheduled for further evaluation if the cause is not readily apparent. There is a third class of symptoms (e.g., dizziness, back pain, palpitations) that, although usually not urgent, may occasionally require more immediate attention, depending on the patient's age, associated symptoms, comorbid conditions, and risk factors.

In this question, *acutely* is the important qualifier. By this we mean symptoms that not only can herald a potentially serious disease but ones that, if not diagnosed promptly, may result in death or serious morbidity in a matter of days or weeks. Cardiopulmonary symptoms, acute abdominal pain, and the occasional "worst headache I've ever had" fall into this category. Other diseases (thyroid disorders, autoimmune diseases, chronic neurologic disorders, most cancers) may be serious, but typically develop in a progressive rather than catastrophic fashion. Unless other signs or symptoms make such disorders prominent considerations, diagnostic evaluation can usually be reserved for those whose symptoms remain unexplained and persist a month or longer.

Clinicians are sometimes concerned about the medicolegal implications of "failure to diagnose," particularly for diseases like cancer. Culpability, however, is more an issue when clinicians tell patients, "nothing is wrong," do not provide adequate follow up, and then the disease becomes manifest many months later. Deferring an extensive work up at the first presentation of an unexplained symptom is not the same as dismissing the symptom entirely. Either schedule a follow-

Figure 15-1

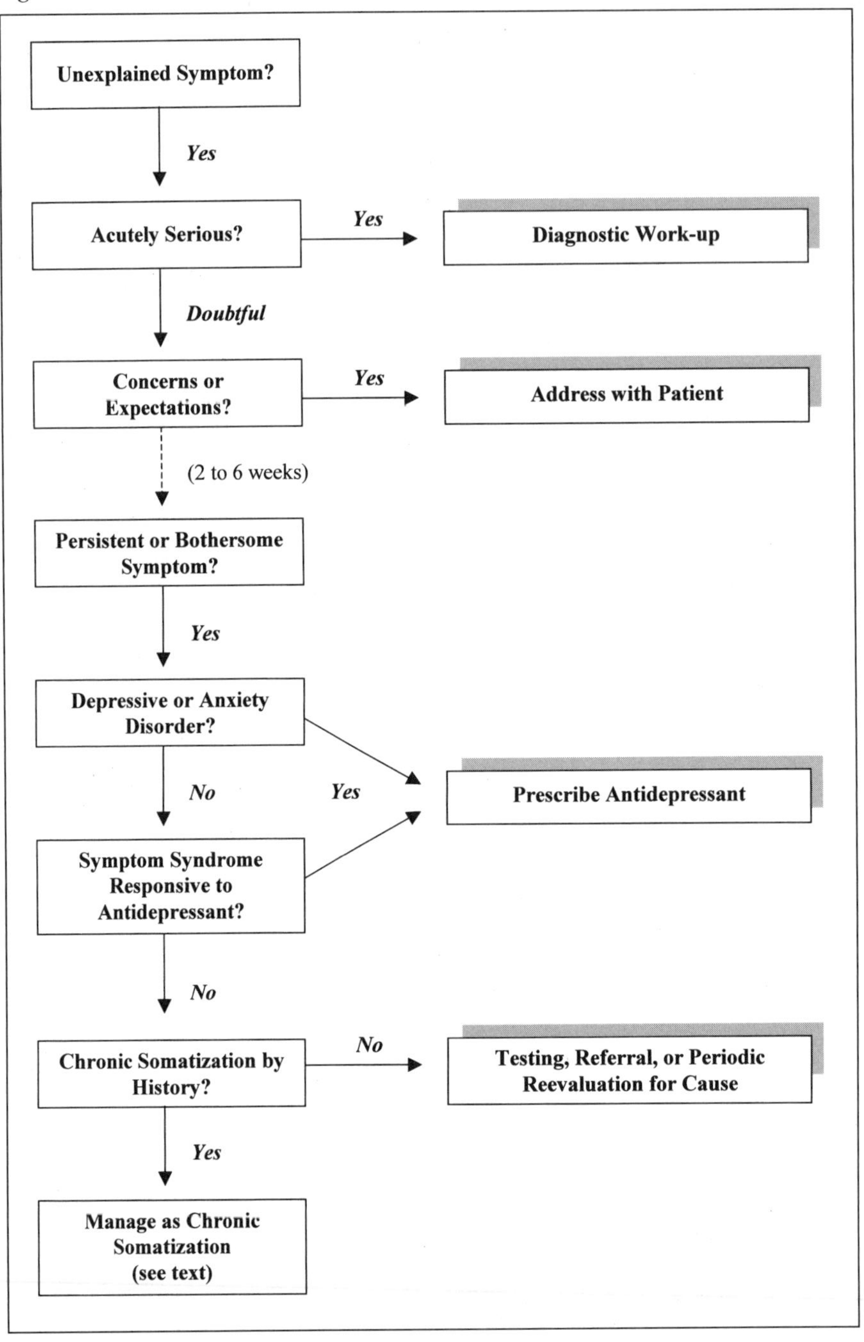

A practical approach to the patient with unexplained symptoms consists of 7 key questions. An affirmative answer may provide a “skip-out” to a specific clinical action or treatment. Diagnostic algorithm for chronic somatization.

up visit (within 1 to 2 months) to reassess the symptom or, alternatively, instruct patients to come back themselves if the symptom does not improve. Patients who may be unreliable candidates for follow up may warrant initial diagnostic evaluation.

Does the Patient Have Specific Concerns or Expectations?

There remains an important proportion (at least 20 to 35 percent) of primary care patients in whom symptoms are neither readily explainable nor acutely serious. In such cases, the clinician might close the encounter with two useful questions: "Was there anything else you were worried about?" and "Was there anything else you thought might be helpful?" The first question is intended to elicit unexpressed concerns; the second, unstated expectations. Concerns may be generic ("Do I have something serious?" "How long will this symptom last?") or specific ("Do I have heart disease? Cancer? An impending stroke?"). Expectations may be for a prescription medication, diagnostic test, subspecialty referral, work excuse, or other clinician action.

If the patient responds, "I don't know; you're the clinician," the clinician can reply, "Often patients have specific concerns or thoughts about what might be helpful." For some symptoms, there are certain disorders that are most commonly feared, in which case the clinician may reveal a patient's hidden agenda through directed inquiry. For example, a clinician may ask a patient with headache or dizziness, "Sometimes, patients are concerned about something more serious, such as a tumor or a stroke. Was there anything you were wondering about?" or, "Sometimes, patients wonder whether an x-ray or other tests are needed. What about you?" Whether on target or not, a brief question or two may invite the patient to disclose unexpressed concerns. The clinician can then provide patient-specific explanations or reassurance: "I can understand why you were worried about your heart. Let me tell you why your chest pain is not the type we see in patients with angina."

Clinicians are often encouraged to ask more open-ended questions so that encounters can be more patient centered. However, time constraints in primary care require a balance between a limited amount of open-ended questions and a larger number of close-ended (yes/no or clarifying) questions. Regarding the patient's agenda, open-ended questions are most appropriate at the beginning and the end of the encounter. At the beginning, it is important to identify the patient's problems or complaints. Although the visit may appear to be a scheduled visit for hypertension follow up or an unscheduled visit for dizziness, the clinician should determine whether there are any other problems the patient would like to discuss. This is to avoid the "Oh, by the way" complaints patients sometimes volunteer as the visit winds to a close. The end of the visit is an appropriate time to briefly inquire about residual concerns or expectations. These are not new problems, but lingering questions or desires related to the problem(s) that you have dealt with during the encounter.

Does the Symptom Remain Persistent and Bothersome?

Follow up is often preferable to a work up for unexplained symptoms. Because one-half to two-thirds of symptoms improve within several weeks of an initial clinic visit, and one-half of those not improved at 2 weeks gradually improve by 3 months, it makes sense to focus more extensive and costly diagnostic efforts on the minority of patients with unexplained symptoms that persist for 2 to 6 weeks or longer. The exact interval for watchful waiting is not a precise time period but is patient and symptom specific. Also, what the clinician provides may vary from education and reassurance to simple empiric treatment.

Does the Patient Have a Depressive or Anxiety Disorder?

Over one-half of patients with medically unexplained physical symptoms will have a coexisting depressive or anxiety disorder. Antidepressants may be effective for many of these patients, particularly those with major depression, dysthymia, and panic disorder. Diagnosis and treatment of depressive, anxiety, and panic disorders are discussed in Chaps. 16, 17, and 18. However, somatizing patients are sometimes reluctant to readily accept a psychological explanation or treatment for their symptoms.

Does the Patient Have a Symptom Syndrome Responsive to Antidepressants?

O'Malley and colleagues report that there are a number of symptom syndromes for which there is some evidence of antidepressant efficacy, including fibromyalgia, migraine and tension headaches, chronic pain disorders, and irritable bowel syndrome. There are also a few studies showing antidepressant efficacy in premenstrual disorder, chronic tinnitus, and noncardiac chest pain. Many of these studies do not clearly distinguish whether the benefits for physical symptoms are related to or independent of medication effects on depression itself. However, the evidence is such that an empiric trial of antidepressants is certainly warranted in selected patients with one of these bothersome symptom syndromes. Most of the studies to date have been conducted with tricyclic antidepressants (TCAs), and it remains to be seen whether selective serotonin reuptake inhibitors (SSRIs) and other newer antidepressants are also effective in symptom syndromes.

Does the Patient Have a History of Chronic Somatization?

One should be cautious in labeling the patient presenting with a first unexplained symptom as somatoform. Chronic somatization is in essence a "cumulative" diagnosis—the longer the duration of symptoms and the larger the number of previous symptoms that languish as unexplained, the greater becomes the circumstantial evidence for a somatoform diagnosis.

Once you have reached the bottom rung of the diagnosis algorithm with a patient, you should focus your efforts on management issues. Our example of Joyce Stillman is helpful for addressing some of the relevant management issues.

Questions to Ask about Chronic Somatization

JOYCE STILLMAN (CONTINUED) *The patient you saw for dizziness, Joyce Stillman, returns 2 months later with continuing symptoms. You refer her to an otolarynogologist, who performs an electronystagmogram (which is normal) and concludes the consult with a diagnosis of "nonspecific dizziness with no vestibular disorder." Joyce now asks you, "What about an MRI? And shouldn't I see a neurologist?" When asked why, she says, "Can't multiple sclerosis present with dizziness?" You say, "That's a good question, and I understand your concerns. Let me tell you why the dizziness you are experiencing is not what we see in MS."*

A month later Joyce returns, asking about applying for disability and bringing you some forms. You reply, "I know your dizziness interferes quite a bit with your ability to function well at work. Let's talk a bit more about what your employer expects and how it most affects you at work."

Additionally, she reports some new palpitations as well as worsening of her chronic fatigue. For the latter she has joined a chronic fatigue syndrome support group and has found St. John's wort and vitamin E partly beneficial. When you ask about her medications she says, "Yes, I need all of them refilled. And by the way, isn't it time for my annual Pap smear?"

The encounters with Joyce illustrate not only the challenges of time management but also several other common themes in caring for the somatizing patient. Once it becomes apparent that a patient is prone to chronic somatization, there are 10 additional issues salient to chronic somatization that you should consider as you think about symptom management.

1. Is there a history of sexual or physical *abuse*? People with unexplained symptoms, particularly chronic and multiple symptoms, are sub-

stantially more likely to have been sexually or physically abused. This is one of those "Pandora's box" questions that many clinicians avoid because they do not know how to handle an affirmative response. For the patient in a currently abusive situation, clinicians may refer to social services, counseling, or support groups. Because psychiatric comorbidity is prevalent among those with a history of abuse, clinicians may focus on treating concurrent depressive or anxiety disorders. Clinicians may consider psychotherapy for those with disabling somatization and a past history of abuse, although the efficacy of such therapy remains to be established. See Chap. 6 for more information on violence and abuse.

2. Is there an aspect of *hypochondriasis*? Patients who are convinced that they have a serious medical disorder that, despite comprehensive evaluation, remains undiagnosed can be particularly difficult to care for. Conviction or phobia of a serious illness related to a single symptom can be more frustrating than multiple symptoms about which the patient is less insistent. In this sense, hypochondriasis can be more clinically frustrating than somatization disorder. Kellner reports that various treatments such as psychotropic medications for comorbid depressive or anxiety disorders, psychotherapy, and other primary care management strategies for somatization (see below) can be used. Clinicians should also be aware that when their own level of irritation with a somatizing patient continues to rise, it may be because the patient has hypochondriacal concerns that prompt repeated evaluations yet remain refractory to reassurance. Being objective about this patient characteristic may partially ameliorate the clinician's irratation.
3. There are some generic *primary care management principles* that have been best studied by Smith in clinical trials of patients with full as well as abridged somatization disorder. These include scheduling regular, brief appointments that are not related to symptom exacerbations, avoiding tests and subspecialty referrals as much as possible, and empathizing with new symptoms but conducting focused evaluations rather than exhaustive work ups. Additional suggestions by Kaplan and colleagues include not disputing the reality of the complaint, recognizing that symptom management rather than cure is the goal, and reassuring the patient that when referral occurs (medical or psychiatric) it is for consultation or comanagement rather than dismissal. More than most other disorders, somatization requires that the primary care provider remain the "captain of the ship."
4. Consider *cognitive-behavioral therapy (CBT) or other psychotherapy* for disabling somatization. Kroenke and Swindle found that CBT has been one of the better studied psychotherapies for somatization, but behavioral therapy, stress reduction, biofeedback, and problem solving therapy have also been shown to have some degree of efficacy. In some studies, as few as 4 to 6 sessions and group rather than individual therapy has proven effective. Because somatization is such a costly condition for practices, managed care systems and other payers might consider making one or more of these nonpharmacologic therapies available.
5. Symptoms, rather than specific diseases, are one of the most common reasons patients use *complementary and alternative medicine* (CAM) according to Eisenberg and associates. Patients may be disappointed with what conventional medicine has to offer for chronic or unexplained symptoms and conventional clinicians are not often eager to care for patients with such complaints. In contrast, CAM clinicians may be more empathetic as well as enthusiastic in providing ongoing care. More evidence is needed to distinguish effective from ineffective CAM therapies, especially because regular use may be costly and often not covered by insurance plans. At the same time, studies have shown that chiropractic, acupuncture, herbal medicine, massage and

other CAM therapies are beneficial for selected symptomatic conditions.

6. Aim for *rehabilitation rather than disability*. A rehabilitative approach is increasingly being advocated for back pain, pain disorders, chronic fatigue syndrome, and other symptom syndromes. Barriers can make this difficult, such as a job that continually aggravates the symptom (e.g., back pain in someone who must do a lot of bending or heavy lifting), patients whose work is unsatisfying or whose limited skills preclude transfer to another job, and employers who for financial or other reasons cannot be sympathetic to reduced work loads or prolonged rehabilitation. Still, one of the toughest yet most consequential decisions the clinician can make is to recommend permanent disability for a patient with chronic symptoms. By refusing to do so, or at least delaying in favor of continued rehabilitation efforts, the patient may perceive the clinician as being unsympathetic to his or her suffering. However, premature assignment of disability status not only has financial consequences for employers and society but, more importantly, it encourages the patient to assume a chronic sick role.
7. *Time management* strategies are essential to prevent the clinician from becoming overwhelmed by the somatizing patient. Various factors conspire to lengthen the visit, including multiple symptoms at the beginning of the visit, "oh, by the way" complaints near the end of the visit, talkative or tangential elaborations on a given symptom, and review of extensive previous evaluations. The clinician can take several steps to control the length of the encounter: (1) Establish all the patient's potential concerns at the beginning of the visit. After an initial, "Has anything been bothering you lately?" do not accept one complaint as the complete list. Ask "Is there anything else?" until the patient says, "No." (2) Prioritize the list. If the symptom list is too long for a single visit, say something like, "You clearly have a number of concerns. Because we only have 15 mins, can you tell me what is bothering you most at this time?" (3) If the patient still inserts "by the way complaints" at the end of the visit, quickly validate them—"I'm glad you mentioned this." Then defer an extended discussion—"We spent most of our time evaluating your headaches, which you said at the beginning of the visit have been very severe lately. However, because the tiredness you just mentioned must also be bothering you I'd like to have adequate time to figure out what might be causing it. Can we schedule another visit in a couple weeks to talk about your fatigue in more detail?" (4) Begin closing the visit earlier than usual. If you typically reserve 1 to 2 min of closure for a nonsomatizing patient, reserve 3 to 5 min for the somatizing patient. Closure will always take longer than you think, even if you established and prioritized an agenda at the beginning.
8. *Reassurance* can be therapeutic in some patients. However, *avoid fighting words:* "There is nothing wrong" Or "Everything is normal." The somatizing patient does have something wrong (bothersome symptoms); and not everything is normal—just the physical examination and laboratory tests. Somatizing patients have an illness rather than a disease, and the perception that their primary provider does not take their afflictions seriously is one reason they may clinician shop or seek out CAM clinicians. Instead use *healing words,* examples of which are captured by the mnemonic, CLING:
    - Let patients know that individuals with symptoms like theirs are *common* in your practice (e.g., one out of every three or four patients). Tell patients that they are not unusual or "abnormal."
    - *Legitimize* the suffering: "Persistent dizziness can be quite disabling. I understand why you want something done about it."
    - Explain that symptoms like theirs are often *idiopathic*. Tell them blood tests, x-rays, and other types of tests are only helpful for certain diseases. Assure them this does not

mean that their discomfort is less real, just that symptoms are poorly measured by current diagnostic tests.

- Assure somatizing patients that the symptoms they have are usually *nonprogressive.* Tell them what they are not, and why. Explain the reasons why their chest pain is not the type seen in heart disease, or why their dizziness does not suggest a tumor or a stroke. Inform them that although their symptoms may wax and wane, many patients may have long periods of symptom reduction or remission, with more good days than bad. This kind of positive message is in fact borne out by studies of chronic somatization and can be therapeutic in some patients.
- Clarify that improvement is typically *gradual.* Too often patients expect to be better a day or two after visiting a clinician. Patience must be part of the prescription, the expectation that symptoms may slowly improve over weeks to months.

William Mayo wrote in 1927 that, "To a considerable extent we leave reassurance to the quack and the cultist, and if we are unable to find physical disease we say that a patient needs no medical attention, although he may be urgently in need of reassurance and mental comfort."

9. *Outcomes* such as mortality or serious morbidity are uncommon in patients with chronic somatization. Also, as with any chronic disease, treatment is not expected to attain a cure (complete and final eradication of the patient's symptoms). Rather, reasonable goals include reduction of one or more "*Ds*": (1) *Discomfort* related to the symptom, including both physical and emotional; (2) *Disability* related to the symptom. Aims would be to improve coping skills as well as occupational and social functioning. The focus might be on living despite the symptom, rather than without it. (3) *Dissatisfaction* with care. Here, the clinician would attempt to identify and address the patient's concerns and expectations, such as serious illness worry and desires for testing and referral. (4) *Debts* of the patient and/or health care system related to excessive prescribing, testing, referral, clinic and emergency room visits, and hospitalization. (5) *Difficulty* experienced by the provider in caring for the somatizing patient. Reducing some of these *Ds* is a reasonable goal for managing a somatizing patient.
10. *External influences* may either benefit or sustain somatization, as illustrated by three examples: *Family* or significant others may sustain or aggravate somatization either through family stress, dysfunction, and conflict or through secondary gain, for example, by fostering a sick role and dependency in the patient. Conversely, family members can be engaged in a therapeutic role by understanding and supporting the clinician's management strategy or, when indicated, family therapy. *Support groups* have sprung up for chronic fatigue syndrome, fibromyalgia, chronic tinnitus, irritable bowel syndrome, temporomandibular joint syndrome, and numerous other symptom syndromes. These groups may provide a mutually supportive environment that individuals may not experience with their family, friends, employers, or health care providers. At the same time, these groups may comprise a more disabled or distressed group of patients and sometimes focus on chronic disability rather than rehabilitation. Some groups also focus exclusively on organic/biological etiologies and resent any mention of psychological factors as contributory factors. The *media* may have a kindling effect, particularly for new syndromes. Television, radio, newspapers, magazines, and books have publicized and popularized chronic fatigue syndrome, Lyme disease, sick building syndrome, multiple chemical sensitivity, and Gulf War illness, to name a few examples. This sometimes has incited mini-epidemics by either amplifying concerns in individuals who already believe they have the syndrome or raising concerns in those with common, nonspecific symptoms.

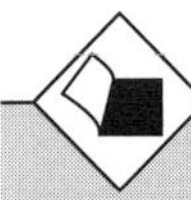

Summary

Unexplained physical symptoms are among the most common problems encountered in outpatient practice and account for considerable patient disability, provider frustration, and health care costs. Physical symptoms as they are encountered in primary care often have a favorable natural history, and only a small proportion become chronic and disabling. Although symptoms related to specific diseases may have targeted treatments, therapy is less developed for symptoms that are idiopathic or part of a symptom syndrome. For these symptoms as well as those that constitute a somatoform disorder, generic management strategies rather than specific treatments may be more realistic. Few disorders pose as great a challenge to the provider-patient relationship, yet few disorders are as dependent on a strong relationship for successful management. Success is more appropriately measured by small steps, not dramatic strides; improved functioning rather than symptom resolution. Clinicians must be aware of their own counterproductive emotions—anger, frustration, and incompetence. Recognizing these as almost ubiquitous reactions to chronic somatization, the clinician can better objectify them as intrinsic to the illness and proceed beyond them to care for and comfort the person afflicted with persistent and disabling somatic symptoms.

Suggested Reading

Bass CB (ed): *Somatization: Physical Symptoms and Psychological Illness.* Oxford, UK: Blackwell; 1990.

A practical review by British experts on the evaluation and management of somatization in general as well as specific entities such as chronic fatigue syndrome, functional abdominal pain, functional cardiorespiratory syndromes, dermatologic symptoms, gynecologic complaints, and conversion symptoms.

Ford CV: *The Somatizing Disorders: Illness as a Way of Life.* New York: Elsevier; 1983.

A classic text that in addition to DSM syndromes provides valuable guidance and perspectives on caring for the somatizing patient.

Kellner R: *Psychosomatic Syndromes and Somatic Symptoms.* Washington, DC: American Psychiatric Press; 1991.

From a clinical scientist who devoted his life to the study of somatization, this reference provides a scholarly review of theoretical mechanisms as well as specific conditions, including fibromyalgia, chronic fatigue syndrome, globus, esophageal disorders, functional gastrointestinal disorders, urethral syndrome, hyperventilation, and chronic pain.

Kirmayer LJ, Robbins JM (eds): *Current Concepts of Somatization: Research and Clinical Perspectives.* Washington, DC: American Psychiatric Press; 1991.

Compilation of chapters by experts on topics such as the psychology of physical symptoms, psychiatric comorbidity, cognitive and social factors, functional somatic syndromes, treatment approaches, a historical perspective, and prospects for research.

Smith GR: *Somatization Disorder in the Medical Setting.* Washington, DC: American Psychiatric Press; 1991.

A concise monograph focusing on the author's expertise in somatization disorder and reviewing its epidemiology, diagnosis, and treatment.

Bibliography

American Academy of Allergy and Immunology: Clinical ecology. *J Allergy Clin Immunol* 78:269, 1986.

American College of Clinicians: Clinical ecology. *Ann Intern Med* 111:168, 1989.

American Medical Association Council on Scientific Affairs: Clinical ecology. *JAMA* 268:3465, 1992.

American Psychiatric Association: *Diagnostic and Statistical Manual of Mental Disorders,* 4th ed: Primary Care Version (DSM-IV-PC). Washington, DC: American Psychiatric Association; 1995.

Banks MH, Beresford SA, Morrell DC, et al: Factors influencing demand for primary medical care in women aged 20–44 years: A preliminary report. *Int J Epidemiol* 4:189, 1975.

Baron RJ: An introduction to medical phenomenology: I can't hear you while I'm listening. *Ann Intern Med* 103:606, 1985.

Barsky AJ, Goodson JD, Lane RS, et al: The amplification of somatic symptoms. *Psychosom Med* 50:510, 1998.

Barsky AJ, Wyshak G, Klerman GL: Transient hypochondriasis. *Arch Gen Psychiatry* 47:746, 1990.

Barsky AJ, Wyshak G, Klerman GL: Psychiatric comorbidity in DSM-III-R hypochondriasis. *Arch Gen Psychiatry* 49:101, 1992.

Bass C (ed): *Somatization: Physical Symptoms and Psychological Illness.* Oxford, UK: Blackwell; 1990.

Beckman HB, Frankel RM: The effect of clinician behavior on the collection of data. *Ann Intern Med* 101:692, 1984.

Bigos S, Bowyer O, Braen G, et al: *Acute Low Back Pain Problems in Adults. Clinical Practice Guideline No. 14.* AHCPR publication no. 95-0642. Rockville, MD: Agency for Health Care Policy and Research, Public Health Service, U.S. Department of Health and Human Services; 1994.

Bock GR, Whelan J (eds): *Chronic Fatigue Syndrome.* Chichester, UK: John Wiley & Sons; 1993.

Brody DS, Miller SM, Lerman CE, et al: Patient perception of involvement in medical care: Relationship to illness attitudes and outcomes. *J Gen Intern Med* 4:506, 1989.

Buchwald D, Garrity D: Comparison of patients with chronic fatigue syndrome, fibromyalgia, and multiple chemical sensitivities. *Arch Intern Med* 154:2049, 1994.

Buchwald D, Pearlman T, Umali J, et al: Functional status in patients with chronic fatigue syndrome, other fatiguing illnesses, and healthy individuals. *Am J Med* 171:364, 1996.

Cahill GF, Soeldner JS: A non-editorial on non-hypoglycemia. *N Engl J Med* 291:905, 1974.

Ciccone DS, Just N, Bandilla EB: Non-organic symptom reporting in patients with chronic non-malignant pain. *Pain* 68:329, 1996.

Cluff LE: Medical aspects of delayed convalescence. *Rev Infect Dis* 13(suppl 1):S138, 1991.

Dawson DM, Sabin TD (eds): *Chronic Fatigue Syndrome.* Boston, MA: Little, Brown and Company; 1993.

Dismukes WE, Wade JS, Lee JY, et al: A randomized, double-blind trial of nystatin therapy for the candidiasis hypersensitivity syndrome. *N Engl J Med* 323:1717, 1990.

Drossman DA: Diagnosing and treating patients with refractory functional gastrointestinal disorders. *Ann Intern Med* 123:688, 1995.

Drossman DA, Talley NJ, Leserman J, et al: Sexual and physical abuse and gastrointestinal illness. *Ann Intern Med* 123:782, 1995.

Eisenberg L: What makes persons "patients" and patients "well?" *Am J Med* 69:277, 1980.

Eisenberg D, Davis RB, Ettner SL, et al: Trends in alternative medicine use in the United States, 1990–1997: Results of a follow-up national survey. *JAMA* 280:1569, 1998.

Escobar JI, Burnam MA, Karno M, et al: Somatization in the community. *Arch Gen Psychiatry* 44:713, 1987.

Escobar JI, Golding JM, Hough RL, et al: Somatization in the community: Relationship to disability and use of services. *Am J Public Health* 77:837, 1987.

Escobar JI, Rubio-Stipec M, Canino G, et al: Somatic Symptom Index (SSI): A new and abridged somatization construct. Prevalence and epidemiological correlates in two large community samples. *J Nerv Ment Dis* 177:140, 1989.

Fry R: Adult physical illness and childhood sexual abuse. *J Psychosom Res* 37:89, 1993.

Fukuda K, Straus SE, Hickie I, et al: The chronic fatigue syndrome: A comprehensive approach to its definition and study. *Ann Intern Med* 121:953, 1994.

Garro LC, Stephenson KA, Good BJ: Chronic illness of the temporomandibular joints as experienced by support-group members. *J Gen Intern Med* 9:372, 1994.

Goodnick PJ, Klimas NG (eds): *Chronic Fatigue and Related Immune Deficiency Syndromes.* Washington, DC: American Psychiatric Press; 1993.

Gothe CJ, Molin C, Nilsson CG: The environmental somatization syndrome. *Psychosomatics* 36:1, 1995.

Hahn SR, Kroenke K, Spitzer RL, et al: The difficult patient in primary care: Prevalence, psychopathology and impairment. *J Gen Intern Med* 11:1, 1996.

Hahn SR, Thompson KS, Wills TA, et al: The difficult clinician-patient relationship: Somatization, personality and psychopathology. *J Clin Epidemiol* 47:647, 1994.

Hudson JI, Goldenberg DL, Pope HG, et al: Comorbidity of fibromyalgia with medical and psychiatric disorders. *Am J Med* 92:363, 1992.

Hyams KC, Wignall FS, Roswell R: War syndromes and their evaluation: From the U.S. Civil War to the Persian Gulf War. *Ann Intern Med* 125:398, 1996.

Iowa Persian Gulf Study Group: Self-reported illness and health status among Gulf War veterans: A population-based study. *JAMA* 277:238, 1997.

Jackson JL, Kroenke K: Difficult patient encounters in the ambulatory clinic: Clinical predictors and outcomes. *Arch Intern Med* 159:1069, 1999.

Jackson JL, Kroenke K, Chamberlin J: Effects of physician awareness of symptom-related expectations and mental disorders. A controlled trial. *Arch Fam Med* 8:135, 1999.

Jensen MC, Brant-Zawadski MN, Obuchowski N, et al: Magnetic resonance imaging of the lumbar spine in people without back pain. *N Engl J Med* 331:69, 1994.

Kaplan C, Lipkin M, Gordon GH: Somatization in primary care: Patients with unexplained and vexing medical complaints. *J Gen Intern Med* 3:177, 1988.

Katon W, Kleinman A, Rosen G: Depression and somatization: A review. Part I. *Am J Med* 72:127, 1982.

Katon W, Lin E, Von Korff M, et al: Somatization: A spectrum of severity. *Am J Psychiatry* 148:34, 1991.

Kellner R: *Psychosomatic Syndromes and Somatic Symptoms*. Washington, DC: American Psychiatric Press; 1991.

Kellner R: Diagnosis and treatment of hypochondriacal syndromes. *Psychosomatics* 33:278, 1992.

Kirmayer LJ, Robbins JM: Three forms of somatization in primary care: Prevalence, co-occurrence, and sociodemographic characteristics. *J Nerv Ment Dis* 179:647, 1991.

Komaroff AL, Fagioli LR, Doolittle TH, et al: Health status in patients with chronic fatigue syndrome and in general population and disease comparison groups. *Am J Med* 101:281, 1996.

Kravitz RL: Patients' expectations for medical care: An expanded formulation based on review of the literature. *Med Care Res Rev* 53:3, 1996.

Kravitz RL, Callahan EJ, Paterniti D, et al: Prevalence and sources of patients' unmet expectations for care. *Ann Intern Med* 125:730, 1996.

Kroenke K: Symptoms and science: The frontiers of primary care research. *J Gen Intern Med* 12:509,1997.

Kroenke K: Patient expectations for care: How hidden is the agenda? *Mayo Clin Proc* 73:191, 1998.

Kroenke K, Arrington ME, Mangelsdorff AD: The prevalence of symptoms in medical outpatients and the adequacy of therapy. *Arch Intern Med* 150:1685, 1990.

Kroenke K, Jackson JL: Outcome in general medical patients presenting with common symptoms: A prospective study with a 2-week and a 3-month follow-up. *Fam Pract* 15:398, 1998

Kroenke K, Jackson JL, Chamberlin J: Depressive and anxiety disorders in patients presenting with physical complaints: Clinical predictors and outcome. *Am J Med* 103:339, 1997.

Kroenke K, Koslowe P, Roy M: Symptoms in 18,495 Persian Gulf War veterans: Latency of onset and lack of association with self-reported exposures. *J Occup Environ Med* 40:520, 1998.

Kroenke K, Lucas CA, Rosenberg ML, et al: Causes of persistent dizziness: A prospective study of 100 patients in ambulatory care. *Ann Intern Med* 117:898, 1992.

Kroenke K, Lucas CA, Rosenberg ML, et al: Psychiatric disorders and functional impairment in patients with persistent dizziness. *J Gen Intern Med* 8:530, 1993.

Kroenke K, Lucas C, Rosenberg ML, et al: One-year outcome in patients with a chief complaint of dizziness. *J Gen Intern Med* 9:684, 1994.

Kroenke K, Mangelsdorff AD: Common symptoms in ambulatory care: Incidence, evaluation, therapy, and outcome. *Am J Med* 86:262, 1989.

Kroenke K, Price RK: Symptoms in the community: Prevalence, classification, and psychiatric comorbidity. *Arch Intern Med* 153:2474, 1993.

Kroenke K, Spitzer RL: Gender differences in the reporting of physical and somatoform symptoms. *Psychosom Med* 60:150, 1998.

Kroenke K, Spitzer RL, deGruy FV, et al: Multisomatoform disorder: An alternative to undifferentiated somatoform disorder for the somatizing patient in primary care. *Arch Gen Psychiatry* 54:352, 1997.

Kroenke K, Spitzer RL, deGruy FV, et al: A symptom checklist to screen for somatoform disorders in primary care. *Psychosomatics* 39:263, 1998.

Kroenke K, Spitzer RL, Williams JBW, et al: Physical symptoms in primary care: Predictors of psychiatric disorders and functional impairment. *Arch Fam Med* 3:774, 1994.

Kroenke K, Swindle R: Cognitive-behavioral therapy for somatization and symptom syndromes: A critical review of clinical trials. *Psychother Psychosom* 69: 205, 2000.

Kroenke K, Wood DR, Mangelsdorff AD, et al: Chronic fatigue in primary care: Prevalence, patient characteristics, and outcome. *JAMA* 260:929, 1988.

Kurt TL: Multiple chemical sensitivities—A syndrome of pseudotoxicity manifest as exposure perceived symptoms. *J Toxicol Clin Toxicol* 33:101, 1995.

Lin EHB, Katon W, Von Korff M, et al: Frustrating patients: Clinician and patient perspectives among distressed high users of medical services. *J Gen Intern Med* 6:241, 1991.

Marple RL, Kroenke K, Lucey CR, et al: Concerns and expectations in patients presenting with physical complaints: Frequency, clinician perceptions and actions, and 2-week outcome. *Arch Intern Med* 157:1482, 1997.

Martina B, Bucheli B, Stotz M, et al: First clinical judgment by primary care clinicians distinguishes well between nonorganic and organic causes of abdominal or chest pain. *J Gen Intern Med* 12:459, 1997.

McCauley J, Kern DE, Kolodner K, et al: The "battering syndrome": Prevalence and clinical characteristics of domestic violence in primary care internal medicine practices. *Ann Intern Med* 123:737, 1995.

McKenzie R, Straus SE: Chronic fatigue syndrome. *Adv Intern Med* 40:119, 1995.

O'Malley PG, Jackson JL, Santoro J, et al: Antidepressant therapy for unexplained symptoms and symptom syndromes. *J Fam Pract* 48:980, 1999.

Pope HG, Hudson JI: A supplemental interview for forms of "affective spectrum disorder." *Int J Psychiatry Med* 21:205, 1991.

Quill TE, Lipkin M, Greenland P: The medicalization of normal variants: The case of mitral valve prolapse. *J Gen Intern Med* 3:267, 1988.

Reidenberg MM, Lowenthal DT: Adverse nondrug reactions. *N Engl J Med* 279:678, 1968.

Robbins JM, Kirmayer LJ, Kapusta MA: Illness worry and disability in fibromyalgia syndrome. *Int J Psychiatry Med* 20:49, 1990.

Rothman AL, Weintraub MI: The sick building syndrome and mass hysteria. *Neurol Clin* 13:405, 1995.

Roy MJ, Koslowe PA, Kroenke K, et al: Signs, symptoms and ill-defined conditions in Persian Gulf War veterans: Findings from the Comprehensive Clinical Evaluation Program. *Psychosom Med* 60:663, 1998.

Schappert SM: National Ambulatory Medical Care Survey: 1989 summary. National Center for Health Statistics. *Vital Health Stat* 13:1, 1992.

Sigal LH: The Lyme disease controversy: Social and financial costs of misdiagnosis and mismanagement. *Arch Intern Med* 156:1493, 1996.

Simon G, Gater R, Kisely S, et al: Somatic symptoms of distress: An international primary care study. *Psychosom Med* 58:481, 1996.

Simon GE, Daniell W, Stockbridge H, et al: Immunologic, psychological, and neuropsychological factors in multiple chemical sensitivity: A controlled study. *Ann Intern Med* 119:97, 1993.

Simon GE, Von Korff M: Somatization and psychiatric disorder in the NIMH Epidemiologic Catchment Area study. *Am J Psychiatry* 148:1494, 1991.

Smith GR: The course of somatization and its effects on utilization of health care resources. *Psychosomatics* 35:263, 1994.

Smith GR, Monson RA, Ray DC: Psychiatric consultation in somatization disorder: A randomized, controlled study. *N Engl J Med* 314:1407, 1986.

Smith GR, Rost K, Kashner TM: A trial of the effect of a standardized psychiatric consultation on health outcomes and costs in somatizing patients. *Arch Gen Psychiatry* 52:238, 1995.

Speckens AEM, van Hemert AM, Bolk JH, et al: Unexplained physical symptoms: Outcome, utilization of medical care and associated factors. *Psychol Med* 26:745, 1996.

Steere AC, Taylor E, McHugh GL, et al: The overdiagnosis of Lyme disease. *JAMA* 269:1812, 1993.

Straus SE, Dale JK, Tobi M, et al: Acyclovir treatment of the chronic fatigue syndrome: Lack of efficacy in a placebo-controlled trial. *N Engl J Med* 319:1692, 1988.

Terr AI: Multiple chemical sensitivities. *Ann Intern Med* 119:163, 1993.

Thomas KB: General practice consultations: Is there any point in being positive? *Br Med J (Clin Res Ed)* 294:1200, 1987.

van Dulmen AM, Fennis JFM, Mokkink HGA, et al: Clinicians' perception of patients' cognitions and complaints in irritable bowel syndrome at an out-patient clinic. *J Psychosom Res* 38:581, 1994.

Verbrugge LM, Ascione FJ: Exploring the iceberg: Common symptoms and how people care for them. *Med Care* 25:539, 1987.

Von Korff MR, Howard JA, Truelove EL, et al: Temporomandibular disorders: Variation in clinical practice. *Med Care* 26:307, 1988.

Walker EA, Katon WJ, Hansom J, et al: Psychiatric diagnoses and sexual victimization in women with chronic pelvic pain. *Psychosomatics* 36:531, 1995.

Wasson JH, Sox HC, Sox CH: The diagnosis of abdominal pain in ambulatory male patients. *Med Decis Making* 1:215, 1981.

White KL: The ecology of medical care. *N Engl J Med* 265:885, 1961.

Wolfe F, Smythe HA, Yunus MB, et al: The American College of Rheumatology 1990 criteria for the classification of fibromyalgia: Report of the Multicenter Criteria Committee. *Arthritis Rheum* 33:160, 1990.

Yunus MB, Masi AT, Aldag JC: A controlled study of primary fibromyalgia syndrome: Clinical features and association with other functional syndromes. *J Rheumatol* 16(suppl 19):62, 1989.

W. Perry Dickinson

Chapter 16

The Management of Depression as a Chronic Disease

Introduction

NADINE DALTON *Nadine Dalton is 43 years old and very tired. She has had fatigue for the past 5 or 6 weeks. She has always had heavy periods, and she also has trouble sleeping sometimes. Her physical exam is unremarkable, except that she appears a bit pale. You finish your interview and exam, reassure her about your findings, and draw blood for thyroid function tests and a CBC. The lab work is completely normal.*

You schedule her to return in 1 week, and upon return she complains of worsening symptoms with the development of intermittent headaches and more trouble sleeping. On closer questioning, she describes going to sleep fairly easily, but she wakes up at 3:00 almost every night, and has great difficulty getting back to sleep.

She initially denies any problems at home but subsequently admits to a great deal of stress taking care of her husband's 79-year-old mother, who has Alzheimer's disease and who moved in with them about 4 months ago. She also works 30 hours a week and takes care of her 10 year-old daughter and 15 year-old son. Her husband does very little to help out; he has also been upset with the situation and has been going out drinking with friends instead of staying at home in the evenings.

As you talk about this situation a bit further, Nadine starts crying and admits that her husband has been verbally and physically abusive of her about once a week for the past 3 months. She defends him, saying that he just can't deal with his mother's illness, but she also admits that she has started being afraid of him. She describes feeling "down" much of the time, experiences decreased pleasure in activities she used to enjoy, poor concentration, and low self-esteem in addition to the fatigue and insomnia. All these symptoms have been present for about 6 weeks, but she has actually felt depressed much of the time and has had poor self-esteem since she was a teenager. Moreover, her stepfather physically abused her numerous times during childhood. You feel somewhat overwhelmed by all of this information, but you make the diagnosis of a major depressive episode, probably superimposed on dysthymia, and discuss management options with her.

Prevalence

Depression is the most common mental health diagnosis in primary care settings and one of the most common diagnoses of any sort. The lifetime prevalence of major depression in the general population is approximately 20 percent in women and 10 percent in men. Many of these patients have a chronic and/or recurrent pattern of depressive symptoms. Because depressed patients visit primary care clinicians about three times more often than nondepressed patients, there are higher rates of depression in primary care than in the general population. Thus, studies have indicated a point prevalence of major depression of between 5 and 10 percent in primary care practices.

Impact

Depression has a major effect on people's lives. The Rand Medical Outcomes Study and the PRIME-MD study both showed that the functional health of people with major depression was worse than that seen in most other chronic medical conditions. Depression is also a major cause of death, particularly from suicide. Between 30,000 and 40,000 Americans commit suicide each year, making it the seventh leading cause of death in the United States. An estimated 60 percent of suicides are associated with depression. Approximately 15 percent of patients with severe depression lasting at least 1 month successfully commit suicide.

Depression also increases morbidity and mortality from coexisting medical conditions. For example, following a myocardial infarction, depressed patients are three times more likely to die within the next year than are nondepressed patients.

Chronic forms of depression may be especially disabling. A study of patients with chronic depression found that 20 percent were unemployed and 37 percent were employed in jobs significantly below their education and training level. Over 75 percent of the patients who were employed outside the home had impaired work functioning. The same study also documented that patients with chronic depression manifested significant impairments in overall social functioning, quality of life, and interpersonal functioning.

Risk Factors

Major depression is twice as likely to occur in women as in men. Family history is also an important risk factor; people with a first-degree relative with depression are about three times more likely to develop a mood disorder during their lifetimes.

Marital status can be a risk factor in several interesting ways. Separated or divorced men and women are more likely to become depressed. Married men have a lower incidence of depression than single men, but married women have a higher incidence than single women.

People with major caretaking responsibilities, those who have suffered recent losses, or those who have experienced a variety of stressful events are at risk for becoming depressed. In addition, a history of previous or ongoing physical or sexual abuse is associated with a greatly increased risk of depression and dysthymia, as demonstrated by Nadine Dalton.

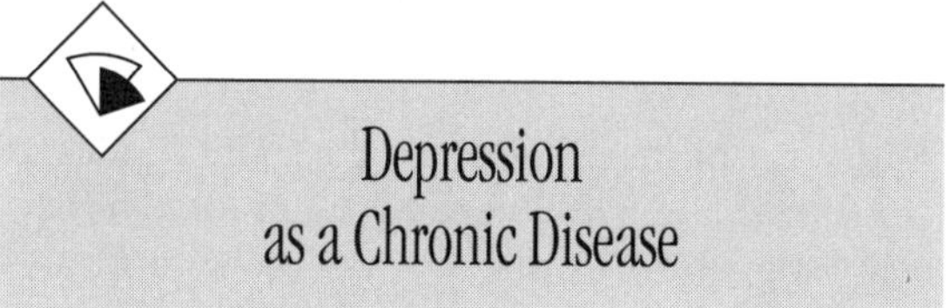

Depression as a Chronic Disease

Many experts on depression are urging that depression be managed as a chronic disease rather than as a one-time episode. This recommendation applies even in the absence of continued depressive symptoms that would meet the criteria for "chronic depression."

This management philosophy is based on a great deal of new information that is available regarding the long-term course of major depression. In an important 10-year prospective study by Keller and colleagues of patients treated for an episode of major depression, it was found that only 18 percent of the patients had a complete resolution of symptoms and remained well for the 10 years after the initial episode. Seven percent had no remission of their symptoms over the entire 10-year period.

Of those patients who were successfully treated for their acute episode, 28 percent had a recurrence within 1 year, 62 percent within 5 years, and 75 percent within the 10-year study period. Because the study only covered 10 years, it is likely that some of the 18 percent of patients who remained well after the initial treatment would have a later recurrence.

Although other studies suggest that primary care patients have less of a problem with chronic depression, it is becoming clear that a minority of patients with depression have a single episode without recurrence. The following sections present new concepts for managing depression as a chronic disease.

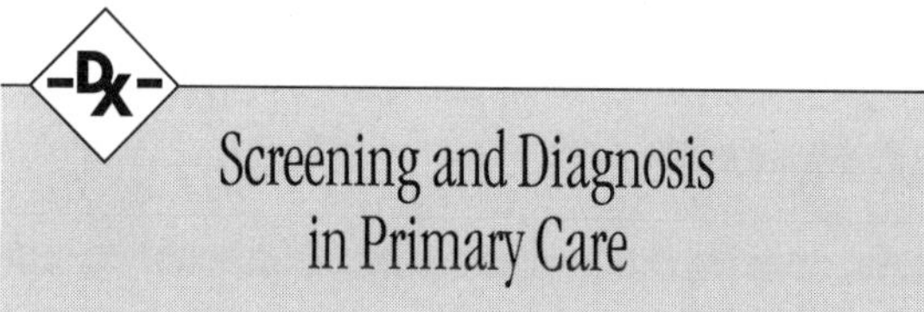

Screening and Diagnosis in Primary Care

Underrecognition and Undertreatment

As described, depression is a very common problem in primary care offices. However, numerous studies indicate that 30 to 70 percent of patients with depression in primary care practices are not diagnosed or treated adequately. Since a flurry of initial studies indicated a problem with underdiagnosis of mood disorders in primary care, other studies of this issue have suggested that many of the patients who are "undiagnosed" actually have less severe symptoms than the patients who are labeled and managed as depressed.

Many primary care clinicians believe that the current system for classifying mood disorders, as well as other mental health diagnoses, does not always work well in primary care. It is possible that further research will help us in the identification and appropriate labeling and management of those patients who need further treatment for their mood disorders.

However, the classification system is clearly not the only problem here. In an excellent study of the management of depression in primary care practices, Rost and colleagues found that almost half of the patients with undetected major depression developed suicidal ideation, and over half continued to meet diagnostic criteria for major depression 1 year later.

Although a number of the patients not formally diagnosed as depressed may be less severe and would respond well to a period of watchful waiting, *we are missing patients who need further treatment.* Furthermore, even those patients recognized and labeled as depressed often receive suboptimal treatment, with poor monitoring of response and adherence, inadequate dosage of medication, and insufficient length of treatment.

Barriers to Recognition

Other than the possible inadequacies of the classification system, what are the reasons why primary care clinicians do not correctly identify patients with mood disorders? One reason is that depressed patients presenting to primary care clinicians usually complain of *somatic symptoms,* which mask the underlying psychosocial issues and mental symptoms. Primary care clinicians are bombarded with issues that are "essential" to be dealt with in increasingly shorter office visits, and these multiple *competing demands* make it extremely difficult to dig through the physical complaints to the underlying depression.

The presence of multiple physical and mental problems that so commonly coexist with depression in primary care patients also makes it difficult to focus on and adequately treat the depression. The diagnosis of depression often carries a social stigma that causes patients to hide the problem or to resist accepting the diagnosis. Clinicians may also hesitate to make the diagnosis because of the problems with subsequent insurability of patients labeled "depressed."

Finally, the reimbursement system often places barriers to the optimal diagnosis and management of depression and other mental diagnoses. Health plans often either refuse to reimburse primary care clinicians for the diagnosis and management of mental disorders or "carve out" mental disorders to be cared for by mental health professionals. Because of this, clinicians may resist labeling the problem as depression, and instead either focus on the presenting physical symptoms or try to manage the symptoms with the biomedical tools that the health plan allows them to use. The effective long-term management of patients with depression by the primary care clinician, providing coordination of care in the context of the continuity relationship with the patient, is made difficult or impossible by this type of health care plan.

The aforementioned list of barriers includes some of the reasons why depression is underrecognized in primary care practice. Tools are available, however, that can assist the primary care clinician in identifying patients who have depression.

Screening Instruments

A number of instruments for the identification of depression and other mental health problems have been suggested for use in primary care offices. Instruments that may be especially useful for this purpose include the depression module of the self-report version of the PRIME-MD, the Beck Depression Scale, and the Hamilton Depression Rating Scale. The Beck, the Hamilton, and the depression module of the PRIME-MD have also been used to track the response of depressed patients to treatment.

Studies implementing screening protocols using such instruments in primary care offices have had mixed results, with some of the patients identified as having depression or other disorders still not receiving adequate treatment. Also, clinicians may resist using these instruments because of the time spent chasing down false-positive responses or dealing with the issues that can arise in discussing these problems with patients who have multiple, chronic problems.

The instruments themselves and the classification system that they reflect need refinement to assist with the identification of cases most likely to respond to treatment. Overall, the screening instruments are potentially useful tools, but their effective implementation in a primary care setting is a complex issue requiring a commitment of time and energy by the clinician and office staff.

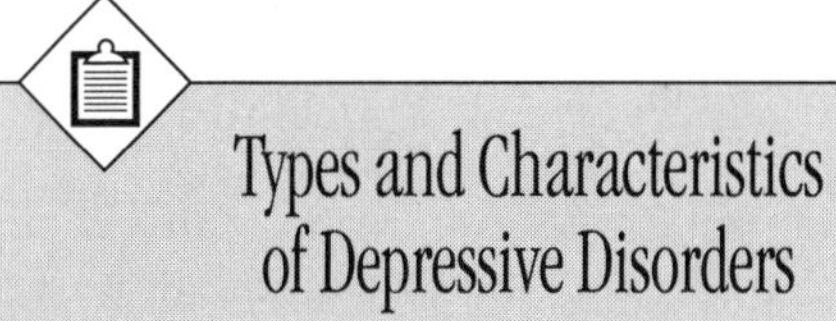

Types and Characteristics of Depressive Disorders

The following sections describe the types of depression most commonly found in primary care practice.

Major Depression

Major depression is the most severe form of depression, and, as related above, it is associated with a significant amount of suffering, cost, and mortality in primary care practices. The DSM-IV criteria for diagnosing major depression require that at least five symptoms from a list of nine be present most of the time for at least 2 weeks. One of the symptoms has to be either (1) a persistently depressed mood or (2) a pervasive loss of interest or pleasure in doing things that arc normally pleasurable. The other seven symptoms include (3) fatigue, (4) psychomotor changes (agitation or vegetation), (5) sleep problems, (6) increased or decreased appetite, (7) guilt or diminished self-esteem, (8) hopelessness, and (9) difficulty concentrating. *Note that a persistently depressed mood is not required for the diagnosis of major depression;* clinicians who use "persistently depressed" as a requisite diagnostic criterion may miss depressed patients who need treatment.

As noted, patients will often present complaining of the physical symptoms associated with depression and not the psychological symptoms. These include the physical symptoms listed in the DSM-IV criteria (sleep problems, change in appetite, fatigue, and psychomotor changes), but other physical symptoms can also serve as *masked*, somatized presentations of depression. These include vague somatic symptoms such as abdominal pain, pelvic pain, headaches, dizziness, dysesthesias, and many others that cause people to seek care from their primary care clinicians. Patients may not readily bring up their emotional symptoms due to embarrassment, stigma issues, lack of knowledge of the role of primary care clinicians in treating mental health problems, or unawareness of their own emotional issues. Primary care clinicians should suspect depression as a cause of somatic symptoms that are vague, difficult to explain, or respond poorly to treatments that should otherwise be effective.

Bipolar Disorder

It is important for primary care clinicians to be alert to the possibility of bipolar disorder in their depressed patients. Studies have indicated that between 20 and 50 percent of all depressed patients in psychiatric practices may have a bipolar disorder. Even though patients with bipolar disorder will generally present with apparent depression, bipolar disorder has some important differences from typical "unipolar" depression that affect management.

The most important diagnostic distinction between unipolar depression and bipolar disorder is that bipolar disorder is characterized by intermittent episodes of mania or hypomania (pathologically elevated mood). Patients may not recognize that the manic periods are a pathologic part of their underlying condition or may be embarrassed or feel guilty about things that happen during the manic phases, leading them to withhold this information from their clinician. Primary care clinicians may find it challenging enough to identify symptoms of depression and tend to not pursue questions regarding previous episodes of manic symptoms. Thus, clinicians diagnose those patients as having depression and place them on antidepressant medications. However, the use of antidepressants in patients with bipolar disorder is fraught with problems and risks.

Antidepressant medications may induce a manic or hypomanic episode in bipolar patients and may lead to more severe recurrences in the future. Additionally, antidepressants can lead to rapid cycling of mania and depression in some bipolar patients, and in others may induce mixed manic and depressive symptoms that are very difficult to manage. Because of these potential problems, primary care clinicians should screen patients with depression for manic symptoms. In most situations, unless primary care clinicians have a great deal of experience and expertise with such problems, they should refer patients with bipolar disorder to a psychiatrist for the initiation of treatment with a mood stabilizing medication such as lithium. Antidepressant medications are used in such patients very cautiously and only if the patient's depressive symptoms do not improve with the mood stabilizer.

Chronic Depression

In earlier versions of the DSM, chronic depression was classified as a personality disorder to be treated by psychotherapy aimed at altering the dysfunctional personality characteristics. However, subsequent studies have consistently indicated that chronic depression is linked physiologically to acute major depression; chronic depression was subsequently reclassified as a mood disorder. The DSM-IV now describes three major subtypes of chronic depression: dysthymia, double depression, and chronic major depression.

Dysthymia

A diagnosis of dysthymia is appropriate when a patient has a depressed mood and at least two of the other eight symptoms of depression on most days for at least 2 years. The lifetime prevalence of dysthymia is estimated at 3 to 5 percent in the general population. The onset of dysthymia tends to be earlier than is seen with most other forms of depression, commonly developing before or in adolescence. Dysthymia seems to have a strong association with childhood abuse and other traumatic experiences. More comorbid conditions are associated with dysthymia than with other mood disorders, perhaps in part because of the common association with childhood abuse. One study of patients with early-onset dysthymia found that the average duration of symptoms in those patients was 30 years, with only 41 percent having ever been treated with an antidepressant.

Dysthymia and the other chronic forms of depression have received increased attention over the past few years due to recognition of the major influence that they can have on quality of life. The negative consequences of dysthymia persist over long periods of time, often despite appropriate treatment. Recent studies of dysthymia indicate that this condition responds to treatment with antidepressant medications with an associated improvement in the level of psychosocial functioning. However, the symptoms usually do not completely remit; residual symptoms are common. In the Medical Outcomes Study, patients with dysthymia actually had worse outcomes and more depressive symptoms upon follow-up than did patients with a major depressive episode only.

Double Depression

Double depression is an episode of major depression superimposed on preexisting dysthymia. Most patients with dysthymia—perhaps over 90 percent—develop major depression at some point in their lifetimes, many with multiple recurrences. Double depression is often difficult to treat, and patients commonly have residual symptoms despite receiving optimal treatment.

Chronic Major Depression

By DSM-IV criteria, chronic major depression is defined as symptoms qualifying for the diagnosis of major depression lasting over 2 years. There are two subtypes: (1) residual major depression, referring to an episode of major depression that only partially improves, with persistent residual symptoms and (2) residual recurrent depression, defined as recurrent episodes of major depression that do not fully remit between episodes. In reality, as will be discussed further, many patients with depression have multiple recurrences, whether or not they qualify as having a type of chronic major depression.

Minor Depression

Minor depression involves depressed mood with fewer symptoms than major depression and shorter duration than dysthymia. The term "minor" is misleading in that minor depression can have a substantial effect on a person's quality of life and level of functioning. In a portion of the Medical Outcomes Study comparing minor depression with major depression, Kessler and associates found that the lifetime patterns of symptoms, recurrence, impairment, comorbidity, and other associated features of minor depression were very similar to those of major depression, primarily differing in degree. Minor depression also has been shown to be associated with an increased lifetime risk for one or more episodes of major depression.

There are few data to guide the management of minor depression in primary care settings. It is possible, and in fact likely, that antidepressants would help with the symptoms and impairment, and might prevent subsequent worsening into a major depression episode, but further study is needed to determine if this is so.

The entire picture of how minor depressive symptoms ebb and flow over the years is not fully understood. Some patients appear to have subthreshold symptoms that flare up into full depression that may or may not recur and that may fully remit, but also may give way to chronic residual symptoms that then flare up again. A longitudinal study of the course of depressive symptoms would have great potential for clarifying some of these patterns and informing management for primary care clinicians.

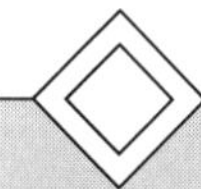

Course of a Major Depressive Episode

NADINE DALTON (CONTINUED) *Ms. Dalton is still in your office, and you carefully discuss the treatment options with her and recommend starting both selective serotonin reuptake inhibitor (SSRI) and psychotherapy for the underlying psychosocial problems. She is very anxious about how her husband would react if he found out she was going for counseling, but eventually agrees to contact a local battered women's shelter, discuss her situation with them, and deal with the issue of psychotherapy at a future visit with you. You talk with her about the possible side effects of the medication, the lag time before she should expect a response, and the possible need for long-term maintenance therapy because of the underlying dysthymia and multiple episodes of major depression. She is hesitant about committing to a prolonged course of treatment, but agrees to try the medication and to call or come in before stopping it.*

The course of major depression can be understood in three phases, marked by five change points—the "Five R's."

Change Points—The "Five R's"

As you navigate the long-term course of an episode of major depression, there are various change points that you will encounter. The terms used to describe these change points were inconsistent prior to the activities of a task force of the MacArthur Mental Health Research Network on the Psychobiology of Depression. This task force proposed a conceptual schema for the change points based on variations in the severity of symptoms and the duration of symptomatic improvement or worsening. This schema resulted in the identification of the "Five R's":

1. *Response* is a significant reduction of symptoms to below the threshold for major depression.
2. *Remission* involves the reduction of symptoms to the point of "wellness."
3. *Recovery* is a sustained period of remission.
4. *Relapse* is the exacerbation of symptoms after a response or remission but before a recovery.
5. *Recurrence* is a new episode of major depression after recovery from a prior episode.

Phases of Treatment

The change points define the three phases in the chronic management of depression. The *acute phase* is the first phase of treatment, moving from the identification of the problem and the beginning of treatment, through the initial response, to the achievement of remission. The *continuation* phase follows the acute phase, after remission is achieved, and aims to prevent a relapse of symptoms and to sustain remission so that recovery can be achieved. Finally, the *maintenance* phase involves treating high-risk patients after the continuation phase and recovery to prevent recurrence. Each of these phases will be further discussed below.

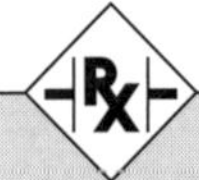

Components of Treatment

There are four major categories of options for actively treating an episode of depression in primary care: psychotherapy, pharmacotherapy, office counseling by the primary care clinician, and psychiatric referral. In most situations a combination of two or more of these options is used. With an episode of minor depression, however, or even a mild episode of major depression, sometimes the best course of action is watchful waiting; if the symptoms soon improve, then active therapy may not be necessary.

Psychotherapy

Psychotherapy has been shown to be effective alone as treatment for patients with mild to moderate major depression, dysthymia, and possibly minor depression, and it can be used as adjunctive treatment for virtually any patient with depression. Forms of therapy that have been shown in various trials to be effective in the treatment of depression include cognitive behavioral therapy and interpersonal therapy. Cognitive behavioral therapy attempts to change the negative and maladaptive patterns of thought, behavior, and attitudes often adopted by depressed patients. Interpersonal therapy focuses more on the various relational problems that can also be associated with depression. Other forms of psychotherapy might also be useful in treating depression, especially when targeting specific problems experienced by particular patients, but have not been proven effective in clinical trials.

A recent study by Keller and co-workers may change the way we think of the potential role of psychotherapy in the treatment of chronically depressed patients. The researchers compared the response of patients to treatment with the drug nefazadone, cognitive behavioral psychotherapy, or both. They found that 48 percent of the patients treated with nefazadone alone or psychotherapy alone had a satisfactory response to treatment, whereas 73 percent of patients treated with both responded satisfactorily. More information is needed regarding which patients might respond better to one form of treatment versus another, but this study suggests that combined therapy should be considered for most if not all patients with chronic forms of depression. The potential value of psychotherapy, either as primary or adjunctive treatment, should be carefully explained to the patient so that it can be considered as a management option. Psychotherapy may have particular value when there are underlying psychosocial issues, including previous or ongoing abuse, family dysfunction, life transitions, various forms of loss, or other stressful or traumatic life issues.

Although the technique of cognitive-behavioral therapy is not difficult to master, it is a time-consuming process and is difficult for most primary care clinicians to fit into their normal patient care routines. This therapeutic option is easiest to incorporate into a primary care regimen when a trained mental health professional is readily available.

Pharmacotherapy

Many medications now exist for treating the various forms of depression. Medication regimens have been demonstrated to be effective for treating major depression and dysthymia and may help with minor depression, although this indication is largely untested.

The monoamine oxidase inhibitors (MAOIs), once a mainstay treatment, are now only rarely used, especially in primary care settings. Similarly, tricyclic antidepressants are still on many formularies and are in widespread use, but their use has been declining with the advent of newer medications. The biggest advantage of tricyclic antidepressants is their low cost. They have consistently been shown to be as effective as newer agents. However, side effects are fairly common and can be very bothersome, so adherence to tricyclics can be a problem, especially with long-term treatment. Also, overdosage can occur at relatively low levels, is difficult to manage, and is commonly lethal. Thus, most primary care clinicians use newer antidepressants as the first line choice for treatment. This trend will probably continue as longer courses of treatment become the norm, because adherence with tricyclics becomes more difficult as the length of treatment increases.

Several types of new antidepressants are available. SSRIs are the most prominent of the newer antidepressants. SSRIs include fluoxetine, citalopram, paroxetine, and sertraline. Other new non-SSRI antidepressants, such as bupropion, mirtazapine, nefazodone, and venlafaxine, each have slightly different profiles of effects, benefits, and side effects. The non-SSRI antidepressants are very useful second line options, with occasional use as first line choices. A suggested protocol for medication treatment of depression is outlined later in this chapter.

Office Counseling by the Primary Care Clinician

The primary care clinician should serve as a primary source of certain types of counseling for patients with depression. This role of the primary care clinician has been underappreciated in the literature, largely addressed in descriptive terms, and not well studied as a part of the therapeutic intervention. There are a number of components of this form of treatment, all of which include support of the patient and family through the difficulties of the depression and its underlying problems. This supportive counseling has at least five benefits (Table 16-1).

In essence, the cornerstone of the long-term management of depression as a chronic disease is a partnership between the primary care clinician, the patient, and the patient's family (except in special circumstances). In various situations or office settings, other people may also be included in this partnership. Office nurses, social workers, and other people from the primary care office can provide or extend many of the services normally delivered by the clinician, including providing support, assisting with monitoring the response to treatment, or assisting in accessing other community resources. Mental health professionals, including psychiatrists, psychologists, or counselors, can also be valued members of the team. Regular close communication between the men-

Table 16-1

Benefits of Office Counseling with a Primary Care Clinician

1. The opportunity for the patient to talk through the problems with a nonreactive person can be very therapeutic. The power of even brief forms of *disclosure* has been shown repeatedly in studies by Pennebaker and others.
2. The effect of a normal, nonjudgmental, *supportive relationship* over time with a clinician also should not be underestimated.
3. Some patients need assistance with *basic problem solving*, and minimal facilitation by the clinician can allow them to find solutions to underlying problems resulting from, causing, or complicating the depression.
4. *Patient education* regarding the nature of the problem, treatment options, the likely course of treatment (including potential side effects of medications), and signs and symptoms of relapse or recurrence results in better-informed patients who are more capable of assisting in their own management.
5. *Shared decision making* regarding management options for the depression can help to further anchor the therapeutic clinician–patient relationship and has been shown to lead to better adherence with treatment regimens and improved outcomes.

tal health professionals and the primary care clinician can greatly improve the coordination of the management plan. Models of care involving joint visits with the primary care clinician and the mental health professional have also been shown to be effective. New interdisciplinary models of practice can be very effective for dealing with depression and other mental health disorders in the primary care setting and should be explored and extended further.

Psychiatric Referral

Most depressed patients can be managed successfully by their primary care clinicians. However, situations occasionally arise in which referral to a psychiatrist may be desirable or necessary. Primary care clinicians should usually refer patients with bipolar disorder, at least for confirmation of the diagnosis and initiation of therapy. Referral may also be helpful when the specific diagnosis is unclear, such as when multiple comorbid conditions cloud the diagnosis and make the optimal management uncertain. Patients with a high degree of suicidality also should be considered for psychiatric referral, often in concert with hospitalization. Primary care clinicians should consider the possibility of referral when patients do not respond to treatment with first- or second-line medications.

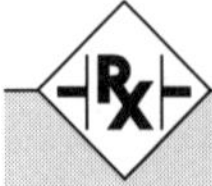

Acute Phase of Treatment

The various stages of treatment will now be discussed, with guidelines for managing each stage. First is the acute phase of treatment, lasting from the time depression is identified and a management plan established until a remission of symptoms is accomplished. The initial management decisions revolve around whether the symptoms need immediate treatment and, if so, what option or combination of treatment options to include. As discussed, clinicians should encourage a shared decision making approach by giving the patient a much larger role in developing the management plan than has traditionally been the case. Patients respond better when the treatment they receive is the treatment they prefer.

For patients with minor depression or milder symptoms of major depression or dysthymia, a course of watchful waiting combined with supportive office counseling by the primary care clinician may be more appropriate than immediate institution of pharmacotherapy or referral for psychotherapy. If watchful waiting is used, it should always be combined with inquiry about associated underlying issues. After a period of time, if the patient is worsening or not improving, if major underlying issues needing counseling are uncovered, or if the chronicity of the depressive symptoms or comorbid conditions becomes a concern, the patient can be started on medication or referred for further counseling.

Many patients, however, will present with more severe symptoms and require immediate institution of a more intensive treatment plan. The guidelines for referral to a psychiatrist have been outlined and should be considered with such patients.

For the great majority of patients who will not need psychiatric referral, referral for psychotherapy should still be discussed as an option, along with pharmacotherapy. If the patient chooses psychotherapy as the primary treatment, the primary care clinician generally makes a referral, but should still follow the patient closely. Some patients will not follow through with the planned psychotherapy, by either not going at all or by dropping out early in treatment. In some cases, this can be the result of a poor match between patient and therapist, and referral to a new therapist will solve the problem. In other situations, the patient may decide to proceed with pharmacotherapy. In addition, some patients may not get full relief of symptoms from the psychotherapy and will need to be placed on medication. Finally, some patients will have a relapse of the depressive symptoms after the initial improvement and may need medication at that point. Regardless, it is important for the primary care clinician to closely monitor the patient's progress with psychotherapy, usually with visits or telephone contact every 2 to 4 weeks. This can be extended to less frequent contacts—every 4 to 8 weeks—after an initial remission of symptoms.

Many patients entering a plan of watchful waiting or psychotherapy will eventually require pharmacotherapy. Usually, this will be instituted by the primary care clinician. Even in situations where the initial treatment is instituted by a psychiatrist, however, the primary care clinician may follow the patient through the continuation and maintenance phases of treatment. Thus, it is vital that primary care clinicians thoroughly understand pharmacotherapy for depression.

Suggested Protocol for Acute Phase Pharmacotherapy

A complete discussion of the various medications that now are available for the treatment of depression is beyond the scope of this chapter. As discussed, however, the primary options fall into four categories. MAOIs are virtually never used as first-line treatment currently, and few primary care clinicians are familiar with them. Tricyclics have been a standby for years, but their side effect profiles have progressively relegated them to a secondary status, except in selected patients. Tricyclics are still useful for patients for whom the cost of the medication is a major barrier to treatment or for patients with coexisting neuropathic or other pain syndromes or with long-term problems with insomnia.

SSRIs are the medications most commonly used as first-line choices currently. The other new non-SSRI agents are occasionally used initially, but are generally reserved for use as second choices for patients with poor responses or side effects with the SSRIs. Therefore, in this chapter we will present a pharmacotherapy protocol that involves the use of an SSRI as the choice for initial treatment.

Initiating an SSRI

Although there are differences among the SSRIs in their pharmacokinetics and metabolic pathways, the choice of the specific SSRI usually makes little difference. The effectiveness and the side effect profiles of the various agents are very similar. However, individual patients definitely respond differently to the various SSRIs. The fact that one SSRI caused problems or did not work does not preclude a favorable response with another. Certainly if the patient has had previous experience with specific agents, the clinician should take that experience into account when selecting a medication for the current episode. An antidepressant that worked well previously with few side effects is likely to behave similarly again. If the medication worked well but had bothersome side effects, changing to a slightly different medication from the same class might reduce or eliminate those side effects. If a particular medication caused serious side effects or was not effective, changing to a different class of medication would be appropriate. Because the response to specific antidepressants often runs in families, gathering information regarding the experiences with antidepressants of close relatives could also assist when selecting a specific agent.

One advantage of the SSRIs over tricyclics is the ability to begin with a full therapeutic dosage of the medication. However, elderly patients or patients with panic disorder or other significant anxiety disorders should be started on a half-dosage level and increased to a full dose as tolerated. This approach reduces the chance that patients with panic and other anxiety disorders with have an unpleasant stimulant reaction to SSRIs. If a half dose produces side effects, further reduce the dosage. In patients who responded to SSRIs with a stimulant reaction in the past, start the agent at an even lower dosage level.

Promoting Adherence

As discussed, using a shared decision making approach is one of the most important interventions that will encourage the patient to adhere to the treatment regimen. The patient should feel in control of the choice of a management approach and should have the information needed to assess his or her response to the therapeutic plan. In addition, a case management approach, as described more thoroughly below, may have a striking influence on patient adherence with treatment. Several specific issues should be covered in regard to pharmacotherapy. The clinician must

1. Explain that it usually takes at 2 to 4 weeks before antidepressants begin to become effective, and longer for the full effect. This will reduce the chance that patients prematurely discontinue the medication because "it's not working."
2. Discuss the most common side effects from the medication. For example, if patients know that their SSRI may cause a little restlessness and difficulty sleeping, but that this will improve with time, then they may be able to endure these side effects that would otherwise cause them to discontinue the medication. Ask the patient to call for any disturbing side effects, letting them know that many can be dealt with or that the medication can be changed if necessary.
3. Tell the patient what to expect in terms of the anticipated length of treatment. Encourage patients not to stop the medication when they start feeling better. Explain the need for the continuation phase of treatment and the risk of stopping the medication too soon.

Nadine Dalton (continued) *Nadine returns for a follow-up visit in 2 weeks. Initially she had some restlessness and difficulty sleeping with the SSRI, but was able to continue the medication, and those symptoms have abated at this point. She thinks that her symptoms of depression have improved somewhat, and she feels a bit more optimistic about the chances of working through her difficult situation. She talked to the counselors at the battered women's shelter and recognizes the need to take action at this point, although she is still not sure what she needs to do. You discuss the possibilities with her, and she agrees to see a counselor whom you know is very good at dealing with domestic violence. You leave her on the same dose of the same medication and schedule another appointment in 2 weeks.*

Monitoring Patients' Responses

Studies of the usual practice standards of primary care clinicians have consistently shown a tendency toward undertreatment of depression, including the use of inadequate dosages of antidepressants in each of the three stages of treatment. The primary aim of the acute phase of treatment for a major depression episode is to rapidly reduce symptoms to the point of remission. The patient should be seen at 2- to 4-week intervals until remission is attained, with visits closer together if there is suicidal ideation or a need for additional office counseling.

If a medication is going to be effective, symptoms should be reduced within 4 weeks after reaching a therapeutic dosage level. In the case of dysthymia or chronic major depression, however, this may take 6 to 8 weeks. If there is not a response or only a minimal response in that time period, the clinician should take several steps:

1. Closely assess the patient's adherence to the treatment regimen.
2. Reevaluate the diagnosis.
3. Adjust the dosage upward if there is a minimal response or if the dosage was started at a relatively low level.
4. Consider changing the patient to a new medication, probably in a different class, if there is no response whatsoever to a full dosage of the medication.
5. Consider adding psychotherapy to the medication regimen as adjunctive therapy.
6. Consider psychiatric consultation if the diagnosis is unclear or the patient continues to be unresponsive to treatment after increasing dosages and/or changing medications.

Acute phase treatment of dysthymia or double depression is similar, except that (1) it may take longer before a response is seen, and (2) it may not be possible to decrease the symptoms to the point of full remission. It still makes sense to increase the dosage of the antidepressant to attempt to completely eradicate the symptoms, but if a further reduction of symptoms is not forthcoming or if side effects become bothersome, the best plan is to proceed to maintenance at the lowest fully effective dosage level. Similarly, making multiple changes in medication to achieve full symptom remission is generally not a good idea.

The acute phase treatment of minor depression should probably proceed as described for major depression, although there are few data to guide the process.

NADINE DALTON (CONTINUED) *You see Nadine back in 2 weeks. She looks much more relaxed and positive, and she states that her depression symptoms have improved quite a bit. She has had two visits with the counselor, and they have discussed ways of dealing with her husband as well as proceeding with cognitive behavioral therapy for the depressive symptoms. You give her a lot of positive reinforcement for the steps that she has taken, leave her on her present medication, and schedule her back in 2 weeks.*

At that point she returns again, indicating that she is feeling about the same as on her last visit, improved from where she started, but with a lot of residual symptoms. You increase her antidepressant dosage and see her back in 3 more weeks. At that point, she reports some mild residual symptoms, but she feels that her outlook is better and more positive than it has been in several years. Her counselor and the patient both indicate that the counseling sessions are going well, with both feeling optimistic about working out the situation.

You would like to see her depression symptoms completely gone, but recognize that that might not be possible, so you leave her on her present dosage of medication, planning to monitor the situation closely and increase the medication further if she worsens. You explain that she needs to continue the medication for at least a year for this acute episode of depression, but also alert her to the probable need for long-term, maintenance therapy. You plan to see her back at 3- to 4-week intervals for the next few months, recognizing the need for ongoing support and monitoring with the difficult issues that she is working on with her home situation.

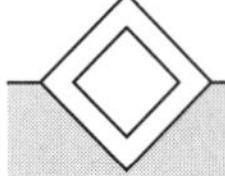

Continuation Phase

The goal of the acute phase is to attain a complete remission of symptoms, which is generally attained in an average of 8 to 12 weeks after the initiation of treatment. Remission marks the transition to the continuation phase, which aims to maintain the remission gained during the acute phase and maximize the probability of a recovery. At the point of remission the patient typically is feeling pretty close to normal, and many patients and some clinicians may be inclined to reconsider whether the medication is really necessary. It most likely is. Studies have shown a greatly increased risk of relapse if the medication is discontinued too soon. One study by Prien and Kupfer indicated a 40 to 60 percent risk of relapse if the antidepressant is stopped in the first few months, with continued treatment reducing this risk to 5 to 10 percent over the same time period. The AHCPR guidelines on depression recommend 4 to 9 months of continuation therapy *in addition to* the typical 2 to 3 months for the acute phase, resulting in a minimum of 6 to 12 months of treatment for most major depression episodes.

Tricyclics and SSRIs have both been studied for continuation therapy and are equally effective, although the side effect profile and compliance are substantially better for SSRIs. During the continuation phase, continue the full dosage of the medication that was successfully used to attain a relapse in the acute phase, unless side effects or other problems require a change.

After the continuation phase the medication should be withdrawn slowly, typically tapered over a 1- to 2-month period. Clinicians should see the patient every 2 to 3 weeks and closely monitor them for symptoms of a recurrence. In addition the patient and family should be reeducated about the early signs and symptoms of a recurrence.

There are almost no data available regarding the need for or optimal length of continuation therapy for minor depression. A total course of treatment of approximately 6–12 months would appear to be appropriate. Although future studies should help to further inform this decision. Most experts currently recommend indefinite maintenance therapy for patients with dysthymia.

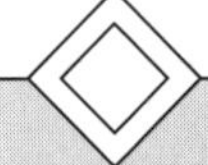

Maintenance Phase

The goal of maintenance phase treatment is to prevent recurrent episodes of major depression in patients at high risk for recurrence.

Risk Factors for Recurrence

The primary risk factor for recurrence is a history of recurrence. The more episodes of major depression a person has, the more likely there will be another recurrence. Among people with at least three prior episodes, 90 percent will have a fourth episode. Thus, upon the third episode, maintenance therapy is recommended. Maintenance is also recommended after a second episode in the following situations:

1. A first episode at age less than 20 or greater than 60.
2. A severe or difficult-to-treat prior episode, especially with a sudden onset.
3. A family history of bipolar disorder or recurrent major depression episodes.
4. Multiple comorbid conditions.
5. Recurrence within 1 year after previously effective medication is discontinued.

Patients are at an increased risk for recurrence when they do not completely recover between episodes (essentially representing a form of chronic depression needing more long-term treatment). Additionally, patients with double depression need maintenance therapy, both to prevent a recurrence of major depression and to treat the underlying dysthymia.

It is important for the clinician to consider and discuss the risk factors for recurrence with the patient early so that maintenance can be incorporated into the overall plan. It is better if the patient plans for a prolonged course of treatment from the beginning rather than discovering the need right before he or she is anticipating completing the continuation phase.

Generally, use the same dose of the medication for the maintenance phase that was effective in inducing a remission during the acute phase. Obviously there can be exceptions to this, including side effects that the patient can tolerate for a short course of treatment but not over the long course of maintenance.

Psychotherapy in Maintenance

Psychotherapy is not effective as the sole therapy during maintenance. Studies have indicated that psychotherapy does not prevent recurrences, although it may delay them. For patients who desire to stay off medication for a period of time, such as during a pregnancy, psychotherapy could be useful to attempt to delay recurrence until the patient can start back on the medication regimen. Psychotherapy can also be useful as an adjunct to drug therapy for patients in the maintenance phase, and this should be considered as a therapeutic option in all patients. As before, this is an especially good option when the patient has significant underlying psychosocial issues.

Length of Maintenance Pharmacotherapy

Currently, there are few data available on the necessary length of maintenance. Over the last few years, progressively longer periods have been recommended, and results are needed from very long-term longitudinal studies to really inform the decision. A study by Thase indicated that across the first 3 to 5 years of maintenance, the risk for failure of the medication is 10 percent per year compared to a risk of recurrence of depression of 30 to 50 percent in the first 6 months after discontinuation. The AHCPR guidelines are somewhat vague regarding the optimal length of maintenance therapy, but suggest a maintenance course of at least 1 year beyond the acute and continuation courses, with especially high-risk patients maintained for longer periods. Currently, however, many experts recommend a course of 4 to 5 years and suggest that lifelong treatment may be needed for a large subset of patients. If and when a decision is made to stop maintenance therapy, there is some evidence that a slow taper of the medication is better than abrupt discontinuation. Once again, the patient and family must be carefully educated about monitoring for early signs and symptoms of recurrence. Also, counseling may be considered to assist with the transition off medication, whether or not the patient had counseling earlier in the course of treatment.

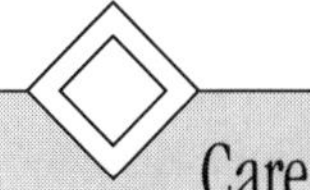

Care Management Strategies

One of the most effective strategies for improving the treatment of patients with depression in primary care has been the use of "care management." Multiple studies have demonstrated the value of various aspects of care management, many in managed care settings but with a growing number in other practice settings. This is consistent with a growing body of literature documenting the value of such strategies in the management of chronic diseases in general.

Typically, there are several elements to care management of depression. The first is that maintenance of a registry of patients with depression is central to any care management strategy. Contacts are made with the patients on the registry according to a protocol to check on progress and deal with any barriers to effective care. For example, a patient who is put on medication for an acute episode of major depression would receive a phone call a few days after the initial office visit. The caller would make sure that the prescription was filled and that the patient has been able to take the medication, encourage the patient to come in for planned follow-up visits, and deal with any other problems that may have arisen. A patient referred for psychotherapy would be contacted to make sure that the appointment was made and the visit carried out, to reinforce follow-up plans, and to deal with barriers or problems. Subsequent contacts would be interspersed among the office visits, monitoring the patient's progress, dealing with problems, and providing an additional contact for the patient, with the frequency of contacts decreasing as the patient improves. These contacts are usually made by existing personnel in the primary care clinician's office, such as an office nurse, with clinician backup to deal with problems. There is a growing literature, however, to suggest that such care management can be done by personnel external to the practice, allowing a group of practices to contract for these services when it is not practical to have individuals within the practice provide them.

A second characteristic of care management is the use of practice guidelines that establish evidence-based protocols for treating patients with depression. Such guidelines can greatly assist with decisions made by everyone involved in the patient's care. The AHCPR guidelines for the management of depression in primary care have commonly been used for this purpose.

A third component of care management is the use of information systems beyond the registry to track patients' responses, to determine whether patients are receiving care consistent with the practice guidelines. Information systems, such as computerized medical records and databases can facilitate quality monitoring and improvement efforts.

Finally, improved systems of communication between the primary care clinician and mental health specialist(s) can greatly improve the coordination of the care for the patient and assist in making certain that the patient does not "fall between the cracks" of the health care system.

Despite the documented success of such interventions in improving the care of patients with depression and other chronic diseases, these strategies have not been implemented in many practices and are not widely used in primary care. Current practice and reimbursement patterns do not necessarily facilitate such changes, and many primary care practices are unable to incorporate care management protocols. Further work is needed to make such innovations practical for most primary care practices. Also, models need to be developed for chronic disease management that can work across multiple disease entities, with varying protocols for specific diseases but an overall system that applies to all.

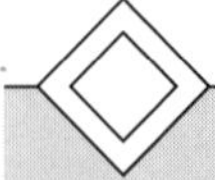

Treatment of Dysthymia

Dysthymia is, by its nature, chronic and requires a long-term management plan. Many patients with dysthymia have the onset of their symptoms during adolescence or early adulthood, and the symptoms often persist for many years—perhaps for life. Superimposed on this base of chronic depressive symptoms, patients with dysthymia often have flare ups of major depressive episodes. This can be a severely disabling, life-long process. Medication does offer some relief, and clinical trials have shown that both tricyclics and SSRIs are effective at reducing symptoms in dysthymic patients. Even so, the symptoms often do not totally disappear.

The utility of psychotherapy for dysthymia, either as monotherapy or adjunctive therapy, has not been definitively studied. However, with dysthymia's high association with psychosocial issues and its major impact on quality of life and relationships, psychotherapy should be helpful for most dysthymic patients. It makes sense to offer and encourage psychotherapy as adjunctive therapy in the long-term management of dysthymia, with the type of counseling depending on the nature of the underlying problems.

There are few data regarding the optimal length of drug treatment for dysthymia. A prudent plan might base the decision regarding the length of treatment on the duration of symptoms and the number of major depressive episodes the patient has had superimposed on the dysthymia. Patients with only a few years of relatively mild symptoms and no episodes of major depression might respond well to a 9- to 12-month course of antidepressants, with a trial discontinuation of medication followed by close monitoring for the return of symptoms. For patients with prolonged symptoms complicated by multiple episodes of major depression, it would seem wise to leave the patient on long-term maintenance therapy, perhaps for life. For some patients, that decision might be affected by successful psychotherapy for difficult underlying problems such as major abuse or trauma. Hopefully, further data will be forthcoming to help inform these management decisions.

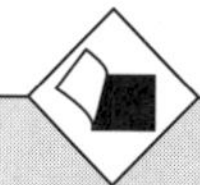

Summary

There is increasing evidence that depression is often a lifelong, simmering process, with multiple recurrences and remissions and with many patients having a pattern of chronic symptoms even between episodes of major depression. Few patients have only one isolated episode of depression.

Thus, management of depression as a chronic disease appears increasingly prudent. Management should include long-term close monitoring for depressive symptoms, careful patient education, psychotherapy and/or pharmacotherapy, and the development of a partnership among the patient, family, psychotherapist, office staff, and others.

Many patients with dysthymia or multiple recurrences of major depression require long-term maintenance therapy to improve their quality of life and prevent the disability and complications that often accompany these conditions.

Suggested Reading

Depression Guideline Panel: *Depression in Primary Care Volume 1: Detection and Diagnosis*. Rockville, MD: Agency for Health Care Policy and Research, U.S. Department of Health and Human Services; 1993.

Although there has been some important work since these were developed, these guidelines provide a standard for the diagnosis of patients with depression in primary care.

Depression Guideline Panel: *Depression in Primary Care, vol. 2: Treatment of Major Depression*. Rockville, MD: Agency for Health Care Policy and Research, U.S. Department of Health and Human Services; 1993.

As Volume 1 does for the diagnosis of depression, this set of guidelines provides the standard for the treatment of depression in primary care. Anyone interested in depression in primary care should familiarize themselves with these sets of guidelines.

Coyne J, Schwenk TL, Fechner-Bates S: Non-detection of depression by primary care physicians reconsidered. *Gen Hosp Psychiatry* 17:3, 1995.

This is a thoughtful response to studies that have been critical of the care that depressed patients receive in primary care settings. It describes some of the difficult factors that complicate the primary care management of depression and gives a primary care perspective on the entire issue.

Thase ME: Long-term nature of depression. *J Clin Psychiatry* 60:3, 1999.

This is an excellent article that discusses the long-term nature of depression in many patients and makes a strong case for the importance of managing depression as a chronic disease.

Wagner E: Organizing care for patients with chronic illness. *Milbank Q* 74:511, 1996.

This is an important, classic article dealing with the reorganization of the way we deliver primary care for patients with chronic disease. It is not specific to depression, but most of the interventions discussed in the article have been shown to be effective in improving care for depression in primary care.

Bibliography

American Psychiatric Association: *Diagnostic and Statistical Manual of Mental Disorders*, 4th ed. Washington, DC: American Psychiatric Association; 1994.

Barraclough B, Bunch J, Nelson B, et al: A hundred cases of suicide: Clinical aspects. *Br J Psychiatry* 125:355, 1974.

Beck AT, Ward CH, Mendelson M, et al: An inventory for measuring depression. *Arch Gen Psychiatry* 4:561, 1961.

Coyne J, Schwenk TL, Fechner-Bates S: Non-detection of depression by primary care physicians reconsidered. *Gen Hosp Psychiatry* 17:3, 1995.

Depression Guideline Panel: *Depression in Primary Care, vol. 1: Detection and Diagnosis*. Rockville, MD: Agency for Health Care Policy and Research, U.S. Department of Health and Human Services; 1993.

Depression Guideline Panel: *Depression in Primary Care, vol. 2: Treatment of Major Depression*. Rockville, MD: Agency for Health Care Policy and Research, U.S. Department of Health and Human Services; 1993.

Dienstfrey H: Disclosure and health: An interview with James W. Pennebaker. *Advances in Mind-Body Medicine* 15:161, 1999.

Frank E, Prien R, Jarrett R, et al: Conceptualization and rationale for consensus definitions of terms in major depressive disorder. Remission, recovery, relapse, and recurrence. *Arch Gen Psychiatry* 48:851, 1991.

Frazure-Smith N, Lesperance F, Talajic M: Depression following myocardial infarction: Impact on 6-month survival. *JAMA* 270:1819, 1993.

Hamilton M: *The Hamilton Rating Scale for Depression.* In: Sartorius TB (ed): *Assessment of Depression.* New York: Springer-Verlag; 1986.

Hirschfeld R, Klerman G, Andreasen N, et al: Psychosocial predictors of chronicity in depressed patients. *Br J Psychiatry* 148:648, 1986.

Katon W, Robinson P, Von Korff M, et al: A multifaceted intervention to improve treatment of depression in primary care. *Arch Gen Psychiatry* 53: 924, 1996.

Katon W, Von Korff M, Lin E, et al: Collaborative management to achieve treatment guidelines: Impact on depression in primary care. *JAMA* 273:1026, 1995.

Keller M, Lavori P, Mueller T, et al: Time to recovery, chronicity, and levels of psychopathology in major depression: A 5-year prospective follow-up of 431 subjects. *Arch Gen Psychiatry* 49:809, 1992.

Keller MB, McCullough JP, Klein D, et al: A comparison of nefazodone, the cognitive behavioral-analysis system of psychotherapy, and their combination for the treatment of chronic depression. *N Engl J Med* 342:1462, 2000.

Kessler RC, Zhao S, Blazer D, et al: Prevalence, correlates, and course of minor depression and major depression in the national comorbidity survey. *J Affect Disord* 45:19, 1997.

McCauley J, Kern D, Kolodner K, et al: The "battering syndrome": Prevalence and clinical characteristics of domestic violence in primary care internal medicine practices. *Ann Intern Med* 123:737, 1995.

Miller IW, Keitner G, Schatzberb A, et al: The treatment of chronic depression, part 3: Psychosocial functioning before and after treatment with sertraline or imipramine. *J Clin Psychiatry* 59:608, 1998.

National Institutes of Mental Health (NIMH) Consensus Development Conference: Mood disorders: Pharmacologic prevention of recurrences. *Am J Psychiatry* 142:469, 1985.

Pennebaker JW: Putting stress into words: Health, linguistic, and therapeutic implications. *Behav Res Ther* 31:539, 1993.

Prien R, Kupfer D: Continuation drug therapy for major depressive episodes: How long should it be maintained? *Am J Psychiatry* 143:18, 1986.

Rost K, Zhang M, Fortney J, et al: Persistently poor outcomes of undetected major depression in primary care. *Gen Hosp Psychiatry* 20:12, 1998.

Scholle SH, Rost KM, Golding JM: Physical abuse among depressed women. *J Gen Intern Med* 13:607, 1998.

Shelton R, Davidson J, Yonkers K, et al: The undertreatment of dysthymia. *J Clin Psychiatry* 58:59, 1997.

Simon G: Can depression be managed appropriately in primary care? *J Clin Psychiatry* 59:3, 1998.

Simon G, Korff MV, Rutter C, et al: Randomised trial of monitoring, feedback, and management of care by telephone to improve treatment of depression in primary care. *BMJ* 320:550, 2000.

Smyth JM, Stone AA, Hurewitz A, et al: Effects of writing about stressful experiences on symptom reduction in patients with asthma or rheumatoid arthritis. *JAMA* 281:1304, 1999.

Spitzer RL, Kroenke K, Linzer M, et al: Health-related quality of life in primary care patients with mental disorders: Results from the PRIME-MD 1000 Study. *JAMA* 274:1511, 1995.

Spitzer R, Kroenke K, Williams J: Validation and utility of a self-report version of PRIME-MD: The PHQ primary care study. *JAMA* 282:1737, 1999.

Stoudemire A, Frank R, Hedemark N, et al: The economic burden of depression. *Gen Hosp Psychiatry* 8:387, 1986.

Thase ME: Long-term nature of depression. *J Clin Psychiatry* 60:3, 1999.

Wagner E: Organizing care for patients with chronic illness. *Milbank Q* 74:511, 1996.

Wells K, Burnam A, Rogers W, et al: The course of depression in adult outpatients: Results from the medical outcomes study. *Arch Gen Psychiatry* 49: 788, 1992.

Wells K, Sherbourne C, Schoenbaum M, et al: Impact of disseminating quality improvement programs for depression in managed primary care: A randomized controlled trial. *JAMA* 283:212, 2000.

Wells KB, Stewart A, Hays RD, et al: The functioning and well-being of depressed patients. *JAMA* 626:914, 1989.

Larry Culpepper

Worries and Anxiety

Overview

The worries in patients' lives often creep into the clinician's office, at times subtly, and at times overwhelmingly. Patients' worries encompass the spectrum of human dilemmas—they might be about events in the external world, job changes, or changes in interpersonal relationships. Factory workers might perceive the movement of jobs overseas or upcoming contract negotiations as a major, realistic threat to the only job they have ever held. Other individuals might be concerned that one of their key relationships has become increasingly distant and argumentative. For others, worries might be related to feared losses of a more personal nature, such as the loss of control, loss of self-esteem, or the loss of ability. These concerns might be related to yet other losses, such as the loss of a job, or to illness. The new diabetic might fear loss of sexual prowess or view the illness as greatly damaging self-image and self-esteem. For others, worries might relate to intimacy and dependency in an interpersonal relationship, with conflicting feelings about autonomy and self-sufficiency and the intense demands of intimacy. Still for others, worry emerges over anticipated events, an upcoming birthday, the start of chemotherapy, or an upcoming move.

At times, such worries are discussed with primary care clinicians simply as part of a normal office visit interaction by patients who find comfort in the nonjudgmental, confidential, and caring context of an ongoing primary care relationship. For many patients, simply being able to briefly share a worry with the clinician is helpful. For those facing major life issues, the clinician's advice related to such worries might be sought and highly valued.

Other patients present for care of symptoms they perceive as emanating from their worries: the woman unable to sleep at nights in anticipation of the successful completion of a major business venture; the mother with tension headaches, back pain, and irritability that she associates with the impending start of a son's trial on drug possession charges. For others, the clinician does not encounter the worry except by probing, if at all. Instead, these patients present the resulting physical symptoms and have no insight into their symptoms being connected with their worries. For example, insomnia, palpitations and chest pain, headache, backache, abdominal pain, episodes of dizziness, and nausea all might bring patients to the clinician's office without the patients being aware that the symptoms are related to their worries.

For the primary care provider, a major task accomplished dozen of times each week is to determine the appropriate response to worried patients. For whom is the simple sharing of the concern all that is desired or necessary? For whom is brief counseling and help in decision making appropriate? For many patients, the clinician is the only trusted counselor and advisor to whom they can turn. For other patients, recognizing and treating the acute situational distress caused by the worry is required. And for some, the right course is recognizing that the worry and resulting symptoms are the presentation of an ongoing anxiety disorder requiring diagnosis, treatment, and follow up.

This chapter discusses all of these, but particularly focuses on generalized anxiety disorder (GAD), the diagnostic and assessment issues involved, and the treatment options available. All of these issues are best considered following review of our current understanding of the various factors leading to the development of anxiety disorders.

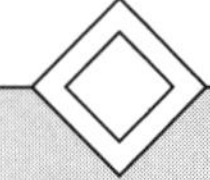

The Origins of Anxiety

Why do some individuals have their lives filled with worries while others do not? Although the occasional patient might recognize that their worries are ill founded, the vast majority identify their current situation and possibly similar past experiences which, at least to them, thoroughly justify their worries. However, in exactly the same situation, other people view the stresses as challenges to be met or even enjoyed. What accounts for these differences?

This section reviews our understanding of genetic and family influences, early childhood influences, and neurobiological and cognitive behavioral theories regarding the origins of anxiety disorders.

Genetics

At least in part, anxiety disorders appear to have a genetic basis. Not all anxiety disorders are the same though, and the genetic influence on the development of panic disorder appears to be much stronger than that on the development of GAD. About 20 percent of relatives of patients with GAD also suffer from GAD, according to Crowe. The rate of panic disorder among relatives with panic disorder however, is 25 to 50 percent, compared to only 2 percent to 4 percent to relatives of normal controls. One study of female twins found that the familial component of GAD is almost all genetic, with a concordance with a rate of about 30 percent. In a small twin study, panic attacks were reported in both of 4 out of 13 monozygotic twins in contrast to 0 out of 16 dizygotic twins. Another twin study also found a significant genetic contribution for panic suggesting that the heritability of the condition is about 30 to 40 percent. To date, the mode of inheritance has not clearly been determined for panic or other anxiety conditions.

Family and Childhood Experience

Anxiety, which often presents clinically for the first time in late adolescence or early adulthood, clearly has its precursors during childhood. Epidemiologic studies by Shaffer and colleagues suggest that 13 percent of the general population of children suffer from a diagnosable anxiety disorder. Sullivan and colleagues propose a model of stress and anxiety in which the evolution of neurohumoral mechanisms is linked to early childhood experience using animal, primate, and human experimental evidence. Sullivan and colleagues found that primate infants raised in unpredictable environments have anxious-like behaviors and become behaviorally inhibited when confronted with unfamiliar circumstances. The primate infants' behavioral inhibition is a major response to stressful situations such as separation, fear stimuli, and placement in new social situations.

Prospective studies by Kagan and co-workers demonstrated that 4-month-old human infants who respond with higher than average distress and motor arousal to unfamiliar stimuli are more fearful and behaviorally inhibited when observed during the early childhood years. This pattern of behavioral inhibition is likely to persist throughout childhood and be a precursor in the development of specific anxiety disorders in late childhood and adolescence. Sullivan suggests that early experiences, such as unpredictable caregiver nurturing, prolonged separations, neglect, and abuse, all might serve as strong environmental influences on the development of anxiety. Prolonged separation disorder also can be a precursor to panic disorder with agoraphobia. Thus, childhood environment interacts with underlying genetic components to lead to the development of neurophysiologic mechanisms predisposing selected individuals to high anxiety responses to stress throughout their lives.

The Stress Response

An understanding of the mechanisms involved in the stress response will provide primary care clinicians with further insight into the development of anxiety disorders. The stress response and stress syndrome were first proposed by Hans Seyle, who built his description of the stress response on the earlier work of Cannon and Claude Bernard. Bernard originally proposed the concept of physiologic equilibrium through which animals, including humans, return to a baseline state following disturbances. Cannon built on this concept, which he termed *homeostasis*, to propose the *fight or flight response* to perceived threats. Seyle extended this concept to propose a framework that includes both adaptive and maladaptive, or pathologic, adaptation to stress.

A key insight of Seyle's was that organisms respond to very diverse stresses in essentially the same manner, and thus the stress response is a basic uniform mechanism of adaptation to what the individual views as threats. Anxiety and fear clearly are a major component of the stress response. He also proposed that the adrenal glands, through hormones they produce, are a central mechanism in the physiologic modulation of stress. Seyle further proposed that a variety of behavioral, metabolic, endocrine, and immune system responses to chronic stress lead to a set of "diseases of adaptation." This fundamental insight is helpful in conceptualizing, at a physiologic level, aspects of the psychosomatic symptomatology that often accompanies anxiety states and anxiety disorders.

More recently, Chrousos and Gold summarized the current conceptualization of the neuroendocrine, neurologic, and behavioral components of the stress response. Worry and anxiety can result in individuals perceiving themselves as threatened, and activate the stress response either acutely or chronically. Higher cortical thought processes involved in perceiving threats lead to activation of the corticotropin-releasing factor (CRF) system and the norepinephrine (NE) system. Through both the NE and CRF systems, the body prepares to respond to threats. Such preparation includes mobilization of fat stores, production of glucose, and diversion of the blood supply preferentially to the brain and large muscles and away from systems not required to respond to threats (such as the digestive and reproductive systems).

The stress response or certain of its components can be involved acutely in producing somatic symptoms in individuals suffering from anxiety. For example, anxiety results in the sympathetic arousal characterized by increased blood pressure, heart rate, and cardiac output. In addition, through the stress response system's chronic activation, anxiety can result in a variety of chronic stress-related symptoms involving target organ systems (see diagnostic section).

Cognitive Processes

Although the stress response, neurohumoral factors, and end-organ mechanisms help to explain the symptoms and physiologic responses to anxiety, they do not provide insight into why the anxiety arises in the first place. This instead requires understanding of why two individuals in very similar life circumstances, faced by similar immediate stresses, may respond very differently, one activating coping strategies that lead to mastery of the situation, the other responding with massive anxiety and decompensation. Clearly, these different responses involve how individuals interpret the world and the degree to which they perceive specific events as being threatening. In addition, given the same interpretation of an external threat, some perceive themselves able to cope, leading to a sense to confidence, whereas others perceive the situation as beyond their cop ing ability with consequent feelings of hopelessness, fear, negative affect, and low self-esteem.

Ultimately, all of the worries listed at the opening of this chapter involve the cognitive appraisal that a situation is a threat and a secondary appraisal that the individual might not be able to cope with the threat in a desirable manner. These threats all either involve the possibility of direct harm, punishment, or a loss of something the individual views as important. The related sense of uncontrollability is cognitive. Two related theories have evolved to explain how individuals respond to their worries and stresses: the transactional model of stress and coping and cognitive theory.

The Transactional Model of Stress and Coping

Lazarus and Folkman's transactional model of stress and coping proposes two related processes. The first is one of *cognitive appraisal,* through which individuals evaluate a perceived threat and its emotional meaning within their life circumstances, values, beliefs, and goals. The second has been termed *secondary appraisal,* which is the cognitive process by which coping potential is determined.

Coping responses can be grouped into two general strategies: *problem focused* and *emotion focused*. Using problem-focused coping, the individual attempts to deal with stresses by actually changing the external environment. Thus, the individual faced with an unexpected financial loss who adopts an aggressive budget to reduce spending is using a problem-focused coping strategy. In emotion-focused strategies, a person faced with the same financial loss responds by denying its importance or simply perceiving it, without developing other plans to deal with it.

COGNITIVE THEORY

The second theory that explains how individuals respond to their worries and stresses is cognitive theory. Cognitive theory was developed by Beck and others as a means of understanding and developing therapeutic approaches to emotional disorders including anxiety and depression. Central to cognitive theory is the concept of *schemata,* which are internal mental representations through which experiences are interpreted. They are built from the individual's past set of encounters with similar experiences. These internal representations of the external world become filters through which individuals perceive and interpret experience with others and information about themselves. Schemata also affect the recall of information about prior events, selectively reinforcing the schemata themselves. Schemata include affective responses, such as fear and distress, and determine the meanings attributed to events. Usually, individuals are not consciously aware of the totality of the past experiences and memories that lead to schemata, making self-reflection difficult.

Within this conceptual framework, worrisome events trigger fear and anxiety leading to a set of responses that might include physical sensations and symptoms (such as heightened sensitivity to headaches or gastrointestinal sensations), affective responses (fear), and meaning (e.g., confirmation of low self-worth). This response includes *automatic thoughts,* by which Beck means thoughts or mental images that, although available to conscious awareness, are systematically not attended to by the individual. These automatic thoughts often reveal the individual's view of the future based on their perception of self and the environment. These thoughts often lead to the way the individual responds (both with overt action and emotionally) to the events triggering a schemata. Thus, attention to these automatic thoughts and images often provides insight into the underlying schemata and associated behaviors. A component of the individual's use of the schemata can be *cognitive distortion* of the way the individual evaluates new information. This can include seeking out and emphasizing evidence that tends to confirm the schemata, while ignoring contradictory new information. It also might involve catastrophically overestimating the perceived likely bad outcomes accruing from a set of worrisome events.

Fear and danger schemata, through which individuals interpret either external events or internal thoughts perceived as dangerous, are of particular relevance in understanding anxiety and anxiety disorders. The cognitive distortions involved make the schemata resistant to change through simple education and counseling. The schemata might lead the individual to interpret bodily sensations, including those stimulated by the stress response, as confirmation of fear and the perception of danger, and to portend catastrophic events themselves.

Thus, the path from an event to worry to anxiety and to an anxiety disorder often involves genetic influences, early childhood experiences, familial and environmental influences, the stress response and its associated bodily sensations, as well as cognitive interpretations, including selective attention and distortion of events occurring to the individual. Together, these influences help explain why one person perceives a situation as a minor worry while another person finds the same situation to be an overwhelming source of anxiety. For the primary care clinician, a critical task is identifying individuals who require professional help with their anxiety or anxiety disorder.

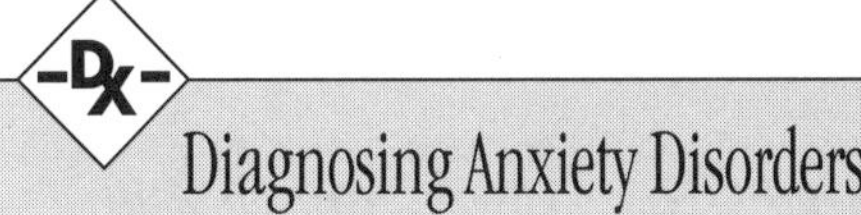

Diagnosing Anxiety Disorders

Our concepts regarding the diagnosis and classification of anxiety disorders have evolved remarkably over the past 150 years, with major advances in the past 20 years. As further insights into the emotional, neurochemical, genetic, and environmental contributions emerge, the approach to diagnosis and classification is likely to continue to advance.

Early Concepts

During the American Civil War, Jacob Mendez DeCosta coined the phrase "irritable heart" to describe a syndrome of chest pain, palpitations, and other cardiac signs without other evidence of cardiac disease. During the Franco-Prussian and Boer wars, irritable heart and the associated syndrome of "neurasthenia" were popularized. Neurasthenia is a syndrome of anxiety, pervasive exhaustion, and depression.

At the turn of the century, Freud proposed that anxiety was central to these conditions and initiated the term "anxiety neurosis" to describe a condition characterized by anxious expectations, generalized irritability, respiratory and cardiac distress (including palpitations and dyspnea), and often sweating, paresthesias, and vertigo. Freud proposed both acute and chronic forms of anxiety neurosis, with the former often manifesting as acute attacks, now regarded as panic attacks. Freud noted that these "anxiety attacks" often were associated with the development of agoraphobia. Although "irritable heart" continued to be viewed as an organic problem involving disordered "neurocirculatory asthenia," by World War II this condition was considered a manifestation of psychiatric distress. Freud's conception of the single condition "anxiety neurosis" with varying manifestations was incorporated into the *Diagnostic and Statistical Manual of Mental Disorders* (DSM) and continued in use until release of third edition of the DSM in 1980.

Generalized Anxiety Disorder in DSM-III

In the DSM-III, GAD and panic disorder replaced anxiety neurosis. For DSM-III, the diagnosis of GAD required persistent high levels of deffuse anxiety for at least 1 month with symptoms from at least three of four categories: vigilance and scanning, apprehensive expectation, autonomic hyperactivity, and motor tension. With release of DSM-III-R in 1987, these criteria were changed to require at least 6 months duration and 6 of 18 potential anxiety symptoms. The DSM-III-R also emphasized the excessive and unrealistic nature of the underlying worry.

Panic Disorders in DSM-III

Until 1980, patients with panic disorders frequently were given a variety of diagnoses, such as irritable heart, neurotachycardia, irritable bowel syndrome, or hyperventilation syndrome, depending on the symptom complex involved. With DSM-III, recurrent panic attacks were defined by a set of inclusion symptoms and frequent recurrence over a specified interval of time. DSM-III also linked panic attacks to agoraphobia, with the latter forming the major diagnostic focus. However, in 1987 this conceptualization was reversed in DSM-III-R with the insight that agoraphobia usually develops as a complication of recurrent panic attacks. Whereas DMS-III divided patients with panic disorder into those with agoraphobia with or without panic attacks, or panic disorder without agoraphobia, DSM-III-R instead classified them into panic disorder with and without agoraphobia, and agoraphobia without a history of panic disorder. DSM-III-R also added categories to describe agoraphobia including mild, moderate, severe, in partial remission, and in full remission based on current severity of agoraphobic avoidance. A similar evolution in nomenclature has occurred for the other anxiety disorders, including social phobia, specific phobias, and obsessive-compulsive disorder (these conditions are not considered in this chapter).

International Classification of Diseases

Although the DSM evolved with the increased understanding of anxiety during the latter part of the twentieth century, the more generally used *International Classification of Diseases,* 9th Revision (ICD-9), first produced in 1978, did not. ICD-9 continues to include a set of generic anxiety states under the single category "neurotic disorders," and provides no guideline for specifically classifying individuals with both panic attacks and agoraphobia.

With ICD-10, however, GAD and panic disorder are recognized as separate categories, but the diagnostic system becomes a bit more complicated: ICD-10 continues the DSM-III approach of giving precedence to agoraphobia (listed under phobic disorders) over panic disorder. It therefore uses panic attacks in phobic situations, including agoraphobia, as an indicator of phobic severity, and restricts the diagnosis of panic disorder to only cases without a phobic component. Unfortunately, ICD-9 continues to be the diagnostic classification required by Medicare and most third-party payers within the United States health care system.

DSM-IV

In 1994, DSM-IV refined the classification of GAD, panic disorders, and agoraphobia. The DSM-IV strategy for diagnosing GAD is presented in Table 17-1. This strategy represents our best current understanding of what constitutes the essential components of GAD.

Table 17-1

Diagnostic Criteria for Generalized Anxiety Disorder Based on DSM-IV

1. Excessive anxiety and worry (apprehensive expectation), occurring more days than not for at least 6 months, about a number of events or activities (e.g., school or work performance).
2. The person finds it difficult to control the worry.
3. The anxiety and worry is associated with at least three of the following (only one required in children), with at least some symptoms present for more days than not for the past 6 months:
   - restlessness or feeling on edge or keyed up
   - easily fatigued
   - difficulty concentrating or mind going blank
   - irritability
   - muscle tension
   - sleep disturbance (difficulty falling or staying asleep, or restless unsatisfying sleep)
4. The anxiety, worry, or physical symptoms cause clinically significant distress or impairment in social, occupational, or other important areas of functioning.
5. The disturbance is not due to the direct effects of a substance (e.g., drug abuse or medication) or medical condition (e.g., hyperthyroidism) and does not occur exclusively during a mood disorder, a psychotic disorder, or a pervasive developmental disorder.
6. The focus of the anxiety and worry is not confined to features of the Axis I disorder, that is, the anxiety is not about
   —having a panic attack [panic disorder]
   —being embarrassed in public [social phobia]
   —being contaminated [obsessive-compulsive disorder]
   —being away from home [separation anxiety disorder]
   —gaining weight [anorexia nervosa]
   —having multiple physical complaints [somatization disorder]
   —having a serious illness [hypochondriasis]
   and the anxiety and worry do not occur exclusively during posttraumatic stress disorder.

SOURCE: Reproduced with permission from The American Psychiatric Association Task Force on DSM-IV: *Diagnostic and Statistical Manual for Mental Disorders: DSM-IV*, 4th ed. Washington, DC: American Psychiatric Association; 1994.

GAD, as defined in DSM-IV, involves excessive worry and anxiety for at least 6 months accompanied by at least three of six somatic symptoms in adults (only one is required in children). DSM-IV thereby simplifies the number of symptoms required, and stresses that the worry must be pervasive and difficult to control over an extended time. In addition, it emphasizes that the excessive anxiety must cause significant impairment in social or occupational functioning. It also acknowledges the childhood origin of GAD for many patients.

DSM-IV defines *panic attacks* as discrete periods of intense fear or discomfort with at least 4 of 13 possible symptoms, and a temporal course of abrupt onset with peak intensity within 10 minutes. However, panic attacks in of themselves are not considered a mental disorder. See Chap. 18 for more information on panic disorder.

Among patients with full-blown anxiety disorders, decreases in functioning are similar to those seen with major depression, and are as great if not greater than decreases with a number of chronic medical diseases including cardiac, respiratory, diabetes, and arthritic conditions.

Limitations of DSM-IV

Although the DSM-IV classification represents a major advance in our ability to evaluate and classify anxiety conditions, it continues to have shortcomings for the primary care clinician. One shortcoming is that many primary care patients present with significant worries and resulting functional limitations but do not meet full criteria for any anxiety disorder. Such patients are said to have *subsyndromal anxiety*. A second shortcoming of DSM-IV is its failure to consider cross-cultural differences in the manifestations of anxiety.

Subsyndromal Anxiety

Depending on the practice setting and the definition of subsyndromal anxiety, patients with subsyndromal anxiety are at least as common as those diagnosed as meeting formal DSM criteria for anxiety disorders. Ormel and colleagues found that among patients with subsyndromal anxiety or mixed subsyndromal anxiety and depression, impairment in social role (40 and 43 percent, respectively) and occupational role (30 and 57 percent, respectively) are frequent. Patients with subsyndromal panic symptoms are particularly likely to be impaired. Patients with subsyndromal anxiety conditions are also common in primary care settings. Even though they do not have a diagnosable anxiety disorder, they would likely benefit from care.

Cultural Limitations

A second limitation of the DSM criteria involves culturally bound symptom complexes. Immigrant groups are particularly likely to present in primary care settings rather than psychiatric settings. Although a discussion of cross-cultural issues involved in the diagnosis and treatment of anxiety disorders is beyond the scope of this chapter, an understanding of cultural issues is valuable.

From a cognitive theory perspective, an understanding of cultural and immigrant family influences on the interpretation of symptoms and perception of self and others can be critical to properly interpreting patient worries. For instance, within a Muslim community, being bound to the home is viewed as a sign of great virtue rather one of severe agoraphobia. In addition, although the DSM language of anxiety and panic has been popularized and broadly understood by the mainstream public in American and Western European societies, the same might not be true for members of other cultures. Some cultures have anxiety-like syndromes with symptom complexes and courses that do not match any established DSM disorder, yet remain major mental health concerns within the culture. Two of these are described here.

ATAQUES DE NERVIOS (NERVE ATTACKS) Latin American and Caribbean Hispanics often report *ataques* *de nervios*, usually involving a loss of emotional control and often occurring at funerals, accidents, or in times of major family conflict or other severe stress. Symptoms include shaking and palpitations, a sense of numbness, episodes of shouting and swearing, pseudoconvulsive movements, and no recollection after the event.

Those reporting *ataques de nervios* also have elevated rates of established psychiatric disorders compared to Latinos who do not report a history of such ataques (63 percent versus 28 percent). Although some patients experiencing *ataques de nervios* meet criteria for panic disorder, such patients report that their panic attacks are at times quite distinct from their *ataques de nervios*. The possibility exists that the popular term is used to describe a heterogeneous set of conditions including panic and other anxiety disorders.

HWA-BYUNG Another example is the Korean folk illness, *hwa-byung*, which is considered a physical illness within the Korean culture. Symptoms include long-standing suppressed anger, somatic complaints including dizziness, insomnia, fatigue, panic attacks, a sense of helplessness and guilt, tension, and a sense of impending doom. From a Western perspective, this condition has elements of GAD and depression, but also elements of panic.

Thus, the primary care clinician must be ready to provide care not only to individuals with diagnosable anxiety disorders, but also to those with subsyndromal symptoms associated with significant functional limitation, and those from cultural groups whose conditions, although debilitating, do not meet any establish DSM diagnostic pattern.

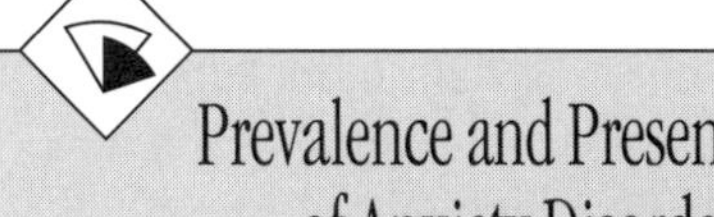

Prevalence and Presentation of Anxiety Disorders

Although the DSM-IV criteria are helpful in defining a set of human conditions, they by no means include all the individuals with the conditions. In primary care settings, it is unusual for an individual to present solely with one of these diagnoses. Instead, primary care patients often have other comorbid conditions of a psychiatric or medical nature. Depression and other concurrent anxiety disorders (e.g., social phobia, GAD, and panic disorder together) are particularly common.

Prevalence in the Community

Community-based studies reported by the Surgeon General have found that 21 percent of individuals have had a mental disorder within the past 12 months. The majority of these have multiple disorders and over half meet criteria for an anxiety disorder, with GAD being the most common. In these community-based studies, GAD has been found to be present within the past year in between 2.5 and 8 percent of the population, with women affected almost twice as often as men. An estimated 10 to 20 percent of those of with anxiety disorders also have a co-occurring substance use disorder. Among those with alcohol abuse or dependence, anxiety disorder is two to three times more likely than among those without such alcohol use. Swendsen and associates found that alcohol abuse is as likely to precede as follow the development of panic disorder. Lifetime prevalence of panic disorder in the community is 3.8 percent. Another 5.6 percent report subthreshold panic attacks (see Chap. 18).

Prevalence in Primary Care

In primary care settings, the prevalence of anxiety disorders is higher than in the community, although few studies are available to precisely quantify their prevalence. Spitzer has reported that 9 percent of primary care patients have GAD or panic with another 9 percent having anxiety disorders not otherwise specified. Sartorious, in a World Health Organization-sponsored international study, found panic, GAD, or agoraphobia to be present in about 10 percent of primary care patients.

LAURA BENDER *Laura Bender is worried about her heart. Rather, she is now also worried about her heart. She has a long string of worries, and the pain in her chest is making all of them worse. She is 25 years old, has a new job as a realtor, and needs to be at her best. She comes to your office and says, "I just can't keep this many balls in the air at once. I have a house mortgage, my friends are all back in my hometown, my mom died last summer, and I'm worried about my dad."*

You find out that Ms. Bender has always been "the nervous type," but only since her move to this town 8 months ago has her worrying been uncontrollable and getting in the way of her normal activities. She now has trouble concentrating, is much more irritable, has trouble falling asleep, and is fatigued.

This is her second visit to you in a month, this time for the new pain that has developed in her chest. She tells you it has been present continuously for over a week, although it is worse with exertion and before she meets a client. You question her further and learn that she is having trouble getting a deep enough breath, and occasionally has episodes of diarrhea that do not seem related to anything at all.

Primary care clinicians should recognize that within their practice patients such as Laura Bender may have an anxiety disorder. Anxiety disorders are likely to be present in patients with specific symptom constellations including cardiac, respiratory, and gastrointestinal symptoms.

CARDIAC PRESENTATIONS

GAD and panic disorders occur commonly among patients with cardiac symptoms who lack angiographic evidence for cardiac pathology, according to Roy-Byrne and Katon. For example, GAD was found in 56 percent of such patients in one study and panic disorder was diagnosed in 40 percent in a second study. Panic disorder is also frequent in patients presenting to emergency rooms with chest pains and other cardiac symptoms who turn out to have no cardiac abnormalities. However, panic disorder also has been found to be more frequent in patients with documented cardiac pathology; three studies documented rates of 9, 16, and 23 percent. Given the stress response mechanisms and their effect on blood pressure and chronic cardiac stress, the association of panic disorder and anxiety with worsening cardiac disease and sudden death are not unexpected.

RESPIRATORY PRESENTATIONS

Respiratory conditions, particularly asthma, also demonstrate complex interactions with anxiety disorders. Five studies found an increased prevalence, ranging from 6.5 to 24 percent, of panic disorder among patients with asthma. Likewise, asthma appears to be more common in those with panic disorder.

Clinically, panic attacks can be differentiated from asthma attacks both by their more rapid onset and shorter duration, and the presence of wheezing, mucus production, and coughing among asthmatics. However, both panic attacks and acute asthmatic attacks involve similar respiratory symptoms of distress and impending doom and fear that may lead to phobic avoidance of situations associated with attacks. Dyspnea can also occur in both asthma and panic disorder.

Notably, among asthmatics, the sensation of panic and fear (including among those not meeting DSM criteria) has been associated with worse outcomes, independent of pulmonary function. Kinsman and colleagues report that *generalized panic-fear* is evaluated in such patients separate from the measurement of *illness-specific panic-fear*. Patients with high generalized panic-fear tend to have the most intensive asthma medication regimens, the longest hospitalizations, and the highest rates of rehospitalization. Patients with low generalized panic-fear underuse asthma treatments and also have a high rate of rehospitalization, according to Dirks and associates. Asthmatics reporting both high generalized and illness-specific panic-fear are most likely to panic during asthma attacks, overmedicate, and demonstrate poor self-management. Those with moderate scores on both panic-fear scales have the best outcomes and most appropriate use of medications. As a corollary of these associations, the care of children with asthma might be complicated by their parents' anxious reactions.

Gastrointestinal Presentations

Gastrointestinal symptoms also occur more frequently in patients with anxiety disorders. Irritable bowel syndrome is the condition most studied. Lydiard and associates found that 31 percent of patients with irritable bowel syndrome reported a history of panic disorder and 34 percent reported GAD. In contrast, Blewett and colleagues found that 19 percent had panic disorder and 14 percent had GAD at the time of evaluation. At a physiologic level, the autonomic system stimulates the gut in response to the norepinephrine component of the stress response. In addition, the locus ceruleus receives input from the gut and has connections to the gut. Through such mechanisms, irritable bowel syndrome and anxiety conditions have complex neurobiological interactions.

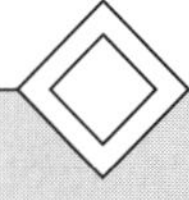

Assessment of the Anxious Patient

As with other mental health problems, anxiety is often unrecognized in primary care practice. For example, in one study by Fifer and co-workers only 44 percent of patients with clinically significant anxiety symptoms were appropriately diagnosed. Thus treatment of anxiety begins with its recognition. After diagnosis, treatment involves the development of a shared understanding by the patient and clinician of its influence on the patient's life, and agreement on an approach to treatment and treatment objectives.

An assessment of worried patients includes identifying the level of anxiety involved, and whether multiple behavioral disorders are involved, including depression and substance abuse. It can be very helpful to identify the symptoms the patients find most troubling and to develop an understanding of the patients' internal explanation of the cause of their anxiety and the illness model through which they view their symptom complex. A brief assessment of the symptoms' effect on patients' performance and ability to function often helps in developing a mutually agreed upon set of treatment goals and assists in motivating patients to adhere to treatment.

Concomitant depression and anxiety are extremely common. Table 17-2 presents the common and differentiating symptoms of depression and anxiety. Substance misuse also is common in patients with anxiety and should not be overlooked. Panic disorder with agoraphobia is associated with an increased risk of suicide attempts, and clinicians should ask patients about suicidal thoughts.

Identifying the symptoms and functional impairment important to the patient also helps in planning treatment. Insomnia and sexual dysfunction, the latter particularly among those with comorbid depression, often are both quite troubling to patients. Patients often volunteer information about insomnia, and with gentle probing by the clinician it is often possible to uncover concerns about sexual performance.

In evaluating insomnia, determining whether the difficulty is falling asleep (often present with anxiety) or early morning awakenings (more often with depression) and the chronicity and perceived severity of sleep difficulties is useful. Of note, Ford and colleagues found that in individuals predisposed to depression (those with prior episodes), insomnia is a significant risk factor for recurrence and its development often leads to the onset of a depressive episode. Thus, even though not associated with a full anxiety disorder, worries deserve attention if they are causing insomnia in the patient at risk for recurrent major depression.

Sexual dysfunction occurs in as many as 80 percent of patients initially presenting with major depression. Because there is an overlap between depression and the anxiety disorders, and because

Table 17-2

Symptoms Differentiating of Anxiety and Depression

Specific Depression Symptoms	Common Symptoms	Specific Anxiety Symptoms
Depressed mood	Apprehension/fear	Hypervigilance
Hopelessness	Panic attacks	Agoraphobia
Weight change	Somatic symptoms	Rituals
Loss of interest or pleasure	Unrealistic worry	More difficulty getting to sleep
Guilt	Agitation	
More early morning wakening	Poor concentration	
	Insomnia	
	Irritability	
	Fatigue	

Source: Reproduced with permission from The American Psychiatric Association Task Force on DSM-IV: *Diagnostic and Statistical Manual for Mental Disorders: DSM-IV*, 4th ed. Washington, DC: American Psychiatric Association; 1994.

selective serotonin reuptake inhibitors (SSRIs) and other medications can cause sexual dysfunction, it is important for clinicians to identify sexual dysfunction before beginning treatment. If dysfunction is present, clinicians should determine whether it was long-standing or developed as part of the symptom complex associated with the depression/anxiety disorder. This knowledge can be very helpful in monitoring a patient's response to treatment. It also facilitates discussion of sexual dysfunction as a possible treatment side effect and in planning treatment. For more about sexual problems, see Chap. 7.

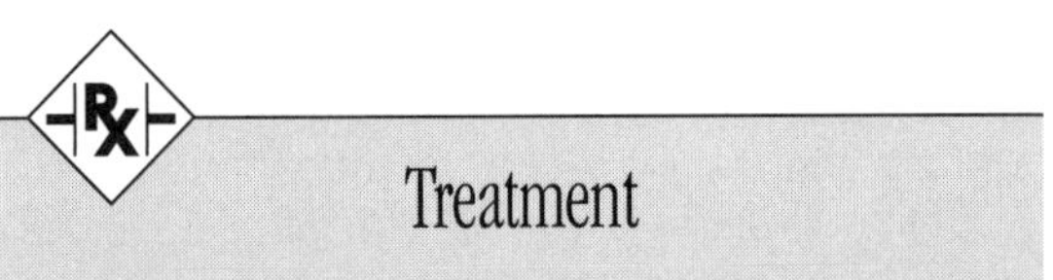

Treatment

LAURA BENDER (CONTINUED) *Ms. Bender is somewhat reassured by her normal physical examination, but is reluctant to accept that her physical symptoms are related to anxiety. But she trusts you—you have learned a great deal about her concerns and how she is dealing with them—and is willing to try a few things aimed at her anxiety before she insists on referral to a cardiologist for a heart evaluation. She is willing to reduce the amount of coffee she drinks from eight cups a day to two. She is willing to begin a program of regular exercise after work each day. She will try to use the time immediately after dinner to rehash the day's problems, and will try for a regular bedtime, with the alarm clock out of sight, and with the day's worries out of her mind.*

For the patient with anxiety disorders or worries affecting function, a comprehensive treatment plan includes education and counseling, life style modification, and specific treatment interventions. For patients voicing worries but not requiring active treatment, an efficient approach to providing support and counseling is helpful. In addition, having an established strategy for evaluating and responding to insomnia is highly useful for the clinician. All of these will be considered next.

Responding to Patients' Worries

Doctors Stuart and Lieberman, in *The Fifteen Minute Hour*, provide an excellent, efficient model for responding to patient worries: the BATHE technique (Table 17-3). This approach involves an interview sequence. Exploring the *background* of the patient's concern is the first step. The clinician then asks the patient about feelings *(affect)* about the worry. This is followed by an inquiry regarding the issues most *troubling* the patient. The clinician follows this by inquiring about how the patient is *handling* the problem. The final step, showing *empathy*, concludes the sequence. The BATHE strategy, which can be completed in 3 to 5 min, is perceived by patients as being very supportive and provides the clinician with a basis for follow up and insight as to whether more intensive investigation and intervention are necessary.

Education and Counseling

An important part of engaging the patient in active treatment involves developing a shared understanding and explanation for the diagnosis and symptoms. For patients lacking insight into the connection between their worries and somatic symptoms, this can be critical to motivating cooperation with treatment recommendations. The genetic, familial, neurobiological, and cognitive-behavioral concepts underlying our professional understanding of anxiety can be tailored to individual patients. Thus, patients reporting a major familial pattern of anxiety and for whom the clinician plans pharmacologic treatment might particularly benefit from an explanation emphasizing the genetic and neurobiological aspects of anxiety. In contrast, individuals whose cognitive associations appear to play a major part in their anxiety disorder might benefit from an abbreviated explanation of cognitive aspects of anxiety in support of referral for cognitive-behavioral therapy. It is also helpful to patients to assist them in developing an approach to explaining their disorder to other family members.

Table 17-3

Components of the BATHE Technique for Counseling Patients

• Background:	"What is going on in your life?"
• Affect:	"How are you feeling about that?"
• Trouble:	"What troubles you the most?"
• Handling:	"How are you handling that?"
• Empathy:	"That must be very difficult."

SOURCE: Reproduced with permission from Stuart MR, Lieberman JA: *The Fifteen Minute Hour.* London, UK: Praeger; 1993.

Life Style Modifications

A brief inquiry into the use of caffeine and other stimulants, as well as alcohol and other sedating agents, can be helpful. The clinician should counsel moderate use of such agents if appropriate. Brief counseling regarding exercise can be therapeutic, particularly for the patient with insomnia or depression. A meta-analysis by Petruzzello and colleagues has demonstrated that regular exercise can be as effective as pharmacologic treatment in improving anxiety. Although similar evidence for its effect on anxiety is not available, clinical experience suggests that exercise can be of considerable value in reducing stress and anxiety as well as in improving sleep.

Treating Insomnia

For the anxious patient, control of insomnia often is a major treatment objective. Improved sleep often leads to improved coping and function. Frequently, patients will accept the association between stresses and insomnia and interventions targeting them, while being unwilling to accept associations between anxiety and other somatic complaints.

In evaluating insomnia, a brief review of contributory factors in addition to anxiety can be helpful. Evaluating contributory medical conditions such as pain, allergies, and respiratory, cardiac, and neurologic abnormalities can be helpful. The restless legs syndrome (in which patients have an irresistible urge to move their legs to relieve pain) and sleep-related apneas should be considered. Stimulants, including weight control medications, prednisone, theophylline, SSRIs, or alcohol are potential drug-related causes of anxiety. Nicotine is a stimulant and its withdrawal a stress. This accounts for the association between heavy smoking and sleep disturbance with the heavy smoker smoking immediately before going to bed or after awakening during the night, and then having difficulty getting to sleep.

A full discussion of the work-up and treatment of insomnia is beyond the scope of this chapter; however, a number of suggestions are helpful to anxious patients. Irregular bed times, attempting to sleep immediately after working without an interval for relaxation, and use of alcohol or coffee after lunchtime all may contribute to poor sleep. Clinical experience suggests that patients who curtail their total time in bed to that required prior to developing insomnia begin to sleep deeper and with fewer awakenings, and become more alert during the day. Psychophysiologic or learned insomnia frequently takes the form of trying too hard to sleep or trying too hard to get back to sleep after mid-night awakenings with various maladaptive behaviors developed due to the anticipation of poor sleep. Environmental factors such as noise, light, or uncomfortable temperature also may contribute.

Daytime exercise helps people fall asleep more easily at night, awaken less often during the night, shift their sleep content from light sleep to more deep sleep (stage 3 and 4), and feel more rested during the day, Kubitz and co-workers report. Such effects are profound and can be particularly beneficial to the anxious depressed patient. Of note, Hauri found that the effects of exercise often develop gradually, with a period of weeks before marked changes in sleep occur. Ideally, because exercise increases metabolism and body temperature followed by a decrease in both several hours later, the ideal time to exercise is 5 to 6 hours before going to bed.

Anxious patients often become overly focused on their inability to get to sleep or their mid-night awakenings. This often takes the form of clock watching and worry about the time lost from sleep. A simple but often effective intervention is to recommend that the alarm clock be placed out of sight and that the patient not look at the time from getting in bed until the alarm goes off. Distracting activities such as reading or watching television might be useful to divert the patient's mind from their worries and promote relaxation before attempting to go to sleep, but overly stimulating material should be avoided. Reading as long as possible, fighting sleep, is often best, promoting the association between reading, turning the light off, and rapidly falling asleep.

Some patients, particularly those with long-standing insomnia, develop learned dysfunctional behaviors that might respond to a defined stimulus-control therapeutic approach. Bootzin and associates proposes steps to improve sleep hygiene, including:

1. Lie down, intending to go to sleep, only when you are sleepy.
2. Do not use your bed for anything but sleep or sexual activity.
3. If unable to fall asleep easily, get up and go to another room. Stay up as long as needed and return to the bedroom only when you feel ready to fall asleep.

Notably, Bootzin advises against reading or watching television in bed. For those who find that reading helps them go to sleep, this rule might be modified based on the clinician's judgment. For patients who continue to have difficulty with insomnia or for whom sleep apnea or other pathologic sleep processes might be at work, referral to a sleep specialist can be helpful.

Life Style and Scheduled Worry Time

Anxious patients often find themselves rehashing the problems and unmet demands in their lives. This rehashing is frequently associated with insomnia and the inability to get beyond repetitive thoughts about unattended tasks and problems.

For some patients, suggesting simple coping strategies, such as setting aside a half an hour during the day or early evening to organize their worries, might be helpful. During this time, patients should sit quietly, briefly review the problems that are preoccupying them, and then let their minds wander. As worries enter their minds, these should be jotted down on note cards. After 5 or 10 min, most patients have reviewed their usual litany of concerns. Their written lists can then be organized into the minor clutter of life—phone calls, making appointments, paying bills—and larger issues such as financial, occupational, or family concerns. Patients can then use the "clutter" list to prioritize their activities for the next few days and to reassure themselves that the items will not be forgotten. For the major issues, it is helpful to advise patients to identify priorities that they are ready to address, and the one or two activities they need to do as an initial step or next step, such as making contact with an individual, or sorting out their monthly financial obligations. For many anxious patients, this exercise, particularly if conducted two or three times a week, leads to an improved sense of coping and self-control. This can be particularly helpful for the individual whose life is overcommitted with responsibilities both at home and at work.

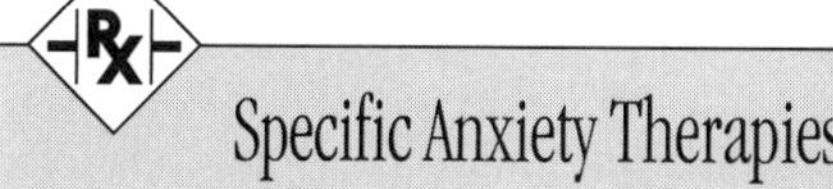

Specific Anxiety Therapies

LAURA BENDER (CONTINUED) *Ms. Bender returns to your office and tells you she is exercising regularly, doing all the other things she agreed to do, and feels better. But she is still not sleeping well, and is still fatigued and irritable. After a short discussion, you prescribe buspirone 5 mg three times a day. She returns in 2 weeks and reports that she is dramatically improved. After a month she reports that she is less nervous than she can ever remember being. She reviews the symptoms that might signify a return of her anxiety, and agrees to come back in 6 months for a follow-up visit.*

For the patient with a true anxiety disorder and for some with significant suffering and functional decline due to subsyndromal disorders, pharmacologic agents, formal counseling, or both should be considered. There is strong evidence of the effectiveness of both pharmacotherapy and cognitive behavioral therapy, and little evidence to indicate that either is better than the other in the treatment of GAD. Nor is there convincing evidence that combined treatment offers substantial additional benefit over either therapy alone.

Given the realities of the primary care setting, financial and insurance limitations, and the resistance of many patients to referral for counseling, pharmacologic treatment accompanied by the educational and counseling interventions already reviewed is a pragmatic initial approach. Referral for formal psychological interventions can be discussed as an option and encouraged for those patients accepting or seeking such care or not fully responsive to treatment.

Pharmacologic Treatment

Like treatment of panic disorders (see Chap. 18), both pharmacologic and cognitive-behavioral therapy treatment modes have been demonstrated effective for treating GAD. For pharmacologic treatment, the benzodiazepines, buspirone, and venlafaxine are the main options, although the SSRIs might have a supportive role. GAD also responds well in many trials to placebo interventions, demonstrating the importance of supportive counseling. Indeed, for mild cases supportive counseling alone may be sufficient treatment. Because GAD is chronic, often initially presenting during childhood or adolescence, long-term treatment options should be considered. Some patients may prefer intermittent pharmacotherapy during times of increased stress and disability.

Because of the relatively immediate onset of action, the benzodiazepines, particularly the long-acting agents, have great utility when immediate control of more severe symptoms are desired. With long-term use, however, dependence occurs. For this reason, clinicians recommend against long-term benzodiazepine therapy.

Buspirone, a partial serotonin 5-HT1a receptor agent is the only agent in its class that is FDA approved for treatment of GAD. It requires a 2- to 4-week treatment interval before significant treatment response emerges, but beyond this initial interval has been demonstrated to be as effective for GAD as a number of the benzodiazepines, including oxazepam, alprazolam, and lorazepam. In higher doses, buspirone also has some antidepressant effect and reduces agitation in patients with dementia.

The SSRI venlafaxine likewise requires several weeks' interval before treatment effect fully emerges but is as effective as buspirone. Particularly for patients with comorbid major depression, the SSRIs may be useful either in combination with other agents or, for some patients, as monotherapy. SSRIs also may be used in cases for which benzodiazepine use is not desired and the patient has failed a trial of buspirone.

Cognitive Behavioral Therapy

Cognitive behavioral therapy is the most studied and most widely accepted psychotherapeutic approach to treating anxiety disorders. There are numerous approaches to cognitive behavioral therapy. In an analysis of these, Brewin identified three fundamental strategies: re-education to correct misconceptions or omissions in a patient's knowledge or understanding, modifying mental representations (schemata), and modifying self-regulation.

For panic, re-education addresses the origins and effect of panic symptoms such as palpitations or dizziness. For many patients, these symptoms are interpreted as having catastrophic complications, such as heart attack, stroke, or similar events. For the agoraphobia, re-education may be required regarding the events leading to restriction of movement. For GAD, such correction of misconceptions involves an analysis of the worries and the interpretation patients make of the underlying events, particularly with regard to perceived potential losses and loss of control.

A second major component of cognitive behavioral therapy is modifying the nonconscious mental representations, or schemata, used by the patient to interpret and to ascribe meaning to events. Insights into these mental representations can be gained by the therapist by having patients investigate their automatic thoughts related to the events. Because these mental representations are strongly ingrained, and themselves bias the interpretation and selective attention to events in a reinforcing manner, simple re-education generally will not lead to substantial change in patient outcomes. Thus, modifying schemata (mental representations) generally requires an experiential therapeutic activity. For patients suffering from panic attacks, this usually involves progressive exposure to cues the patient has begun to avoid as a way of limiting panic attacks. These cues may be physical—locations, events, and people—or internal thoughts. Through prolonged and repeated therapeutic exposure, the patient reliably internalizes the recognition of their erroneous thoughts and mental representations, and modifies them with associated reduction in anxiety. They also develop an improved sense of self-efficacy and willingness to encounter the source of anxiety.

A third component of cognitive behavioral therapy is modifying self-regulation of thoughts, feelings, and behaviors. Through this component, the therapist helps the patient learn and practice new coping strategies. For panic, these might include learning new interpretations of their symptoms—that they are not catastrophic—and new coping strategies such as breathing techniques, and self-talk to reinforce the patient's recollection of the limited and benign course of panic attacks.

These three core strategies often are combined with other modalities such as relaxation techniques or breathing training. Interpersonal couple therapies might be used to restructure relations that have become dysfunctional because of responses to panic and other anxiety symptoms.

A key role for the primary clinician with the patient for whom cognitive behavioral therapy is the desired therapeutic approach is the selection of an experienced therapist expert. Furthermore, for some patients it is desirable to combine cognitive behavioral therapy with pharmacotherapy, particularly for those with severe symptoms during the early phases of treatment. For panic disorder and GAD, such combined therapy has been found both to lead to greater early improvement, although the long-term (1- to 2-year) outcomes show little difference. In such cases, the clinician might manage medication while the therapist deals with the cognitive behavioral therapy. In such cases, communication and coordination between clinician and therapist is important.

Another important role of the primary care clinician is the long-term follow up of patients with anxiety disorders. The anxiety disorders are all chronic and have a high likelihood of recurrence over the course of the patient's life. Continuing treatment for at least 6 to 12 months after good control of symptoms is attained is advisable for many patients. For those with multiple past episodes or whose symptoms have not completely resolved, continuing treatment indefinitely might be best. For those terminating pharmacotherapy, gradual withdrawal over a period of weeks to months might then be advisable, with careful monitoring to detect recurrence. Educating patients to be alert for signs of recurrence is important. For those who have benefited from cognitive behavioral therapy, refreshing their learned skills during times of stress might be therapeutic.

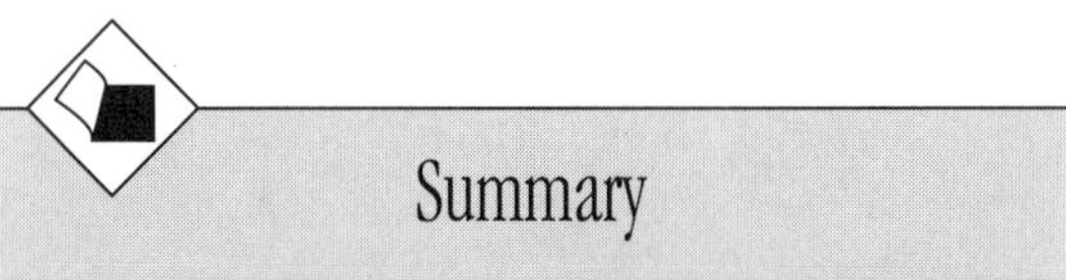

Summary

The anxiety disorders, although common in primary care, are often unrecognized. Kirmayer and colleagues report that 50 to 80 percent of primary care patients with such disorders do not have them diagnosed properly, particularly when patients present primarily with somatic signs and symptoms. Even when diagnosed, only about one out of four patients receives treatment either with appropriate medications or referral for psychotherapy, according to Meredith and co-workers. This underrecognition and undertreatment in primary care has serious consequences through the perpetuation of increased disability and high rates of using medical services.

Over the last decade, very effective pharmacologic and cognitive behavioral therapies have been developed that hold great promise for alleviating the suffering of patients with anxiety disorders. Given this increasing capacity to improve the lives of patients with anxiety, primary care clinicians have an increased responsibility to recognize and respond to the anxious patient, and to care for the worried patient to minimize progression to major anxiety disorders.

Suggested Reading

Chrousos GP, Gold PW: The concepts of stress and stress system disorders. Overview of physical and behavioral homeostasis. *JAMA* 267:1244, 1992 [published erratum appears in *JAMA* 268:200, 1992].

This landmark article provides an overview of the concept of stress, and how it affects humans at both the somatic and psychological levels. It provides a useful framework for the primary care clinician in caring for patients in our stressed society.

Lazarus RS: Coping theory and research: Past, present, and future. *Psychosom Med* 55:234, 1993.

This article excellently conceptualizes the dimensions of coping and the limits of coping. It provides a helpful framework for understanding the patient and family who turn to primary care clinicians when they have exhausted their own coping mechanisms.

Beck JS: *Cognitive Therapy: Basics and Beyond.* New York: The Guilford Press; 1995.

This reference provides an introduction to the concepts and practice of cognitive therapy. The text is useful for the clinician who needs to determine which patients might benefit from cognitive therapy. When the clinician has patients who benefited in the past from cognitive therapy but are now facing new stresses, this book will help the clinician reinforce the gains made through cognitive therapy.

Mental Health: A Report of the Surgeon General. Rockville, MD: Department of Health and Human Services, US Public Health Service; 1999.

This well-written report provides an excellent overview of not only anxiety disorders but the entire mental health field. It summarizes prevalence data, identifies populations at special risk, reviews our understanding of the pathophysiology and treatment of mental health disorders, and reviews recent research breakthroughs.

American Psychiatric Association, Work Group on Panic Disorder: Practice guideline for the treatment of patients with panic disorder. *Am J Psychiatry* 155 (Suppl 5):1, 1998.

This reference provides a helpful framework for considering pharmacotherapy for anxiety disorders.

deGruy FV 3rd: Mental health care in the primary care setting. In: Donaldson MS (ed): *Primary Care: America's Health in a New Era.* Washington, DC: National Academy Press; 1996, p 285.

This landmark report captures the issues facing primary care clinicians as they care for patients in daily practice. It articulates the inseparable nature of somatic and behavioral problems, and the special opportunities and challenges of providing integrated care.

Bibliography

American Psychiatric Association Task Force on DSM-IV: *Diagnostic and Statistical Manual of Mental Disorders: DSM-IV,* 4th ed. Washington, DC: American Psychiatric Association; 1994.

Barlow DH, Chorpita BF, Turovsky J: Fear, panic, anxiety, and disorders of emotion. In: Hope DA (ed): *Perspectives on Anxiety, Panic, and Fear.* Lincoln: Nebraska University Press; 1996, p 251.

Beck JS: *Cognitive Therapy: Basics and Beyond.* New York: The Guilford Press; 1995.

Blewett A, Allison M, Calcraft B, et al: Psychiatric disorder and outcome in irritable bowel syndrome. *Psychosomatics* 37:155, 1996.

Bootzin RR, Epstein D, Wood JM: Stimulus control instructions. In: Hauri PJ (ed): *Case Studies in Insomnia.* New York: Plenum; 1991, p 19.

Brewin CR: Cognitive change processes in psychotherapy. *Psychol Rev* 96:379, 1989.

Chrousos GP, Gold PW: The concepts of stress and stress system disorders. Overview of physical and behavioral homeostasis. *JAMA* 267:1244, 1992.

Crowe RR: The genetics of panic disorder and agoraphobia. *Psychiatr Dev* 3:171, 1985.

deGruy FV 3rd: Mental health care in the primary care setting. In: Donaldson MS (ed): *Primary Care: America's Health in a New Era.* Washington, DC: National Academy Press; 1996, p 285.

Dirks JF, Schraa JC, Brown EL, et al: Psycho-maintenance in asthma: Hospitalization rates and financial impact. *Br J Med Psychol* 53:349, 1980.

Fifer SK, Mathias SD, Patrick DL, et al: Untreated anxiety among adult primary care patients in a health maintenance organization. *Arch Gen Psychiatry* 51:740, 1994.

Ford DE, Kamerow DB: Epidemiologic study of sleep disturbances and psychiatric disorders. An opportunity for prevention? [see comments]. *JAMA* 262:1479, 1989.

Freud S: Inhibitions, symptoms, and anxiety. In: *Standard Edition of the Complete Psychological Works of Sigmund Freud.* London, UK: Hogarth Press; 1966.

Friedman S: *Cultural Issues in the Treatment of Anxiety.* New York: The Guilford Press; 1997.

Hauri P: Effects of evening activity on early night sleep. *Psychophysiology* 4:266, 1968.

Hirshfeld DR, Rosenbaum JF, Biederman J, et al: Stable behavioral inhibition and its association with anxiety disorder. *J Am Acad Child Adolesc Psychiatry* 31:103, 1992.

Kagan J, Reznick JS, Snidman N: The physiology and psychology of behavioral inhibition in children. *Child Dev* 58:1459, 1987.

Katon W, Von Korff M, Lin E, et al: Distressed high utilizers of medical care. DSM-III-R diagnoses and treatment needs. *Gen Hosp Psychiatry* 12:355, 1990.

Kinsman RA, Dirks JF, Dahlem NW, et al: Anxiety in asthma: Panic-fear symptomatology and personality in relation to manifest anxiety. *Psychol Rep* 46:196, 1980.

Kirmayer LJ, Robbins JM, Dworkind M, et al: Somatization and the recognition of depression and anxiety in primary care. *Am J Psychiatry* 150:734, 1993.

Kubitz KA, Landers DM, Petruzzello SJ, et al: The effects of acute and chronic exercise on sleep. A meta-analytic review. *Sports Med* 21:277, 1996.

Lazarus RS, Folkman S: *Stress, Appraisal, and Coping.* New York: Springer; 1984.

Lazarus RS: Coping theory and research: past, present, and future. *Psychosom Med* 55:234, 1993.

Lehrer PM: Emotionally triggered asthma: A review of research literature and some hypotheses for self-regulation therapies. *Appl Psychophysiol Biofeedback* 23:13, 1998.

Lydiard RB, Brawman-Mintzer O, Ballenger JC: Recent developments in the psychopharmacology of anxiety disorders. *J Consult Clin Psychol* 64:660, 1996.

Lydiard RB, Fossey MD, Marsh W, et al: Prevalence of psychiatric disorders in patients with irritable bowel syndrome. *Psychosomatics* 34:229, 1993.

Marcus SC, Olfson M, Pincus HA, et al: Self-reported anxiety, general medical conditions, and disability bed days. *Am J Psychiatry* 154:1766, 1997.

Meredith LS, Sherbourne CD, Jackson CA, et al: Treatment typically provided for comorbid anxiety disorders. *Arch Fam Med* 6:231, 1997.

National Institute of Mental Health: *Genetics and Mental Disorders: Report of the National Institute of Mental Health's Genetics Workgroup.* Rockville, MD: Department of Health and Human Services; 1998.

Ormel J, Oldehinkel T, Brilman E, et al: Outcome of depression and anxiety in primary care. A three-wave 3½-year study of psychopathology and disability. *Arch Gen Psychiatry* 50:759.

Petruzzello SJ, Landers DM, Hatfield BD, et al: A meta-analysis on the anxiety-reducing effects of acute and chronic exercise. Outcomes and mechanisms. *Sports Med* 11:143, 1991.

Roy-Byrne PP, Katon W: Anxiety management in the medical setting: Rationale, barriers to diagnosis and treatment, and proposed solutions. In: Mostofsky DI, Barlow DH (eds): *The Management of Stress and Anxiety in Medical Disorders.* Boston: Allyn and Bacon; 2000, pp xiv, 418.

Salman E, Liebowitz MR, Guarnaccia PJ, et al: Subtypes of ataques de nervios: The influence of coexisting psychiatric diagnosis. *Cult Med Psychiatry* 22:231, 1998.

Sartorius N, Ustun TB, Lecrubier Y, et al: Depression comorbid with anxiety: Results from the WHO study on psychological disorders in primary health care. *Br J Psychiatry Suppl* (30):38, 1996.

Shaffer D, Fisher P, Dulcan MK, et al: The NIMH Diagnostic Interview Schedule for Children Version 2.3 (DISC- 2.3): Description, acceptability, prevalence rates, and performance in the MECA Study. Methods for the Epidemiology of Child and Adolescent Mental Disorders Study. *J Am Acad Child Adolesc Psychiatry* 35:865, 1996.

Spitzer RL, Kroenke K, Linzer M, et al: Health-related quality of life in primary care patients with mental disorders. Results from the PRIME-MD 1000 Study. *JAMA* 274:1511, 1995.

Stuart MR, Lieberman JA: *The Fifteen Minute Hour.* London, UK: Praeger; 1993.

Sullivan GM, Kent JM, Coplan JD: The neurobiology of stress and anxiety. In: Mostofsky DI, Barlow DH (eds): *The Management of Stress and Anxiety in Medical Disorders.* Boston, MA: Allyn and Bacon; 2000, p 15.

Swendsen JD, Merikangas KR, Canino GJ, et al: The comorbidity of alcoholism with anxiety and depressive disorders in four geographic communities. *Compr Psychiatry* 39:176, 1998.

US Department of Health and Human Services: *Mental Health: A Report of the Surgeon General.* Rockville, MD: Department of Health and Human Services, US Public Health Service; 1999.

David A. Katerndahl

Panic Disorder

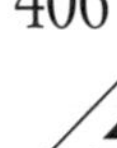

Overview

Panic disorder has been recognized as a unique entity since the publication of the third edition of the *Diagnostic and Statistical Manual of Mental Disorders* (DSM-III) in 1980. "Panic attacks" are discrete episodes of tension or fear that quickly peak in intensity and are associated with at least four autonomic symptoms during the attack (Table 18-1). Panic attacks tend to be consistent phenomena within and between patients. The DSM system offers specific criteria for the diagnosis of panic disorders, but patients with panic symptoms that fail to meet these criteria may also suffer the emotional devastation characteristic of the disorder.

Table 18-1

Criteria for Panic Attack*

A discrete period of intense fear or discomfort, in which four (or more) of the following symptoms developed abruptly and reached a peak within 10 min:
1. palpitations, pounding heart, or accelerated heart rate
2. sweating
3. trembling or shaking
4. sensations of shortness of breath or smothering
5. feeling of choking
6. chest pain or discomfort
7. nausea or abdominal distress
8. feeling dizzy, unsteady, lightheaded, or faint
9. derealization (feelings of unreality) or depersonalization (being detached from oneself)
10. fear of losing control or going crazy
11. fear of dying
12. paresthesias (numbness or tingling sensation)
13. chills or hot flushes

*A panic attack is not a codable disorder. Code the specific diagnosis in which the panic attack occurs (e.g., 300.21 Panic Disorder with Agoraphobia).

SOURCE: Reprinted with permission from the American Psychiatric Association: *Diagnostic and Statistical Manual of Mental Disorders*, 4th ed. Washington, DC: American Psychiatric Association; 1994.

Panic disorder is particularly important in primary care settings because it is common, associated with significant morbidity, and treatable. Panic disorder presents in a variety of settings in a variety of ways, and is often misdiagnosed. This chapter begins by emphasizing the importance of panic disorder as based on its prevalence, morbidity, and treatability. After describing how and where such patients present for health care, the chapter discusses its recognition and diagnostic criteria. Discussion of management addresses educational, dietary, behavioral, and pharmacologic issues. Prognosis and risk factors are reviewed, and controversies are then discussed.

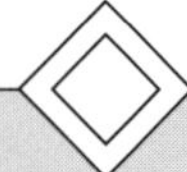

Importance of Panic Disorder

As generalists, primary care clinicians often perceive every medical condition as important. However, if we use prevalence, consequences, and treatability to identify those disorders that are critical for the primary care clinician, then knowledge of panic disorder is essential.

Panic disorder is a prevalent condition in many settings. In a community-based study, Katerndahl and Realini found the lifetime prevalence of panic disorder and subthreshold panic was 3.8 and 5.6 percent, respectively. In a primary care setting, Katon and colleagues found the incidence of current panic disorder and current subthreshold panic was 13 percent and 9 percent, respectively. The incidence of new cases of panic attacks in one private practice was 0.015 cases per patient-year (Katerndahl, unpublished data). Hence, if a practice cares for 3000 patients each year, 45 patients will suffer new onset of panic attacks.

Not only is panic disorder a prevalent condition in primary care settings, but it is associated with significant consequences. In particular, psychiatric comorbidity is common in panic disorder. Panic disorder is so closely linked to agoraphobia (Table 18-2) that the DSM-IV makes a diagnostic distinction between panic disorder with and without agoraphobia. When fear of another panic attack is attributed to a particular place or activity, some patients fear that activity and avoid it. When such avoidance becomes generalized, agoraphobia has developed. Up to 65 percent of people with panic disorder have some degree of phobic avoidance, according to Starcevic and associates.

Panic disorder is also frequently associated with depression. Not only do panic attacks develop in patients with major depressive episodes, but unresolved panic can cause patients to become depressed as well. In addition, the presence of panic in a depressed patient often leads to a poor response to either psychotherapy or pharmacotherapy for depression. Irrespective of the presence of depression, panic disorder is also associated with suicide attempts. Weissman and colleagues report that suicidal ideation and attempts occur in 19 and 8 percent, respectively, of patients with panic disorder; these rates are higher than for patients with major depression.

Other psychiatric conditions are also associated with panic disorder. Although the relationship is complex, panic disorder is often associated with substance abuse. Not only can self-medication of panic lead to substance abuse, but the direct effects of stimulants or the kindling phenomenon of withdrawal from psychoactive substances can lead to panic disorder. Both panic disorder and subthreshold panic are associated with social phobia, generalized anxiety disorder, and obsessive-compulsive disorder.

In addition to psychiatric comorbidity, panic disorder results in higher health care utilization rates owing to the panic symptoms themselves (e.g., emergency department visits for evaluation of chest pain). Finally, panic disorder leads to

Table 18-2

Criteria for Agoraphobia*

A. Anxiety about being in places or situations from which escape might be difficult (or embarrassing) or in which help may not be available in the event of having an unexpected or situationally predisposed Panic Attack or panic-like symptoms. Agoraphobic fears typically involve characteristic clusters of situations that include being outside the home alone; being in a crowd or standing in a line; being on a bridge; and traveling in a bus, train, or automobile.

Note: consider the diagnosis of Specific Phobia if the avoidance is limited to one or only a few specific situations, or Social Phobia if the avoidance is limited to social situations.

B. The situations are avoided (e.g., travel is restricted) or else are endured with marked distress or with anxiety about having a Panic Attack or panic-like symptoms, or require the presence of a companion.

C. The anxiety or phobic avoidance is not better accounted for by another mental disorder, such as Social Phobia (e.g., avoidance limited to social situations because of fear of embarrassment), Specific Phobia (e.g., avoidance limited to a single situation like elevators), Obsessive-Compulsive Disorder (e.g., avoidance of dirt in someone with an obsession about contamination), Posttraumatic Stress Disorder (e.g., avoidance of stimuli associated with a severe stressor), or Separation Anxiety Disorder (e.g., avoidance of leaving home or relatives).

*Agoraphobia is not a codable disorder. Code the specific disorder in which the agoraphobia occurs (e.g., 300.21 Panic Disorder with Agoraphobia or 300.22 Agoraphobia Without History of Panic Disorder.

SOURCE: Reprinted with permission from the American Psychiatric Association: *Diagnostic and Statistical Manual of Mental Disorders*, 4th ed. Washington, DC: American Psychiatric Association; 1994.

work-related disability and a poorer quality of life. Wittchen and Essau found that overall, panic disorder results in the worst outcomes and most psychosocial impairment of any anxiety disorder. The importance of and distinction between subthreshold panic and panic symptoms is controversial. Nonetheless, although panic symptoms and subthreshold panic are associated with psychiatric comorbidity, full panic disorder results in more disability and health care utilization.

The final characteristic of an important condition is that it must be treatable. As we will discuss, there are a variety of treatment modalities available for the management of panic disorder. With studies by Buigues and Vallejo reporting response rates of over 90 percent, panic disorder is considered by Liebowitz and colleagues to have the "most favorable prognosis of any major psychiatric condition."[1] Hence, because of its prevalence, consequences, and treatability, panic disorder is an important condition in primary care settings.

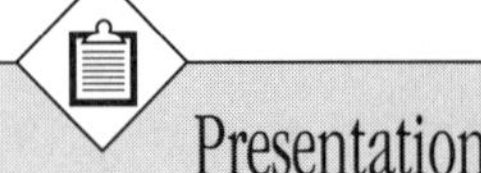

Presentation for Health Care

MARLA ALBERS *Marla Albers is a 25-year-old woman who comes into your office visibly upset. She says she suddenly had an attack of chest pain last night while she was watching television. At the time she was terrified. The pain was associated with palpitations, dyspnea, hot/cold sensations, and a feeling that something was seriously wrong. She tells you that this has never happened before. While experiencing the pain, she felt the need to escape from the room. Even though she thinks it is unrelated, she also tells you that she has had occasional crying spells over the past 2 months and recently has been under increased stress from her family.*

An understanding of how and where patients with panic disorder present for health care is essential if the condition is to be recognized and treated. About 60 percent of people with panic attacks seek medical care for their symptoms according to Realini and Katerndahl. People with panic disorder seek care earlier in its course than those with other psychiatric disorders. Although it is not uncommon for patients to seek care in multiple sites in an attempt to get relief, the most common site is the primary care clinician's office, with the emergency department almost as frequent (Table 18-3). When initially seeking care for their symptoms, 85 percent of patients with panic attacks seek care in a medical, not a mental health, setting. Katerndahl and Realini found that only 26 percent of people with panic will ever seek care in a mental health setting. Patients who seek care from primary care clinicians for their panic attacks have less severe disease and present earlier in its course than do patients seeking care from psychiatrists. This emphasizes the need for primary care and emergency clinicians to be alert to the diagnosis.

Over half of the people who seek care for their panic symptoms do so for their first panic attack. In one study by Realini and Katerndahl, 18 of the 57 patients initially presenting for care thought they were dying or having a heart attack. Ten patients thought they were going crazy. When asked why they sought care when they did, 39 of the patients reported seeking care due to the somatic symptoms or the resulting fears. Thus, it is not surprising that patients with panic attacks tend to present to primary care settings with somatic complaints. In a study by Katerndhal, 8 out of 10 patients seeking care for unexplained panic-related symptoms met criteria for panic attacks. Most of the research has centered on patients presenting with chest pain. The prevalence of panic disorder in patients presenting with chest pain to the emergency room is 16 to 47 percent, and the prevalence in patients referred for esophageal motility studies for chest pain is 34 to 49 percent. In cardiology settings, 10 to 58 percent of patients with chest pain but with normal coronary angiograms meet criteria for panic disorder, and 31 percent of patients admitted to a cardiac care unit for chest pain have panic disorder. In primary care settings, half the patients presenting with chest pain have panic attacks. In fact, the presence of chest pain

[1]Liebowitz MR, Fyer AJ, Gorman J, et al: Lactate provocation of panic attacks. *Arch Gen Psychiatry* 41:764, 1974.

Table 18-3

Sites Selected by Patients Seeking Treatment for Panic Attack

Treatment Site	Patients Presenting at Any Time (%) (N = 97)	Patients Presenting for Episode of Initial Contact (%) (N = 53*)
Medical health care settings	49	85
Emergency department	32	43
Minor emergency center	11	7
Clinic	9	7
Physicians' office		
General/family physician	35	35
General internist	3	6
Cardiologist	9	6
Otolaryngologist	3	6
Ambulance	19	15
Mental health care settings	26	35
Psychiatrist	24	22
Psychologist	10	13
Social worker	5	4
Mental health clinic	11	7
Alternative care settings	13	19
Telephone help line	10	6
Clergy	8	7
Folk healer/*curandero*	8	7
Chiropractor	6	6

Note: Subjects may have presented to more than one site so percentages may not total 100.
*Only the 57 patients who presented to at least one site were included. Four of these subjects did not respond to this question.
Source: Reprinted from Katerndahl DA, Realini JP: Where do panic attack sufferers seek care? *J Fam Pract* 40:237, 1995.

during panic attacks is a predictor of seeking care from a primary care clinician.

Other physical symptoms may also serve as the initial presentation for panic disorder. In patients referred for Holter monitoring for complaints of palpitations, the prevalence of panic disorder is 19 percent; the prevalence in those with syncope is 24 percent. Overall, the prevalences of panic disorder and subthreshold panic in primary care patients with unexplained panic-related symptoms are 42 and 16 percent, respectively. Recent research has found that panic disorder is also commonly seen in patients with asthma and irritable bowel syndrome.

Patients with panic attacks often seek care from general medical settings after only one attack, usually complaining of somatic symptoms rather than anxiety. This presentation makes recognition difficult and the consequences of nonrecognition significant.

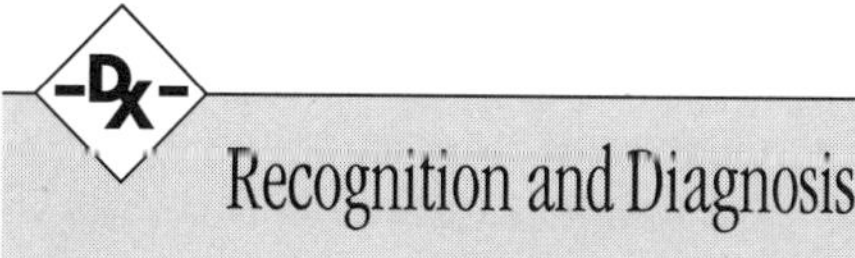

Recognition and Diagnosis

Because patients with panic disorder present with somatic symptoms, it is important for the

Table 18-4

Diagnostic Criteria for 300.01 Panic Disorder without Agoraphobia

A. Both (1) and (2):
   1. Recurrent unexpected Panic Attacks
   2. At least one of the attacks has been followed by 1 month (or more) of one (or more) of the following:
      a. Persistent concern about having additional attacks
      b. Worry about the implications of the attack or its consequences (e.g., losing control, having a heart attack, "going crazy")
      c. A significant change in behavior related to the attacks

B. Absence of Agoraphobia

C. The Panic Attacks are not due to the direct physiological effects of a substance (e.g., a drug of abuse, a medication) or a general medical condition (e.g., hyperthyroidism).

D. The Panic Attacks are not better accounted for by another mental disorder, such as Social Phobia (e.g., occurring on exposure to a specific phobic situation), Obsessive-Compulsive Disorder (e.g., on exposure to dirt in someone with an obsession about contamination), Posttraumatic Stress Disorder (e.g., in response to stimuli associated with a severe stressor) or Separation Anxiety Disorder (e.g., in response to being away from home or close relatives).

SOURCE: Reprinted with permission from the American Psychiatric Association: *Diagnostic and Statistical Manual of Mental Disorders*, 4th ed. Washington, DC: American Psychiatric Association; 1994.

clinician to recognize the disorder. Studies conducted in primary care settings suggest that although clinicians may recognize that a patient has a mental illness, they may not correctly identify the specific disorder. This lack of recognition is particularly true for panic disorder. In a community-based sample, Realini and Katerndahl found that less than one half of patients who sought care for panic symptoms were told that they had panic attacks. Studies of patients presenting with new-onset chest pain who have panic attacks were rarely recognized as such by either emergency room clinicians or primary care practitioners.

Failure to recognize the presence of panic attacks has significant consequences. Not only is lack of recognition associated with fewer mental health referrals and lower prescription rates for psychotropic medications, but patients with unrecognized panic received significantly more laboratory testing and had more ambulatory visits to medical settings than did patients who were correctly diagnosed. Patients with unrecognized panic disorder also had significantly higher costs for referrals and follow-up visits.

The diagnosis of panic disorder is based on DSM-IV criteria (Table 18-4) and requires the presence of recurrent panic attacks associated with at least 1 month of fear or other consequences. Physical examination during a panic attack may reveal sinus tachycardia and mild elevation of systolic blood pressure. The significance of panic symptoms failing to meet criteria for panic disorders or subthreshold panic is still unclear. Patients with such symptoms have more psychiatric comorbidity and receive more laboratory testing than those without panic symptoms, but whether the panic symptoms themselves are the cause of the differences is uncertain. Clinicians demonstrate more confidence in their diagnosis of panic when the duration of attacks is consistent, and when symptom abatement patterns are consistent.

Screening Instruments

Two mental illness screening instruments have been developed for primary care settings: Primary Care Evaluation of Mental Disorders (PRIME-MD) and Symptom Driven Diagnostic System (SDDS).

Both instruments include a screen for the presence of panic disorder. Based on the sensitivities and specificities reported by the instruments' developers, positive likelihood ratios (LRs) for the PRIME-MD and the SDDS are 57 and 3.16 to 3.96, respectively. The negative LRs for the PRIME-MD and the SDDS are 0.43 and 0.27 to 0.70, respectively. Because LRs greater than 5.0 and less than 0.2 are needed to produce moderate changes in posttest probability, there is controversy over the value of these screening tools.

Ancillary Tests

Panic symptoms can be associated with a variety of medical conditions (Table 18-5). A thorough history and physical examination is important to rule out these disorders as the cause of the panic symptoms. Assessment of thyroid function has been recommended, but routine testing during research studies rarely uncovers previously unsuspected hyperthyroidism. Similarly, echocardiography and exercise treadmills have been advocated in the work up of patients with panic attacks, but research has failed to show any benefit to either test. There may be some rationale to the use of drug screening in young adults presenting with panic symptoms to exclude the use of recreational drugs that can cause panic symptoms, such as marijuana, cocaine, and other stimulants. Routine, extensive laboratory testing should be discouraged in patients with panic disorder because it may reinforce the patients' belief in an "organic" cause for their symptoms.

Mavissakalian and associates found a 15 percent prevalence of mitral valve prolapse among a sample of 46 female patients with agoraphobia. The authors of the study conclude that although panic disorder is associated with mitral valve prolapse, the presence of this condition does not alter either the clinical course of or treatment response to panic attacks.

Other Screening Methods

Once the diagnosis of panic disorder is made, the patient should be screened for secondary consequences such as depression, substance abuse, agoraphobia, and suicidal ideation. In addition to treating the panic attacks, management must target comorbid conditions as well, if they are present.

If an associated disorder (see Table 18-5) is found, therapy should be directed at this disorder

Table 18-5

Conditions Associated with Panic Symptoms

Psychiatric disorders
Major depression
Agoraphobia
Specific phobia
Social phobia
Generalized anxiety disorder
Obsessive-compulsive disorder
Substance abuse
Posttraumatic stress disorder
Cardiovascular disorders
Mitral valve prolapse
Paroxysmal supraventricular tachycardia
Endocrine disorders
Hyperthyroidism
Hypoglycemia
Menopause
Pheochromocytoma
Carcinoid syndrome
Neurologic disorders
Temporal lobe epilepsy
Cerebral tumor
Parkinson's disease
Sleep disorders
Narcolepsy
Sleep apnea
Drug-related disorders
Antidepressant withdrawal
Sedative-tranquilizer withdrawal
Stimulant (cocaine, cannabis, PCP) use
Metronidazole use
L-Dopa use
Neuroleptic use
Organic solvent exposure
Miscellaneous
Wilson's disease
Acute intermittent porphyria
Hyperventilation syndrome

SOURCE: Reprinted with permission from Katerndahl DA: Panic attacks and panic disorder. *J Fam Pract* 43:275, 1996.

first. Only after associated disorders have been ruled out or taken into account can therapy directed at panic disorder be properly implemented. Although the prognosis for treated panic disorder is good, the presence of comorbid psychiatric disorders (e.g., depression, agoraphobia) often decreases treatment response.

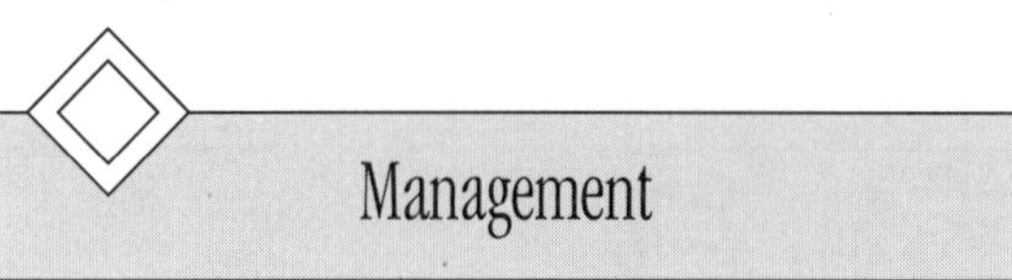

Management

Management of panic disorder is complex, and may include patient education, life style changes, family issues, psychotherapy, drug therapy, and possibly referral to mental health settings.

Patient Education

Patient education is particularly important when dealing with patients who have panic disorder. Because of the striking physical symptomatology associated with panic attacks, these patients and their clinicians are often initially convinced that there is a physical cause for the symptoms. Consequently they may seek care from numerous clinicians in search of a physical explanation. Initially, they may be resistant to accepting a psychiatric explanation. If patients do accept the diagnosis (and primary care clinicians report that they usually do), they may fail to comply because they feel "crazy," as if it is "all in their head" and that they should be able to "snap out of it." These perceptions can lead to "doctor shopping" and interfere with adherence to the treatment plan. Patient education can address these perceptions, facilitating appropriate management.

Labeling symptoms as "panic disorder" may reassure the patient that their symptoms are not imagined, that they are not "crazy," and that there is reason to hope. An explanation of the role of neurotransmitters in psychiatric disease may let patients know that the diagnosis of panic disorder has a physical dimension as much as diabetes, and that "snapping out of it" is simply not possible. Finally, patient education should include a discussion of the treatability of panic disorder to provide the patient with hope and maximize compliance. The National Institute of Mental Health has a hotline to assist people with panic disorder (1-800-64-PANIC).

MARLA ALBERS (CONTINUED) *After conducting a careful initial evaluation, which included particular attention to the heart, you tell Marla that she had a panic attack. You reassure her that her heart is healthy and that, although her symptoms were terrifying, she is not in imminent danger of dying. She asks many questions about the meaning and significance of this attack and the relationship to her stress and crying spells, but seems to be reassured by the answers you provide. You advise her to reduce her caffeine intake, begin exercising daily, and report back if the symptoms recur.*

Life Style Issues

Dietary changes may be helpful in patients with panic disorder. Stimulants, including caffeine, nicotine, tobacco, chocolate, and tyramine (e.g., cheese, red wines, avocado, nuts) should be avoided. Patients frequently reduce their caffeine intake prior to seeking care because they have noticed that it exacerbates their panic symptoms. Cannabis (marijuana) has been linked to panic attacks, as well.

Inositol (a sugar involved in neurotransmitter metabolism) may reduce panic symptoms. Normally found in poultry, fish, and dairy products, dietary inositol in doses of 12 grams per day reduces the severity and frequency of panic attacks and phobias, according to Benjamin and colleagues. Although inositol probably cannot be used as monotherapy, it may be a helpful adjunct.

Some patients are sensitive to environmental conditions such as fluorescent lighting, sleep deprivation, and emotional conflict according to Roy-Byrne and Uhde. If so, these factors should be minimized. Regular aerobic exercise may also be beneficial. Not only can it lower general levels of stress and improve coping, but Broocks and colleagues found that exercise reduces panic frequency over controls. Exercise is usually well tolerated by patients with panic disorder. However, patients with panic disorder occasionally report that exercise triggers panic attacks, presumably due to symptomatic cues produced by the exertion. In this case, such exercise should be curtailed until other measures have suppressed the panic attacks. Although life style changes can reduce panic symptoms, these changes rarely eliminate the attacks completely. Therefore, these measures cannot be used alone in the management of panic disorder.

Family Issues

Because both panic disorder and agoraphobia are familial disorders, the clinician is in the position to recognize new cases early in their course. Factors within the family have been linked to panic disorder, and domestic violence may be a key issue for patients. Not only is panic disorder more common in adults that were victims of sexual abuse as children, but adults with panic attacks report more household violence within the previous year. In addition, avoidance behavior in parents with panic disorder is associated with behavioral problems in their children, according to Silverman and colleagues. Families of people with panic symptoms often exhibit high levels of dysfunction and stress with low levels of support. Katerndahl and Realini found that in some instances this family dysfunction may be related to comorbid substance abuse in the person with panic.

The family can also be a strong source of support for people experiencing panic attacks. Both panic disorder and agoraphobia are stressful for the marital relationship; yet families frequently adapt to patients' fears. Family members may be particularly helpful in improving treatment adherence, such as assisting the agoraphobic patient to perform "homework" assignments as part of their systematic desensitization therapy. It is important to realize, however, that successful therapy will produce change in the family situation and dynamics, which may itself result in a new source of family stress.

Psychotherapy

Although individual psychoanalysis and insight therapy are not helpful in panic disorder, other forms of psychotherapy are effective. Relaxation therapy can sometimes help patients to use relaxation techniques to abort or decrease the impact of panic episodes. Respiratory training can assist patients in slowing their respiratory rates during attacks, assisting in relaxation and decreasing hyperventilation. Exposure therapy, in which patients are encouraged to expose themselves to phobic situations for progressively longer periods of time, is advocated for all patients with panic disorder and can be instituted during a patient's initial visit, even if that occurs in the emergency room. Patients with agoraphobia should begin this systematic desensitization as soon as their panic attacks are under control. Swinson and associates report that desensitization can be initiated via telephone if necessary. These patients will need exposure therapy if the phobic symptoms of agoraphobia are to resolve.

Cognitive behavioral therapy (CBT) is as effective as pharmacotherapy and may have a lower relapse rate. Barlow and Lehman found that overall, about 80 percent of patients become panic free with CBT. During individual or group CBT sessions, patients train themselves to reexperience their worst panic attack, but without the sense of impending doom, to eliminate the catastrophic cognitions that accompany attacks. In addition, particular symptoms that seem to herald an impending panic attack are recreated in the office setting. For example, dizziness may be recreated by turning patients around on a swivel stool; dyspnea may be recreated by having patients use a stair stepper. Once experienced in a "safe" setting, patients can learn the difference between a panic attack and symptoms caused by normal physiologic mechanisms. The patients can thus learn that it is possible to experience symptoms without developing a panic attack.

Primary care clinicians who feel confident in their counseling skills can provide counseling to their patients with panic disorder. In addition, family and community support groups can be helpful, particularly to patients with co-existent phobias.

Drug Therapy

Although no medication will abort a panic attack once it has begun, a variety of medications will reduce the frequency of attacks (Table 18-6).

Table 18-6

Drugs Used for Treating Panic Disorder

Drug	Dosage Range (mg/day)
Tricyclic antidepressants	
Imipramine (Tofranil)	50–300
Clomipramine (Anafranil)	25–250
Nortriptyline (Pamelor)	25–100
Desipramine (Norpramin)	25–300
SSRIs	
Fluoxetine (Prozac)	20–80
Paroxetine (Paxil)	10–50
Sertraline (Zoloft)	50–200
Fluvoxamine (Luvox)	50–300
MAOIs	
Phenelzine (Nardil)	45–90
Tanylcypromine (Parnate)	30–60
Benzodiazepines	
Alprazolam (Xanax)	2–10
Lorazepam (Ativan)	2–6
Clonazepam (Klonopin)	1–3

Abbreviations: MAOIs, monoamine oxidase inhibitors; SSRIs, selective serotonin reuptake inhibitors.

Source: Reprinted with permission from Saeed SA, Bruce TJ: Panic disorder: Effective treatment options. *Am Fam Physician* 57:2405, 1998.

Selective Serotonin Reuptake Inhibitors

The selective serotonin reuptake inhibitors (SSRIs) are effective in panic disorder. Although all of the SSRIs that have been tested appear to be effective, only paroxetine and sertraline have Food and Drug Administration (FDA) approval for the treatment of panic disorder. Venlafaxine may be effective, but has not been adequately studied to date. Treatment response can be expected after 3 to 6 weeks of therapy. Many patients experience an initial excitatory period when placed on an SSRI, resulting in agitation, insomnia, and many of the symptoms of a panic attack. Because this reaction is especially common in patients with panic disorder, SSRIs should be started at a low dose and increased gradually. Headaches, sexual dysfunction in men, and gastrointestinal symptoms are the most common side effects.

Tricyclic Antidepressants

Although none of the tricyclic antidepressants (TCAs) have FDA approval for use in panic disorder, TCAs are effective in 90 percent of patients. Imipramine is the most studied of the TCAs, but desipramine and clomipramine are also effective in panic disorder. As with the SSRIs, the initial dose should be low to minimize transient excitation, and at least 3 weeks of therapy are required to see a response. Mavissakalian and Perel report that imipramine shows a plasma level-response relationship up to plasma levels of 140 ng/mL. Cardiotoxicity and anticholinergic side effects are the primary concerns with the use of TCAs.

Benzodiazepines

Although neuroleptic agents are contraindicated in panic disorder, high-potency benzodiazepines (BDZs) are as effective as TCAs and produce a more rapid response. Although the psychiatry literature recommends high doses, experience in primary care settings suggests that lower doses may be effective. Carter and colleagues found that the new sustained-release alprazolam derivative, adinazolam-SR, may also be effective with once per day dosing. Low-potency BDZs such as diazepam may be effective, but require excessive doses. Alprazolam and clonazepam are the only BDZs with FDA approval for use in panic disorder.

Sedation, physical dependence, and cognitive impairment are the major side effects of BDZs. Clonazepam may have less sedation and fewer withdrawal symptoms. Alprazolam-related memory impairment may continue even after the medication is discontinued. Although abuse of BDZs is a concern, abuse of alprazolam has been limited to patients with a prior history of substance abuse.

Monoamine Oxidase Inhibitors

Monoamine oxidase inhibitors (MAOIs) may be more effective in panic disorder than TCAs. However, the possibility of a hypertensive crisis in reaction to ingesting tyramine-containing foods is a major concern, limiting the use of MAOIs to second-line agents. The new reversible monoamine oxidase-A inhibitors may represent a safer alternative.

Other Drugs

Although clonidine and verapamil have some antipanic activity, they do not completely suppress attacks and require doses that produce significant side effects. Sodium valproate may be effective in panic disorder, but beta blockers, buspirone, and carbamazepine are not effective. These agents are only helpful in dealing with comorbid social phobia and generalized anxiety disorder. Preliminary work by Berigan and associates suggests that nefazodone may be effective in panic disorder.

Combination Treatment

Combination therapies have also been attempted. Combining a BDZ with an antidepressant has been advocated to produce rapid reduction in attacks, after which the BDZ can be withdrawn. The effectiveness of this regimen has not been shown, and empirical data suggest that patients are reticent to discontinue the BDZ once they have responded. Marks and colleagues found that combining alprazolam and exposure therapy produces benefit over either alone. However, Barlow and Lehman report that combining short-course alprazolam and cognitive therapy sequentially may be beneficial. Exposure therapy and either imipramine or fluvoxamine are synergistic in reducing phobias.

Because a variety of treatment options exist, the approach to a particular patient with panic disorder should be individualized based on the patient's age, comorbid conditions, and concurrent medications. Because patients with panic disorder often undermedicate themselves, patient input into the therapeutic plan should be sought as a means of maximizing cooperation.

Elderly patients often do not tolerate tranquilizers or the anticholinergic and cardiotoxic side effects of TCAs. Consequently, BDZs and TCAs should be avoided in the elderly. Patients with comorbid depression should probably receive an SSRI or TCA. However, patients with a history of substance abuse should not be started on a BDZ. Cognitive therapy may be the best approach for pregnant women and for patients who do not tolerate medications. In addition, other patient symptoms and common drug side effects need to be considered when choosing a particular agent.

Cox and associates' comparison among treatments reveals that psychological treatments produce the most consistent effects followed by combination drug therapies. Although exposure therapy was most efficacious for phobic symptoms, pharmacotherapy was most beneficial for panic symptoms. Differences between antidepressants and BDZs were inconsistent.

The use of a panic diary recording the frequency of panic attacks and levels of fear may be helpful in management. The goal of therapy in panic disorder is for the patient to be panic free. Once this is achieved, therapy should be continued for 6 to 12 months. Medications should be tapered due to the possibility of withdrawal symptoms. Relapse after pharmacotherapy is common and may be severe enough to warrant reinstitution of medication. Three-year follow up data suggest that most patients continue to do well after short-term alprazolam, imipramine, or group therapy.

Referral to Mental Health Settings

Although mental health professionals may feel that all patients with panic disorder should be referred for specialized care, this is controversial. Mental health managed care "carve outs" may dictate referral, but primary care clinicians are in the optimal position to recognize panic disorder and are capable of managing it if they choose. Primary care clinicians tend to refer these patients when they lack confidence and when the local mental health system is adequate to ensure the patient's care.

Referral should be considered in the presence of comorbid substance abuse or suicidal ideation. In addition, referral is appropriate when the patient fails to respond or when the clinician is unfamiliar with an indicated therapy. Finally, patients with full-blown agoraphobia or with a history of childhood sexual abuse will need more intensive counseling than a primary care clinician can usually provide. The role of psychiatric liaison services within primary care settings is an attractive option that is still controversial.

MARLA ALBERS (CONTINUED) *Despite following your recommendations, Marla experiences three more attacks in the next week. She calls your office Monday morning asking that something be done to stop these terrible attacks. You prescribe paroxitine and refer her to a psychologist for CBT.*

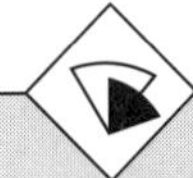

Prediction and Prevention

Panic disorder and agoraphobia, left untreated, can produce a lifetime of disability. Not only are the panic attacks and phobias emotionally traumatic as they occur, but they cause alteration in the patient's life style, which can produce long-term disability. Factors have been identified that may predict the onset and consequences of panic disorder. Although this knowledge may not lead to prevention of panic disorder, it may allow us to diagnose and intervene at an earlier stage, reducing the ultimate morbidity.

Panic disorder usually begins during early adulthood, but it has been reported to begin in children as young as 5 and in elders. The notion of a group of patients with "late-onset panic" is controversial. These patients report the onset of panic attacks after age 50 and appear to have milder disease than those with an earlier onset, according to Raj and associates.

Classically, panic attacks begin during times of stress and hormonal change, or as a result of stimulant use or depressant withdrawal. The effect of pregnancy on panic disorder is variable. Although panic attacks may begin during pregnancy or immediately postpartum, some women with panic report improvement during pregnancy.

Factors during childhood can predict which children are at risk for the eventual development of panic disorder. In addition to a family history of panic disorder suggesting a genetic link, behavioral aspects in children may assist in identifying at-risk children. Children demonstrating behavioral inhibition (reluctance to engage in unfamiliar activities) and extreme separation anxiety are more prone to develop panic disorder as adults. Finally, as mentioned, children that have been victims of sexual abuse are also at risk for panic disorder.

Other more controversial risk factors may be important. Hoffman and associates report that people with a particular personality—phobic anxious temperament—may be at risk for panic disorder. However, abnormal scores on personality scales tend to improve as the panic disorder responds to either CBT or imipramine, according to Lelliott and colleagues.

Patients with panic attacks differ from age-related controls in illness beliefs, behaviors, and coping. Patients with panic disorder generally exhibit less healthy illness attitudes and behaviors as well as being more interpersonally sensitive. In addition, they more frequently use negative coping mechanisms to deal with stress. However, whether these differences represent personality characteristics or are due to childhood trauma is unclear. Although it has been suggested that panic symptoms may precede the development of panic disorder, there is little evidence to support this.

Knowledge of these risk factors can be useful clinically. With the help of an ongoing doctor–patient relationship, knowledge about childhood and family history as well as assessment of beliefs and coping skills can identify patients at risk for development of panic disorder. If these patients are advised to avoid stimulants and depressants, perhaps panic disorder can be prevented. Similarly, if clinicians increase their sensitivity to the possibility of panic disorder when these patients are undergoing stress or hormonal changes (e.g., pregnancy), perhaps the development of panic disorder can be diagnosed at an earlier stage.

Most experts believe that uncontrolled panic attacks can lead to agoraphobia, although this is not universally accepted, because the lag time between the onset of panic and the onset of agoraphobia is short. Although a variety of predictors for the development of agoraphobia have been identified, the most important may be the spontaneity of the panic attack and the patient's cognitive assessment. This suggests that if the clinician can see the patient and recognize the panic attack early, the patient's cognitive assessment can be dealt with and perhaps the development of agoraphobia can be averted.

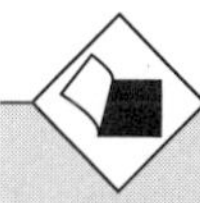

Summary

Panic attacks and panic disorder are common and commonly crippling conditions in primary care. By knowing the risk factors, common presenting symptoms, and diagnostic criteria, the clinician can identify most patients affected and institute treatment. In most cases, panic can be managed in the primary care setting.

Suggested Reading

American Psychiatric Association: Practice guidelines for the treatment of patients with panic disorder. *Am J Psychiatry* 155(Suppl):1, 1998.

A psychiatry-derived set of guidelines focusing on treatment alternatives, factors influencing treatment, and individualizing therapy.

Katerndahl D, Dresser JG (eds): *Advances in the Recognition and Treatment of Panic Disorder.* Springfield, NJ: Scientific Therapeutics Information, Inc.; 1997.

Oriented toward primary care providers, pharmacists, and nurses, this monograph provides a more in-depth look at the epidemiology, presentations, and pathophysiology of panic disorder in addition to a discussion of treatment.

Rosenbaum JF, Pollack MH (eds): *Panic Disorder and Its Treatment.* New York: Marcel Dekker; 1998.

Written by psychologists and psychiatrists for clinicians in general medical settings, this volume provides an overview of panic disorder, including a discussion of the role of managed care in the management of patients with panic disorder.

Roy-Byrne P, Stein M, Bystrisky A, et al: Pharmacotherapy of panic disorder: Proposed guidelines for the family physician. *J Am Board Fam Pract* 11:282, 1998.

Guidelines for pharmacotherapy and monitoring progress developed for primary care clinicians written by four psychiatrists and reviewed by two clinicians.

Saeed SA, Bruce TI: Panic disorder: Effective treatment options. *Am Fam Physician* 57:2405, 1998.

Written by a psychiatrist and a psychologist, a thorough overview of treatment options including patient education handout.

Bibliography

American Psychiatric Association: *Diagnostic and Statistical Manual of Mental Disorders,* 3rd ed. Washington, DC: American Psychiatric Association; 1980.

American Psychiatric Association: *Diagnostic and Statistical Manual of Mental Disorders,* 4th ed. Washington, DC: American Psychiatric Association; 1994.

Andersen SM, Harthorn BH: Recognition, diagnosis and treatment of mental disorders by primary care physicians. *Med Care* 27:869, 1989.

Bakish D, Saxena BM, Bowen R, et al: Reversible monoamine oxidase-A inhibitors in panic disorder. *Clin Neuropharmacol* 16(suppl 2):S77, 1993.

Bakker A, van Balkom A, Spinhoven P: Follow-up on the treatment of panic disorder with or without agoraphobia. A quantitative review. *J Nerv Ment Dis* 186:414, 1998.

Barlow DH, Lehman CL: Advances in the psychosocial treatment of anxiety disorders. *Arch Gen Psychiatry* 53:727, 1996.

Barsky AJ, Cleary PD, Coeytaux BA, et al: Psychiatric disorders in medical outpatients complaining of palpitations. *J Gen Intern Med* 9:306, 1994.

Barsky AJ, Cleary PD, Sarnie MK, et al: Panic disorder, palpitations and the awareness of cardiac activity. *J Nerv Ment Dis* 182:63, 1994.

Beitman BD, Mukerji V, Lamberti JW, et al: Panic disorder in patients with chest pain and angiographically normal coronary arteries. *Am J Cardiol* 63:1399, 1989.

Benjamin J, Levine J, Fux M, et al: Double-blind, placebo-controlled, crossover trial of inositol treatment for panic disorder. *Am J Psychiatry* 152:1084, 1995.

Berigan TR, Casas A, Harazin J: Nefazadone and the treatment of panic. *J Clin Psychiatry* 59:256, 1998.

Borus JF, Howes MJ, Devins NP, et al: Primary health care providers' recognition and diagnosis of mental disorders in their patients. *Gen Hosp Psychiatry* 10:317, 1988.

Boulenger JP, Uhde TW, Wolff EA, et al: Increased sensitivity to caffeine in patients with panic disorder. *Arch Gen Psychiatry* 41:1067, 1984.

Breier A, Charney DS, Heninger GR: Agoraphobia with panic attacks. Development, diagnostic stability, and course of illness. *Arch Gen Psychiatry* 43:1029, 1986.

Broadhead WE, Leon AC, Weissman MM, et al: Development and validation of the SDDS-PC screen for multiple mental disorders in primary care. *Arch Fam Med* 4:211, 1995.

Broocks A, Bandelow B, Pekrun G, et al: Comparison of aerobic exercise, clomipramine, and placebo in the treatment of panic disorder. *Am J Psychiatry* 155:603, 1998.

Brown C, Schulberg HC, Madonia MJ, et al: Treatment outcomes for primary care patients with major depression and lifetime anxiety disorders. *Am J Psychiatry* 153:1293, 1996.

Buigues J, Vallejo J: Therapeutic response to phenelzine in patients with panic disorder and agoraphobia with panic attacks. *J Clin Psychiatry* 48:55, 1987.

Carter CS, Fawcett J, Hertzman M, et al: Adinazolam-SR in panic disorder with agoraphobia. *J Clin Psychiatry* 56:202, 1995.

Carter C, Maddock R, Amsterdam E, et al: Panic disorder and chest pain in the coronary care unit. *Psychosomatics* 33:302, 1992.

Chignon JM, Lepine JP, Ades J: Panic disorder in cardiac outpatients. *Am J Psychiatry* 150:780, 1993.

Clum GA, Clum GA, Surls R: Meta-analysis of treatments for panic disorder. *J Consult Clin Psychol* 61:317, 1993.

Cox BJ, Endler NS, Lee PS, et al: Meta-analysis of treatments for panic disorder with agoraphobia. *J Behav Ther Exp Psychiatry* 23:175, 1992.

Curran HV, Bond A, O'Sullivan G, et al: Memory functions, alprazolam and exposure therapy. *Psychol Med* 24:969, 1994.

DeBuers E, van Balkom AJLM, Large A, et al: Treatment of panic disorder with agoraphobia. *Am J Psychiatry* 152:683, 1995.

Dumas C, Katerndahl DA, Burge SK: Familial patterns in patients with infrequent panic. *Arch Fam Med* 4: 863, 1995.

Edlund MJ, Swann AC: Economic and social costs of panic disorder. *Hosp Community Psychiatry* 38: 1277, 1987.

Fava GA, Grandi S, Canestran R: Prodromal symptoms in panic disorder with agoraphobia. *Am J Psychiatry* 145:1564, 1988.

George DT, Nutt DJ, Dwyer BA, et al: Alcoholism and panic disorder: Is the comorbidity more than coincidence? *Acta Psychiatr Scand* 81:97, 1990.

Geracioti TD Jr, Post RM: Onset of panic disorder associated with rare use of cocaine. *Biol Psychiatry* 29: 403, 1991.

Hendryx MS, Doebbeling BN, Kearns DL: Mental health treatment in primary care: Physician treatment choices and psychiatric admission rates. *Fam Pract Res J* 14:127, 1994.

Hoffman SG, Shear MK, Barlow DH, et al: Effects of panic disorder treatments on personality disorder characteristics. *Depress Anxiety* 8:14, 1998.

Jaeschke R, Guyatt GH, Sackett DL: Users guides to the medical literature: III. How to use an article about a diagnostic test: B. What are the results and will they help me in caring for my patients? *JAMA* 271(90): 703, 1994.

Jensen CF, Cowley DS, Walker RD: Drug preferences of alcoholic polydrug abusers with and without panic. *J Clin Psychiatry* 51:189, 1990.

Kane FJ Jr, Strohlein J, Harper RG: Noncardiac chest pain in patients with heart disease. *South Med J* 84: 847, 1991.

Katerndahl DA: Panic is panic. *Fam Pract Res J* 9:147, 1990.

Katerndahl DA: Relationship between panic attacks and health locus of control. *J Fam Pract* 32:391, 1991.

Katerndahl DA: Intrapatient agreement in phenomenology of panic attacks. *Psychol Rep* 79:219, 1996.

Katerndahl DA, Realini JP: Lifetime prevalence of panic states. *Am J Psychiatry* 150:246, 1993.

Katerndahl DA, Realini JP: Where do panic attack sufferers seek care? *J Fam Pract* 40:237, 1995.

Katerndahl DA, Realini JP: Comorbid psychiatric disorders in subjects with panic attacks. *J Nerv Ment Disord* 185:669, 1997.

Katerndahl DA, Realini JP: Family characteristics of subjects with panic attacks. *Fam Med* 29:563, 1997.

Katerndahl DA, Realini JP: Use of health care services by persons with panic symptoms. *Psychiatr Serv* 48:1027, 1997.

Katerndahl DA, Realini JP: Patients with panic attacks seeking care from family physicians compared with those seeking care from psychiatrists. *J Nerv Ment Dis* 186:249, 1998.

Katerndahl DA, Realini JP: Associations with subsyndromal panic and the validity of DSM-IV criteria. *Depress Anxiety* 8:33, 1998.

Katerndahl DA, Trammell C: Prevalence and recognition of panic states in Starnet patients presenting with chest pain. *J Fam Pract* 45:54, 1997.

Katon W, Hall ML, Russo J, et al: Chest pain: Relationship of psychiatric illness to coronary arteriographic results. *Am J Med* 84:1, 1988.

Katon W, Vitaliano PP, Russo J, et al: Panic disorder: Epidemiology in primary care. *J Fam Pract* 23:233. 1986.

Kessler RC, Olfson M, Berglund PA: Patterns and predictors of treatment contact after first onset of psychiatric disorders. *Am J Psychiatry* 155:62, 1998.

Klein DF: Anxiety reconceptualized. In: Klein DF, Rabkin JG (eds): *Anxiety*. New York: Raven; 1981.

Lelliott P, Marks I, McNamee G, et al: Onset of panic disorder with agoraphobia. *Arch Gen Psychiatry* 46:1000, 1989.

Lepola UM, Rimon RH, Riekkinen PJ: Three-year follow-up of patients with panic disorder after short-term treatment with alprazolam and imipramine. *Int Clin Psychopharmacol* 8:115, 1993.

Liebowitz MR, Fyer AJ, Gorman J, et al: Lactate provocation of panic attacks. *Arch Gen Psychiatry* 41:764, 1974.

Linzer M, Felder A, Hackel A, et al: Psychiatric syncope. *Psychosomatics* 31:181, 1990.

Lydiard RB, Fossey M, Marsh W, et al: Prevalence of psychiatric disorders in irritable bowel syndrome. *Psychosomatics* 34:229, 1993.

Manicavasagar V, Silore D, Hadzi-Pavlovic: Subpopulations of early separation anxiety. *J Affect Disord* 48: 181, 1998.

Margraf J, Taylor CB, Ehlers A, et al: Panic attacks in the natural environment. *J Nerv Ment Disord* 175;558, 1987.

Markowitz JS, Weissman MM, Ouellette R, et al: Quality of life in panic disorder. *Arch Gen Psychiatry* 46:984, 1989.

Marks IM, Swinson RP, Basoglu M, et al: Alprazolam and exposure alone and combined in panic disorder with agoraphobia. *Br J Psychiatry* 162:776, 1993.

Mateos JLA, Perez CB, Carrasco JSD, et al: Atypical chest pain and panic disorder. *Psychother Psychosom* 52:92, 1989.

Mavissakalian M: Combined behavioral therapy and pharmacotherapy of agoraphobia. *J Psych Res* 27 (Suppl 1):179, 1993.

Mavissakalian M, Salerni R, Thompson ME, et al: Mitral valve prolapse and agoraphobia. *Am J Psychiatry* 40:1612, 1983.

Mavissakalian MR, Perel JM: Imipramine treatment of panic disorder with agoraphobia. *Am J Psychiatry* 152:673, 1995.

McNally RJ: Psychological approaches to panic disorder. *Psychol Bull* 108:403, 1990.

Nagy LM, Krystal JH, Charney DS, et al: Long-term outcome of panic disorder after short-term imipramine and behavioral group treatment. *J Clin Psychopharmacol* 13:16, 1993.

Perna G, Bertani A, Politi E, et al: Asthma and panic attacks. *Biol Psychiatry* 42:625, 1997.

Perugi G, Toni C, Benedetti A, et al: Delineating a putative phobic-anxious temperament in 126 panic-agoraphobic patients. *J Affect Disord* 47:11, 1998.

Raj BA, Corvea MH, Dagon EM: Clinical characteristics of panic disorder in the elderly. *J Clin Psychiatry* 54:150, 1993.

Realini JP, Katerndahl DA: Factors affecting threshold for seeking care: The Panic Attack Care-Seeking

Threshold (PACT) Study. *J Am Board Fam Pract* 6:215, 1993.

Reznick JS, Hegeman IM, Kaufman E, et al: Retrospective and concurrent self-report of behavioral inhibition and their relation to adult mental health. *Dev Psychopathol* 4:301, 1992.

Ross CA, Walker JR, Norton GR, et al: Management of anxiety and panic attacks in immediate care facilities. *Gen Hosp Psychiatry* 10:129, 1988.

Roy-Byrne P, Uhde TW: Exogenous factors in panic disorder. *J Clin Psychiatry* 49:56, 1988.

Salvador-Carulla L, Segui J, Fernandez-Cano P, et al: Costs and offset effect in panic disorders. *Br J Psychiatry* 166(Suppl 27):23, 1995.

Schweitzer E, Rickels K: New and emerging clinical uses for buspirone. *J Clin Psychiatry* 12:46, 1994.

Sheehan DV, Raj BA, Trehan RR, et al: Serotonin in panic disorder and social phobia. *Int Clin Psychopharmacol* 8(Suppl 2):63, 1993.

Sholomskas DE, Wickramaratne PJ, Dogolo L, et al: Postpartum onset of panic disorder. *J Clin Psychiatry* 54: 476, 1993.

Silverman WK, Cerny JA, Nelles WB, et al: Behavior problems in children of parents with anxiety disorders. *J Am Acad Child Adolesc Psychiatry* 27:779, 1988.

Spitzer RL, Williams JBW, Kroenke K, et al: Utility of a new procedure for diagnosing mental disorders in primary care. *JAMA* 272:1749, 1994.

Starcevic V, Uhlenhuth EH, Kellner R, et al: Comorbidity in panic disorder. *Psychiatry Res* 46:285, 1993.

Stein JM, Papp LA, Klein DF, et al: Exercise tolerance in panic disorder patients. *Biol Psychiatry* 32:281, 1992.

Swinson RP, Fergus KD, Cox BJ, et al: Efficacy of telephone-administered behavioral therapy for panic disorder with agoraphobia. *Behav Res Ther* 33:465, 1995.

Telch MJ, Lucas JA, Schmidt NB, et al: Group cognitive-behavioral treatment of panic disorder. *Behav Res Ther* 31:279, 1993.

Van Balkom AJLM, Bakker A, Spinhoven P, et al: Meta-analysis of the treatment of panic disorder with or without agoraphobia. *J Nerv Ment Dis* 185:510, 1997.

Villeponteaux VA, Lydiard RB, Laraia MT, et al: Effects of pregnancy on pre-existing panic disorder. *J Clin Psychiatry* 53:201, 1992.

Walker EA, Katon WJ, Hansom J, et al: Medical and psychiatric symptoms in women with childhood sexual abuse. *Psychosom Med* 54:658, 1992.

Weissman MM, Klerman GL, Markowitz JS, et al: Suicidal ideation and suicide attempts in panic disorder and attacks. *N Engl J Med* 321:1209, 1989.

Williams SL, Falbo J: Cognitive and performance-based treatments for panic attacks in people with varying degrees of agoraphobic disability. *Behav Res Ther* 34:253, 1996.

Wittchen HU, Essau CA: Epidemiology of panic disorder. *J Psychiatry Res* 27(Suppl 1):47, 1993.

Wulsin LR, Hillard JR, Geier P, et al: Screening emergency room patients with atypical chest pain for depression and panic disorder. *Int J Psychiatric Med* 18:315, 1988.

L. Miriam Dickinson
W. Perry Dickinson

Post-Traumatic Stress Syndromes in Primary Care Patients

Introduction

Traumatic experiences are commonplace in modern society. Individuals who experience physical or psychological trauma can suffer both short- and long-term effects on their health. Many develop a characteristic set of post-traumatic symptoms that can endure for years after the original trauma. People with post-traumatic stress may have comorbid psychiatric diagnoses, substance abuse, undetected physical injuries, changes in health behavior, unexplained physical symptoms, adverse effects on immune system functioning, and stress-related health problems. The wide range of symptoms and high levels of comorbidity can obscure the presence of underlying trauma and its consequences, making it difficult for clinicians to accurately diagnose and effectively manage these problems.

The existing studies of post-traumatic stress disorder (PTSD) have been carried out in specialty practices in military populations, the general community, and post-disaster situations. Thus, we do not yet know the prevalence of post-traumatic stress among patients in the primary care medical setting. However, the evidence is sufficient for some experts to believe that there is an epidemic of PTSD that primary care physicians are not detecting in their patients.

SUSAN MILLER *Susan, a 32-year-old divorced mother of two young children, comes to your office for persistent severe headaches. She has a history of urinary infections and had a hysterectomy 2 years ago. Other symptoms include abdominal pain, insomnia, nausea, and fatigue. Susan's headaches began after a serious head injury in a car accident at age 16. You question her further and discover that she had post-traumatic stress symptoms for about 2 years following the accident, including recurrent intrusive thoughts and nightmares about the accident, avoiding riding in cars, feeling numb most of the time, insomnia, and generalized anxiety. Although most of these symptoms abated over time, her headaches have continued. Further psychosocial history was remarkable for domestic violence in her second marriage, which caused a flare of her previous PTSD symptoms until after her divorce 6 months ago. She still is having insomnia and some generalized anxiety symptoms, along with occasional intrusive thoughts about both the car accident and the domestic abuse.*

After a discussion of the possible causes of her headaches, you and Susan jointly decide to proceed with a medical evaluation looking for a possible source of the headaches. However, you also tell Susan that the headaches and other symptoms may be part of a post-traumatic stress syndrome and discuss the possibility of counseling to deal with residual issues from both the accident and the domestic violence. She agrees, and you refer her for counseling in addition to the planned medical evaluation. You also schedule her for a follow-up office visit in 2 weeks.

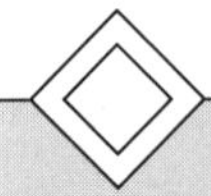

Post-Traumatic Stress Syndromes in Primary Care Medical Settings

Trauma-related physical and psychological symptoms seem relatively common in primary care patients, cutting across diagnostic categories and often producing confusing symptom constellations. Patients with post-traumatic syndromes often have associated physical symptoms and thus are more likely to seek care from medical professionals than from mental health professionals. Post-traumatic symptoms and comorbid psychiatric and medical conditions may persist for years after the initial trauma, significantly impairing health-related quality of life. Actually, some patients with past PTSD have few, if any, residual psychiatric symptoms but may continue to have lingering physical symptoms and impairment, for which they may visit their primary care clinicians.

Patients with post-traumatic stress symptoms may have experienced accidental trauma, as in the case of natural disasters, or intentional trauma, as in the case of interpersonal violence. Post-traumatic responses tend to be more severe and longer lasting in response to interpersonal violence than in response to a natural disaster or an accident, especially when the trauma occurred before adolescence. Additionally, patients suffering from life-threatening medical illnesses commonly exhibit post-traumatic symptoms. This is especially true for patients undergoing surgery or other invasive therapies, cancer chemotherapy, intensive care, or other prolonged, traumatic treatments. People may also develop post-traumatic stress from dealing with such difficult or life-threatening clinical situations in their children, spouses, or other close family members.

A substantial number of patients in the primary care medical setting have experienced interpersonal violence at some point in their lives, and many of these patients suffer from a variety of current physical and psychological symptoms arising from this previous trauma exposure. Although it may not necessarily produce symptoms, previous trauma can increase a person's vulnerability to subsequent stress, and exposure tends to have a cumulative effect. People who have experienced multiple traumas or severe prolonged trauma may develop a more complex form of PTSD, which may include somatization, dissociation, long-lasting personality changes, vulnerability to revictimization, a tendency to become easily upset or irritable, and difficulty controlling anger or excessive anger, in addition to post-traumatic symptoms.

History of Post-Traumatic Stress Disorder

Early systematic observations of post-traumatic syndromes come from Pierre Janet, a psychiatrist in the late nineteenth century. Janet described a group of patients who displayed uncontrollable emotions, psychosomatic symptoms, disturbances in memory and information processing, and violent outbursts, all linked to past frightening events. Subsequently, in a published work on hysterics in 1896, Freud hypothesized that the current psychological problems of these patients originated in childhood sexual trauma. Freud later renounced this position in favor of his psychoanalytic theory, which dominated psychiatry through much of the twentieth century and resulted in abuse-related symptoms being ascribed to fantasies and internal conflict surrounding psychosexual developmental issues.

Until recent years, the study of post-traumatic responses largely dealt with combat stress reactions in men, and few studies focused on post-traumatic stress in women and children. Clinicians and researchers gradually noticed that there were common elements in the response to trauma, regardless of the nature of the trauma or gender of the individual. Recently, post-traumatic syndromes have been studied in a variety of civilian populations and situations. These studies have broadened and refined our understanding of post-traumatic responses and syndromes.

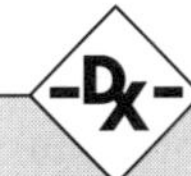

Diagnostic Criteria

PTSD was formally recognized and included as a diagnosis in the DSM-III and subsequently in the DSM-III-R and DSM-IV. The essential diagnostic criterion is an individual's exposure and response to a traumatic event or stressor (criterion A). The DSM-IV describes a traumatic stressor as a "direct personal experience of an event that involves actual or threatened death or serious injury, or other threat to one's physical integrity; witnessing an event that involves death, injury, or a threat to the physical integrity of another person; or learning about unexpected or violent death, serious harm, or threat of death or injury experienced by a family member or other close associate."[1] The DSM-IV specifies that the individual must respond to the event with "intense fear, helplessness, or horror," or, in children, disorganized or agitated

[1]American Psychiatric Association: *Diagnostic and Statistical Manual of Mental Disorders,* 4th ed. Washington, DC: American Psychiatric Association, 1994, p 424.

behavior.[2] Specific symptoms required for the diagnosis of PTSD include at least one symptom that involves re-experiencing of the trauma (criterion B), three symptoms of avoiding stimuli associated with the trauma or numbing of general responsiveness (criterion C), and two symptoms of anxiety or hyperarousal (criterion D). All these symptoms must persist for at least 1 month. They may begin immediately after the traumatic event or may have a delayed onset. The course is considered acute if symptoms persist for less than 3 months or chronic if symptoms last for more than 3 months. Table 19-1 displays common symptoms of PTSD and their corresponding DSM diagnostic criteria.

Some individuals have post-traumatic symptoms that are clinically significant but are not sufficient to meet DSM-IV criteria for the diagnosis of PTSD. Such individuals may be considered to have subthreshold or partial post-traumatic stress, the significance of which is not yet fully understood. Survivors of prolonged, severe trauma may have a complex post-traumatic syndrome that involves a more "complex, diffuse, and tenacious" symptom picture, often including problems with relationships and repeated victimization.[3] These patients have somatoform, depressive, and dissociative symptoms along with the classic PTSD symptoms and are a subgroup of the PTSD patients found in primary care populations.

Table 19-1

Common Symptoms of Post-Traumatic Stress Disorder

A patient with post-traumatic stress disorder may have (Criterion B)
- Recurrent and intrusive distressing memories of the event.
- Recurrent distressing dreams about the event.
- Intense psychological distress and/or physiologic reactivity when exposed to cues that remind the person of aspects of the event.

A patient with post-traumatic stress disorder may (Criterion C)
- Act or feel as if the event were happening again.
- Avoid thoughts, feelings, or conversations associated with the trauma.
- Avoid activities, places, or people that bring memories of the trauma.
- Not be able to remember important aspects of the trauma.
- Feel detached or estranged from others.
- Not be able to have loving feelings.
- Not expect to have a career, marriage, children, or normal life span.

A patient with post-traumatic stress disorder may have symptoms of increased arousal, such as (Criterion D)
- Difficulty falling or staying asleep.
- Outbursts of anger or irritability.
- Difficulty concentrating.
- Hypervigilance.
- Exaggerated startle response.

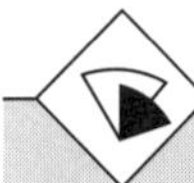

Prevalence

The first studies of PTSD in community samples were undertaken in the late 1980s using the Diagnostic Interview Schedule (DIS) with DSM-III criteria. Lifetime prevalence rates for PTSD were estimated at 2.9 percent for men and 3.3 percent for women in one study, and only about 1 percent in the other study, leading many to believe that the disorder was uncommon in the general population. Evidence from later investigations, however, suggests that DSM-III criteria and the DIS tend to underestimate the true prevalence of post-traumatic stress syndromes. Reported lifetime prevalence of PTSD from later studies, using

[2]American Psychiatric Association: *Diagnostic and Statistical Manual of Mental Disorders,* 4th ed. Washington, DC: American Psychiatric Association, 1994, p 424.

[3]Herman JL: Complex PTSD: A syndrome in survivors of prolonged and repeated trauma. *J Trauma Stress* 5:377, 1992.

DSM-III-R criteria, ranged from 7.8 to 12.3 percent in the general population. Estimated prevalence of PTSD in the Somatization in Primary Care study in three family practice clinics was 9.6 percent, which was higher than the prevalence of generalized anxiety disorder, bulimia, panic disorder, or somatization disorder.

Subthreshhold syndromes may have an even greater influence in a primary care population than cases that meet formal DSM criteria, largely due to their greater prevalence of subthreshold syndromes. Lifetime prevalence rates for subthreshold or partial post-traumatic stress have ranged from 6.6 to 15 percent in the general population in the Epidemiological Catchment Area studies and 21.2 to 22.5 percent in Vietnam veterans. In the Somatization in Primary Care study, in which two-thirds of the sample had multiple unexplained physical complaints, 31 percent of the patients had a qualifying traumatic event and three or more post-traumatic symptoms but did not meet criteria for the full diagnosis. In Canada, Stein and associates carried out a community telephone survey to examine the current prevalence of full and partial PTSD using DSM-IV criteria. Partial PTSD was defined as having had a qualifying event plus at least one symptom from each DSM criterion. Both full and partial PTSD were more prevalent in women. Full PTSD was present within the past month for 2.7 percent of women and 1.2 percent of men with somewhat higher rates for partial PTSD—3.4 percent for women and 1.5 percent for men.

Trauma Exposure

Exposure to traumatic stressors was once thought rare and out of the range of normal human experience; however, we now know that such exposure is quite common. Evidence suggests that 39 to 84 percent of the population has been exposed to at least one traumatic event during their lives, and many have multiple exposures. Norris surveyed 1000 adults from four southeastern cities and examined how many people experienced robbery, physical assault, sexual assault, fire, other disaster, other hazard, tragic death, motor vehicle crash, and combat. Sixty-nine percent of the subjects reported that they had experienced at least one of the targeted events during their lifetimes (21 percent within the past year).

Studies in the primary care setting have generally focused on particular types of trauma, rather than the broad spectrum of traumatic stressors. For example, there have been several recent studies of the prevalence of sexual victimization, childhood physical abuse, and domestic violence among women in primary care medical settings. Reported prevalence rates of exposure to traumatic stressors in these studies are shown in Table 19-2.

As many as 22 percent of the women in a primary care practice experienced multiple forms of childhood abuse. A major limitation of these studies is that only a few have included men. In a study that included 84 male primary care patients, reported prevalences of childhood physical and sexual abuse were 22 and 12 percent, respectively, for men. In a survey of randomly selected family practice patients by Gould and co-workers, 21 percent of males reported childhood physical abuse, 14 percent of males reported childhood sexual abuse, and 28 percent of males reported violent behavior by family members with a drug or alcohol problem during childhood. When all three types of abuse or violence were considered, overall exposure to abuse or violent behavior during childhood was 44 percent for both males and females.

Overall, studies from the primary care medical setting indicate that a substantial proportion of patients have experienced interpersonal violence at

Table 19-2

Prevalence of Traumatic Stressors in Primary Care Patients

• Lifetime sexual victimization	46%
• Rape or attempted rape	29%
• Childhood sexual abuse	40%
• Childhood physical abuse	29%
• Lifetime physical abuse	39%
• Domestic violence involving battery or sexual violence	38%

some point in their lives, and many of these patients suffer substantial impairment in health and psychosocial functioning. We have little information regarding the exposure to other types of traumatic stressors or its effects in a primary care population.

Reactions to Traumatic Experiences

The risk of developing post-traumatic stress symptoms for individuals exposed to traumatic experiences is highly variable and depends on a number of factors, including the nature and severity of the trauma. In community-based studies, 8 to 14 percent of men and 18 to 30 percent of the women who had been exposed to at least one traumatic stressor had a lifetime history of PTSD, but rates were as high as 75 percent for trauma involving interpersonal violence. The risk of developing PTSD is higher when the person suffers physical injury or direct threat to life. Blanchard and colleagues found that PTSD has been reported in as many as 40 percent of victims seeking medical attention following a motor vehicle accident, with another 35 percent demonstrating partial PTSD. Individual or family factors may affect a person's vulnerability or resilience following traumatic exposure, including the severity of the traumatic exposure, comorbid medical or psychiatric conditions, prior exposure to traumatic events, current psychosocial stress, childhood adversity, coping styles, family support and functioning, social support, and spirituality.

Course of Post-Traumatic Symptoms

Post-traumatic symptoms may begin immediately after the traumatic event or may be delayed. The course of PTSD can be acute, with symptoms lasting up to 3 months, or chronic, lasting greater than 3 months. In addition, the longitudinal course of post-traumatic symptoms may wax and wane, with some patients having multiple recurrences of full PTSD, interspersed periods of remission or with symptoms intermittently subsiding to a subthreshold level. In many cases, patients who have had complete or partial resolution of their PTSD will have a reactivation of their symptoms in response to a new traumatic or stressful event. Finally, some patients will have prolonged residual symptoms even after their symptoms have subsided to levels below the threshold for diagnosis. As mentioned, physical symptoms may especially persist even after the resolution of the psychiatric symptoms.

The National Comorbidity Survey found the median time to remission of post-traumatic symptoms was 64 months for those not receiving treatment and 36 months for subjects receiving treatment. Only about 25 percent had achieved remission 12 months after onset of symptoms, and about one-third were symptomatic after 10 years.

Many of the patients in the primary care medical setting who have a history of post-traumatic stress will have a chronic, residual, or recurrent type of syndrome. Although underlying trauma exposure can cause or significantly contribute to the patient's current distress, often neither the patient nor the clinician recognizes the relationship. Compared with patients who have no history of post-traumatic stress syndromes, patients who do have such a history have more stress-related medical problems and tend to seek care for unexplained somatic complaints, such as pain, fatigue, and irritable bowel syndrome.

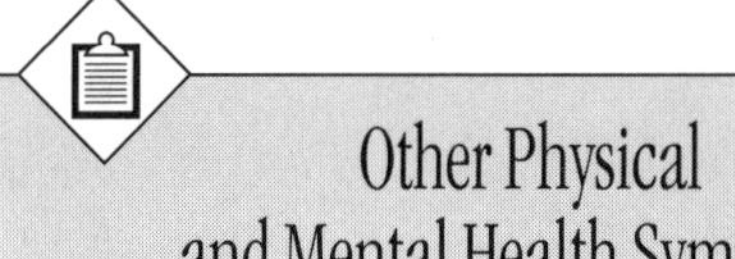

Other Physical and Mental Health Symptoms

The combination of PTSD and other mental health conditions results in significant comorbidity, especially for PTSD accompanied by anxiety, depression, panic disorder, phobic disorder, conduct disorder, alcohol or substance abuse, or somatization. The pattern of comorbidity differs between men and women. Patients with post-traumatic stress syndromes can have a variety of physical and mental health symptoms and clinically significant functional impairment even if they do not meet the diagnostic criteria for additional disorders.

Childhood abuse (physical and/or sexual) appears to be a vulnerability factor for an increased risk of developing post-traumatic stress in adulthood, as well as a direct risk factor in PTSD. Furthermore, an elevated risk of chronic post-traumatic stress has been associated with childhood adversity, separation from parents in childhood, a family history of anxiety, and a family history of antisocial behavior, according to Breslau and Davis.

SAM CONNERS *Sam, age 43, comes into the clinic with chest pain, but no organic pathology can be found. Medical history includes depression, alcoholism, rosacea, and fibromyalgia. Sam was a Vietnam veteran and has had chronic post-traumatic stress since his military experience. He continues to have nightmares about events that happened in Vietnam and has chronic difficulty with insomnia and anxiety. Sam also reports that there was a history of physical violence and alcoholism in his family of origin, and he thinks that the abuse that he suffered during his childhood may have contributed to his reaction to combat. He has not been taking antidepressants for the past 2 years, but he agrees that because of his continued PTSD symptoms he should consider resuming counseling and going back on an SSRI. You restart the SSRI that he previously was taking and schedule him for a return visit in 2 weeks. He will meanwhile make an appointment with his counselor in the Veterans Hospital system.*

Physical symptoms are often a significant component of post-traumatic symptoms. PTSD has been associated with more medical problems, poorer health status, more visits to clinicians, and increased levels of disability. PTSD is also accompanied by higher rates of explained and unexplained physical symptoms of virtually every type. In one study, firefighters who were exposed to a major bush fire in Australia were interviewed and medical records reviewed at 4, 11, 29, and 42 months after the disaster. McFarlane and colleagues found that firefighters who developed PTSD reported more cardiovascular, respiratory, musculoskeletal, and neurologic problems than did those who did not develop PTSD. Although the firefighters with PTSD had more visits to a doctor than did those without PTSD, clinicians tended not to recognize the PTSD or the relationship between physical symptoms and traumatic exposure. Furthermore, there was a poor correlation between patients' and clinicians' reports of physical symptoms.

In a number of studies, PTSD has been associated with somatization. In a prospective study of young adult HMO members in the Detroit area, Andreski and associates found that individuals with a history of PTSD were more than three times as likely than those without PTSD to have some degree of somatization and were at increased risk of new onset of conversion symptoms and pain symptoms.

Why Is There a Relationship Between Physical Symptoms and Post-Traumatic Symptoms?

Several hypotheses have been suggested to explain the relationship between physical symptoms and post-traumatic stress symptoms. These include increased biological sensitivity to a variety of stimuli, long-term neurophysiologic changes, overreporting of symptoms, neuroticism, stress-related vulnerability, trauma-related injury, deficits in information processing, and misinterpretation of somatic sensations. Hurricane Andrew victims with post-traumatic stress symptoms were found to have decreased immune functioning, suggesting a possible immunologic source for some of their somatic symptoms.

Many people with post-traumatic stress syndromes preferentially seek treatment in medical rather than mental health care settings, possibly because they have more somatic symptoms and medical problems or because of other factors. Clinicians in medical settings rarely associate physical symptoms with a history of trauma.

Trauma Exposure and Post-Traumatic Stress in Adolescents

Recent surveys indicate that exposure to traumatic stressors and associated post-traumatic symptoms is a serious problem in adolescents. In a study of students from four geographically and sociodemographically diverse high schools, Singer and colleagues found that as many as 10 percent of men and 31 percent of women reported being beaten at home within the past year. Among the females, up to 17 percent reported being sexually abused or assaulted within the past year. Additionally, many more students experienced violence in their school or community or were witnesses to violence. In this study, recent and past exposure to violence was associated with post-traumatic symptoms, anxiety, dissociation, stress, depression, and anger.

Similar findings have been reported by Giaconia and colleagues, who found that over 25 percent of adolescents experience at least one DSM-III-R trauma by the time they reach age 14 and 40 percent by age 18, with a lifetime prevalence of PTSD of over 6 percent by age 18. Adolescents with PTSD had more health problems, suicidal behavior, academic failure, and interpersonal problems than did youths without PTSD. Adolescents with trauma exposure and post-traumatic symptoms who did not meet all the criteria for PTSD were also at higher risk for suicide ideation or attempts, poorer health, and poorer academic performance than those with no trauma exposure. Of those with PTSD, 80 percent had at least one other DSM-III-R disorder. The primary gender difference found in these studies was differential exposure to physical assault (higher in boys) and sexual assault (higher in girls). Sexual assault in girls was associated with much higher rates of PTSD than any other type of trauma. In general, higher socioeconomic class did not protect youths from trauma exposure or PTSD. Studies such as these emphasize the need to screen adolescents for exposure to violence and psychological and physical effects during routine health visits.

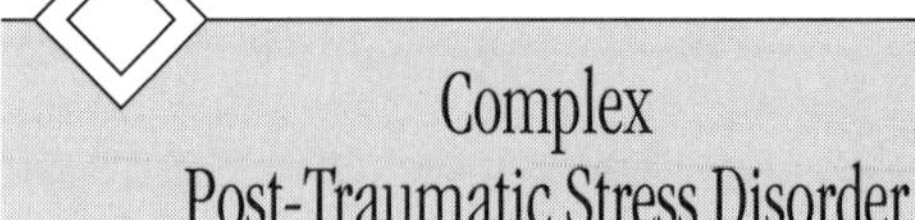

Complex Post-Traumatic Stress Disorder

The heterogeneity of post-traumatic stress symptoms has led many researchers to question whether the diagnosis of PTSD, alone, sufficiently captures the complexity and variety of symptoms. Some investigators have theorized that PTSD is a spectrum disorder that can range from subthreshold to complex.

Researchers and clinicians have described a complex post-traumatic syndrome in survivors of severe, prolonged trauma, which includes symptoms outside the usual PTSD construct. Cited in the DSM-IV as associated features of PTSD, these include impaired affect modulation (difficulty controlling feelings), somatic complaints, dissociative symptoms, shame, despair, hopelessness, and impaired relationships. A structured interview based on specific criteria for complex PTSD (also referred to as disorders of extreme stress) has been developed and tested as part of the DSM-IV PTSD field trials. In one report from these field trials, Roth and associates found that 63 percent of subjects with preadolescent onset of interpersonal abuse and 38 percent of those reporting later onset of interpersonal abuse met the criteria for complex PTSD, as opposed to only 10 percent of subjects exposed to a disaster.

DARLA HARRIS *Darla Harris, age 31 and divorced mother of three, sees you for the first time complaining of dizziness, shortness of breath, and blurred vision. Her medical history includes hypertension, depression, anxiety, pelvic adhesions, and two laparoscopies to explore reasons for abdominal pain. She had multiple visits to other physicians within the past year for severe headaches, chest pain, gastrointestinal complaints, and joint pain.*

Darla thought that her previous primary care clinician was getting tired of dealing with her and decided to switch. She has also had problems with alcohol and drugs and made a serious suicide attempt a few years ago. Darla admits that she has had problems with depression and "stress" for many years, but she never has received counseling or been treated with antidepressants. She reports that it started at age 10 when her father sold her into prostitution. She ran away from home several times. She says that her siblings also were severely abused and neglected. In addition to severe sexual abuse, Darla was physically abused by her father. Darla tells you that she has never been asked about previous abuse or trauma by any of her previous clinicians, and she never volunteered the information, although she thought that her previous abuse probably was somehow related to a lot of her problems. You suggest a trial of medication, and she readily agrees. She is also willing to consider the possibility of counseling, although she wants to wait to see if the medication will help.

Recognizing Post-Traumatic Stress Disorder

Many people with post-traumatic stress syndromes preferentially seek treatment in medical rather than mental health care settings, possibly due to their preponderance of somatic symptoms associated with PTSD. Yet, the association of physical symptoms with a history of trauma is rarely identified by clinicians, who often do not recognize the ways in which trauma has affected their patients' health, and who rarely ask about trauma history. Almost 60 percent of a sample of 144 patients surveyed by Dickinson and co-workers in an academic family practice reported a lifetime history of exposure to interpersonal violence. However, clinicians in that practice estimated that fewer than 20 percent of their patients had ever been exposed to interpersonal violence or abuse. Most subjects said they would be willing to discuss their history of exposure to abuse or violence with a doctor or other health care clinician, but few had ever been asked about their abuse history. In a study by Hamberger and colleagues of more than 300 women in a family practice clinic in a Midwestern community, 38.8 percent reported being physically abused at some time in their lives by a partner. Although 6.5 percent of the women reported that their clinicians asked them about relationship problems, fewer than 2 percent reported their clinicians had ever asked about physical assault.

The cues that a patient might have a post-traumatic stress syndrome are quite diverse. One approach to finding patients who might have a post-traumatic stress syndrome is to include screening questions about trauma as part of the routine information gathered on all patients. As is discussed in more detail in Chap. 6, many patients seen in primary care settings have been victimized by either past or present violence and abuse. A question, such as "Has anything really bad or traumatic ever happened to you?" followed by more specific questions regarding abuse and victimization, would be appropriate for all patients. For patients with a history of trauma or victimization, the clinician should ask further questions to determine whether the patient meets the criteria for PTSD as described. In addition, other possible effects of the trauma should be explored, including other mental health or physical problems that might be linked to the patient's traumatic experience.

Beyond the initial screening questions, clinicians should be aware of the potential influence that various traumatic experiences might have on their patients. Patients can have significant post-traumatic stress reactions to invasive procedures or serious illness, automobile or other accidents, or the death or serious illness of a close friend or family member. Clinicians should ask any patient who experiences an event that might be construed as traumatic about the patient's reaction to the event. The clinician should counsel such patients to discuss the event with supportive family or friends or with the clinician, and should monitor the patient for further symptoms or problems related to the event.

Clinicians who do not ask every patient about traumatic experiences should be particularly alert for signs and symptoms that specific patients might be experiencing problems related to current or past trauma. In the primary care setting, recognition of PTSD in patients with predominantly somatic complaints is particularly important. Patients presenting with somatization or with mental health problems such as anxiety, panic, or depression should be screened for traumatic experiences.

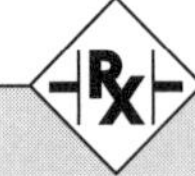

Treatment

It is estimated by Kessler that only 38 percent of the people in the United States with current PTSD receive treatment in a given year. Of those who did not seek treatment, 66 percent of men and 60 percent of women did not perceive a need for treatment. Over half of women and two-thirds of men wanted to solve the problem on their own: 43 percent of the women and 67 percent of the men thought the problem would get better by itself. In general, individuals with PTSD "perceive themselves as unlucky people who were in the wrong place at the wrong time," and such opinions are characteristic of the PTSD population that does not seek treatment.[4]

Although previous research on treatment of PTSD has yielded mixed results, there is now sufficient evidence to support treatment recommendations for PTSD. Treatment goals for PTSD should be directed toward several domains, including reducing the core symptoms of PTSD, dealing with the psychiatric comorbidity, improving coping and stress management, improving quality of life, reducing adverse practices such as violence and excess alcohol consumption, and reducing disability. The two primary treatment approaches are pharmacotherapy and psychotherapy, supplemented by psychosocial support and psychoeducation.

[4]Davidson J: Discussion (Pharmacotherapy of posttraumatic stress disorder: Treatment options, long-term follow-up, and predictors of outcome). *J Clin Psychiatry* 61(Suppl 5):57, 2000.

Pharmacotherapy

The selective serotonin reuptake inhibitors (SSRIs), specifically fluoxetine and sertraline, have been shown to reduce post-traumatic symptoms, reduce disability, and improve functioning. Many of the trials of these medications have been short term, generally ranging from 5 to 14 weeks, and studies suggest that some patients require a longer treatment regimen for improvement. Trials of longer-term pharmacotherapy with fluoxetine (6 months or more) indicate that more prolonged treatment regimens have potential benefit for some patients. At this point, the general recommendation is to treat patients with acute episodes of PTSD for 12 months or more, although data regarding the optimal length of treatment are somewhat lacking. Patients with more chronic or recurring forms of PTSD may need more prolonged treatment than patients with an acute reaction to a recent trauma, but that level of distinction has not yet shown up in published trials. An important task will be to determine how to motivate patients to continue treatment.

Other pharmacologic treatments shown to be effective in clinical trials include tricyclic antidepressants, the monoamine oxidase inhibitor phenelzine, and the anticonvulsant lamotrigine. However, these agents are not recommended as first-line treatments for PTSD.

Psychosocial Treatments

The other primary treatment modality for PTSD is psychosocial treatment, including cognitive behavioral therapy, psychodynamic therapy, group therapy, family therapy, and eye movement desensitization reprocessing (EMDR). Etten and colleagues' meta-analysis of 39 studies of treatments for PTSD indicated that psychosocial therapies such as cognitive behavioral therapy tend to be slightly more effective than drug therapies, but treatment adherence is more of a problem with pharmacotherapy.

Psychosocial treatment modalities for PTSD generally share many common elements, including a reappraisal of the threat experienced during the trauma, overcoming avoidance of reminders of the trauma, working through the meaning of the traumatic experience, and achieving mastery over intrusive memories. It is useful for primary care clinicians to have some understanding of the types of counseling that are effective, especially to inform the selection of appropriate counseling resources for specific patients.

Cognitive Behavioral Therapy

Among the psychosocial treatments, empirical support seems to be greatest for cognitive-behavioral therapy, in particular exposure therapy, used either as the primary treatment or as a key element in a multifaceted approach. Exposure therapy was used successfully in combat veterans early in the course of investigating possible treatments, and has been extended to a range of other traumas, including sexual assault, incest, and motor vehicle accidents. This approach uses techniques to help patients confront their fears around memories or images of the traumatic event. This may involve such tasks as recounting the experiences verbally or in writing and confronting physical situations that are related to the trauma. Lange and associates' recent pilot of an innovative, computer-based cognitive behavioral therapy intervention for post-traumatic stress symptoms involving 10 structured writing sessions produced significant improvement in general psychological functioning and reduction in post-traumatic symptoms, with clinical recovery in 19 out of 20 subjects. Many cognitive behavioral interventions for PTSD have exposure therapy as an important component. Exposure therapy has been shown to be very effective for patients with a variety of traumas, and it is relatively easy to train therapists in its use.

Other approaches that have been used either alone or in conjunction with exposure therapy include cognitive therapy, which is based on changing thinking patterns that are dysfunctional and unrealistic. Anxiety management, aimed toward developing or improving skills needed to cope with anxiety or stressful situations, also is useful adjunctive therapy.

Disclosure Therapy

Another psychosocial approach that appears promising is disclosure therapy, which has some elements of exposure therapy. A number of experts have cited the importance of allowing victims to "tell their story" in some way, and state that "the more articulate the story, the less PTSD they are going to have." In a study of somatization and PTSD in immigrants and refugees in primary care medical settings, Waitzkin and Magana report reduction in somatic symptoms using verbal disclosure techniques that empower patients "to express more coherent narratives of their prior traumatic experiences."[5]

The disclosure intervention used in most studies involves a simple writing exercise. Subjects are instructed to write about the most stressful thing that has happened to them, letting the story flow out onto paper as freely as possible. This is usually done for 30 min or so, with one or two follow-up sessions that are structured similarly. Positive effects of this type of disclosure intervention have been observed in college students, patients with asthma or rheumatoid arthritis, Holocaust survivors, and primary care medical patients with somatization, producing improvements in health, illness behavior, job and school performance, and immune function. Disclosure therapy has not been adequately tested as an intervention for PTSD; however, it is possible that this type of simple intervention can be modified for use in primary care settings. In addition, research about the importance of disclosure may partially explain the therapeutic effect that is often seen when a patient simply tells the story of past trauma to a receptive and supportive clinician. Diagnosis is treatment; uncovering the trauma and exploring it with the patient has therapeutic benefit.

[5]Waitzkin H, Magana H: The black box in somatization: Unexplained physical symptoms, culture, and narratives of trauma. *Soc Sci Med* 45:811, 1997.

Role of Primary Care Clinicians

Primary care clinicians are being increasingly recognized as important in the detection and management of mental health problems, including PTSD. Current treatment recommendations for primary care practice are based on approaches that have been used in mental health inpatient and outpatient settings and will need to be adapted for primary care. Some authors believe that "primary care practitioners are uniquely placed to identify [PTSD] and initiate effective therapy,"[6] and "management in a primary care setting may be the treatment of choice."[7] Suggestions for primary care interventions include providing a supportive environment and opportunities for victims to talk about their experiences. Clinicians need to be aware that symptoms of post-traumatic stress can persist for months or years. Even after the individual recovers, reminders can be triggered many years later and cause distress. Furthermore, this distress may be experienced physically as well as emotionally.

The treatment of PTSD may need to be multifaceted, incorporating both pharmacologic and psychosocial interventions. Clinicians should provide emotional support and offer information, targeting mood, coping skills, and social support. Patients should be empowered to become partners with their clinicians in taking responsibility for their health and encouraged to set their own achievable goals. The heterogeneity of post-traumatic syndromes may necessitate a more individualized approach to treatment of post-traumatic syndromes than of many mental health problems. There may be a need to treat concomitant conditions such as depression, insomnia, or substance abuse. There should be periodic assessments of current life stresses, such as family or marital problems, work difficulties, and financial difficulties, which can produce fluctuation of PTSD symptoms.

Consideration of social support and other interpersonal factors is important when weighing treatment options. Social support can be a significant protective factor during and after periods of extreme stress; however, people often become isolated from their support systems after a traumatic experience. Clinicians should encourage patients to use their available sources of support, discussing their experiences and reactions with the people who would be the most receptive.

A thorough investigation of risk and protective factors, along with careful assessment of the broader spectrum of post-traumatic responses, is needed to determine who may benefit from which treatments. This should include exploring prior traumatic experiences, specifically abuse and victimization. A discussion of the patient's response to prior experiences, including previously successful coping strategies, can greatly assist in developing a management strategy for the current episode.

Primary care clinicians should be alert to situations in which patients may be prone to develop post-traumatic symptoms. For example, patients who have experienced previous traumatic exposure often may have exacerbation of their symptoms or develop new post-traumatic reactions when faced with new stressors such as illness, the birth of a child, the death of a loved one, or marital problems. Furthermore, the possibility of post-traumatic stress responses among patients suffering from life-threatening medical illnesses should be considered. In this way, the clinician can anticipate potential problems, alert the patient to the possibility, and intervene earlier in the process, before symptoms become as severe.

PTSD symptoms tend to fluctuate, possibly reflecting successive phases of the disorder. There may be a need to first identify and treat concomitant conditions such as depression, anxiety, insomnia, or substance abuse. Then, if necessary, the patient can be referred for psychotherapy. Patients should be counseled to avoid overuse of alcohol or other drugs to control symptoms. Anxiety management can involve physically oriented interventions to counteract the physiologic component of anxiety and provide alternative adaptive coping strategies, for example, using relaxation techniques, moderate aerobic exercise, and reducing the use of stimulants such as caffeine and nicotine. It is important to deal with the patient's emo-

---

[6]Tiller J, Kyrios M, Bennett P: Post traumatic stress disorder. *Australian Family Physician* 25:1569, 1996.

[7]Rosser R: Post-traumatic stress disorder. *Practitioner* 238:393, 1994.

Table 19-3

Guidelines for Treatment of Post-Traumatic Stress Disorder

- Early response to *acute trauma exposure:*
  - Educate about normal stress responses.
  - Encourage victims to talk to family and friends about their experience.
  - Provide one or two primary care counseling sessions within 2 weeks after exposure.
- To deal with distress:
  - Create a sense of safety.
  - Evaluate need for specialized interventions.
- If no clinical improvement after 3 weeks:
  - Prescribe drug therapy.
  - SSRIs are first-line medication.
  - Continue for 12 months or longer.
- Refer to mental health professional for psychotherapy.
- Special considerations:
  - Acute sleep disturbance for 4 consecutive nights.
  - Provide symptomatic relief (nonbenzodiazepine hypnotics).
  - Avoid benzodiazepines in treating PTSD.
- Referral to psychiatrist if:
  - Unresponsive to initial drug therapy at 3 months.
  - Complicating comorbid conditions (e.g. severe depression) are present.

SOURCE: Adapted from Ballenger J, et al: Consensus statement on posttraumatic stress disorder from the International Consensus group on depression and anxiety. *J Clin Psychiatry* 61(suppl 5):60.

tional responses with skills of listening, empathy, and reframing, and taking a long-term view—it can take time for post-traumatic responses to resolve. The chronicity of the problem is one reason that a long-term relationship with a supportive primary care provider may be the most appropriate healing environment for patients with PTSD.

In April of 1999, members of the International Consensus Group on Depression and Anxiety, along with several invited PTSD experts, developed a consensus statement with treatment guidelines for PTSD based on empirical evidence, primarily from mental health settings. A primary objective of this effort was to provide primary care clinicians with "a better understanding of management issues in posttraumatic stress disorder (PTSD) and guide clinical practice with recommendations on the appropriate management strategy."[8]

Guidelines for the management of PTSD by primary care clinicians were developed, with three major components: (1) pychoeducation/psychosocial support, (2) psychotherapy, and (3) pharmacotherapy. The treatment guidelines are primarily directed toward individuals with recent trauma exposure, but many aspects of the management should be appropriate for chronic PTSD. Further study of the applicability of the guidelines for primary care patients is needed. The specific guidelines developed by the International Consensus Committee can be found in Table 19-3, followed by additional management recommendations in Table 19-4.

[8]Ballenger J, et al: Consensus statement on posttraumatic stress disorder from the International Consensus Group on Depression and Anxiety. *J Clin Psychiatry* 61(Suppl 5):60, 2000.

Table 19-4

Additional Recommendations for Primary Care Management of Post-Traumatic Stress Disorder

Comprehensively evaluate patient's medical and mental health problems

- Because post-traumatic stress syndromes rarely exist in isolation, it is essential to address coexisting medical and mental health problems.
- Particular attention should be paid to management of physical symptoms and medical problems and their possible association with trauma history and psychosocial factors.
- This information can then be used to jointly develop a comprehensive treatment plan by the primary care health team and patient.

Provide patient education and activation

- Provide written educational materials on post-traumatic stress disorder for the patient to take home.
- Review educational materials and answer patient's questions.
- Areas of focus for patient education should include the effects of and normal reactions to trauma; especially focus on effects on mental and physical health, experience of physical symptoms, experience of stress; also cover to some extent the effect on relationships, families.
- Skill training
  - Medical shared problem solving—empowerment
  - Stress reduction—relaxation, exercise
  - Goal setting—specific homework assignments to be completed in between visits
- Exercise program
- Increasing social interaction
- Community resources—be familiar with community resources

Formulate an active treatment plan based on recommendations in Table 19-3 to include any or all of the following.

- Medication management
  - Initiate pharmacotherapy with SSRIs, if needed, for depression or panic disorder.
  - Monitor medications for chronic diseases and symptom management.
- Refer for psychotherapy—
  - Identify experienced professionals (family therapists, counselors, psychologists), know something about their style of treatment, and be able to inform and support the patient in choosing among possible options.
  - Assist the patient in making the initial appointment and provide encouragement to follow through with the process.

Provide a supportive environment

- Emotional support
  - Provided by physician, health care team
  - Regular visits, phone calls to check in
  - Model normal interpersonal relationships (especially important for victims of childhood abuse or family violence)
- Expression and putting into context the story of the trauma
  - Allow the patient to tell his or her story
  - Help put it into some sort of context; may need to encourage the patient to write the story out; patient may need to go through it more than once.
  - Deal with guilt, self-blame
  - Normalize the response to the trauma
- Establish physician's office as safe place; medical home
- Shared decisions
- Special care with invasive procedures, hospitalization
- Appropriate access to physician and health care team

SOURCE: Adapted from Ballenger J, et al: Consensus Statement on posttraumatic stress disorder from the International Consensus group on depression and anxiety. *J Clin Psychiatry* 61(suppl 5):60.

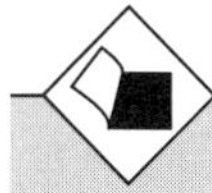

Summary

Most of our patients are affected by trauma at some point in their lives. There is great variability in the types and level of impact of the trauma, but many patients develop post-traumatic stress syndromes that may cause them to present for care. It is often hard to connect the patient's symptoms to the trauma that is the root cause, especially when the patient presents at a time that is fairly distant from the trauma, and we often miss the diagnosis. We need to be more alert to the harmful impact of trauma in our patients' lives and watch and screen more actively in our patients for traumatic events and their sequelae. Effective treatment options are available, including pharmacotherapy and psychotherapy, although the optimal treatment protocols are still being worked out.

However, the central core of an effective treatment plan for a patient with post-traumatic stress is a relationship with a primary care clinician who can identify the problem, allow the patient to disclose and process the problem in a supportive environment, provide helpful information, develop and implement an individualized treatment plan, and monitor the patient's response over the long haul. PTSD is a very important primary care problem, and it is incumbent on us to become masters of its management.

Suggested Reading

Journal of Clinical Psychiatry, volume 61, supplement 5, 2000.

This entire issue is devoted to post-traumatic stress disorder. In April of 1999, members of the International Consensus Group on Depression and Anxiety, along with several invited experts in the area of post-traumatic stress, met and developed a consensus statement with evidence-based treatment guidelines for PTSD. A key objective of this effort was to provide primary care clinicians with "a better understanding of management issues in post-traumatic stress disorder (PTSD) and guide clinical practice with recommendations on the appropriate management strategy." Although few studies have actually been carried out with primary care patients, this is a good start toward developing evidence-based guidelines for the management of PTSD by primary care clinicians. All of the articles in this issue are excellent, but the following will be of particular interest to the clinician.

Ballenger J, et al: Consensus statement on posttraumatic stress disorder from the International Consensus Group on Depression and Anxiety. *J Clin Psychiatry* 61(Suppl 5):60, 2000.

Davidson J: Pharmacotherapy of posttraumatic stress disorder: Treatment options, long-term follow-up, and predictors of outcome. *J Clin Psychiatry* 61(Suppl 5): 52, 2000.

Foa E: Psychosocial treatment of posttraumatic stress disorder. *J Clin Psychiatry* 61(Suppl 5):43, 2000.

Kessler RC: Posttraumatic stress disorder: The burden to the individual and to society. *J Clin Psychiatry* 61(Suppl 5):4, 2000.

McFarlane AC: Discussion (Posttraumatic stress disorder: A model of the longitudinal course and the role of risk factors). *J Clin Psychiatry* 61(Suppl 5):15, 2000.

Herman JL: Complex PTSD: A syndrome in survivors of prolonged and repeated trauma. *J Trauma Stress* 5:377, 1992.

In this article, Herman discusses the range of symptoms that often accompany PTSD in individuals who have been exposed to chronic trauma. This syndrome often includes medical problems and somatization, and thus should be of particular interest to primary care clinicians.

Waitzkin H, Magana H: The black box in somatization: Unexplained physical symptoms, culture, and narratives of trauma. *Soc Sci Med* 45:811, 1997.

This is a very interesting and provocative account of Waitzkin and Magana's experiences with trauma as a root cause of somatization in some primary care patients. The authors discuss issues around processing of traumatic events and offer evidence to suggest that allowing patients to "tell their story" in a coherent way may be a powerful way to reduce suffering and disability.

Bibliography

American Psychiatric Association: *Diagnostic and Statistical Manual of Mental Disorders*, 3rd ed. Washington, DC: American Psychiatric Association; 1980.

American Psychiatric Association: *Diagnostic and Statistical Manual of Mental Disorders,* 3rd ed, revised. Washington, DC: American Psychiatric Association, 1987.

American Psychiatric Association: *Diagnostic and Statistical Manual of Mental Disorders,* 4th ed. Washington, DC: American Psychiatric Association, 1994.

Andreski P, Chilcoat H, Breslau N: Post-traumatic stress disorder and somatization symptoms: A prospective study. *Psychiatry Res* 79:131, 1998.

Andrykowski M, Cordova MJ: Factors associated with PTSD symptoms following treatment for breast cancer: Test of the Andersen model. *J Trauma Stress* 11:189, 1998.

Antoni MH: Empirical studies of emotional disclosure in the face of stress: A progress report. *Adv Mind-Body Med* 15:163, 1999.

Baker D, Brady K, Goldstein S, et al: Double-blind flexible dose multicenter study of sertraline and placebo in outpatients with post-traumatic stress disorder. *Eur Neuropsychopharmacol* 8(Suppl 2):S261, 1998.

Ballenger J, Davidson J, Lecrubier Y, et al: Consensus statement on posttraumatic stress disorder from the International Consensus Group on Depression and Anxiety. *J Clin Psychiatry* 61(Suppl 5):60, 2000.

Ballenger JC: Introduction: Focus on posttraumatic stress disorder. *J Clin Psychiatry* 61(Suppl 5):3, 2000.

Barlow DH, Lehman CL: Advances in the psychosocial treatment of anxiety disorders: Implications for national health care. *Arch Gen Psychiatry* 53:727, 1996.

Beckham JC, Moore SD, Feldman ME, et al: Health status, somatization, and severity of posttraumatic stress disorder in Vietnam combat veterans with posttraumatic stress disorder. *Am J Psychiatry* 155:1565, 1998.

Beebe DK, Gulledge KM, Lee CM, et al: Prevalence of sexual assault among women patients seen in family practice clinics. *Fam Pract Res J* 14:223, 1994.

Berton MW, Stabb SD: Exposure to violence and post-traumatic stress disorder in urban adolescents. *Adolescence* 31:489, 1996.

Blanchard EB, Hickling EJ, Vollmer AJ, et al: Short-term follow-up of post-traumatic stress symptoms in motor vehicle accident victims. *Behav Res Ther* 33: 369, 1995.

Booth R: Language, self, meaning, and health. *Adv Mind-Body Med* 15:171, 1999.

Borkan J, Schvartzman P, Reis S, et al: Stories from the sealed rooms: Patient interviews during the Gulf War. *Fam Pract* 10:188, 1993.

Bravo M, Rubio-Stipec M, Canino GJ, et al: The psychological sequelae of disaster stress prospectively and retrospectively evaluated. *Am J Community Psychol* 18:661, 1990.

Bremner JD, Southwick SM, Johnson DR, et al: Childhood physical abuse and combat-related posttraumatic stress disorder in Vietnam veterans. *Am J Psychiatry* 150:235, 1993.

Breslau N, Davis GC, Andreski P, et al: Traumatic events and posttraumatic stress disorder in an urban population of young adults. *Arch Gen Psychiatry* 48:216, 1991.

Breslau N, Davis GC: Posttraumatic stress disorder in an urban population of young adults: Risk factors for chronicity. *Am J Psychiatry* 149:671, 1992.

Breslau N, Davis GC, Andreski P: Risk factors for PTSD-related traumatic events: A prospective analysis. *Am J Psychiatry* 152:529, 1995.

Ciccone PE, Greenstein RA: Dr. Ciccone and associates reply. *Am J Psychiatry* 146:812, 1989.

Connor K, Sutherland S, Tupler L, et al: Fluoxetine in post-traumatic stress disorder: Randomised, double-blind study. *Br J Psychiatry* 175:17, 1999.

Davidson J: Pharmacotherapy of posttraumatic stress disorder: Treatment options, long-term follow-up, and predictors of outcome. *J Clin Psychiatry* 61 (Suppl 5):52, 2000.

Davidson J: Discussion (Pharmacotherapy of posttraumatic stress disorder: Treatment options, long-term follow-up, and predictors of outcome). *J Clin Psychiatry* 61(Suppl 5):57, 2000.

Davidson J, Kudler H, Smith R, et al: Treatment of posttraumatic stress disorder with amitriptyline and placebo. *Arch Gen Psychiatry* 47:259, 1990.

Davidson J, Fairbank J: The epidemiology of posttraumatic stress disorder. In: *Posttraumatic Stress Disorder: DSM-IV and Beyond.* Washington, DC: American Psychiatric Press; 1990.

Davidson JRT, Weisler RH, Malik M, et al: Fluvoxamine in civilians with posttraumatic stress disorder. *J Clin Psychopharmacol* 18:93, 1998.

Decoufle P, Holmgreen P, Boyle CA, et al: Self-reported health status of Vietnam veterans in relation to perceived exposure to herbicides and combat. *Am J Epidemiol* 135:312, 1992.

Devilly G, Spence S: The relative efficacy and treatment distress of EMDR and a cognitive-behavior trauma protocol in the amelioration of posttraumatic stress disorder. *J Anxiety Disord* 13:131, 1999.

Dickinson L, de Gruy FV, Dickinson WP, et al: Complex posttraumatic stress disorder: Evidence from the primary care setting. *Gen Hosp Psychiatry* 20: 214, 1998.

Dickinson LM, de Gruy FV, Dickinson WP, et al: Health-related quality of life and symptom profiles of female survivors of sexual abuse in primary care. *Arch Fam Med* 8:35, 1999.

Dickinson WP, Dickinson LM, Adams M, et al: Abuse and violence in primary care patients. Presented at the annual meeting of the Society for Teachers of Family Medicine. Chicago, IL: April 1998.

Dienstfrey H: Disclosure and health: An interview with James W. Pennebaker. *Advan Mind-Body Med* 15: 161, 1999.

Dumas CA, Katerndahl DA, Burge SK: Familial patterns in patients with infrequent panic attacks. *Arch Fam Med* 4:863, 1995.

Elliott BA, Johnson MMP: Domestic violence in a primary care setting. *Arch Fam Med* 4:113, 1995.

Escobar JI, Canino G, Rubio-Stipec M, et al: Somatic symptoms after a natural disaster: A prospective study. *Am J Psychiatry* 149:965, 1992.

Etten MV, Taylor S: Comparative efficacy of treatments for posttraumatic stress disorder: A meta-analysis. *Clin Psychol Psychother* 5:125, 1998.

Fairbank J, Keane T: Flooding for combat-related stress disorders: Assessment of anxiety reduction across traumatic memories. *Behav Ther* 13:499, 1982.

Foa E: Psychosocial treatment of posttraumatic stress disorder. *J Clin Psychiatry* 61(Suppl 5):43, 2000.

Foa E, Dancu C, Hembree E, et al: A comparison of exposure therapy, stress inoculation training, and their combination for reducing posttraumatic stress disorder in female assault victims. *J Consult Clin Psychol* 67:194, 1999.

Foa E, Rothbaum B: *Treating the Trauma of Rape*. New York: Guilford Press; 1997.

Foa E, Meadows E: Psychosocial treatments for posttraumatic stress disorder: A critical review. *Annu Rev Psychol* 48:449, 1997.

Friedman MJ: Posttraumatic stress disorder. *J Clin Psychiatry* 58(Suppl 9):33, 1997.

Friedman MJ, Charney DS, Deutch AY (eds): *Neurobiological and Clinical Consequences of Stress: From Normal Adaptation of PTSD*. New York: Lippincott-Raven; 1995, p 507.

Friedman MJ, Schnurr PP: The relationship between trauma, PTSD, and physical health. In: Giaconia RM, Reinherz HZ, Silverman AB, et al (eds): Traumas and posttraumatic stress disorder in a community population of older adolescents. *J Am Acad Child Adolesc Psychiatry* 34:1369, 1995.

Giaconia RM, Reinherz HZ, Silverman AB, et al: Traumas and posttraumatic stress disorder in a community population of older adolescents. *J Am Acad Child Adolesc Psychiatry* 34:1369, 1995.

Gould DA, Stevens NG, Ward NG, et al: Self-reported childhood abuse in an adult population in a primary care setting. *Arch Fam Med* 3:252, 1994.

Greenwood CL, Tangalos EG, Maruta T: Prevalence of sexual abuse, physical abuse and concurrent traumatic life events in a general medical population. *Mayo Clin Proc* 65:1067, 1990.

Hamberger LK, Saunders DG, Hovey M: Prevalence of domestic violence in community practice and rate of physician inquiry. *Fam Med* 24:283, 1992.

Helzer JE, Robins LN, McEvoy L: Post-traumatic stress disorder in the general population. *N Engl J Med* 317:1630, 1987.

Herman JL: Complex PTSD: A syndrome in survivors of prolonged and repeated trauma. *J Trauma Stress* 5:377, 1992.

Hertzberg M, Butterfield N, Feldman M, et al: A preliminary study of lamotrigine for the treatment of posttraumatic stress disorder. *Biol Psychiatry* 45:1226, 1999.

Horowitz M: Stress response syndromes, character style and dynamic psychotherapy. *Arch Gen Psychiatry* 31:768, 1974.

Ironson G, Wynings C, Schneiderman N, et al: Posttraumatic stress symptoms, intrusive thoughts, loss, and immune function after Hurricane Andrew. *Psychosom Med* 59:128, 1997.

Keane T, Fairbank J, Caddell J, et al: Implosive (flooding) therapy reduces symptoms of PTSD in Vietnam combat veterans. *Behav Ther* 20:245, 1989.

Kessler RC, Sonnega A, Bromet E, et al: Posttraumatic stress disorder in the national comorbidity survey. *Arch Gen Psychiatry* 52:1048, 1995.

Kessler RC: Posttraumatic stress disorder: The burden to the individual and to society. *J Clin Psychiatry* 61(Suppl 5):4, 2000.

Klein NA, Dow BM, Brown SA, et al: Sertraline efficacy in depressed combat veterans with posttraumatic stress disorder [letter]. *Am J Psychiatry* 151:621, 1994.

Koss MP, Koss PG, Woodruff WJ: Deleterious effects of criminal victimization on women's health and medical utilization. *Arch Intern Med* 151:342, 1991.

Kosten T, Frank J, Dan E, et al: Pharmacotherapy for posttraumatic stress disorder using phenelzine or imipramine. *J Nerv Ment Dis* 179:366, 1991.

Kulka RA, Schlenger WE, Fairbank JA, et al: *Trauma and the Vietnam War Generation.* Report of Findings from the National Vietnam Veterans Readjustment Study. New York: Brunner/Mazel; 1990.

Lange A, van de Ven JP, Schrieken BA, et al: Internet-mediated, protocol-driven treatment of psychological dysfunction. *J Telemed Telecare* 6:15, 2000.

Lechner ME, Vogel M, Garcia-Shelton LM, et al: Self-reported medical problems of adult female survivors of childhood sexual abuse. *J Fam Pract* 36:633, 1993.

Lemieux AM, Coe CL: Abuse-related posttraumatic stress disorder: Evidence for chronic neuro-endocrine activation in women. *Psychosom Med* 57: 105, 1995.

Leskin G, Kaloupek D, Keane T: Treatment for traumatic memories: Review and recommendations. *Clin Psychol Rev* 18:983, 1998.

Lindy JD, Green BL, Grace M: Somatic reenactment in the treatment of posttraumatic stress disorder. *Psychother Psychosom* 57:1806, 1992.

Loewenstein RJ: Somatoform disorders in victims of incest and child abuse. In: Kleuft RP (ed): *Incest-Related Syndromes of Adult Psychopathology.* Washington, DC: American Psychiatric Press; 1990.

Marks I, Lovell K, Noshirvani H, et al: Treatment of posttraumatic stress disorder by exposure and/or cognitive restructuring: A controlled study. *Arch Gen Psychiatry* 55:317, 1998.

Marshall RD, Schneier FR, Fallon BA, et al: An open trial of paroxetine in patients with noncombat-related, chronic posttraumatic stress disorder. *J Clin Psychopharmacol* 18:10, 1998.

Mazza D, Dennerstein L, Ryan V: Physical, sexual and emotional violence against women: A general practice-based prevalence study. *Med J Aust* 164:14, 1996.

McCauley J, Kern D, Kolodner K, et al: Clinical characteristics of women with a history of childhood abuse. *JAMA* 277:1362, 1997.

McFarlane A: Individual psychotherapy for posttraumatic stress disorder. *Psychiatr Clin North Am* 17:393, 1994.

McFarlane AC: Discussion (Posttraumatic stress disorder: A model of the longitudinal course and the role of risk factors). *J Clin Psychiatry* 61(Suppl 5):15, 2000.

McFarlane AC, et al: Physical symptoms in posttraumatic stress disorder. *J Psychosom Res* 38:715, 1994.

McFarlane AC, Papay P: Multiple diagnoses in posttraumatic stress disorder in the victims of a natural disaster. *J Nerv Ment Dis* 180:498, 1992.

Norris FH: Epidemiology of trauma: Frequency and impact of different potentially traumatic events on different demographic groups. *J Consult Clin Psychol* 60:409, 1992.

Pelcovitz D, van der Kolk B, Roth S, et al: Development of a criteria set and a structured interview for disorders of extreme stress (SIDES). *J Trauma Stress* 10:3, 1997.

Pelcovitz D, Libov BG, Mandel F, et al: Posttraumatic stress disorder and family functioning in adolescent cancer. *J Trauma Stress* 11:205, 1998.

Pennebaker JW: Putting stress into words: Health, linguistic, and therapeutic implications. *Behav Res Ther* 31:539, 1993.

Pennebaker JW, Barger SD, Tiebout J: Disclosure of traumas and health among Holocaust survivors. *Psychosom Med* 51:577, 1989.

Pennebaker JW, Colder M, Sharp LK: Accelerating the coping process. *J Pers Soc Psychol* 58:528, 1990.

Petrie KJ, Booth RJ, Pennebaker JW, et al: Disclosure of trauma and immune response to a Hepatitis B vaccination program. *J Consult Clin Psychol* 63:787, 1995.

Petrie KJ, Booth RJ, Pennebaker JW: The immunological effects of thought suppression. *J Pers Soc Psychol* 75:1264, 1998.

Pitman R, Orr S, de Jong J, et al: Prevalence of posttraumatic stress disorder in wounded Vietnam veterans. *Am J Psychiatry* 146:667, 1989.

Radomsky NA: The association of parental alcoholism and rigidity with chronic illness and abuse among women. *J Fam Pract* 35:54, 1992.

Resick P, Schnicke M: Cognitive processing therapy for sexual assault victims. *J Consult Clin Psychol* 55:317, 1992.

Resnick HS, Kilpatrick DG, Dansky BS, et al: Prevalence of civilian trauma and posttraumatic stress disorder in a representative national sample of women. *J Consult Clin Psychol* 61:984, 1993.

Rime B: Expressing emotion, physical health, and emotional relief: A cognitive-social perspective. *Adv Mind-Body Med* 15:175, 1999.

Robins LN, Helzer JE, Croughan J, et al: National Institute of Mental Health Diagnostic Interview Schedule. *Arch Gen Psychiatry* 38:381, 1981.

Rosser R: Post-traumatic stress disorder. *Practitioner* 238:393, 1994.

Roth S, Newman E, Pelcovitz D, et al: Complex PTSD in victims exposed to sexual and physical abuse: Results from the DSM-IV field trial for posttraumatic stress disorder. *J Trauma Stress* 10:359, 1997.

Rothbaum B: A controlled study of eye movement desensitization and reprocessing in the treatment of posttraumatic stress disordered sexual assault victims. *Bull Menninger Clin* 61:317, 1997.

Selley C: Post-traumatic stress disorder. *Practitioner* 235:635, 1991.

Shalev A: Measuring outcome in posttraumatic stress disorder. *J Clin Psychiatry* 61(Suppl 5):33, 2000.

Shalev A, Bleich A, Ursano RJ: Posttraumatic stress disorder: Somatic comorbidity and effort tolerance. *Psychosomatics* 31:197, 1990.

Shalev A, Omer B, Spencer E: Treatment of post-traumatic stress disorder: A review. *Psychosom Med* 58:165, 1996.

Sherman J: Effects of psychotherapeutic treatments for PTSD: A meta-analysis of controlled clinical trials. *J Trauma Stress* 11:413, 1998.

Shore JH, Vollmer WM, Tatum EL: Community patterns of posttraumatic stress disorders. *J Nerv Ment Dis* 177:681, 1989.

Silva C, McFarlane AC, Soeken K, et al: Symptoms of post-traumatic disorder in abused women in a primary care setting. *J Women Health* 6:543, 1997.

Singer MI, Anglin TM, Song LM, et al: Adolescents' exposure to violence and associated symptoms of psychological trauma. *JAMA* 273:477, 1995.

Smyth JM: Written disclosure: Evidence, potential mechanism, and potential treatment. *Adv Mind-Body Med* 15:179, 1999.

Smyth JM, Stone AA, Hurewitz A, et al: Effects of writing about stressful experiences on symptom reduction in patients with asthma or rheumatoid arthritis. *JAMA* 281:1304, 1999.

Solomon Z: Somatic complaints, stress reaction, and posttraumatic stress disorder: A three-year follow-up study. *Behav Med* 14:179, 1988.

Solomon Z, Bleich A, Koslowsky M, et al: Post-traumatic stress disorder: Issues of co-morbidity. *J Psychiatr Res* 25:89, 1991.

Solomon Z, Mikulincer M: Combat stress reactions, post traumatic stress disorder and somatic complaints among Israeli soldiers. *J Psychosom Res* 31: 131, 1987.

Solomon Z, Mikulincer M, Habershaim N: Life-events, coping strategies, social resources, and somatic complaints among combat stress reaction casualties. *Br J Med Psychol* 63:137, 1990.

Solomon Z, Mikulincer M, Kotler M: A two year follow-up of somatic complaints among Israeli combat stress reaction casualties. *J Psychosom Res* 31:463, 1987.

Springs FE, Friedrich WN: Health risk behaviors and medical sequelae of childhood sexual abuse. *Mayo Clin Proc* 67:527, 1992.

Stein MB, Walker MR, Hazen AL, et al: Full and partial posttraumatic stress disorder: Findings from a community survey. *Am J Psychiatry* 154:1114, 1997.

Suedfeld P, Pennebaker JW: Health outcomes and cognitive aspects of recalled negative life events. *Psychosom Med* 59:172, 1997.

Tarrier N, Pilgrim H, Sommerfield C, et al: A randomized trial of cognitive therapy and imaginal exposure in the treatment of chronic posttraumatic stress disorder. *J Consult Clin Psychol* 67:13, 1999.

Tiller J, Kyrios M, Bennett P: Post traumatic stress disorder. *Aust Fam Physician* 25:1569, 1996.

Traue HC, Deighton R: Inhibition, disclosure, and health: Don't simply slash the Gordian knot. *Adv Mind-Body Med* 15:184, 1999.

van der Kolk BA, Dreyfuss D, Michaels M, et al: Fluoxetine in posttraumatic stress disorder. *J Clin Psychiatry* 55:517, 1994.

van der Kolk BA, Pelcovitz D, Roth S, et al: Dissociation, somatization, and affect dysregulation: The complexity of adaptation to trauma. *Am J Psychiatry* 153:83, 1996.

van der Kolk DD, Michaels M, Shera D, et al: Fluoxetine in posttraumatic stress disorders. *Yearbook Psychiatry Appl Ment Health* 7:276, 1996.

Veronen L, Kilpatrick D: Stress management for rape victims. In: Meichenbaum D, Jaremko M (eds): *Stress Reduction and Prevention.* New York: Plenum; 1983, p 341.

Wagner PJ, Mongan P, Hamrick D, et al: Experience of abuse in primary care patients. *Arch Fam Med* 4:956, 1995.

Waitzkin H, Magana H: The black box in somatization: Unexplained physical symptoms, culture, and narratives of trauma. *Soc Sci Med* 45:811, 1997.

Walch AG, Broadhead WE: Prevalence of lifetime sexual victimization among female patients. *J Fam Pract* 35:511, 1992.

Walker EA, Katon WJ, Hanson J, et al: Medical and psychiatric symptoms in women with childhood sexual abuse. *Psychosom Med* 54:658, 1992.

Walker EA, Torkelson N, Katon WJ, et al: The prevalence rate of sexual abuse in a primary care clinic. *J Am Board Fam Pract* 6:465, 1993.

Weinstein HM, Dansky L, Iacopino V: Torture and war trauma survivors in primary care practice. *West J Med* 165:112, 1996.

Zaidi LY, Foy DW: Childhood abuse and combat-related PTSD. *J Trauma Stress* 4:325, 1991.

Frank Verloin deGruy, III

Mental Symptoms

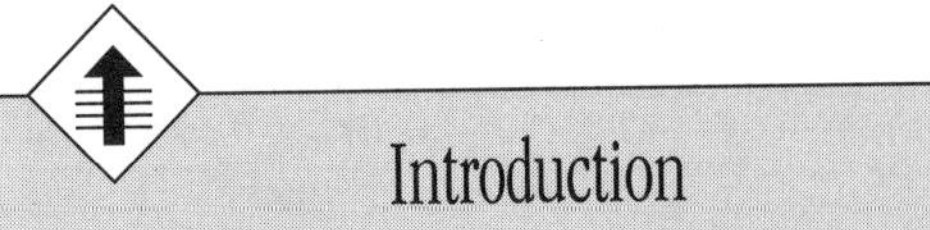

Introduction

Several chapters in this book deal with mental disorders in the primary care setting—depression, panic, anxiety, somatoform disorders, and alcohol and tobacco abuse. Mental disorders as they are described in these chapters might be defined as the DSM-IV manual defines them: distinct psychological or behavioral syndromes or patterns that are associated with distress or impaired function, or the risk of pain, disability, loss of freedom, or death. For most mental health providers, the diagnostic criteria for mental disorders that are spelled out in the DSM-IV manual are accepted as the gold standard. But mental symptoms have significant effects on primary care patients and their clinicians long before the symptoms accumulate and consolidate into a pattern that meets DSM criteria as a mental disorder. In addition, mental *symptoms* may become important long before they cluster into syndromes. Even a single mental symptom can be disabling.

Mental symptoms are part of virtually all primary care visits, and their presence can have a pronounced effect on the outcomes of those visits. A successful medical encounter depends on the adequacy with which clinicians identify and address these mental symptoms.

Think about mental symptomatology along a continuum of severity with minor symptoms at one end of the spectrum and mental disorders at the severe end of this continuum. Although many chapters in this text addressed mental disorders, this chapter will address the rest of the continuum, from so-called subthreshold conditions all the way down to single mental health symptoms. Subthreshold conditions are important in primary care by virtue of their high prevalence, the cost of care, and the burden of suffering associated with their presence. The further one moves down the continuum from mental disorders toward simple symptoms, the more important are the personal meaning of the symptoms, their functional consequence, their context, their association with other symptoms or medical problems, their behavior over time, and the response people have to them. The remainder of this introductory section will describe these aspects of mental symptoms and patients' reactions to the symptoms.

What Is a Symptom?

Perhaps the least controversial way to define a mental symptom would be to count any symptom that appears in the DSM-IV. There are over 250 diagnoses in the DSM-IV manual, some of which require a half dozen or more symptoms to meet criteria; thus, there are well over 1000 symptoms in the this manual. Essentially all primary care patients have at least one of these symptoms. In fact, virtually all *people*, whether or not they are patients, will sometimes report at least one of the symptoms found in the DSM manual. There is neither the space in this chapter nor the supporting research to justify looking at this enormous set of symptoms one by one—nor would it make any sense to a primary care clinician—so we will confine ourselves to a few of the most common symptoms. The symptoms in the somatoform section were dealt with in Chap. 14. The most important symptoms of substance abuse were addressed in Chap. 6. Within Axis II of the DSM-IV, which includes personality disorders, much of the relevant material has been covered in Chap. 11 and will not be dealt with in detail here. Thus, in this chapter we will be considering the few mood and anxiety symptoms listed in Table 20-1, with only passing reference to somatoform and other symptoms.

Meaning of Symptoms Vary

Patients may come to a primary care office because of a medical problem or a physical symptom to which they are having an incidental psychological reaction, or they may come in because a mental symptom has itself become the focus of concern and a source of impairment. A mental symptom

Table 20-1

Mood and Anxiety Symptoms

During the past two weeks, have you experienced a lot of any of these?
Feeling down or depressed most of the day?
Losing interest or pleasure in things previously interesting or pleasurable?
Lost or gained a lot or weight, or lost or gained your appetite?
Insomnia or sleeping too much?
Being slowed down or agitated?
Fatigued?
Feeling worthless or very guilty?
Trouble concentrating or making decisions?
Thoughts of death or suicide?
Having an attack of intense fear or panic?
Palpitations or heart pounding or racing?
Trembling or shaking?
Sweating?
Smothering or choking?
Chest pain or discomfort?
Nausea or abdominal discomfort?
Dizziness or faintness?
Fear of dying or going crazy?
Numbness?
Chills or hot flashes?
Excessive worry about a lot of things?
Being restless or on edge?
Being irritable?
Having muscle tension?

may actually be a solution to a problem rather than the problem itself, such as when mild anxiety motivates a person to do an unpleasant task. Sometimes a symptom is perfectly understandable and fitting, such as guilt at forgetting a daughter's wedding. Sometimes a symptom's meaning is obscure, or it has no meaning, such as the mysterious appearance of nocturnal awakening with fear that appears out of the blue. The following three cases illustrate some of these distinctions.

LAURA BANNOCK *Laura Bannock has returned as you requested to follow up on her diabetes mellitus. Two weeks ago you first made this diagnosis and instituted a regimen of diet, exercise, an oral hypoglycemic agent, and home monitoring of her blood glucose levels. She returns today with a number of new questions about her dietary requirements and an incomplete home monitoring log. When you ask her how she is adjusting to the diagnosis of diabetes, she bursts into tears and tells you that she is very sad about having this condition and thinks it means the end of the good health she has enjoyed up to this point. She does not see much point in making all the adjustments in her life that you have requested, because the diabetes cannot be cured anyway.*

ARTHUR BLANFORD *Arthur Blanford has returned 2 two weeks before his scheduled follow up for hypercholesterolemia, which you diagnosed 2 weeks ago during a routine check for cardiac risk factors. He reports that he is taking his medication and following his diet and exercise regimen faithfully, but that he is "worried sick" about this new problem. He believes that this means he will die young of heart disease, as his father did, and he cannot sleep because of worry. In fact, he's been sleeping so poorly at night that he has begun to fall asleep at work and during his commute home, and this has added to his worries, which are in a worsening spiral. He wants you to give him something to help with his sleep.*

DONALD MOORE *Donald Moore is in the office to have an ingrown toenail treated. During the procedure, you ask how he is doing, and he tells you that for the past month he has been waking up at 3 AM in a panic. You are concerned and ask him to tell you more about it. It turns out that he was getting up and writing a business plan that was due, but that he had been unable to complete during the workday. He finished 3 days ago and has been sleeping normally since.*

It is easy to see that these symptoms have entirely different meanings and call for different responses from the clinician. In the first case, one might understand the symptom of pessimism or despair as a normal way of adjusting to a chronic disease that has serious consequences. All that might be necessary is to increase the level of supportive counseling and patient education, or simply monitor her closely. In the second case, one might prescribe a regimen of sleep hygiene and possibly prescribe a hypnotic medication for a short time. In the third case, one would not view the symptom as a problem requiring intervention and would simply monitor for recurrence. As these three cases demonstrate, the meaning of a symptom—from both the clinician's and the patient's perspectives—affect how we should think about and address the symptom.

Functional Consequences Differ

In addition to understanding the meaning of the symptom, the clinician should also seek to understand the functional consequences the symptom has on a patient. As part of learning whether a mental symptom is incidental or has itself become a primary problem, the clinician should learn the extent to which the symptom is causing harm to the patient's health or welfare. For example, insomnia has one meaning if it is simply causing mild fatigue but it has a very different meaning if it is causing a measurable impairment in work productivity or driving safety. These two extremes would call for different interventions on the part of the primary care clinician.

Symptom severity is more important than diagnostic specificity. As we will see when we review subthreshold syndromes later in this chapter, there are instances in which diagnostic specificity breaks down, and patients cluster more in terms of their symptom severity, while the symptoms themselves cut across the normal diagnostic categories.

Context Is Important

A given symptom can have an entirely different meaning and require an entirely different response depending on the context in which it arises. Consider the two different presentations of the same symptom in the case of Marla Toover versus that of Carla Rubin.

MARLA TOOVER *Marla Toover cannot even go to the grocery store without looking over her shoulder to see if anyone is following her. She reports that this constant vigilance is getting old, but it is appropriate for her to behave this way; her former husband threatened to kill her if she left him, which she did. In fact, last month he caught her in the parking lot and split her lip with his fist. She has secured a restraining order and next week intends to move to another state.*

CARLA RUBIN *Carla Rubin cannot even go to the grocery store without looking over her shoulder to see if anyone is following her. This began a month ago and does not seem to be related to any recent or past danger, trauma, or harm. In her calmer moments she knows she has nothing to fear, that nobody is following her, but this problem is getting worse and is profoundly disturbing—she has stopped going out into public places unless she absolutely has to. She thinks she must be going crazy.*

Ms. Toover's hypervigilance occurs in a context of real threat and danger and is thus a rational and reasonable response—a symptom that represents normal behavior. The clinician should be most concerned for her physical safety. Ms. Rubin has the same mental symptom, but her symptom occurs in a drastically different context. She is not under the threat of physical danger, and her clinician should be more concerned with her psychological condition than her physical safety.

Mental Symptoms Are Associated with Other Symptoms

Another important characteristic of mental symptoms is their relationship to other mental symptoms. Psychological symptoms almost always have "company," and the presence of one symptom should prompt a search for other mental symptoms or disorders, physical symptoms, medical diseases, or impairment of some other sort. The comorbid conditions that will likely be found can change the significance of the first symptom. For example, jitteriness and anxiety associated with hyperthyroidism could be understood as a consequence of the thyroid condition and could actually be used to monitor the adequacy of treatment. Jitteriness and anxiety associated with alcohol use might be understood as a symptom that points to a more important behavioral problem that requires attention. We will examine this issue of comorbidity more closely in the section on subthreshold conditions.

Duration Is Significant

Finally, when considering the significance of a symptom, clinicians must consider the duration or time course of the symptom. A symptom that has been present for years is different from the same symptom that recently arose; a symptom that is improving is different from the same symptom, of the same intensity, that is worsening. Many mental symptoms wax and wane, and profiling their time course can provide very useful information. For example, in someone who has had a previous major depressive episode, the onset of a loss of interest in previously interesting things might represent the first evidence of a recurrence, whereas an equivalent lack of interest in someone who is recovering from a major depressive episode, and in whom the anhedonia was previously much more severe, is a somewhat reassuring finding.

Considering the characteristics of symptoms described (meaning, functional consequences, context, associated symptoms, and time course) will help a clinician gain a useful perspective regarding the relative significance of mental symptom. In the next section, subthreshold syndromes are described. Compared to the patient who has one or two mental symptoms, patients with subthreshold syndromes may be more impaired and require more attention and intervention from their clinician.

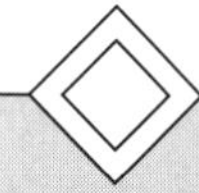

Subthreshold Syndromes

On the continuum between mental disorders and solitary mental symptoms lies the subthreshold syndrome. A *subthreshold syndrome* is an aggregate of symptoms that leans toward a disorder, but does not quite get there. Whereas one patient with a diagnosed mental disorder has symptoms that meet the diagnostic criteria, a second patient with a subthreshold syndrome has numerous symptoms but does meet the diagnostic criteria for a disorder. Even without a distinct diagnosis, however, the second person may be very impaired. In 1990, Broadhead and associates reported that subthreshold or minor depression was associated with significant impairment. Since that time, subthreshold depression and many other subthreshold conditions have come under investigation. In general, these conditions turn out to be as common as or more common than their full-blown counterparts and are generally associated with impairment or disability somewhere between patients meeting full diagnostic criteria and unaffected patients.

Subthreshold mental diagnoses, at least in the primary care setting, rarely exist in pure form. Classification of patients with subthreshold syndromes has been somewhat problematic because of the extensive comorbidity with other mental diagnoses. Several investigators have explored the nature of this comorbidity and have used cluster analysis, grade of membership analysis, and other strategies to search for alternative classifications. Nevertheless, for the sake of building a model of the phenomenology of psychological symptomatology in primary care, I will first describe them as if they were discrete entities, and then explore ways that they coexist, intersect, and interact with one another.

Depression

Subthreshold, or minor depression, is the best studied of the subthreshold conditions and has recently been reviewed by Williams. Although there is no universally accepted definition of subthreshold depression, most have agreed on the presence of just two or more of the symptoms from the DSM schedule for major depression as the diagnostic criteria. It occurs at least as frequently as major depression and is almost as disabling. Currently, there is insufficient evidence to conclude that antidepressants are an effective treatment, but as many as half of these patients will progress to major depression, at which time pharmacotherapy is usually indicated. Consider the presentation of Eugenia Lightfoot.

EUGENIA LIGHTFOOT *Eugenia Lightfoot is in the office with an ankle sprain, and she seems inordinately depressed to you. When asked, she admits that she has been very sad and blue for the last month. She acknowledges that her appetite has fallen off in the last month. This is unrelated to her ankle injury, and she has no other depressive symptoms. Ms. Lightfoot believes these symptoms are hurting her work performance, and her husband is both worried about her change in appetite and irritated that she seems to be withdrawing from him. These symptoms remind Ms. Lightfoot of similar symptoms she experienced 5 years ago, except that time she became severely depressed.*

This is a disturbing presentation, and the clinician would be well advised to take Ms. Lightfoot's symptoms seriously. Even though the preponderance of evidence is against prescribing antidepressant medication for minor depression, office counseling is indicated, close monitoring for worsening is definitely indicated, and a search for other mental and medical conditions may be revealing.

Panic

Subthreshold panic might consist of a single full-blown panic attack, attacks at a lower frequency than necessary for the full diagnosis, or panic disorder with fewer attack symptoms than the requisite for a panic attack as described in DSM-IV. All of these potential presentations of subthreshold panic are associated with increased health care utilization and functional impairment. In at least one study, utilization and impairment among patients with subthreshold panic were more severe than among patients meeting the full criteria for panic disorder. The most likely reason for this is the extremely high comorbidity, which itself is associated with functional impairment, as discussed at the end of this section.

EUGENIA LIGHTFOOT (CONTINUED) *Ms. Lightfoot returns to see you in a month, as you requested. She reports that her sad mood is about the same, but all in all she is worse. She has no new depressive symptoms, but when she was driving to work one day last week, she was overcome with a sudden wave of desperate fear. She thought she was going to die, her heart was racing, she became nauseated, she almost passed out, and she pulled off the road onto the shoulder for half an hour and rode out the panic attack inside her car. A full attack has not happened again, but since then she has experienced headaches, shoulder pain, and waves of nausea similar to symptoms she had during her panic attack. She is asking you for medication to help with all these symptoms before she loses her job.*

Ms. Lightfoot's subthreshold depression is now compounded by subthreshold panic as well as several somatoform symptoms. Her functional impairment is becoming very pronounced. This is not an unusual presentation of subthreshold panic. In one study in a family practice setting by deGruy and colleagues, no patients were identified as having subthreshold panic alone; all had a concurrent mental or subthreshold diagnosis. Patients with multiple subthreshold diagnoses may be profoundly impaired. There is no research evidence testing the effectiveness of either pharmacotherapy or psychotherapy in such situations, but a clinician would be hard pressed to do nothing in the face of such obvious distress. Certainly supportive counseling would be appropriate, and eventually we may learn that medication, psychotherapy, or both is beneficial in such cases.

Post-Traumatic Stress Disorder

If subthreshold post-traumatic stress disorder (PTSD) is defined as the occurrence of an extreme, distressing event, plus one symptom of persistent reexperiencing of the event, or two symptoms of avoidance or numbing, or three symptoms of hyperarousal, then this disorder is more common than PTSD and just as incapacitating. As with panic, the extent of comorbidity may account for much of this disability: over 80 percent of primary care patients with subthreshold PTSD have a somatoform disorder, and almost 60 percent have minor or major depression.

Generalized Anxiety Disorder

The diagnosis of generalized anxiety disorder (GAD) requires the presence for at least 6 months of at least three symptoms such as feeling restless or on edge, irritability, difficulty concentrating, muscle tension, being easily fatigued, or having trouble with sleep. Many people, however, do not wait 6 months before seeking help. Subthreshold GAD can be defined as the full symptom requirement specified in DSM-IV, but without the duration requirement being met. More primary care patients fit this subthreshold category than meet the full criteria. Like somatization and depression, their functional health is between those with the full syndrome and those below the subthreshold cutoff. John Hanes is a good example of a patient presenting with subthreshold GAD.

JOHN HANES *John Hanes has slept through his alarm twice in the last week and is worried that he will get fired. That is not his only worry. In fact, he worries all the time. For the past 6 weeks, he has noticed a worsening muscle tension, irritability, and trouble falling asleep. Even when he finally falls asleep, he tosses and wakes frequently. He works as a school bus driver and lately has been almost unable to drag himself to work. He cannot say whether he is more worried about what has gone wrong or what might go wrong, but he is plenty worried about both. He comes in asking for something for sleep and some advice about the tension in his shoulders. Despite this story, his hypertension is under good control, and his plantar fasciitis has stabilized since it was injected 2 weeks ago. You eventually discover that Mr. Hanes also has lost his interest in woodcarving, which used to be his favorite hobby, and has begun thinking that the world would be better off without him.*

Comorbidity

Perhaps the most striking feature of the subthreshold conditions is the extent to which they overlap with one another. Fig. 20-1 summarizes the extent of overlap of subthreshold conditions in the Somatization in Primary Care dataset. The dataset shows that

- Seventy-five percent of patients with depression also have somatization.
- Of the patients with subthreshold PTSD, 80 percent have a somatizing syndrome and 60 percent have at least minor depression
- Eighty percent of subthreshold GAD patients have at least minor depression and 75 percent have a somatoform disorder
- Eighty percent of the patients with subthreshold panic have at least minor depression and 80 percent have a somatoform condition.

In other words, patients who have one subthreshold conditions have many additional conditions, so much so that the concept of comorbidity is hardly adequate to describe what they have.

Using several analytic approaches, Piccinelli and associates found a large group of patients with mixed anxiety-depression, and Nease and colleagues described four clusters of patients with mixed anxiety-depression that differed from one another principally on the basis of the severity of their symptoms. The two intermediate clusters were moderately severe, differing from one another only in the severity of their depressive symptoms. Analyses of this sort most likely expose only the

Figure 20-1

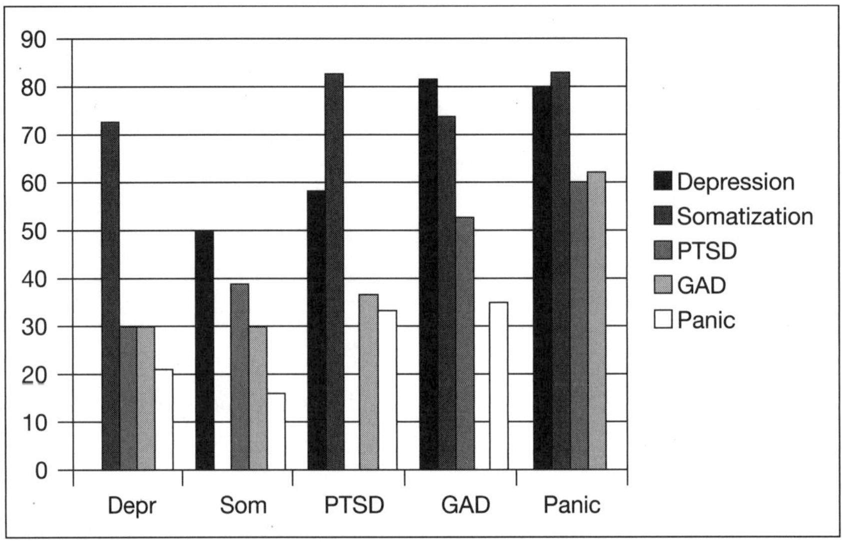

The graph shown here summarizes the extent of overlap of subthreshold conditions in the Somatization of Primary Care data set. Patients who have one diagnosis have many diagnoses, so much so that the concept of comorbidity is hardly adequate to describe these patients' conditions.

beginning of the comorbidity associated with subthreshold syndromes; we have just begun to learn how to sort these mental symptoms and syndromes into meaningful groupings. The ICD-10 has created a diagnostic category called mixed anxiety-depression, and the DSM-IV includes this entity in the appendix as a diagnosis worthy of further research. What is clear is that our primary care practices are full of patients who harbor a large number of mental symptoms, and they suffer as a result; however, we hardly know what to do to relieve their suffering.

One aspect of comorbidity deserves an additional comment. I have chosen to call it the "pile-up factor," because it has to do with the additive and perhaps even exponential effect of additional symptoms on a preexisting syndrome or symptom. It is generally understood that the severity of a diagnosis can be measured by the number of criterion symptoms and the associated degree of impairment or level of distress. Observe, for example, that the DSM-IV grades a major depressive episode as mild, moderate, or severe by exactly these criteria. By the same logic, as symptoms accumulate within primary care patients, they may (and often do) fall outside a single category, instead accumulating across several symptom categories. This means that a patient can be extremely symptomatic, bearing 15 or 20 symptoms, but still not meet the criteria for any single DSM-IV diagnosis.

We have identified just such a subset of patients in the Somatization in Primary Care Study. We found patients who have subthreshold somatization and depression and who have panic and PTSD symptoms, but who meet no diagnostic criteria. These patients show severe functional impairment and are highly distressed. Another example of this extreme symptom accumulation across diagnostic categories might be complex PTSD, in which certain victims of early severe abuse manifest some but not all of the symptoms of PTSD, some symptoms of depression, many somatic symptoms, symptoms of panic, a tendency to dissociate, and personality traits that make relationships difficult. Finally, distress or functional impairment can be affected by the accumulation of stressors as much as the accumulation of symptoms. For example, subthreshold panic might be far more disabling for someone who is going through a divorce, has acting-out adolescents, and whose car was recently stolen than for someone who is going through no serious life stressors.

The point of all this is simply to say that if one searches for symptoms of depression among primary care patients, one will find them. If one searches for symptoms of panic, GAD, or PTSD, one will find them. But often, one will find them in the same patients. In primary care, as elsewhere, symptomatic patients tend to be symptomatic across diagnostic categories, and too hard a focus on "making the diagnosis" of one specific disorder can blind one to this range of symptoms. Clinicians must broaden their inquiry to accommodate this phenomenon. Patients usually come to us when they pass a certain threshold of distress; we should not insist that they pass a threshold of diagnostic criteria before we accord them the care they are seeking.

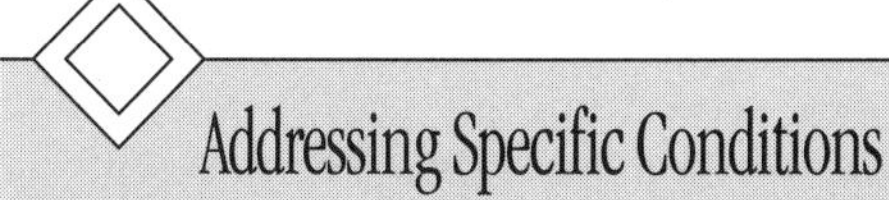

Addressing Specific Conditions

We have covered a number of characteristics that make mental symptoms important to primary care patients and the clinicians, even without a diagnosis of a mental disorder. At this point, we will turn our attention to the usual business of primary care. Most patients who appear for care in this setting do so because they have a chronic disease, or an acute problem, for health maintenance reasons, or because they need help sorting out a symptom. In nearly every case, the "medical" reason for the visit is associated with at least one mental symptom. The following sections describe the kinds of symptoms associated with each of these kinds of visits.

Two caveats are in order: The first is that, although there do seem to be associations between particular medical conditions and specific symptoms, mental symptoms do not discriminate very well between one medical condition and another, and the reader should not be misled into thinking that certain symptoms are associated *only* with particular diseases. Mental symptoms can be found associated with all medical problems, and the clinician should adopt a strategy of broad-based inquiry. The second caveat is that there is little research to support much of the discussion that follows. In preparing this chapter, we have run secondary analyses on several datasets to test clinical suspicions, but there is almost no published literature that addresses the association between specific medical conditions and specific mental symptoms. This material is too important to omit from this chapter and this book, but the reader should take these observations and recommendations as preliminary, in need of corroboration or revision by empirical research. We begin with the symptoms frequently associated with visits for chronic diseases.

Chronic Diseases

In some ways, the presence of mental symptoms in patients with chronic diseases is not surprising. The loss of an important function as a result of a chronic illness, such as losing the ability to swallow or walk following a stroke, is often profoundly disturbing, particularly if this function was central to the maintenance of the patient's identity or self-esteem. Such a loss can be expected to be associated with depressive symptoms. Anticipating such a loss might produce symptoms of depression, but it might also produce anxiety symptoms. In certain patients, any of the above problems that result from chronic disease might be associated with somatization.

A chronic disease represents a long-term or permanent condition usually characterized by pain or loss of function. In the most general terms, the presence or prospect of pain makes one anxious, and severe pain can precipitate a panic attack. There are data to suggest that people with chronic medical diseases have a 30 to 40 percent greater likelihood of having an anxiety, mood, or substance abuse *disorder* than do patients without chronic disease. It follows from this that patients with chronic medical conditions have a much higher likelihood of mental *symptoms*, but such analyses have not yet been published. Data from the same community-based sample suggests that anxiety disorders appear earlier in the course of a chronic illness than do mood disorders. Again, this *suggests* but does not prove that such a pattern also exists for mental symptoms.

Long-standing pain is frequently associated with symptoms of depression. The overuse of narcotics, which may be prescribed for control of pain, is sometimes associated with a worsening of depressive symptoms. People also may use alcohol as a way of deadening or coping with pain, with resultant dependency and possible depression. We are beginning to learn that the presence of depression complicates the course of many medical diseases and is associated with a worse outcome. As stated, it is reasonable to assume that depressive symptoms might likewise be associated with an adverse outcome, but we must await further empirical verification of this assumption. This is an area that needs much more investigation.

Are specific mental symptoms associated with particular chronic diseases? As mentioned, the evidence is very sparse. Wells and co-workers have shown that "persons with current (i.e., active) arthritis, heart disease, or high blood pressure had a significantly increased prevalence of recent (6-month) anxiety disorder, whereas those with current chronic lung disease had an increased prevalence of recent affective and substance use but not anxiety disorder." To elucidate the question of whether there are chronic, disease-specific mental symptoms, Miriam Dickinson reanalyzed the National Comorbidity Survey (NCS) and the Somatization in Primary Care (SPC) datasets. The results are presented below.

Chronic Pulmonary Disease

In the NCS, chronic lung disease increased the likelihood of having a depressive diagnosis by more than threefold. It also increased the likelihood of an anxiety disorder by about threefold. In the SPC sample, about three-quarters of the patients with chronic obstructive pulmonary disease (COPD) had at least one depressive symptom, and about one-half had an anxiety symptom. Although this suggests that depressive symptoms might be more frequent than anxiety symptoms, both are extremely common. For now, the most prudent conclusion is that mental symptoms are extremely common among patients with lung diseases, and these symptoms cut across diagnostic classes.

Diabetes

In the SPC sample, about 90 percent of the subjects with diabetes had one or more depressive symptoms, and over one-half had an anxiety symptom. Until more discriminating data are available, the safest conclusion is that diabetes is associated with a range of mental symptoms affected by the symptom modifiers discussed in the first part of the chapter.

LAURA BANNOCK (CONTINUED) *Ms. Bannock's most conspicuous response to her diabetes is sadness and a sense of loss. After probing more closely, you also discover that she is intensely anxious that she might go blind or lose one of her feet. Both of these happened to her sister, a long-time diabetic. She is worried that she will not live to see her daughters get married, and that as she becomes disabled, someone will have to take care of her. Her anxiety symptoms are muscle tension in her neck, a lump in her throat, trouble catching her breath, and difficulty concentrating. These symptoms are so intense right now that they are interfering with her diabetic self-care. You know Ms. Bannock well and have seen her react to adversity before. She will most likely be very symptomatic for the next week or two and then will actively seek informa-*

tion, organize a plan, mobilize support from her family, and conscientiously follow a regimen. At that point you can anticipate many questions, repeated requests for reassurance, a more realistic reappraisal of her actual and prospective condition, and a dramatic lowering of her anxiety level.

Arthritis

From the NCS we know that the presence of arthritis confers about a threefold greater likelihood of having a depressive or anxiety disorder, and from the SPC data we know that well over one-half the subjects having arthritis have at least one anxiety or depressive symptom. There is little evidence that arthritis predisposes to particular symptoms, other than the Wells and associates study already referenced, which suggests that anxiety in particular is associated with arthritis.

NED CAMBER *Ned Camber has severe osteoarthritis in both knees and his left hip. He lists the three worst things about this arthritis as the constant pain, his inability to play tennis, and the prospect of surgery next year. He tells you that he has always been a high-strung guy, which has helped him succeed in his business, but now his pain is making him so irritable that his associates are avoiding him. Moreover, he awakens every time he turns over in bed, and the resulting sleep deprivation, together with his lack of exercise, makes him feel like he has to fight to keep his edge. He thinks a surgery will further set him back, even if it eventually reduces his pain. His wife made this appointment because he is driving her crazy. He wants you to make the pain stop.*

Arthritis hurts. Mr. Camber is coping with his pain by fighting it, to the misery of those around him. If his distress and irritability can be redirected, perhaps his overall suffering can be lessened.

Coronary Artery Disease

We now know that heart disease increases the likelihood of depression (by about threefold in the NCS), and that the presence of depression worsens the outcome of the heart disease. Indeed, analysis of the SPC sample confirms that about three-quarters of patients with heart disease have at least one depressive symptom. What has not been so well addressed is the high association of heart disease with anxiety symptoms. The presence of heart disease increases the likelihood of panic or generalized anxiety disorder by 3.2 and 5.5, respectively, and almost one-half the patients in the SPC sample with heart disease had at least one anxiety symptom. These symptoms are especially problematic early on, when uncertainty about the future is high, fear of death or disability is fresh, and pain is active. Panic attacks in patients with heart disease can cause a great deal of unnecessary concern, medical evaluation, and hospitalization.

Acute Conditions

Like the chronic diseases discussed, acute diseases are often associated with mental symptoms. Acute diseases by their nature appear suddenly and can be expected to improve or resolve quickly. They may be associated with pain, which is sometimes severe, and may disrupt life's routines. A patient suffering from an acute disease may be temporarily incapacitated and dependent on others. In Chap. 3, the case of Angela Ruiz, who broke her leg in a gymnastics accident, offers a beautiful description of the mental symptoms associated with acute disease. She is irritable and sad about the loss of her newfound independence. Even though this loss is temporary, its effects are tremendous, and her reaction is strong.

Mental symptomatology has at least three dimensions in acute diseases: it is a reflection of severity, it defines the nature of the coping, and it is sometimes the focus of a direct intervention. Thus, the clinician must inquire about and evaluate any mental symptoms associated with acute diseases, no matter how minor or temporary.

Patients may expect their clinicians to respond differently to an acute disease, and any attendant symptoms, than to a chronic one. With acute disease, the patient may feel suddenly helpless and overwhelmed by a new, unpleasant situation, and is usually looking for someone who understands the situation and knows what to do. The patient may respond well to simple explanations and clear prescriptions. Mental symptoms may respond dramatically to reassurance. In the case of chronic disease, the patient is much more responsible for coping with the disease and may respond to a supportive, problem solving partnership.

Health Maintenance

To my knowledge, there is no literature on the mental symptomatology associated with health maintenance visits. Nevertheless, such visits are often motivated by concerns that can provoke such symptoms, and inquiry into such concerns is indicated. Consider, for example, the case of Roger Dushane.

ROGER DUSHANE *Roger Dushane is a 52-year-old grocer whom you are meeting for the first time. You know his family well, but he has not been to see a doctor since he injured his eye 20 years ago. As soon as you walk into the exam room, he says, "No offense, but I don't like doctors. I don't want to be here. The only reason I'm here is because my brother had a stroke a month ago and can't talk now. It looks like he's gonna be useless from here on out. His doctor told my wife that it runs in families, and when she told me that I nearly came out of my skin. I'm not an easy guy to get upset, but this has got me spooked—I keep thinking about what would I do if I ended up like that. It's a horrible thought, and it might be too late to do anything. Is it too late, Doc? Is there anything I can do to avoid that?" You learn that Mr. Dushane smokes a pack of cigarettes a day, never exercises, eats a high-fat diet, and drinks about three beers a night. He is 40 lb overweight. His blood pressure is normal, and it turns out that he is mildly hypercholesterolemic. His blood glucose is normal.*

Mr. Dushane is anxious. In fact, anxiety is his predominant symptom. He is worried about his health, his future ability to provide for his family, and his debts if he got sick. His brother's stroke precipitated a whole cascade of concerns that culminated in this visit, during which Mr. Dushane seeks reassurance and a plan for better health. The most constructive way you can relieve Mr. Dushane's anxiety is not to address the symptoms directly, but to address the concerns that engender them—by reassurance, education, a clear stepwise plan, and reinforcement. The anxiety will most likely take care of itself once these measures have been implemented. Anxiety about possible underlying disease often motivates patients to seek preventive health care. In managing such anxiety, clinicians may walk a fine line between relieving the anxiety when it becomes dysfunctional and using the anxiety to help to motivate patients to make necessary life style or other changes.

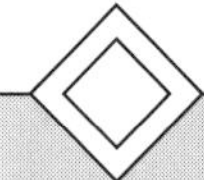

The Clinician's Response

Clinicians can intervene to help patients deal with troublesome mental symptoms. This section describes a number of steps that clinicians should take in every patient encounter to help identify and address mental symptoms. Most of these steps you likely already know about—you either learned them as part of gaining standard interviewing skills, or you read about them in earlier chapters in this text. The key here is to incorporate these steps into your regular visits with each patient. The ideas described are easy to implement and should fit seamlessly into most encounters with patients. The first step is a focused inquiry of mental symptoms.

Inquiry

Mental symptoms do not always require specific action, but whatever the reason for a visit and whatever the problems at hand, the clinician's action should be informed by the accompanying mental symptomatology. The protocol described by Stuart and Lieberman is useful for determining the context of every patient visit. This protocol goes by the acronym BATHE:

Background
Affect
Trouble
Handling
Empathy

This protocol will serve as the basis for the discussion of inquiry in this section. The first step is to identify mental symptoms that are problematic for the patient. The first two letters of BATHE are useful here. The *B* stands for *background* and is intended to elicit anything relevant to the presenting problem. This might be accomplished by simply asking, "What is going on in your life?" or "How does this affect everything else in your life?" or "What else is going on?" The point here is to learn a little something about the context in which the presenting problem exists.

The second letter, *A*, stands for *affect.* This is where the clinician probes directly for mental symptoms using a simple two- or three-question exchange. It should be a part of every primary care visit. The first question should be something like, "How do you feel about that?" or "What kind of feelings are you having?" Depending on the reply, the question may need to be followed up with specific questions about depressive or anxiety symptoms, or physical symptoms that may be related to the problem at hand. The clinician should periodically review the symptoms in the criterion lists for major depressive episode, panic disorder, GAD, and PTSD. At least one of these symptoms will almost always be present.

Once the presence of a symptom is established, it needs to be characterized. For the most part, this conforms to symptom characterization as we learned during our training.

At the beginning of this chapter, a few of the most important dimensions of mental symptoms as they occur in the primary care setting were discussed: the meaning of the symptoms, the functional consequences, the context in which they occur, the association with other symptoms, and the time course of the symptoms. The following sections describe a process for characterizing mental symptoms, beginning with assessing their severity. After you assess the severity, you should learn about other associated symptoms, and the patient's previous experience, coping response, and social support. Each is described in detail.

Assess the Severity of the Symptom

First, learn how severe the symptom is. Ask, "How much trouble are you actually having with your concentration? Can you read technical material if there are no distractions? Can you read pleasure material, such as a good novel? Can you watch a movie or television? Can you follow a conversation? Is it like that every day?" As mentioned at the beginning of this chapter, sometimes a symptom is present but has no particular consequence or is even having a positive effect, whereas sometimes it is so severe that it becomes the focus of an intervention in its own right. Severity is one of the most important dimensions of assessment. In general, mild symptoms warrant monitoring and severe symptoms warrant treatment.

Learn About the Associated Symptoms

Discovering other symptoms associated with the primary mental symptom is necessary for identification of subthreshold syndromes. Ask questions such as, "Since you first noticed that you had lost interest in your woodcarving hobby, have you noticed anything else? Tell me about that. Have you felt sad? Have you had trouble concentrating? Has your appetite changed? Your sleep? Have you felt irritable? Nervous? Are there any physical symptoms that have come up at this time? Anything else you think might be related?" The idea here is to learn whether the symptom occurs in isolation or is part of a meaningful constellation, particularly a subthreshold syndrome. With subthreshold depression, for example, a high proportion of patients will progress to a major depressive episode, and some may benefit from psychotherapy or pharmacotherapy. One could hardly make such a case for the symptom of loss of interest in previously interesting things if that were the only symptom present.

Find Out about the Patient's Previous Experience

As with nearly any symptom, previous experience predicts current experience. A familiar symptom may still be intensely uncomfortable, but previous experience removes some of the anxiety of uncertainty about what is likely to happen. Ask, "Has this ever happened before? Tell me about that. When was that? How many times? Did it come out of the blue, or did something seem to trigger it then? How bad was it that time? How long did it last?"

Ask About the Patient's Coping Response

This is the *H* in the BATHE acronym—*handling*. It serves to trigger inquiry about coping. "How are you handling this? When this first came up, how did you deal with it then? Tell me about that. How did that work? Did that cause other problems? What else did you try? When this happened before, what did you do? How well did that work? How did your wife react? Was that helpful? Tell me about that." As described in Chap. 4, the effectiveness of a given coping response depends on the individual patient, the stage of the symptom or illness, the context in which the coping strategy is employed, and the particular strategy used. Some patients do not think of their reaction to a symptom or an illness as a coping response at all, and have not considered that there is anything they can do to alter how they feel.

Assess the Patient's Social Support

Social support can be a complex phenomenon, but some of its aspects almost always have a bearing on the consequences of a mental symptom. Learn about the patient's social support by asking, "Do you have anyone you are talking to about this? Is there anyone you can talk to about this? Who is helping you with this? Can you get help? How is your family dealing with this? Your friends?" Social isolation is a major risk factor for almost all health outcomes, and a healthy social network protects health. It is important to assess for the depth of the social support, the kinds of things people are willing to help with, and the costs associated with mobilizing this help. At a minimum, the clinician should learn whether the patient has a confidant, any source of emotional support, and help with practical matters like transportation, childcare, or food preparation.

Interventions

The first half of this section on the clinician's response focused on inquiry—identifying and characterizing mental symptoms or subthreshold syndromes in primary care patients. Now the focus switches to what to do for these patients once you have identified them. The first step is to provide supportive counseling to patients who are experiencing problematic mental symptoms.

Provide Supportive Counseling

By the time a clinician has characterized a mental symptom, the clinician has already acted therapeutically. Emotional reactions to illness often begin as inchoate dysphoric states, and the process of eliciting from the patient an orderly description of these reactions serves to resolve them into something more understandable and manageable. It is enormously helpful for a patient to feel understood, and characterizing a patient's reaction serves exactly that purpose. Therefore, the clinician should strive to understand the patient's feelings as clearly as possible, and should regard the effort to do so as the first stage of supportive counseling. Thus, simply inquiring about and clarifying mental symptoms serves as the first aspect of supportive counseling.

A second aspect of supportive counseling is *empathy*, the *E* in BATHE. Empathy is the process whereby the clinician makes it clear that the patients' feelings have been understood, and that the clinician appreciates the difficulty of the patient's situation. Sometimes showing empathy takes no more than making a statement such as, "That must be very difficult for you," or "I can see how hard that must be."

A third aspect of supportive counseling is to reassure the patient that even though the symptoms may seem strange and even frightening, they are not unusual and can be managed. If possible, reassure the patient that his symptoms are a normal reaction to such a situation. You can use statements such as these:

> I can see that your trouble with concentrating is alarming to you, and you are worried that something serious is wrong. Well, this is a serious problem, yes, but not in the sense that you might have a brain tumor or Alzheimer's disease. No, not at all. This trouble you are having is actually a pretty normal reaction to everything you are dealing with. Many people who have a new diagnosis like diabetes have symptoms like this. I see this often. It will most likely quiet down pretty soon. If not, we will look into it more closely, but for now you can count this as a normal reaction.

These first three aspects of supportive counseling—clarification, normalization, and empathy—rarely take more than a few minutes and are enormously therapeutic. For many symptoms at the lower end of the severity spectrum, this counseling and expression of interest might be all that is required. But within the 10 or 15 min allotted for a visit, the clinician can do more, and for more intense presentations should do more. Specifically, the clinician can begin to help the patient act to reduce the symptom severity.

Additional Steps That Help Patients Reduce Symptom Severity

Recall from the inquiry section of this chapter that clinicians should assess their patients' social support. In the course of learning about the patient's social support system, it often becomes apparent that there are members of the patient's family, circle of friends, church group, or neighbors who wish to be helpful but who have not been asked to help. Once you have assessed a patient's level of social support, encourage him or her to take advantage of the support he or she has or that which she may easily get. People may be willing to help if they are simply asked, and the clinician's role is to help the patient to identify helpful others and to encourage the patient to ask for help.

Another intervention you can consider for patients with troublesome symptoms is family counseling. The family is usually the most important part of a patient's social network, and also the part most affected by the patient's symptom status. Remember that the most likely source of care will be members of a patient's family, and that family members will often raise important concerns that the patient will not. Look first to family members for help, and ask about the effects the patient's condition is having on the rest of the family. Sometimes a brief interview with key family members yields critical information. Often this information can be acquired by simply inviting family members who are in the waiting room into the examination room for part of the visit. There may be complicated family issues that require time to sort out or that require the expertise of a family therapist or other mental health professional. Several chapters in this book describe techniques for engaging the family in the process of care (e.g., Chaps. 1, 2, 5, and 12).

Cognitive Behavioral Therapy

Cognitive behavioral therapy (CBT) is an option for helping to reduce the severity of mental symptoms. Evidence of the benefits of CBT for mental symptoms and subthreshold syndromes is sparse. CBT is known to be effective for major depression, a number of anxiety disorders, and even somatization disorder. It has not been demonstrated to be effective for subthreshold syndromes, with the possible exception of subthreshold depression, and very few primary care clinicians acquire skill as cognitive behavioral therapists.

Despite the absence of across-the-board benefit of CBT, elements of this kind of therapy may be helpful in dealing with certain varieties of symptomatic subthreshold syndromes and severe mental symptoms. For example, the feeling of worthlessness sometimes associated with minor depression can lead patients to neglect other medical problems or avoid seeking lifesaving social support. CBT techniques offer a straightforward way to address this problem. Another example is the phobic avoidance that so often follows a panic attack, which can progress to a full DSM diagnosis of panic disorder with agoraphobia. Early desensitization therapy can preempt this serious downward spiral.

PROBLEM SOLVING THERAPY Although a collaborative relationship with a mental health professional skilled in CBT is extremely helpful, primary care clinicians can use elements of behavioral therapies in their ordinary office practice. We often use "Problem Solving Therapy" to help patients partition an overwhelming tangle of distress into discrete problems. Problem solving therapy is analogous to our asking patients to select their most important one or two problems for us to deal with at a given visit, and then going to work on those problems to the (temporary) exclusion of the others.

Stuart and Lieberman structure problem solving therapy into three core questions:

1. How do you feel?
2. What do you want?
3. What can you do?

The first question helps to identify the most salient or pressing mental symptoms and gives the clinician an opportunity to acknowledge the reality and legitimacy of the patient's feelings. Patients often answer the second question with what they do *not* want or they simply cannot answer the question at all. Answering this question may require the clinician to repeatedly ask the question or to schedule another visit when patients have had time to think about the answer. The importance of this second question is that it creates a goal for the patient and establishes the patient's control of the agenda. The answer to the third question is often an insufficiently developed set of options. Here the clinician can clarify the options that are available, emphasize those elements of the problem that are most manageable, and challenge assumptions that limit the patient's choices. It may be that there is nothing that can be done, and this is important to recognize and accept.

PHARMACOTHERAPY

Pharmacotherapy may be an option for lessening the severity of some mental symptoms. In general, the less severe the mental symptomatology, the less beneficial medication is likely to be; thus, pharmacotherapy is not likely to be helpful for symptoms or subthreshold syndromes. That being said, three exceptions to this generalization that relate to subthreshold symptoms of depression, panic, and anxiety are discussed next.

DEPRESSION First is the problem of subthreshold depression. As mentioned, there are only a few published clinical trials of antidepressants in minor depression, and at most they show a marginal benefit. The literature does not support the use of antidepressants for this group of patients; however, within this group of patients, there are some individuals who may warrant a different consideration. The principal risk to patients with minor depression is that they will cross the threshold and develop a major depressive syndrome, for which antidepressants are effective. If you are following a patient's depressive symptoms, particularly a patient who has had a previous major depressive episode, and the symptoms are worsening, it is not necessary to wait until your patient falls into the abyss of major depression to initiate pharmacotherapy. Begin treatment early.

Within this same group of patients, there may be individuals who do not meet full criteria for major depression, but whose symptoms are nevertheless severe and disabling. Some of these patients are likely to respond to medication. For example, a patient who comes to see you because of severe insomnia, but who also feels depressed and is having trouble concentrating, may find that an antidepressant restores her sleep pattern to normal, and relieves the other symptoms as well.

PANIC The second exception is patients who have full-scale panic attacks, but who do not otherwise meet the criteria for panic disorder. There may be a place for treating such people with antipanic medication, even though there is not yet literature to support such treatment. There is no question that antipanic medication is effective at reducing or eliminating the panic attacks, and if you detect a patient whose symptoms are worsening, you need not stand by and wait until the patient's suffering reaches the diagnostic threshold for panic disorder before initiating pharmacologic treatment.

ANXIETY The third exception is certain instances of disabling anxiety symptoms. Antianxiety medications, for all their problems, are quite effective for anxiety symptoms. We frequently see patients who manifest severe anxiety, but who do not meet criteria for GAD because the symptoms have not been present for 6 months. It is somewhat difficult to justify standing by for 4 or 5 months, waiting for a severely symptomatic patient to meet the duration criterion before initiating treatment.

Such "off-label" prescribing should not be undertaken lightly, particularly with psychoactive medications. The three exceptions cited above, and perhaps others like them, represent a particular kind of clinical behavior that requires special safeguards and limits. Clinical trials are conducted on groups of patients, some of whom respond to the intervention and some of whom do not. The effectiveness of our individual clinical decisions is only as good as the fit between our individual patient and the responders within the group studied. In each of the three exceptions described, we know that our patient is in a group not yet shown to respond to an intervention, but we think our patient resembles in some way the group of patients who do respond. We are at risk for erroneous inferences here, and we should maintain a level of observation and monitoring to judge the effects of our off-label clinical decisions.

When to Consult or Refer

There are situations when a primary care clinician may need to consult others or refer a patient with mental symptoms to a specialist. Table 20-2 provides a partial listing of the circumstances under which consultation or referral might be helpful.

Table 20-2

Reasons to Consider Referral to a Behavioral Health Specialist of Patients with Subthreshold Symptoms

- When the diagnostic picture is very complicated or confusing.
- When simple interventions do not work or are not possible.
- When major family work appears necessary.
- When formal CBT or other psychotherapy is indicated.
- When you face a difficult pharmacotherapy decision.
- When the patient requests it.

Primary care is best practiced as a collaborative enterprise, and patients with mental symptoms are especially likely to benefit from the expertise of other members of the primary care team. For the problems discussed in this chapter, it may be useful to collaborate with a family therapist, clinical psychologist, psychiatrist, social worker, or case manager.

Monitoring

The nature of many primary care problems is such that the passage of time yields important diagnostic information. Primary care clinicians often make the decision to "wait and see," and are accustomed to setting schedules for follow-up evaluations. At no time is this more important than with the problems discussed in this chapter. Three examples will illustrate the importance of repeated assessment.

First, a subthreshold condition is often the early stage of a full-blown mental disorder, and one of the clinician's principal responsibilities is to intervene early in this progression. Serial evaluations are the only way to determine whether symptoms are crossing the threshold.

Second, many problems complicated by mental symptoms respond to simple office counseling, but many do not, and it is difficult to predict which will respond. One of the most effective means of determining whether a problem can be handled with simple interventions during routinely scheduled primary care visits is to try it and see what happens. If the patient responds and gets better, a relaxed surveillance schedule is in order. But if the patient is unable to make the changes or if the intervention is not effective, then a different or additional intervention will be required.

Third, many of the problems described in this chapter do not fit comfortably into established diagnostic categories, and some of the interventions, particularly pharmacotherapies, are off-label. The responsible use of such therapies requires careful serial evaluation-close follow-up.

Thus, one can see that monitoring the progress of mental symptoms and subthreshold conditions is critical, and should be incorporated into every diagnostic and management plan.

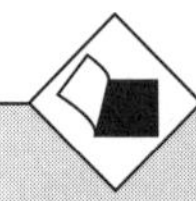

Summary

Mental symptoms are ubiquitous in primary care. They color every visit, and their presence and effect should be accounted for at every visit. Sometimes the effects of symptoms are subtle and require little more than sensitive inquiry and acknowledgement. Sometimes the effect is more pronounced, and affects the management of other problems. Sometimes these symptoms are so prominent that they must be dealt with as problems in their own right. Occasionally, mental symptoms cluster into syndromes that begin to resemble mental disorders, and they must be evaluated, followed, and managed as serious, potentially disabling conditions.

This chapter has taken the reader through this continuum, describing how mental symptoms present and behave at various levels of severity. It underscores the incompleteness of our literature describing how a clinician should proceed on all these points. A number of the recommendations found here will undoubtedly be revised as systematic clinical observation and trials fill in our understanding of how to help with these most common and important of problems.

Suggested Reading

Stuart MR, Lieberman JA: *The Fifteen Minute Hour: Applied Psychotherapy for the Primary Care Physician,* 2nd ed. Westport, CT: Praeger; 1993.

This is the definitive book on how to do office counseling in the context of a busy primary care practice. The advice is practical, detailed, realistic, and effective.

Spitzer RL, Williams JB, Kroenke K, et al: Utility of a new procedure for diagnosing mental disorders in primary care. The PRIME-MD 1000 Study. *JAMA* 272:1749, 1994.

For those who wish to have an efficient means to screen for mental symptoms in the primary care setting, the PRIME-MD is the gold standard. Incidentally, the PRIME-MD also can quickly diagnose the most common mental disorders in this setting.

Goldberg D: A classification of psychological distress for use in primary care settings. *Soc Sci Med* 35:189, 1992.

An evidence-based classification scheme for emotionally distressed primary care patients, together with recommendations about how one might manage them.

Nease DE, Volk RJ, Cass AR: Investigation of a severity-based classification of mood and anxiety symptoms in primary care patients. *JABFP* 12:21, 1999.

Piccinelli M, Rucci P, Ustun B, et al: Typologies of anxiety, depression, and somatization among primary care attenders with no formal mental disorder. *Psychol Med* 29: 677, 1999.

These two papers offer the best evidence that mental symptoms hang together in ways not captured by the DSM system. The papers also offer instances of advanced statistical techniques for getting at these differences.

Bibliography

American Psychiatric Association: *Diagnostic and Statistical Manual of Mental Disorders,* 4th ed. Washington, DC: American Psychiatric Press; 1994.

Broadhead WE, Blazer DG, George LK, et al: Depression, disability days, and days lost from work in a prospective epidemiologic. *JAMA* 264:2524, 1990.

deGruy FV, Dickinson L, Dickinson W, et al: NOS: Subthreshold conditions in primary care. Proceedings of the eighth annual NIMH International Research Conference on Mental Health Problems in the

General Health Sector. Tyson's Corner, VA: September 7–9, 1994.

Dickinson LM, deGruy FV, Dickinson WP, et al: Complex PTSD: Evidence from the primary care setting. *Gen Hosp Psychiatry* 20:214, 1998.

Frasure-Smith N, Lesperance F, Talajic M: Depression following myocardial infaction: Impact on 6-month survival. *JAMA* 270:1819, 1993.

Goodnick PJ, Henry JH, Buki VM: Treatment of depression in patients with diabetes mellitus. *J Clin Psychiatry* 56: 128, 1995.

Katerndahl DA: Infrequent and limited symptom panic attacks. *J Nerv Ment Dis* 178:313, 1993.

Kroenke K, Spitzer RL, deGruy FV, et al: Multisomatoform disorder: An alternative to undifferentiated somatoform disorder for the somatizing patient in primary care. *Arch Gen Psychiatry* 54: 352, 1997.

Lavorie KL, Fleet RP: The impact of depression on the course and outcome of coronary artery disease: Review for cardiologists. *Can J Cardiol* 16:653, 2000.

Mancuso CA, Peterson MGE, Charlson ME: Effects of depressive symptoms on health-related quality of life in asthma patients. *J Gen Intern Med* 15:301, 2000.

Nease DE, Volk RJ, Cass AR: Investigation of a severity-based classification of mood and anxiety symptoms in primary care patients. *JABFP* 12:21, 1999.

Olfsun M, Broadhead E, Weissman MM, et al: Subthreshold psychiatric symptoms in a primary care group practice. *Arch Gen Psychiatry* 53: 880, 1996.

Ormel J, VonKorff M, Ustun B, et al: Common mental disorders and disability across cultures. Results from the WHO collaborative study on psychological problems in general health care. *JAMA* 272:1741, 1994.

Piccinelli M, Rucci P, Ustun B, et al: Typologies of anxiety, depression, and somatization among primary care attenders with no formal mental disorder. *Psychol Med* 29: 677, 1999.

Robins LN, Regier DA: *Psychiatric Disorders in America: The Epidemiologic Catchment Area Study*. New York: The Free Press; 1991.

Spitzer RL, Williams JB, Kroenke K, et al: Utility of a new procedure for diagnosing mental disorders in primary care. The PRIME-MD 1000 Study. *JAMA* 272: 1749, 1994.

Stuart MR, Lieberman JA: *The Fifteen Minute Hour: Applied Psychotherapy for the Primary Care Physician,* 2nd ed. Westport, CT: Praeger; 1993.

Wells KB, Golding JM, Burnham MA: Psychiatric disorder in a sample of the general population with and without chronic medical conditions. *Am J Psychiatry* 145:976, 1988.

Wells KB, Golding JM, Burnam MA: Chronic medical conditions in a sample of the general population with anxiety, affective, and substance use disorders. *Am J Psychiatry* 146:1440, 1989.

Wells KB, Golding JM, Burnam MA: Affective, substance use, and anxiety disorders in persons with arthritis, diabetes, heart disease, high blood pressure, or chronic lung conditions. *Gen Hosp Psychiatry* 11: 320, 1989.

Wells KB, Stewart A, Hayes RD, et al: The functioning and well-being of depressed patients. Results from the Medical Outcomes Study. *JAMA* 262:914, 1989.

Williams JW, Barrett J, Oxman T, et al: Treatment of dysthymia and minor depression in primary care: A randomized controlled trial in older adults. *JAMA* 284: 1519, 2000.

Williams JW, Mulrow CD, Chiquette C, et al: A systematic review of newer pharmacotherapies for depression in adults: Evidence report summary: Clinical guidelines, part 2. *Ann Internal Med* 132:743, 2000.

Zinbarg RE, Barlow DH, Liebowitz M, et al: The DSM-IV field trial for mixed anxiety-depression. *Am J Psychiatry* 151:1153, 1994.

Index

Page numbers followed by "t" indicate tables; page numbers in *italic* indicate figures.

D

Notes

Notes

Notes

Notes

Notes

Notes

Notes

Notes